Immunology for Surgeons

Springer-Verlag London Ltd.

Andrew P. Zbar, Pierre J. Guillou, Kirby I. Bland
and Konstantinos N. Syrigos (Eds)

Immunology for Surgeons

With a Foreword by Sir Gustav Nossal

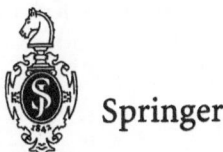 Springer

Andrew P. Zbar
Head of Colorectal Surgery
Senior Consultant Colorectal Surgeon,
Kaplan Medical Center, PO Box 23273,King George PO Branch,
61231 Tel Aviv, Israel

Pierre J. Guillou
St James's University Hospital, School of Medicine, Division of Surgery,
University of Leeds, Clinical Sciences Building, Leeds LS9 7TF, UK

Kirby I. Bland
University of Alabama School of Medicine,
Department of Surgery, Boshell Diabetes Building,1808 7th Avenue South,
Birmingham AL 35233, USA

Konstantinos N. Syrigos
Associate Professor of Medical Oncology,
Head, Oncology Unit 3rd Department Medicine,
Athens Medical School Sotiria General Hospital, Athens, Greece

British Library Cataloguing in Publication Data
Immunology for surgeons
  1. Immunology 2. Surgery - Complications
  I. Zbar, Andrew P.
  617'.01
  ISBN 978-1-85233-482-6

Library of Congress Cataloging-in-Publication Data
Immunology for surgeons / [edited by] Andrew P. Zbar ... [et al.].
    p. ; cm.
  Includes bibliographical references and index.

  ISBN 978-1-85233-482-6   ISBN 978-1-4471-0201-4 (eBook)

  DOI 10.1007/978-1-4471-0201-4

    1. Clinical immunology. 2. Surgery--Immunological aspects. 3. Wounds and
  injuries--immunological aspects. 4. Transplantation immunology. 5. Tumors--Immunological
  aspects. I. Zbar, Andrew P., 1955-
    [DNLM: 1. Immunity. 2. Gastrointestinal System--immunology. 3. Immunotherapy. 4.
  Neoplasms--immunology. 5. Surgical Procedures, Operative. 6. Transplantation Immunology.
  QW 540 I324 2002]
  RC582.15 .I47 2002
  616.07'9--dc21

ISBN 978-1-85233-482-6

http://www.springer.co.uk

Originally published by Springer-Verlag London Limited 2002

Typeset by Q3 Bookwork, Loughborough, Leicestershire, England

28/3830-543210

Dedication

This book is dedicated to my parents and my brother, whose encouragement throughout life to strive for knowledge is a constant source of inspiration and of course, to Mary.

Andrew Zbar
July 2001

Foreword

Can a book be both monumental and accessible? It would appear so, because this is what Andrew P Zbar and colleagues have achieved in their work *Immunology for Surgeons*. This multi-author compendium is authoritatively written, richly referenced and intelligently illustrated, but at the same time it is not overwhelming and its readability is much enhanced by commentaries at the end of each section which not only summarise the highlights of the subject materials covered by the authors, but also give a small number of up-to-date references for those who want to delve further.

It is worth remembering that microbiology and surgery were closely related early on, with Joseph Lord Lister really ushering in the modern era of surgery. Immunology in its turn was initially really a branch of medical microbiology assuming an independent life of its own only in the twentieth century. It is therefore most apposite to see emphasis given early in the book to the immunology of trauma and of sepsis. These two chapters are within the first section on surgical aspects of immunology and follow an overall outline of the broad principles of immunology, which fortunately includes an entire section on the innate immune system where the valuable insight has recently emerged that evolution built strongly on this very ancient set of effector mechanisms to create the vertebrate adaptive immune system. Then follows an outline of the importance of immune deficiency syndromes, inherited or acquired, for surgical practice. How wise to remember that immunodeficiency can be secondary to malnutrition, major trauma, malignancy or immunosuppressive drugs as well as just to HIV/AIDS!

Many would date the close relationship between immunology and surgery from 1953, when Sir Peter Medawar's team discovered immunological tolerance, thus creating an intellectual framework for the eventual development of organ transplantation. What an irony, however, that the early giants of transplantation immunobiology, such as Medawar and Burnet, did not themselves believe that organ transplantation was a realistic possibility. Fortunately, all has been forgiven and forgotten and it is quite appropriate that the second section of the book is devoted to transplant immunology with respect to the fundamentals of allo-recognition, the basis of immunosuppressive therapy, the clinical aspects of transplantation and organ rejection, and finally the still controversial subject of xenotransplantation. Having lived through some of the early verbal skirmishes and also having seen some of the truly disastrous early surgical results, it is a never ending source of satisfaction to me to see organ transplantation still improving with respect to clinical outcomes and having become such a mainstream part of modern surgical practice.

The third section of the book deals with principles of tumour immunology, where of course the news is not quite so good. Despite the immense effort that has gone into tumour immunology and immunotherapy, the successes are still relatively few and far between. Nevertheless, there are success stories both with respect to the vaccine approach and in the newer field of monoclonal antibodies and immunotoxins. It is very satisfying to see this section, too, attack the subject from its very roots with no fewer than ten chapters dealing with basic principles and applied endeavours across a wide front. There is no question that integrated management of the cancer patient will increasingly require the role of tumour immunology to be properly considered and defined.

The last section deals with the important question of immunology and the gastrointestinal tract. The gastrointestinal immune system, as a part of the mucosal immune system, is a wondrous thing with far more lymphocytes present within it than most students of medicine would realise. Therefore we have to consider the function of the mucosal immune system, and how it can go wrong both in inflammatory bowel disease and with respect to lymphoproliferative malignancies of the gastrointestinal tract. Once again, basic and applied science come together very well in this section.

It was a great joy to me to see Andrew Zbar referring to my own mentor Sir Macfarlane Burnet in his Preface. This Nobel Laureate evidently made the field of immunology accessible and exciting to the Editor and now Andrew Zbar is repaying the debt by outlining so many facets of the great science of immunology in a surgical context and doing so in a manner that is both focussed and inclusive.

This volume is a serious piece of scholarship and deserves to be widely read by surgical trainees and practitioners for its timely reminder of how pervasive this great discipline has become. It surely reflects the effort and care that have gone into its preparation.

Sir Gustav Nossal
Department of Pathology
The University of Melbourne
Victoria 3010, Australia

Preface

To the practising surgeon and the postgraduate surgical trainee entertaining the idea of doing a surgical immunology thesis, the field of immunology is daunting. Given the profusion of in vitro immunologic testing, monitoring in particular the humoral and cell-mediated responses to passive and active immunotherapy directed against well-characterized tumor-associated antigens expressed on the surface of many solid tumor cell types, there appears today to be a bewildering array of approaches. The advances which have occurred over the last 10 years have been fascinating, with the routine use now of transgenic technology where animals can manufacture human antibodies to "natural" and novel genetically-engineered antigens and haptens or where dynamic in vivo assessment of cytotoxic activity against xenogeneic tumors transduced with human antigens, can be readily assessed. As a result of this rapidly developing technology, it is difficult to appreciate an overview of the immune system and how knowledge in one area such as tolerance and its clinical impact on transplant immunosuppression for example, is linked to our understanding of mechanisms which tumors employ to escape elimination by potentially competent immunocytes.

This book is an attempt to draw together experts in their field in order to assess the role of immunology in the clinic. In section 1 the immunologic response to sepsis and the trauma of surgery is discussed as well as the interaction between the surgeon and the immunocompromised patient. Section 2 defines the changes in and future direction of transplantation and the burgeoning field of xenotransplantation which has already irrevocably changed our lives. Section 3 discusses the main tumors encountered by the surgeon for which immunotherapy has had a major impact not only in our understanding of complex tumor immunobiology and the presiding conditions required for metastasis development, but in the complex functional derangements of infiltrating lymphocytes which appears to prevent tumor eradication. Section 4 broadly considers the complex area of mucosal immunology and its influence on mucosal disorders such as inflammatory bowel disease and lymphoproliferative disease of the gastrointestinal tract.

This book is not intended to be a complete discussion of surgical immunology, but rather it aims to draw together broad concepts of a discipline which normally requires a massive amount of reading. For the busy surgeon it is hoped that the book provides an idea of the future direction of immunological research likely to affect our understanding of the pathogenesis of complex surgical disease and of the trends in anti-tumor immunotherapy and clinical immunosuppression.

I am particularly indebted to one person during my formative training as a medical student who made the field of immunology accessible and exciting and who encouraged me to undertake postgraduate immunologic research. It is hard to imagine the impact that immunology can have on a medical student when he received weekly lectures from the Nobel prize winner Sir Frank MacFarlane Burnet, but our association fired in me a fascination with immunology and its importance in surgery from a very early period in my surgical development. Although some of the concepts which he espoused and held so dear, now seem dated and do not explain the broad sweep of immunologic findings, I will always be eternally grateful for exposure to the great man when it was not necessary for him to trouble himself with the mundanity of lecturing medical students. In the words of Sir William Temple: "none can be said to know things well who do not know them in their beginnings" and it is a salutary lesson not only in immunology but in surgery in general, that a detailed knowledge of the history of development of a discipline is just as invaluable as familiarity with the latest paper.

I am also grateful to my co-editors for their advice and support during the development of this project and to the editorial staff of Springer-Verlag, most notably Melissa Morton, Eva Senior and Nick Mowat who all pushed me to complete the book on time and whose continuous enthusiasm for the subject matter was essential to the project. Without their help, it simply would not have been done and would have remained as one of those good ideas that we all wish we had seen through.

Andrew Zbar

Contents

xi

Contributors

Professor T.G. Allen-Mersh
Professor of Gastrointestinal Surgery
Imperial College School of Medicine Science
  and Technology
Department of Academic Surgery
Chelsea & Westminster Hospital
London, UK

Dr Martin Béhé
University of Marburg
Marburg/Lahn, Germany

Professor Thomas M. Behr
Professor and Chairman of the Dept of
  Nuclear Medicine — Philipps
University of Marburg
Marburg/Lahn, Germany

Professor Kirby I. Bland
Professor and Chairman Dept of Surgery
University of Alabama
Birmingham, AL, USA

Professor J. Andrew Bradley
Professor of Surgery,
University of Cambridge
Department of Surgery
Cambridge, UK

Dr Nicholas Chadwick
Biochemichal Sciences
UMIST
Manchester
UK

Dr David K.C. Cooper
Associate Professor of Surgery (Immunology)
Transplantation Biology Research Center
Massachusetts General Hospital
Boston, MA, USA

Dr I. Correa
Research Fellow
ICRF Breast Cancer Biology Group
Thomas Guy House
Guy's Hospital
London, UK

Professor Demetrios Demetriades
Professor of Surgery, Director of Trauma/
  SICU
Department of Surgery
Keck School of Medicine
Los Angeles, CA, USA

Dr Lindy G. Durrant
Senior Lecturer Department of Surgery
Cancer Research Campaign
Academic Department of Clinical Oncology
Nottingham University, City Hospital
Nottingham, UK

Professor Isaiah H. Fidler
Professor and Department Chairman
Department of Cancer Biology
University of Texas MD Anderson Cancer
  Center
Houston, TX, USA

Dr Soldano Ferrone
Department of Immunology
Roswell Park Cancer Institute
New York, NY, USA

Professor John J. Fung
Professor of Surgery and Chief
  Division Transplant Surgery
Falk Clinic
Pittsburgh, PA, USA

Dr Reginald Y. Gohh
Division of Transplant Services
Rhode Island Hospital
Transplant Services,
Brown University
Providence, RI, USA

Dr Martin Gore
Consultant Oncologist
Department of Medicine
Royal Marsden Hospital
London, UK

Mr Andrew Huang
Surgical Research Fellow
Department of Academic Surgery
Chelsea & Westminster Hospital
London, UK

Professor Derek P. Jewell
Professor of Gastroenterology
Gastroenterology Unit
Radcliffe Infirmary
Oxford, UK

Dr Anastasios J. Karayiannakis
Associate Professor of Surgery
2nd Dept Surgery
Democritus University of Thrace, Medical
   School
Alexandroupolis, Greece

Dr Martin S. Karpeh Jr.
Associate Attending Surgeon (MSKCC)
Professor of Clinical Surgery Cornell
   Medical Center NY
Dept Surgery
Memorial Sloan-Kettering Cancer Center
New York, NY, USA

Dr Jerald J. Killion
Department of Cancer Biology
University of Texas MD Anderson Cancer
   Center
Houston, TX, USA

Dr Christoph Knosalla
Transplantation Biology Research Center
Massachusetts General Hospital
Boston, MA, USA

Professor Ignazio R. Marino
Professor of Surgery
University of Pittsburgh Medical Center
Pittsburgh, PA, USA

Dr David W. Miles
Consultant Medical Oncologist
ICRF Breast Cancer Biology Group
Guy's Hospital
London, UK

Dr Anthony P. Monaco
Division of Transplant Services
Rhode Island Hospital
Transplant Services,
Brown University
Providence, RI, USA

Dr Paul E. Morrissey
Transplant Surgeon
Division of Transplant Services
Rhode Island Hospital
Transplant Services,
Brown University
Providence, RI, USA

Dr Isha A. Mustafa
Assistant Professor of Surgery Tufts
   University School of Medicine
Division of Surgical Oncology Baystate
   Medical Center
Springfield, MA, USA

Paul D. Nathan
Specialist Registrar in Medical Oncology
The Department of Oncology
Royal Free Hospital
London, UK

Dr Steve Nicholson
St George's Hospital Medical School
London, UK

Dr Susanna Nikolaus
First Medical Department
University Hospital Kiel
Kiel, Germany

Dr Dorothy Pan
Fellow in Medical Oncology
Dept Surgery
Memorial Sloan-Kettering Cancer Center
New York, NY, USA

Mr Stephen J. Parker
Surgical Specialist Registrar
DERA Porton Down
Salisbury, UK

Dr Timothy A. Plunkett
Clinical Research Fellow
ICRF Breast Cancer Biology Group
Guy's Hospital
London, UK

Dr Carol S. Portlock
Attending Physician Dept Medicine
Dept Surgery
Memorial Sloan-Kettering Cancer Center
New York, NY, USA

Dr Judith M. Ramage
Postdoctoral Research Associate
Cancer Research Campaign
Academic Department of Clinical Oncology
Nottingham University
Nottingham, UK

Professor Stefan Schreiber
Professor of Gastroenterology
Universitätsklinikum Kiel
Kiel, Germany

Dr William C. Shoemaker
Department of Surgery
Keck School of Medicine
Los Angeles, CA, USA

Dr D. Speiser
Ludwig Institute
Lausanne
Switzerland

Dr Ian Spendlove
Lecturer
Cancer Research Campaign
Academic Department of Clinical Oncology
Nottingham University
Nottingham, UK

Konstantinos N. Syrigos
Associate Professor of Medical Oncology
Head Oncology Unit, 3rd Dept Medicine
Athens Medical School
Athens, Greece

Dr Nick Torpey
Specialist Registrar
Department of Nephrology
Addenbrooke's Hospital
Cambridge, UK

Dr George C. Velmahos
Department of Surgery
Keck School of Medicine
Los Angeles, CA, USA

Mr Alastair C.J. Windsor
Consultant Colorectal Surgeon
St Mark's Hospital
Harrow, UK

Dr Theresa L. Whiteside
Professor of Pathology
Director of Immunologic Monitoring and
  Cellular Products Laboratory
Departments of Pathology and
  Otolaryngology
University of Pittsburgh Cancer Institute
  IMCPL
Pittsburgh, PA, USA

Mr Andrew P. Zbar
Head of Colorectal Surgery
Senior Consultant Colorectal Surgeon
Kaplan Medical Center (Affiliated with the
Hebrew University, Jerusalem)
Rehovot, Israel

SECTION I

SURGICAL ASPECTS OF IMMUNOLOGY

1. Principles of Immunology

Timothy A. Plunkett, I. Correa and David W. Miles

Introduction

It is not possible to provide a comprehensive review of a burgeoning discipline such as immunology, in a single chapter. Instead we have assumed the reader has a basic understanding of immunology and have endeavored to provide an update of recent advances that we consider important. A short reading list of research papers and reviews that we have found helpful is included at the end of the chapter.

In recent years, the processes involved in generating an immune response have become better understood. Many immunologists, (most notably Matzinger), have advocated a so-called "danger theory" for the immune system. The basic tenet of this theory is that the immune response is not based solely on the discrimination of self from non-self. The immune response to a foreign antigen, or potentially to a self-antigen, (an inherently important event in the fight against malignant transformation), depends on the context in which the immune system encounters the antigen. In the presence of so-called "danger signals", e.g. inflammation or tissue necrosis, antigen recognition by cells of the immune system induces an immune response. In the absence of such "danger signals", the antigen may be ignored or even tolerised.

This theory is intuitively attractive and has been supported by recent advances in our understanding of the innate immune system, antigen-presenting cells (APCs), T and B cell activation and immunological tolerance. These and other developments are the subject of this chapter.

The immune response against infections and tumors is broadly divisible into an innate and an adaptive component.

1. The Innate Immune System

The innate immune system includes complement, polymorphonuclear leukocytes (PMNs), macrophages and natural killer (NK) cells. Since there is a delay of 4–5 days before the adaptive immune response takes effect, the innate immune system has a critical role in controlling infection.

Although individual components of the innate immune system act in different ways, a common result of their activation is inflammation. Clinically this is manifest as redness, swelling, warmth, pain and loss of function. At a cellular level, there is dilation and increased permeability of blood vessels which, combined with endothelial expression of adhesion molecules, results in margination and then extravasation of circulating cells into the damaged tissues. Leukocytes and other effector cells are drawn to the site of inflammation by chemokines released by macrophages and other inflammatory cells, as well as by components of the complement cascade. Inflammation therefore results not only in direct cytotoxicity towards pathogens, but also influences lymphocyte homing and the activation of APCs which secondarily determines the effectiveness of the adaptive immune response.

a) The Alternative Pathway for Complement Activation

The terminal activation of the C3 complement component may be achieved by the classical pathway or by stabilization of the alternate complement pathway. When this activity occurs on a cell or a basement membrane, it proceeds via the membrane attack pathway (activated C5b-9 complex) with the production of lytic lesions (the membrane attack complex — MAC). The end products here (most notably C5a) act as potent anaphylotoxins to activate nearby PMNs.

The alternative pathway of complement activation is an integral component of the innate immune system and can proceed in the absence of specific antibody on many, although not all, microbial surfaces. Therefore, the alternative pathway triggers anti-microbial activity without the delay of 5 to 7 days required for antibody production and complement activation via the classical pathway. The alternative pathway of complement activation has been well described and ultimately results in the production of C3a, which mediates local inflammation and the activation of C5. The latter factor initiates the complement lytic pathway and releases the potent inflammatory peptide C5a.

In this alternate system, a level of C3 conversion may occur in the absence of classical pathway activation, often enhanced by circulating proteases such as plasmin and other inflammatory by-products. Microbial polysaccharides, (most notably endotoxin) and some subclasses of IgG may assist in the stabilization of C3b complexes, preventing its dissociation and supplementing its interaction with other stabilizing factors such as properdin.

b) Cellular Recognition in the Innate Immune System

The innate immune system identifies infectious agents by germline-encoded pattern-recognition receptors (PRR). There are 3 classes of PRR: signaling receptors, endocytic receptors and secreted proteins (the latter bind to microorganisms and target them for phagocytosis or complement-mediated destruction). The ligands for PRR have been termed pathogen-associated molecular patterns (PAMPs), and many examples have been reported (Table 1.1). They are often shared by large groups of pathogens and are generally conserved products of microbial metabolism. As the overall effect of immune recognition is destruction of the target, the recognized structures require to be distinct from self-antigens.

There is striking conservation of signaling pathways involved in innate host defense in organisms as diverse as man, the fruit fly and even to a certain extent,

Table 1.1.   Pattern recognition receptors and their ligands in the innate immune system

Receptor	Ligand	Site of expression	Function
Mannose receptor	Terminal mannose	Macrophage, DC	Phagocytosis
NKR-P1	Unknown carbohydrate	NK cells	Cytolysis
CD14	LPS	Macrophages	Cell signalling
TLR	Unknown	Macrophages	Cell signalling
C-reactive protein	Phosphatidyl choline	Plasma protein	Opsonisation, complement activation
LPS-binding protein	LPS	Plasma protein	Binds LPS for transfer to CD14

plants. In the fruit-fly (*Drosophila*), the signalling pathways involve the Toll protein. Five mammalian homologues to the *Drosophila* protein Toll have been identified and are referred to as Toll-like receptors (TLR1-5). Although the ligands for most TLR are not known, TLR2 is involved with responsiveness to bacterial lipopolysaccharide (LPS) and plays a key role in the pathogenesis of septic shock.

TLR proteins contain a cytoplasmic portion that is homologous to the interleukin-1 receptor. TLR activation triggers intracellular signalling pathways which ultimately activate nuclear factor-κB (NF-κB) and results in the expression of cytokines, anti-microbial peptides and the co-stimulatory molecules CD80 (B7.1) and CD86 (B7.2) necessary for T cell activation.

In *Drosophila*, Toll proteins discriminate between classes of pathogens and induce different effector responses to each. It is possible that TLRs in man have the same capability and emphasize an evolutionary conservation in the interaction between the innate and adaptive immune systems.

c) Effector Cells of the Innate Immune System

Polymorphonuclear Leukocytes (PMNs)

Like macrophages, PMNs respond to infective stimuli via a sequential series of activities; namely chemotaxis, target recognition, ingestion, killing and degradation. Chemotactic responses are via directed movements along concentration gradients (under the activity of anaphylotoxins, eicosanoids and cytokines) as well as by microbially-derived attractant peptides. Target recognition occurs via specific sugar residues (mannose and glycan) or via specific LPS receptors. This occurs in the presence of bound specific IgG and/or complement (a phenomenon known as opsonization) via specific Fc and complement receptors located on the neutrophil surface.

Neutrophils are able to phagocytose microbes directly, or as a result of their being coated with either antibody or complement components. A combination of reactive oxygen intermediates, proteases, phospholipases and defensins are able to eliminate pathogens. Oxygen-dependent bacterial lysis occurs via free radical production through neutrophil myeloperoxidases, superoxide dismutases, catalases and NO-dependent mechanisms with non-oxygen-dependent mechanisms of lysis achieved by lysosomal basic catioinic proteins and serpocidins (including elastase, cathepsins and azurocidin).

Eosinophils have a central role in defense against parasitic infection and have also been demonstrated to have activity against tumors in experimental models.

The role of basophils is probably similarly to mast cells and is mainly in the protection of mucosal surfaces.

NK Cells

These cells are able to inflict fatal damage on bacteria, protozoa, foreign graft tissue and tumor cells. These large granular lymphocytes (LGLs) are called NK cells because of their spontaneous killing against a variety of target cells without the prior need for antigen-specific activation (as normally required by cytotoxic lymphocytes). NK cells lack antigen-specific receptors, but they have carbohydrate-binding lectins on their cell surface as well as MHC class I binding motifs and Fc receptors for IgG1 and IgG3 (so-called FcγRIII).

The mechanisms employed for killing involve cytoplasmic cytotoxins (perforins and granzymes). The perforins are similar in structure to the C6-9 complement proteins which form the MAC, polymerizing at the site of membrane lipid layers to create local membrane destruction. Granzymes are serine proteases which enter the cell with activation of intrinsic endonucleases for the induction of apoptosis via the Fas-FasL pathway.

NK cells are bone marrow-derived lymphocytes. In NK cells, unlike T and B cells, the antigen receptor genes do not undergo somatic recombination. They represent a small percentage of human peripheral blood lymphoid cells and were originally described on a functional basis according to their ability to lyse tumor cell lines without prior immunization and in a non-MHC restricted manner. They also lyse cells infected by virus or intracellular bacteria, mediate potent antibody-dependent cellular cytotoxicity (ADCC) and are able to mediate rejection of bone-marrow allografts.

Some of the specific receptors employed by NK cells for recognition and activation have been identified recently and include both triggering and inhibitory molecules. The effector function of the NK cell will depend on the outcome of these signals. Inhibitory signals for human NK cells are transduced by two families of receptors recognizing MHC class I molecules: the C-type lectin CD94/NKG2 receptors and the killing inhibitory receptors (KIR). After interaction with MHC class I molecules, a common pathway of the inhibitory signal is provided by immunoreceptor tyrosine-based inhibition motif (ITIM) sequences in the cytoplasmic domains of these receptors. This results in a transient inhibition of NK cell-mediated cytotoxicity and cytokine expression. MHC class I molecules consist of a complex of a polymorphic heavy chain, the non-covalently associated light chain β2-microglobulin (β2m), and a short peptide derived from a degraded intracellular protein. Mouse NK cells recognize assembled class I molecules independently of the peptide. For some human KIRs, recognition of class I molecules can be influenced by the composition of the peptides, but not to the extent of T cell recognition and the major role of class I-bound peptides in NK recognition may be to stabilize the MHC class I molecule. This would suggest that the role of class I-inhibition of NK cells is in protection against autologous cells that lose expression of some or all class I molecules, which could allow these cells (most notably malignant cells) to escape "normal" recognition by circulating cytotoxic T cells.

These inhibitory NK cell receptors are members of a novel larger superfamily containing ITIM motifs and include inhibitory receptors for monocytes, macrophages, dendritic cells, B cells, T cells and mast cells. These new inhibitory receptors may regulate many types of immune responses and their specific function has yet to be characterized.

The best-characterized NK triggering receptor is CD16, the low affinity Fc receptor for IgG. Engagement of the CD16 receptor mediates ADCC reactivity and cytokine secretion via immunoreceptor tyrosine-based activation motif (ITAM) sequences in the cytoplasmic tail. Some of the members of the KIR and CD94/NKG2 families also bear these ITAM sequences and may therefore either trigger or inhibit NK cell activation. This is likely to be a ligand-dependent phenomenon. The stimulatory ligand for one of these triggering receptors (CD94/NKG2D) has been identified as the non-classical MHC class I molecule MICA, which is expressed on tumors and by cells under stress, e.g. virally-infected cells. Although NK cells kill tumor cells in vitro, their role in vivo is not clear, as it has not been established whether or not they actively migrate into tissues.

Macrophages

Macrophages mature continuously from circulating monocytes and leave the circulation to migrate into tissues. These phagocytic cells play a role in all phases of the immune response (see antigen-presenting cells).

2. The Adaptive Immune Response

The recognition capacity of the innate immune system is limited by the specificity of germline-encoded PRRs. The recognition system used by cells of the adaptive immune system has evolved to overcome these shortcomings and has two advantages: antigen specificity and memory.

Adaptive immunity comprises humoral and cellular responses via B and T cells respectively. T and B lymphocytes each bear cell surface receptors of a single specificity. The specificity of these receptors is determined by a process of genetic recombination that operates during development.

a) Antigen Recognition Receptors — Generation of Diversity

The T cell receptor (TCR) and B cell receptor (immunoglobulin) generate the diversity necessary in the adaptive immune response by somatic recombination of germline-encoded genes. The antigen-binding site for T cell and B cell receptors is encoded by a series of different genes: variable (V), diversity (D) and joining (J) genes. There are many germline-encoded V, D and J genes for both the TCR and the B cell receptor. Primitive B and T cells possess copies of all these germline-encoded genes. During development each T or B cell undergoes a process of somatic recombination involving the genes encoding the TCR or B cell receptor, respectively. The random recombination of different single V, D and J genes results in great diversity of antigen specificity. This process occurs for the heavy and light chains of the B cell receptor, and for the α and β, or γ and δ, chains of the TCR. The random association of these different chains further increases diversity. There are many other factors which contribute to the antibody repertoire, notably junctional diversity (of light and heavy V, D and J segments), N-region diversity, palindromic sense and anti-sense nucleotide insertions and antigen-driven somatic point mutations in the Ig genes. The latter mechanism occurs as a T helper cell response in the germinal centers of lymphoid tissue to generate clones of B cells with a higher avidity for antigen than the parent B lineage. Immunoglobulin class switch is an irreversible phenomenon and also occurs as part of an antigen-driven T-cell dependent response to produce a B cell with the same antigenic specificity but with a different class and different effector functions. This occurs by evolutionarily conserved switch introns adjacent to the constant regions genes of the basic immunoglobulin motif.

The lymphocyte-specific components for the recombination machinery are encoded by the recombination-activating genes, *RAG1* and *RAG2*. These proteins initiate recombination by recognizing and cleaving chromosomal DNA at specific recombination sites. Mature T cells do not express these proteins. Mature B cells, however, may be induced by antigen to re-express RAG1 and RAG2. This could explain the affinity maturation of antibody observed during some humoral immune responses

b) The T Cell Receptor Complex

In most T cells the antigen recognition receptor consists of two different polypeptide chains (α and β), bound by a disulphide bond. In other T cells the receptor consists of a γ and a δ chain. Fewer than 10 percent of peripheral lymphoid cells bear the γδ receptor and their function is not clear.

T Cell Receptor (TCR)

Each of the α and β polypeptide chains comprises two immunoglobulin-like domains of about 110 amino acids (variable (V) and constant (C) domains), anchored in the membrane and with a short cytoplasmic tail. The sequence variability within the chains resides in the NH_2-terminus and is encoded by a series of genes similar to those in immunoglobulin (V, D and J gene segments for the α chain and V and J gene segments for the β chain). Analysis of the TCR V domain sequences has demonstrated areas of relatively greater variability which correspond to immunoglobulin-like hyper-variable regions. The V domains of each chain associate such that these 6 sites come together to form the antigen-binding site of the TCR.

T Cell Receptor Signal Transduction Apparatus

For both αβ and γδ T cells, the receptor is physically associated with a series of polypeptides, which are required for signal transduction. The TCR complex comprises the invariant CD3-γ, -δ, -ε and TCR ζ chains. The first 3 of these components are products of closely linked genes and are members of the immunoglobulin super-family. The cytoplasmic tails of these polypeptides are highly conserved and the transmembrane regions contain negatively-charged amino acids. The ζ chains have a short 9 amino acid extra-cellular domain, a negatively-charged amino acid within the transmembrane region and a long cytoplasmic tail. The negatively charged residues within the transmembrane region of components of CD3 are essential for the assembly and expression of the TCR complex at the cell surface. The TCR and CD3 have complementary basic and acidic residues respectively and presumably hydrogen bonds form between them within the plasma membrane.

Table 1.2. Immunoglobulin effector functions

	IgG1	IgG2	IgG3	IgG4	IgM	IgA1	IgA2	IgD	IgE
Complement activation									
classical pathway	++	+	+++	–	+++	–	–	–	–
alternative pathway	–	–	–	–	–	+	–	–	–
Placental transfer	–	+	–	+	–	–	–	–	–
Binding to macrophages	+	–	+	–	–	–	–	–	+
Binding to mast cells and basophils	–	–	–	–	–	–	–	–	+++
Reactivity with Staphylococcal protein A	+	+	–	+	–	–	–	–	

During antigen-specific T cell activation, protein kinases associate with the TCR complex. CD3-γ, -δ, -ε each contain one ITAM and TCR-ζ contains 3 such sequences. The phosphorylation of these sites results ultimately in the transcriptional activation of multiple genes, leading to T cell proliferation, differentiation and effector function.

c) B Cell Receptor Complex

There are 5 distinct classes of immunoglobulin in higher mammals: IgM, IgA, IgG, IgD and IgE. They have a basic unit of 2 identical light and 2 identical heavy chains, linked by disulphide bonds. The heavy chains differ between classes and mediate the different antibody effector functions (Table 1.2).

Immunoglobulin Structure

The heavy and light chains are folded into discrete domains. There are 2 domains in light chains (V_L and C_L) and 4 domains in most heavy chains (V_H, CH1, CH2 and CH3). These domains have intra-chain disulphide bonds enclosing a loop of 60–70 amino acids. There is considerable homology between different individuals in the amino acid composition of these loops. Similar structures are found in other molecules, e.g. T cell receptor, MHC class I and II and have given rise to the designation of the immunoglobulin super-family.

Immunoglobulin Antigen-binding Site

The variable regions (V_H and V_L) are at the NH_2 terminus of both chains. Within each of these regions there are 3 areas of exceptional variability. These have been termed hyper-variable regions. The heavy and light chains fold such that the hypervariable regions are brought together to form the antigen-binding site. As a result the hypervariable regions are also known as complementarity-determining regions (CDRs). Antibody recognizes whole antigen with high affinity, in contrast to the T cell receptor which recognizes with low affinity a peptide fragment in association with MHC.

B Cell Receptor Signal Transduction

Membrane-bound immunoglobulin has a cytoplasmic tail of 3 amino acids. This is too short to initiate the intracellular events that occur following antigen binding. Instead, intracellular signaling occurs via the immunoglobulin-associated proteins CD79a (Igα) and CD79b (Igβ), which are encoded by the mb-1 and B29 genes respectively. These transmembrane accessory proteins exist as disulphide-linked heterodimers and are non-covalently associated with the components of the B cell receptor complex which contain ITAM sequences.

d) Structure and Function of the Major Histocompatibility Complex (MHC)

B cells directly recognize conformational determinants on antigenic molecules via specific immunoglobulin molecules expressed at the cell surface. T cells do not recognize antigen directly. Instead, they recognize specific peptide sequences derived from the antigen that are bound to MHC class I or class II molecules. MHC class I and class II have distinct cellular distributions. MHC class I is expressed by almost all nucleated cells, although the level of expression may vary, whereas MHC class II is expressed by cells of the immune system.

MHC Gene Complex

In man, the region encoding the MHC extends over about $4 \ 10^6$ base pairs and contains at least 50 genes. The genes encoding the α chain of MHC class I and the α and β chains of MHC class II, are linked within the complex.

In humans, there are three class I α chain gene families, HLA-A, -B and -C, and three pairs of MHC class II α and β chain gene families, called HLA-DP, -DQ and -DR. There are more than 100 alleles for some MHC class I and class II loci. Therefore, it is statistically unlikely that the loci on both chromosomes will encode the same allele. MHC gene expression is co-dominant and so both alleles are present on the plasma membrane. As the MHC is both polygenic and poly-morphic, an individual is able to potentially bind a greater range of peptides than if only one MHC protein of each class was expressed at the cell surface.

Not all genes within the complex encode MHC class I or II molecules. The LMP and TAP gene products are involved in antigen processing and presentation of peptide with MHC class I. When cells are treated with interferon-α, -β, or -γ, the expression of these molecules, as well as MHC class I, is markedly increased. The HLA-DM gene product is central to peptide presentation with MHC class II. There is co-ordinate regulation of the MHC class II, HLA-DM and the invariant chain (another molecule necessary for effective class II peptide loading) via the MHC class II transactivator (CIITA). CIITA is inducible by interferon-γ.

MHC class Ib molecules (non-classical MHC class I molecules) were originally distinguished by their limited polymorphism and lower levels of cell surface expression. In humans, these include HLA-E, -F, -G and -H and MHC class I-related-A and -B (MICA and MICB). Functions for many of these are now emer-ging. For example, HLA-E plays a role in NK cell function. Others genes within the MHC encode complement factors C2, C4 and factor B or the cytokines tumor necrosis factors α and β.

Structure of MHC Class I and Class II

The MHC class I and class II gene products are cell-surface glycoproteins. They are closely related in overall structure and function, although they have different sub-unit structures. MHC class I consists of an α chain and a separate β2-micro-globulin domain which is encoded by genes outside of the MHC complex. The α chain spans the membrane and consists of 3 domains; the α3 and the β2-micro-globulin domains resemble those of the immunoglobulin super-family. The α1 and α2 domains have a different structure from the other components of MHC class I. They fold together into a single structure consisting of two segmented α helices lying upon a sheet of 8 anti-parallel β strands to create a narrow cleft to which peptide antigens bind.

MHC class II consists of two non-covalently bound α and β chains. Each of these chains has 2 separate domains. The structure of MHC class II is similar to that of class I, except that the peptide-binding groove (formed by the α1 and β1 domains) is more open and extended in MHC class II. As a result the ends of a peptide bound to MHC class II are exposed, whereas those bound to MHC class I are essentially buried. Both MHC class I and class II are unstable when not bound to peptide.

In both MHC class I and class II, the allelic variability resides mostly in residues that form the peptide binding groove. For MHC class I the variability is clustered in 3 regions of the α1 and α2 domains. In class II, the extent of variability differs between polypeptide chains. DRα chains are almost invariant, whereas others vary widely. For the MHC class II, the number of different gene products may be increased further by the combination of α and β chains from different chromosomes (although not all α and β chains form stable dimers).

MHC-binding Peptide Motifs

The ontogeny of MHC division in the processing of foreign protein appears to relate to the immune system recognizing endogenous foreign antigen by cytotoxic lymphocyte (CTL) production (such as in viral replicants or tumor cells) and by endocytic uptake and antibody attack for non-replicating exogenous proteins. Knowledge of the intricate mechanisms involved in foreign antigen presentation will permit the development of potential genetic targets to overcome hetero-geneity in relatively non-immunogenic tumors like colorectal cancer.

Peptides bound to MHC class I are usually 8–10 amino acids in length. The binding is stabilized at the carboxy- and amino-termini as well as invariant sites in the peptide-binding groove. The peptide lies in an extended conformation along the groove but the ends do not protrude; in most cases, variations in peptide length appear to be accommodated by kinking of the peptide backbone.

Different MHC class I alleles have different peptide specificity; different peptides that bind to the same class I allele have been demonstrated to have the same or similar amino acid sequences at 2 or 3 specific positions along the peptide sequence. The amino acids at these points insert into pockets in the MHC molecule. These amino acids have been termed anchor residues. The anchor residues within different peptides are not necessarily identical but are always related, e.g. aromatic amino acids or hydrophobic amino acids. As a result, it is possible to predict potential class I-binding epitopes from the amino acid sequence of antigens.

Peptides that bind to MHC class II are at least 13 amino acids in length. The peptide lies in an extended conformation, and the ends (unlike MHC class I-binding peptides) protrude from the binding groove. It is held in the groove by side chains that protrude into shallow and deep pockets lined by residues that vary between MHC class II molecules. The available data suggest that amino acid residues 1,4,6 and 9 of a minimal MHC class II-bound peptide are held in these binding pockets. These pockets are more permissive than those of the MHC class I molecules and therefore it is more difficult to predict binding sequences.

Non MHC-antigen Presentation: The CD1 Family

Recent investigation has identified molecules that participate in antigen presentation that are encoded by genes outside of the MHC region. CD1 proteins are conserved in all mammalian species so far examined and are expressed on APCs. The human CD1 family is encoded by five non-polymorphic and closely linked genes on chromosome 1 (*CD1A-E*). They show an intron/exon structure similar to MHC class I genes and encode polypeptides with significant homology to MHC class I and class II proteins.

CD1a, CD1b and CD1c are involved in presentation of foreign lipid and glycolipid antigens and generate highly specific interactions with T cell receptors. The first examples of CD1-restricted T cells were CD4⁻CD8⁻ (double-negative) T cells, but it is now apparent that CD1 recognition or restriction is more broadly distributed among T cell subsets. CD8$^+$ T cells expressing the $\alpha\beta$ T cell receptor have been identified that demonstrate CD1-restricted recognition of Mycobacterial antigens

CD1d is found on all bone marrow-derived cells. CD1d molecules bind lipids and may also bind to peptides. CD1d-reactive T cells have been described in man and in mice. A subset of Cd1d-reactive T cells has been well characterized in mice: the NK T cells. NK T cells are so-called because of their expression of cell-surface proteins previously associated with the NK cell lineage. The function of these cells is unclear, but there appears to be marked evolutionary conservation of this subset between mice and humans.

e) Recognition of Antigens by T Cells

Once T cells have completed their development in the thymus, they enter the bloodstream, from which they migrate through the peripheral lymphoid organs, returning to the blood stream to re-circulate until they encounter antigen. To participate in an adaptive immune response, these naïve T cells must be activated to induce their proliferation and differentiation into effector T cells. After the immune response is no longer required, most of the effector cells die and only a few of the activated cells will remain in circulation as memory cells. Memory cells can remain for years in a resting state, but will be able to induce a faster and stronger response if they encounter antigen again.

Activation of T cells entails recognition of antigenic peptides bound to MHC molecules and the simultaneous delivery of a co-stimulatory signal by a specialized APC. Only so-called "professional" APCs are able to express both classes of MHC molecules as well as the co-stimulatory molecules that drive the clonal expansion of naïve T cells and their differentiation into armed effector T cells.

Antigen Processing

MHC molecules present antigenic peptides recognized by the TCR (Fig 1.1). Antigenic peptides that bind class I molecules are mostly derived from endogenous proteins degraded in the cytosol, although specialized APCs can also introduce

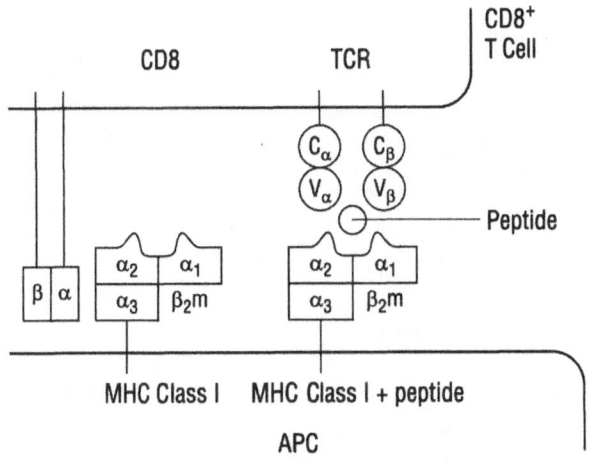

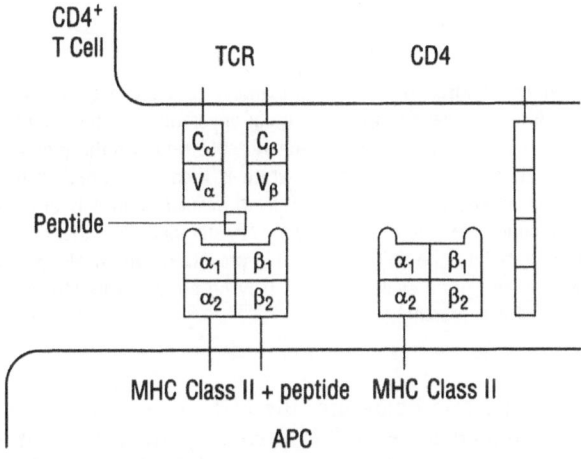

Figure 1.1. Schematic view of the TCR: MCH-peptide complex. The interaction between CD8 and MHC class I and between CD4 and MHC class II (neither of which are antigen-specific) are important in maintaining iner-cellular contact, and ensure that MHC class I presents peptide to CD8+T cells and MHC class II presents peptide to CD4+ T cells.

exogenous proteins into the cytosol and process them following the same pathway as intracellular antigens. MHC class II binds to peptides derived from proteins degraded within intracellular membrane-bound vesicles. These proteins can be endogenous, or more importantly, exogenous antigens engulfed or internalized by APCs.

MHC Class I Antigen Processing Pathway

MHC class I molecules are synthesized in the cytosol and translocated into the endoplasmic reticulum (ER). In the ER, antigenic peptides assemble with MHC class I heavy chains and β2-microglobulin to form stable and functional class I molecules which are then transported and expressed on the cell surface. In the

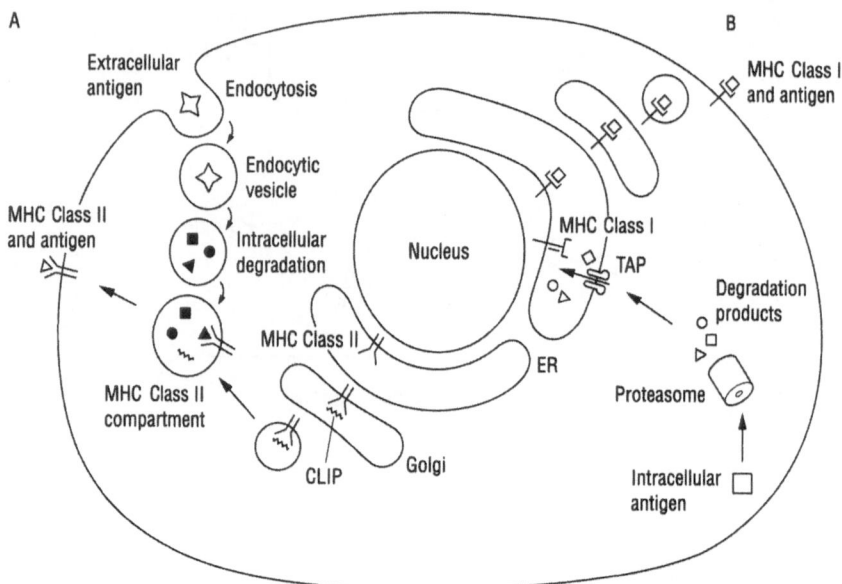

Figure 1.2. (A) Antigen endocytosed by antigen presenting cells are degraded in acidic intracellular vacuoles. The endosomes fuse with vesicles from the Golgi apparatus containing MHC class II molecules. In the resulting MHC class II compartment, the enzyme HLA-DM catalyses the removal of CLIP from the class II molecules. Antigen then binds to the class II which is then transported to the cell surface. This process occurs in specialised antigen-presenting cells. (B) Intracellular antigen is degraded by the proteasome. The degradation products pass into the ER via TAP and bind to MHC class I. The MHC class I/peptide complex is transported to the cell surface. This process occurs in all cells. In reality there is cross-over between the 2 systems; intracellular antigens may be presented by MHC class II and extra-cellular antigen by MHC class I (cross-priming).

absence of peptides or β2-microglobulin, the MHC class I molecule is retained in the ER in a partially folded state and is then degraded. The antigenic peptides that bind to MHC class I molecules are generated in the cytosol and introduced into the ER by two resident proteins of the ER membrane: TAP1 and TAP2 (transporters associated with antigen processing). The main cytosol protease involved in the generation of MHC class I-binding peptides is the proteasome, a non-lysosomal proteinase complex that plays an important role in intracellular protein degradation (Fig 1.2). The 20S proteasome is a cylindrical particle of 700 kDa, composed of 4 stacked rings. The outer rings are each made up of seven α subunits, while the inner rings are each composed of seven β subunits. Only β subunits are catalytically active. In mammalian proteasomes, three constitutively active subunits (delta, MB1 and Z) can be replaced by another three active β subunits (LMP2, LMP7 and MECL-1, respectively) whose transcription is induced by IFNγ. Interestingly, IFNγ-inducible subunits are also highly expressed in lymphoid tissues.

Although most antigens presented by MHC class I molecules are intracellular proteins, some APCs are able to present exogenous antigens for class I presentation in a process known as cross-priming. Macrophages and DCs are able to uptake exogenous antigens by receptor-mediated endocytosis, phagocytosis or micropinocytosis and through a pathway not completely understood, these antigens are translocated into the cytosol and join the main antigen processing pathway for class I molecules. Since professional APCs are responsible for priming of T cells, the process of cross-priming is very important for the initiation of immune responses against pathogens and tumor antigens. Only a minor proportion of antigens follow an alternative MHC class I antigen processing pathway which is TAP and proteasome-independent.

MHC Class II Antigen Processing Pathway

MHC class II molecules are synthesized and translocated into the ER where they associate with a specialized protein known as the invariant chain (Ii). The Ii ensures correct folding of the MHC molecules and prevents the binding of peptides to the MHC class II molecules in the ER. It also targets MHC class II molecules to the acidic endosomes where proteolysis of ingested material occurs. In these acidic compartments Ii is partially degraded. The portion of the Ii binding the peptide groove of the nascent class II molecule is known as CLIP (for class II-associated invariant-chain peptide). CLIP peptide dissociates from class II molecules to be replaced by antigenic peptides (Fig 1.2). This process requires the interaction of HLA-DM. HLA-DM is found in the putative MHC class II binding compartments (MIIC) and catalyses the removal of CLIP. In the absence of HLA-DM molecules, CLIP peptide remains in the groove of MHC class II molecules and antigen presentation by class II molecules is blocked.

Exogenous proteins are introduced into the cell by endocytosis and are degraded in intracellular membrane-bound vesicles by proteases. This pathway is crucial in the processing of proteins that bind to surface immunoglobulin on B cells or are internalized by endocytosis in other APCs.

T Cell Activation

The initial interaction of naïve T cells with antigen takes place in peripheral lymphoid tissues, on the surface of a professional APC. The interaction of TCR with the MHC-peptide complex is of itself not sufficient to stimulate naïve T cells. For proliferation and differentiation into effector T cells, T cells require a second signal. The second signal is provided by co-stimulatory molecules on the APC through interaction with CD28 on the T cell (Fig 1.3). The best characterized co-stimulatory molecules on APC are the glycoproteins B7.1 and B7.2 (CD80 and CD86, respectively). They are homodimeric members of the immunoglobulin super-family. Both molecules are constitutively expressed on DCs and are upregulated on DCs, monocytes, macrophages and B cells following activation. The upregulation on cells activated with various stimuli differs in terms of both the kinetics and density of expression. The complex regulation of CD80 and CD86 expression is consistent with these co-stimulatory ligands functioning as critical regulatory molecules for control of immune responses.

The requirement for simultaneous delivery of both antigen-specific and co-stimulatory signals by the same professional APC plays a crucial role in preventing immune responses to self-antigens. This is important because not all potentially self-reactive cells are deleted in the thymus and it would be possible to generate auto-reactive T cells if naïve T cells could recognize self-antigens on tissues and then be separately co-stimulated by a functional APC.

Binding of the TCR to MHC-peptide complex in the absence of co-stimulation

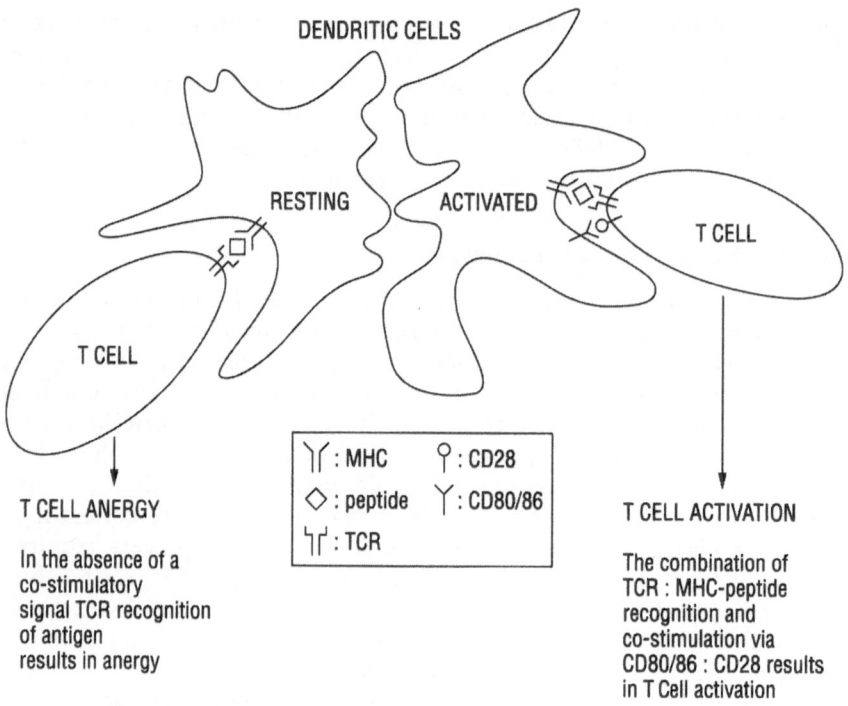

Figure 1.3. T Cell co-stimulation: activation or anergy

not only is insufficient for T cell activation, but may actually anergise the T cell (Fig 1.3). Anergic T cells do not differentiate into effector cells and cannot be stimulated further by APCs. Thus, the presence or absence of co-stimulation during the engagement of the TCR of a naïve T cell will determine antigen-specific immune response or tolerance, respectively.

f) Antigen Presenting Cells

There are three types of antigen presenting cells able to deliver co-stimulatory signals; dendritic cells (DCs), macrophages and B cells. All of them are able to stimulate memory T cells, but DCs may be the only ones able to activate naïve T cells.

Dendritic Cells

DCs are specialized APCs derived, (with the exception of follicular DCs), from the bone marrow. They are found in most tissues where they function as sentinels capturing and processing antigens. DCs found in lymphoid and non-lymphoid tissues represent two different functional subsets of cells. DCs in non-lymphoid tissues are in a so-called "immature" state, because they are unable to stimulate T cells. Immature DCs are mostly residents of the tissue and few of them migrate to lymphoid organs. However, they are very efficient at capturing extracellular products by phagocytosis, macropinocytosis, or receptor-mediated endocytosis through Fc receptors or PRRs.

Maturation of DCs is crucial for the initiation of immunity. It can be influenced by a variety of factors, notably microbial and inflammatory products (both "danger signals" and integral to the innate immune response). During maturation, DCs lose the ability to uptake antigen. They migrate to lymphoid tissues, where they complete maturation and up-regulate co-stimulatory molecules (CD80 and CD86) as well as CD40, MHC class II and adhesion molecules. The mature DC in the lymphoid tissue is then able to activate naïve T cells. Mobilization and migration of DCs are processes mediated by chemokines, some of which are starting to be identified.

DCs also play an important role in the induction of peripheral T cell tolerance, although it is not clear whether tolerogenic DCs represent a specialized lineage or a different state of activation

Macrophages

Macrophages are scavenger cells that express few MHC class II molecules on their surface and do not normally express CD80 or CD86. As part of the innate immune system, macrophages express a variety of receptors (PRRs) that recognize bacterial carbohydrates and other microbial components (PAMPs). After binding to these receptors, macrophages are able to ingest the micro-organisms and degrade them to generate antigenic peptides. The interaction with microbial components concurrently up-regulates the expression of MHC class II as well as co-stimulatory molecules. Thus, macrophage receptors function in innate immunity and play a role in the initiation of adaptive immune responses. The capability of bacterial components to induce co-stimulation has been utilized in immunological adjuvants to induce immune responses against purified proteins. In addition to receptors for bacterial components, inflammatory cytokines may also induce co-stimulatory molecules on macrophages.

B Cells

B cells bind soluble proteins through their surface immunoglobulin. The complex of immunoglobulin and antigen is then internalized and degraded. Resting B cells do not express co-stimulatory molecules. However, as with all other professional APCs, exposure to microbial polysaccharide results in the expression of co-stimulatory molecules. Although they activate resting memory cells, it is not clear that they activate naïve T cells

g) Clonal Expansion of Activated T Cells

Following antigen recognition, interaction of CD28 with either of its ligands, CD80 or CD86, results in enhanced T cell proliferation and IL-2 secretion. During activation, TCR interaction alone is sufficient to induce expression of the high affinity receptor for IL-2. Binding of IL-2 to this receptor allows progression through the cell cycle. The most important function of the co-stimulatory signal is to promote the synthesis of IL-2, probably by stabilizing IL-2 mRNA. IL-2 is crucial to start the immune response and blocking its synthesis or its effect is the mode of action of some immunosuppressive drugs (Cyclosporin A and FK506 block IL-2 synthesis by disrupting signaling through the TCR, and rapamycin inhibits signaling through the IL-2 receptor itself). After proliferation, activated

T cells differentiate into effector cells, able to synthesize all the molecules required for their function. In addition, several surface molecules involved in cell homing and interaction with other cells also change. Activated T cells stop re-circulating through lymph nodes and instead, they express integrins that allow them to migrate to sites of inflammation. Among other changes, activation of CD4$^+$T cells also causes the expression on the cell surface of CD40 ligand (CD154), an important molecule for the helper function of these cells.

h) Effector T Cells

CD4$^+$ effector T cells can be divided into two distinct subsets based on their functional capabilities and the profile of cytokines they produce (Table 1.3). The Th1 subset secretes cytokines usually associated with inflammation, such as IFN-γ and TNF-α and induces cell-mediated immune responses. The Th2 subset produces cytokines such as IL-4 and IL-5 that help B cells to proliferate and differentiate and it is associated with humoral-type immune responses. The selective differentiation of either subset is established during priming and can be significantly influenced by a variety of factors, including the transcription factors induced during activation, the cytokine environment where the CD4$^+$T cell is primed, the co-stimulatory stimuli used to generate the response and the nature of the MHC-peptide ligand.

CD4$^+$Th2 cells activate naïve B cells which recognize the same antigenic complex. Antigens binding the immunoglobulin of a B cell are then internalized, processed and presented by MHC class II molecules on the surface of the B cells. These MHC-peptide complexes can be recognized by an effector Th2 cell and the interaction induces the secretion of cytokines, mainly IL-4, by the T cell. In addition, the CD40 ligand on the effector T cell interacts with the CD40 on the B cell, driving the resting B cell into cell cycle and triggering B cell proliferation and differentiation into antibody-secreting plasma cells. Additional cytokines produced by the helper T cell contribute to this differentiation. One of the main features of an activated B cell is the isotype switching of its immunoglobulin from IgM to IgG, already discussed as a method of altering the specificity of effector function.

Table 1.3. Th1 and Th2 T cell functions

	Th1	Th2
Cytokines	IL-2 IFN-γ TNF-α/β	IL-4 IL-5 IL-6 IL-10 IL-13
Functions	DTH Macrophage activation Cytotoxicity	B cell help Eosinophil stimulation Mast cell activation
Associated isotypes	IgG2a (in mouse)	IgG1 IgE

These observations are largely based on work in animal models, but a similar if not quite so polarised pattern, is likely in man. DTH: delayed-type hypersensitivity.

This process is dependent on the T helper cell through interaction of the CD40 and CD40 ligand molecules. Different cytokines produced by the T cell seem to determine the final immunoglobulin isotype.

CD4$^+$Th1 cells are effector cells involved in activation of macrophages and naïve CD8$^+$T cells. During activation of macrophages, the process is very similar to that in B cells. MHC class II molecules on the macrophage surface can be recognized by the T cell. The macrophage effector functions are activated through CD40–CD154 interactions and the cytokines secreted by the T cell, mainly IFN-γ,

Activation of naïve CD8$^+$T cells also requires the intervention of effector CD4$^+$Th1 cells. CD8$^+$T effector cells are able to kill target cells expressing the specific MHC class I-peptide complex recognized by their TCR. Since this effect can be so destructive, they seem to require more co-stimulatory activity than CD4$^+$T cells and the "help" of CD4$^+$Th1 cells able to recognize peptide derived from the same antigen on the same APC. The nature of this "helper" effect has been elusive for years. On theoretical grounds, Matzinger and colleagues have suggested that by recognizing antigen on APCs, T helper cells deliver a signal that directly activates the APC. The molecular nature of this signal has been defined and it is the interaction of CD40 on the DC with the CD40 ligand on the helper T cell. This interaction activates the DC, up-regulating the co-stimulatory molecules required for the priming of naïve CD8$^+$T cells. In some cases, activation of the DC can also be obtained by inflammatory cytokines, microbial byproducts, or direct infection thus bypassing the necessity of T helper cells. This new view of the "helper" function reconciles experimental observations of T helper dependency and independency during priming of CD8$^+$T cells and opens the possibility of manipulating the activation of DC's particularly for tumor vaccination and therapy.

As already mentioned, effector CD8$^+$T cells recognize antigens bound to MHC class I molecules on the target cells. This recognition induces the secretion of cytokines (mainly IFN-γ and TNF-α) and cytotoxins by the T cell, or the expression of surface molecules like Fas ligand. The binding of Fas ligand to Fas on the target cell results in destruction of the target cell. (vide supra)

i) Memory T Cells

After an effector response has subsided, resting memory T cells are found. Immunological memory can be defined as the faster and stronger response of the adaptive immune system that follows re-exposure to the same antigen. It is unclear how or where memory cells arise. However, once generated they have different pathways of re-circulation and homing from naïve cells. They may derive either from effectors or from some cohort of the activated population either pre-committed to become memory cells or driven by a stochastic or directive process into the memory cell pool.

The requirements for the activation of memory cells for proliferation and cytokine production are not as restricted as those of naïve cells, but co-stimulation is required for optimal responses and for responses to sub-optimal antigen concentrations. The most striking differences in the function of naïve and memory T cells are not in their requirements for stimulation but in the great diversity of cytokines which can be produced in different patterns by memory T cells. Recent investigations have demonstrated two distinct subsets of human memory T cells. Memory T cells not expressing the chemokine receptor CCR7, instead express receptors for migration to inflamed tissues and display immediate effector functions on re-exposure to antigen. In contrast, CCR7$^+$ memory T cells home to lymph nodes on re-exposure to antigen and stimulate DCs. The CCR7$^+$ memory T cells, which have been termed central memory cells, can then generate further antigen-specific T cells and provide additional "help" to B cells.

j) B Cell Activation

Each B cell expresses a different immunoglobulin at the cell surface and this acts as the B cell antigen receptor. Each immunoglobulin gene has 2 exons that encode a transmembrane and cytoplasmic tail for cell surface expression, and a separate sequence that encodes the carboxy-terminus of the secreted form. Differential mRNA splicing following transcription results in expression of the 2 forms. All B cells initially express the transmembrane form of IgM, but may undergo isotype switching, (as already discussed), following activation.

Antigen binding activates the B cell by cross-linking antibody at the cell surface, leading to clonal proliferation and expansion. Although some antigens directly stimulate B cells, most require specialized interaction with other cells that provide additional signals.

T Cell-dependent and -independent B Cell Responses

In many cases antibody cross-linking alone is insufficient to trigger B cell proliferation and antibody secretion. Instead, additional signals are required. Commonly, these are provided by helper T cells. Helper T cells recognize peptide antigens in association with MHC class II on the surface of APCs. Interaction between T helper cells and B cells is essential for isotype switching and for affinity maturation. As a result, T cell-independent antigens, such as bacterial polysaccharides, although able to directly activate B cells to secrete antibody, generate antibodies that are less variable and less versatile than those induced by T cell-dependent antigens.

It is rare for the B cell to prime the helper T cell. Instead, the helper T cell is most likely primed by an activated DC and then interacts with the B cell, with DC-helper T cell binding taking place in lymph nodes. Circulating T cells specific for the relevant antigen are trapped in the lymph nodes by interaction with the DC. B cells migrating through the lymph node first pass through the T cell zone; it seems that B cells specific for the same antigen are trapped, whilst other B cells move quickly through this region where B cells bind to antigen with high affinity. Following endocytosis and intracellular processing, peptide epitopes are presented at the cell surface bound to MHC class II. The activated T helper cells recognize the specific epitopes and stimulate B cell proliferation and antibody secretion.

B Cell Co-receptors

As described for T cell activation, B cell activation requires more than antigen-immunoglobulin binding. The interaction between CD40 on the B cell and CD40 ligand on the T cell is especially important for B cell activation. A similar interaction between DC and helper T cell has been demonstrated for effective CTL induction. CD40 ligand is essential for isotype switching, although cytokines released by the helper T cells influence which isotypes are ultimately produced.

Other co-receptors have been demonstrated to play a role in B cell responses. Studies in mice suggest that they regulate B cell receptor signaling either positively or negatively and reduce or increase the signaling threshold for B cell activation, respectively.

CD22 and FcγRIIB1 both inhibit B cell activation following B cell receptor ligation. These co-receptors contain ITIM sequences in their cytoplasmic tails. CD22 constitutively associates with the B cell receptor and may set a threshold for B cell activation. CD22 binds with high affinity to the trisaccharide sialyl α galactosyl β1-4 N-acetylglucosamine which is found on various glycoproteins, including CD45RO and IgM. Mice deficient in the enzyme necessary to synthesize this trisaccharide show defects in B cell activation. These observations have led to the hypothesis that interaction of CD22 with its ligands may facilitate B cell activation either by dissociation from the B cell receptor (removing the inhibitory signal) or by transmission of an activation signal independent of the B cell receptor. FcγRIIB1 down-regulates B cell receptor signaling only when it is co-ligated to the B cell receptor by antigens complexed with IgG, resulting in negative feedback regulation of IgG production. The co-ligation of the complex with the B cell receptor reduces the threshold for B cell activation and this is one mechanism which provides a link between the innate and humoral immune systems.

k) Tolerance

An understanding of lymphocyte ontogeny and the mechanisms involved in tolerance may assist in improving biologic therapy directed against tumors and explain the defenses some tumor cells employ to evade immunological attack. Mechanisms for thymic negative selection of T cells have been established as part of mature T cell development and as an explanation for the elimination of self-reactive repertoires and knowledge of the peripheral induction of T cell tolerance as it applies to self-MHC recognition may provide clues to the immune anergy and deletion of potentially immunocompetent lymphocytes when repeatedly exposed to tumor antigen. Unlike the B cell system, most but not all of the T cell repertoire must be formed intrathymically with no diversification of the TCR gene once developed. Potentially dangerous antigen may elude the immune system in the periphery if presented in an immunologically privileged site such as the CNS (or the eye), but other more complex mechanisms of peripheral T cell tolerance towards tumors must exist.

Much work has recently been reported using animals transgenic for tissue-specific promoters exposed to extrathymic Class I and Class II molecules. These elegant experiments have shown peripheral T cell tolerance of specific "antigen-ignorant" clones as well as clonal deletion and there is evidence that this state of affairs is somewhat dependent upon local cytokine production. Importantly, relatively high density antigen, exposure (as may occur in some tumors which shed surface tumor-associated antigen, such as gastrointestinal cancers) has been shown in these models to induce TCR and co-receptor down-regulation or apoptosis.

B cell tolerance is obviously important in the avoidance of auto-antibody development for potentially cross-reactive antigen. It is unknown whether similar mechanisms are involved in the failure by tumor-associated antigens to initiate B cell presentation. Auto-antibodies to such naturally occurring but over-expressed antigens may perhaps be produced but be transient, of low affinity or the wrong isotype. Experimentation with hapten-specific B cell populations has shown that tolerance may either lead to clonal deletion (so-called negative selection or clonal abortion) when exposed to high dose antigenic load, or to clonal hapten-specific anergy when much smaller antigen loads are employed. The evidence provided by animals transgenic for both a given antigen and a monoclonal B cell receptor specific for that antigen has shown that early presentation to developing B cells in the bone marrow results in maturation arrest with V region genetic editing for recognition immunoglobulins.

This may have considerable relevance for B cell repertoire development against oncofetal antigens like CEA and α-foetoprotein and will govern the antigenic dose necessary to induce optimal B cell responsiveness during monoclonal antibody therapy directed against the relevant tumor-specific antigen. It is likely that high affinity antibody with a high molarity of presentable antigen favors anergy and this phenomenon may play an important part in the poor responsiveness to membrane-bound ubiquitous tumor-associated antigen which is merely over-represented on solid epithelial tumors. The state of pre-ordained immunotolerance to these tumor antigens which are expressed in low density on normal tissues is probably established early on in the ontogenic lineage of immunocytes and controls their cytokine-mediated receptor/responder phenotype when primary tumors expressing higher density non-mutated surface self-antigens develop.

It is also debatable how important the continuous presence of antigen is in the induction of both B and T cell memory. This may have relevance in cancers where tumor antigen is intermittently shed from the main tumor mass and affects the need for repeated dosing with anti-tumor monoclonal antibodies. Other potential mechanisms for immunological escape by tumor cells include changes in the structure of crucial molecules such as MHC activation ligands, regulators of complement activation, lytic enzyme neutralizers and adhesion molecule receptors. In this sense the immune system contributes to the phenotypic heterogeneity of the tumor.

In general, there are a number of factors that determine tolerance to a specific antigen:

1 antigenic structure
2 stage of development when lymphocytic recognition occurs
3 anatomical site of antigen recognition
4 nature of the cell presenting the antigen
5 the presence or absence of co-stimulatory factors

T Cell Tolerance

T cell tolerance to specific antigens can be broadly divided into central and peripheral mechanisms. Central tolerance occurs in the thymus, whilst peripheral tolerance occurs in the tissues.

Central Tolerance

Although it was previously thought that thymic function declined with age and that by the third decade the periphery was seeded with a full complement of antigen-reactive T cells, recent evidence suggests that the thymus continues to produce naïve, newly differentiated functional T cells throughout adult life. T cells develop within the thymus from pre-cursors that have undergone T cell receptor re-arrangement. The thymus is divided into discrete subcapsular, cortical and medullary areas that contain distinct populations of epithelial cells and other stromal constituents. T cell progenitor cells entering the thymus progress from the subcapsular region via the cortex to the medulla. Early stages of T cell development thought to occur in the subcapsular and cortical zones include expansion of the progenitor pool and expression of pre-TCR, which in turn selects thymocytes with a functional β chain to undergo further maturation and to become $CD4^+CD8^+$ (double positive) thymocytes expressing low levels of TCR. The majority of $CD4^+CD8^+$ thymocytes die within the thymus either because of failure to generate a useable TCR (leading to death by neglect), or because of negative selection or a failure of positive selection.

Positive Selection

In positive selection, $CD4^+CD8^+$ T cells bearing a TCR with some binding avidity for the polymorphic region of the MHC are selected for survival. The T cells recognize the MHC-peptide complex on cells within the thymic cortex; this process is believed to protect the T cells from apoptosis. T cells expressing TCR that cannot interact with MHC are deleted. It is likely that multiple TCRs can be selected by a single peptide-MHC complex. Double-positive thymocytes expressing a T cell receptor of appropriate specificity for the MHC-peptide ligands exhibit some phenotypic characteristics of activation and down-regulate expression of either CD4 or CD8 (depending on whether the cell bound to MHC class I or class II) to yield mature $CD4^+$ or $CD8^+$ T cells (single positive T cells). Concurrent with this process, the T cells undergo the process of negative selection.

Negative Selection

Negative selection is the clonal deletion of self-reactive T cells. The anatomic setting for this process is variable, but probably involves the cortico-medullary and medullary regions of the thymus. At first sight it is difficult to reconcile the distinct functions of positive and negative selection, since both require the binding of TCR to peptide-MHC complexes. The difference between the two is most likely related to the avidity of the interaction between the TCR and peptide-MHC complex. Avidity is a product of both receptor affinity and antigen concentration; T cells with a high avidity for peptide-MHC ligands are deleted, whereas those with lower avidity progress to normal development. These differences also provide an explanation why the interaction between CD4 or CD8 and MHC is essential for positive selection, but is not required for negative selection.

A significant constraint on the process of negative selection, is the requirement for thymic APCs to present the relevant peptide-MHC complex, either as a consequence of their expression of the self-antigen or as a result of endocytosis, processing and subsequent presentation of the antigen from the circulation. In particular, this would pose difficulty in deleting T cells reactive for self-antigens expressed in developmentally, temporally, or spatially regulated patterns. Although it has been proposed that T cells reactive to such auto-antigens are inactivated in the periphery, alternative mechanisms have been recently proposed. Studies have demonstrated expression of a wide variety of molecules expressed by other organs and tissues of endodermal or ectodermal origin in the thymic medulla, indicating thymic expression of genes previously considered "tissue-specific". The expression of such genes in the thymus provides a mechanism for central tolerance. It is uncertain whether such expression reflects a depression of transcriptional control within the thymus, or instead whether there is epithelial differentiation of some thymic medullary cells.

Peripheral Tolerance

It is clear that not all auto-reactive T cells are deleted, as otherwise there would be no auto-immune disease. Auto-reactive T cells may escape negative selection if the relevant antigen is not presented by thymic APCs or if the avidity of TCR for the MHC-peptide complex was low. In such instances, peripheral tolerance has been postulated as a means of preventing T cell auto-reactivity.

Fundamentally, antigen-specific T cell activation requires the binding of antigen in association with MHC to the TCR. However, co-stimulatory signals delivered to the T cell via accessory molecules, which are receptors for specific ligands on APCs, are essential for effective T cell activation. The expression of co-stimulatory molecules by APCs is enhanced by inflammatory stimuli generated by, for example, the innate immune system in response to pathogens. The co-stimulatory molecules CD80 (B7.1) and CD86 (B7.2) already mentioned, are expressed by APCs and bind to CD28 on T cells. Interaction with CD28 encourages T cell activation by lowering the T cell activation threshold (number of TCR that need to be triggered for T cell activation). In the presence of co-stimulation, antigen-binding to the TCR results in a more productive immune response. However, antigen presentation and binding to the TCR in the absence of appropriate co-stimulation (e.g. in the absence of active inflammation) results in anergy and antigenic tolerance.

Therefore, self-antigens presented by APCs in undamaged tissues are likely to enter a tolerising pathway rather than a T cell activating pathway. As a result, self-reactive T cells which might have escaped central tolerance may be anergised through guarding peripheral tolerance mechanisms. A second T cell ligand for CD80 and CD86 is CTLA-4. Binding of CTLA-4 to CD80 or CD86 on APCs also inhibits T cell activation (perhaps by raising the activation threshold), playing an important role in peripheral tolerance. Potential self-reactive T cells may escape peripheral tolerance, however, if they enter the tissue expressing the relevant self-antigen, if the antigen was expressed at low levels or by cells that expressed no MHC ligands.

Peripheral Positive Selection

There is increasing evidence that positive selection in the thymus is not sufficient to ensure survival of naïve T cells in the periphery. In animal models, the survival of naïve T cells requires interaction between the TCR and the self-peptide:self-MHC complexes. Memory T cells do not require such an interaction for long-term survival in the periphery.

B Cell Tolerance

The majority of antibody responses are T-cell dependent. Therefore, T cell tolerance provides an explanation for non-reactivity of some B cells. However, some micro-organisms have both foreign T-cell-reactive epitopes and other epitopes that resemble self-antigens and are capable of stimulating B cells. Such antigens could provoke a response to self, and since antigenically-stimulated B cells undergo hypermutation within the complementarity-determining regions, they may acquire self-reactivity following activation. Tolerance therefore needs to be exerted both during development and following antigenic stimulation.

B cells that bind to membrane-associated self-antigens with high avidity undergo apoptosis during development in the bone marrow. B cells specific for soluble self-antigens are rendered anergic if the self-antigen is present at high concentrations. Such B cell anergy may be reversible, as the B cells can respond to antigen-independent CD40-mediated activation. Chronic T cell activation, for example by infectious agents, can also result in non-specific so-called "bystander" B cell activation and may explain some of the auto-immune antibody reactivity seen in chronic inflammatory conditions.

3. Summary

The aim of this chapter was to up-date readers already acquainted with immunology on some of the recent advances and provide a platform for further reading. Our understanding of the processes of T cell recognition and activation provide new opportunities for treatment of sepsis, wound healing, organ transplantation and cancer.

Further Reading

Journal Articles

Innate Immunity

Medzhitov R, Preston-Hurlburt P, Janeway CA Jr. A human homologue of the Drosphila Toll protein signals activation of innate immunity. Nature 1997,388:394–7.
Yang RB, Mark, MR, Gray A, et al. Toll-like receptor 2 mediates liposaccharide-induced cellular signalling. Nature 1998;395:284–8.
Janeway CA Jr. The road less travelled by: the role of innate immunity in the adaptive immune response. J Immunol 1998;160:539–44.
Kopp EB, Medzhitov R. The toll-receptor family and control of innate immunity. Curr Opin Immunol 1999;11:13–8.

Complement

Wetsel RA. Structure, function and cellular expression of complement anaphylotoxin receptors. Curr Opin Immunol 1995;7:48–53.
Walport MJ, Lachmann PJ. Complement. In: Lachmann PJ, Peters DK, Rosen FS, Walport MJ. Editors. Clinical aspects of immunology. 5th Edn. Oxford: Blackwell Scientific Publications, 1993.
Tomlinson S. Complement defense mechanisms. Curr Opin Immunol 1993;5:83–9.
Brown EJ. Complement receptors and phagocytosis. Curr Opin Immunol 1991;3:76–82.

NK Cells

Lanier, LL. NK cell receptors. Ann. Rev. Immunol 1998;16:359.
Long, E.O. Regulation of immune responses through inhibitory receptors. Ann Rev Immunol 1999;17: 875.

Yokoyama WM. Natural killer cell receptors. Curr Opin Immunol 1995;7:110–20.
Lewis CE, McGee JOD. editors. The natural killer cell. IRL Press Oxford. 1992.

MHC Class I and Class II

Bjorkman, P, Saper M, Samraoui B, Bennett W, Strominger J, Wiley D. Structure of the human class I
histocompatibility antigen HLA-A2. Nature 1987;329:506–12.
Brown, J, Jardetzky T, Gorga J, Stern L, Urban R, Strominger J, Wiley D. Three-dimensional structure
of the human class II histocompatibility antigen HLA-DR1. Nature 1993;364:33–9.

Non-classical MHC Molecules

Braud VM, Allan DSJ, McMichael AJ. Functions of nonclassical MHC and non-MHC-encoded class I
molecules. Curr Opin Immunol 1999;11:100–8.
Porcelli SA, Modlin RL. The CD1 system: antigen-presenting molecules for T cell recognition of lipid
and glycolipid. Annu Rev Immunol 1999;17:297–329.

Antigen Processing

Rock KL. Goldberg AL. Degradation of cell proteins and the generation of MHC class I-presented peptides. Ann Rev Immunol 1999;17:739.
Schumacher TNM. Immunology: accessory to murder. Nature 1999;398:26.

T Cell Activation

Matzinger P. Tolerance, danger, and the extended family. Ann Rev Immunol 1994;12:991.
Bennet SRM, Carbone FR, Karamalis F, Flavell RA, Miller JFAP, Heath WR. Help for cytotoxic-T cell
responses is mediated by CD40 signalling. Nature 1998;393:478.
Lanzavecchia A. Immunology: Licence to kill. Nature 1998;393: 413.
Ridge JP, DiRosa F, Matzinger P. A conditioned dendritic cell can be a temporal bridge between a
CD8+T-helper and a T-killer cell. Nature 1998;393:474.
Schoenberger SP, Toes R.E.M, van der Voort EI, Offringa R, Melief CJM. T-cell help for cytotoxic T
lymphocytes is mediated by CD40-CD40L interactions. Nature 1998;393:480.

Antigen-presenting Cells

Bancherau J, Steinman RM. Dendritic cells and the control of immunity. Nature 1998;392:245.
Sallusto F, Lanzavecchia A. Mobilizing Dendritic cells for tolerance, priming and chronic inflammation.
J Exp Med 1999;189:611.

Memory T Cells

Dutton RW, Bradly LM, Swain SL. T cell memory. Ann Rev Immunol 1998;16:201.
Sallusto F, Lenig D, Forster R, et al. Two subsets of memory T lymphocytes with distinct homing
potentials and effector functions. Nature 1999;401:708–12

B Cell Activation

Campbell KS. Signal transduction from the B cell antigen receptor. Curr Opin Immunol 1999;11:256–
64.
Yancopoulos GD, Alt FW. Regulation of the assembly and expression of variable-region genes. Annu
Rev Immunol 1986;4:339–68.
Alt FW, Blackwell TK, Yancopoulos GD. Development of the primary antibody repertoire. Science
1987;1079–87.
Mayforth RD. Designing antibodies. San Diego:Academic Press, 1993.

Tolerance

Alam SM, Travers PJ, Wung JL, et al. T-cell receptor affinity and thymocyte positive selection. Nature 1996:616–20.

Jameson SC, Bevan MJ. T-cell selection, Curr Opin Immunol 1998;10:214–9.

Klein L, Klein T, Ruther U, Kyewski B. CD4 T cell tolerance to human C-reactive protein, an inducible serum protein, is mediated by medullary thymic epithelium. J Exp Med 1998, 188:5–16

Rocha B, von Boehmer H. Peripheral selection of the T cell repetoire. Science 1991;251:1225–8.

Jamieson BD, Douek DC, Killian S, et al. Generation of functional thymocytes in the human adult. Immunity 1999;10:569–75.

Janeway CA Jr, Kupfer A, Viret C, et al. T cell development, survival and signalling: a new concept of the role of self-peptide:self-MHC complexes. Immunologist 1998;6:5–12.

Janeway CA Jr. Thymic selection: two pathways to life and two to death. Immunity 1994;1:3–6.

Miller JFAP, Morahan G. Peripheral tolerance. Annu Rev Immunol 1992;10:51–69.

Miller JFAP, Morahan G, Allison J, Hoffman M. A transgenic approach to the study of peripheral T-cell tolerance. Immunol Rev 1991;122:103–16.

Nossal GJV. Cellular mechanisms of immunological tolerance. Annu Rev Immunol 1983;1:33–62.

Nossal GJV, Pike BL. Clonal anergy: persistence in tolerant mice of antigen-binding B lymphocytes incapable of responsding to antigen or mitogen. Proc Natl Acad Sci USA 1980;77:1602–6.

Goodnow CC, Crosbie J, Adelstein S, Lavoie TB, Smith-Gill SJ, Brink RA, et al. Altered immunoglobulin expression and functional silencing of self-reactive B lymphocytes in transgenic mice. Nature 1988;334:676–82.

Hartley SB, Crosbie J, Brink R, Kantor AB, Basten A, Goodnow CC. Elimination from peripheral lymphoid tissues of self-reactive B lymphocytes recognizing membrane-bound antigen. Nature 1991;353:765–9.

Gray D, Skarvall H. B cell memory is short-lived in the absence of antigen. Nature 1988;336:70–2.

Gray D, Matzinger P. T cell memory is short-lived in the absence of antigen. J Exp Med 1991;174:969–74.

Lau LL, Jamieson BD, Somasundaram R, Ahmed R. Cytotoxic T cell memory without antigen. Nature 1994, 369:648–652.

2. The Immunology of Trauma and Its Sequelae

Demetrios Demetriades, Geoge C. Velmahos and
William C. Shoemaker

Introduction

Trauma and other acute illnesses begin with an initiating stress which may have both psychological and physiological/inflammatory components. The physiological part begins with the sympathetic adrenal stress response and may escalate to various inter-related immunochemical responses that are phylogenetically protective against foreign proteins and microorganisms. In the process of fulfilling their role, these physiologic responses can be maladaptive mechanisms which can lead to multi-organ failure and death. Since sepsis is a common lethal complication of trauma, these clinical entities widely overlap and cannot be entirely divorced, but in many respects, they must be considered together.

The inflammatory cascades cause changes in the expression and intravascular activity of a wide variety of chemical substances including catecholamines, nitric oxide, glucocorticoids, the complement-coagulation cascade, the kinin-bradykinin system, cytokines, (including tumor necrosis factor -[TNF] and interleukins), eicosanoids (arachidonic acid and its derivatives; leukotrienes, prostaglandins, and thromboxanes), endothelins, heat-shock proteins, platelet activating factor, macrophage migration inhibitory factor and other by-products such as oxygen free radicals. These mediators play key roles in trauma, surgery, burns, the systemic inflammatory response syndrome and septic shock. These cascades interact by stimulating and aggravating various other mechanisms of the inflammatory response, producing circulatory dysfunction and leading to multiple end-organ failures.

Specific and Nonspecific Responses to Trauma

1. Stress Responses to Injury

Initiation of the Stress Responses to Injury

The wide array of responses to injury and other forms of stress include both physiological as well as psychological reactions including immobilization, withdrawal, hostility and aggressive behavior. The stress responses may be minimal after minor operations or injuries, but extensive after major accidental or surgical trauma. This finely honed and appropriately balanced array of compensatory responses to injury and acute critical illnesses is thought to be protective or possibly necessary for recovery. After moderately severe injury, these mechanisms are essentially protective in nature, but when pushed beyond certain limits, in extenuating critical illness, they may become "overcompensations" which can jeopardize survival [1]. Organ failures and death may result from exaggeration or imbalance of physiologic compensations to stress and trauma. It is appropriate to ask when and under what circumstances a given compensation may be advantageous with survival value and when it is potentially harmful to the organism.

Sympathetic Stress Response

The sympathetic (adrenomedullary) stress response may be provoked by psychological stressors such as fear, pain, anxiety and fright as well as by physical factors such as trauma, hypovolemia, tissue hypoxia and hypothermia. These psychological responses may be initiated by the conscious or unconscious perception of danger or the anticipation of pain or injury; they include psychological protective withdrawal and immobilization or antagonistic behavior. Fright, pain, local trauma, or other stressors initiate the neural arcs that increase sympathetic tone by stimulating the release of norepinephrine from peripheral nerve endings. The responses are proportional to the extent of shock and injury. Neural signals initiated in injured and ischemic tissues as well as chemoreceptors communicate systemically the extent of the injury [2].

When the sympathetic nervous system is stimulated, the splanchnic sympathetic effector neurons synapse directly with adrenal medullary cells and stimulate medullary secretion of epinephrine and norepinephrine [1,3,4]. As much as 60-fold increases in adrenal medullary catecholamine output have been reported after pain, hemorrhage, surgery and trauma [5–7]. Evidence of sympathoadrenal axis activation by assay of urinary catecholamines following trauma and with hypercarbia has been well documented; with plasma catecholamine levels being related to the severity of injury [5,7].

The Post-stress Macrocirculatory Patterns

The stress response results in tachycardia, hypertension (or partial correction of hypotension), increased cardiac output, cardiac contractility, minute ventilation and peripheral vasomotor tone as well as reduced urine output. The increased cardiac output effect of these sympathetic stress responses may be limited by hypovolemia. Arterial pressures, however, tend to be maintained even in the presence of decreasing blood flow, until a point is reached when both pressure and flow abruptly fall [8,9].

Elevated cardiac index, tachycardia and hypotension, (with reduced tissue perfusion observed in the monitored patients), reflect the status of acutely traumatized patients with peripheral vasoconstriction from post-traumatic sympathetic neural and adrenergic humoral stimulation. These changes represent the response of trauma which is usually accompanied by concurrent hypovolemia. When hypovolemia is appreciable, low cardiac output is present; when blood volume is corrected, cardiac output rises above the normal range. The onset of consistently high cardiac output in the late stage heralds the post-traumatic hyperdynamic, hypermetabolic state.

Microcirculatory Response to Stress

Prolonged excessive sympathetic stimulation leads to severe uneven metarteriolar vasoconstriction. The intense uneven vasoconstriction collapses some metarterioles while other metarterioles in the same arterial tree remain widely open with nearly adequate capillary flow. The patchy localized vasoconstriction leads to slowing of capillary blood flow, red cell aggregation and stasis in increasing proportions of metarterial-capillary networks. Impaired tissue oxygenation of these localized areas limits the rate of tissue metabolism [8–11]. When the microcirculation is shut off in severe sepsis, microorganisms may flourish in the hypoxic acidotic capillaries plugged with cellular aggregates or "sludge". Other deleterious factors include cell-endothelial adherence which increases resistance to flow, loss of fluid through abnormal capillary exchange, vascular resistance changes and relative resistance to the normal neurohumoral regulatory control of various microcirculatory beds. During septic shock, endothelial cells moderate vascular tone, control local blood flow, activate leukocytes, modulate the margination and extravasation of leukocytes and influence the rate of fluid and protein leakage into tissues [12–14]. With prolonged capillary stasis, hypoxemia, acidosis, inadequate flow and factors released from injured cells, the microcirculation becomes a trap for uncontrolled bacterial growth. Humoral factors released by leukocytes, macrophages, platelets and endothelial cells produce further changes in rheology, coagulation and hematopoiesis [15].

After initial resuscitation, these plugged capillaries may become reperfused. In the meantime, however, the hypoxic acidotic capillary endothelium of poorly perfused capillaries activates macrophages and leukocytes, produces cytokines, platelet activating factor, intravascular coagulation and oxygen free radicals. With resuscitation and reperfusion of hypoxic capillaries, the products of these activated cellular and immunochemical cascades are washed into the venous circulation and lead to the systemic inflammatory response syndrome (SIRS), end-organ dysfunction, and multiple vital organ failures [7–12]. Along with other pathophysiologic mechanisms, this leads to progressive downhill patterns, unremitting hypotension refractory to vasopressor therapy, collapse, shock and death. Between the initial stress response and the final downhill cycle, 15 or more cascades precipitated by the initiating stress and the patient's interacting protective physiologic response mechanisms fall into disarray.

Survivors, however, may have had superior physiologic reserve capacity and ability to generate effective cardiac responses, i.e., the increased cardiac index and vascular responses needed to provide adequate tissue oxygenation and perfusion in the presence of increased metabolic need [7–12] In addition, survivors more often have less blood loss or less severe injury that require compensatory responses of lesser magnitudes. In the late period, the high cardiac index may be explained by increased responses to more severe injury or entry into a hypermetabolic state associated with early SIRS or sepsis not present in the survivors.

Hypothalamic-pituitary-adrenal Axis

Fear, pain, tissue injury, hypotension, hypovolemia and the sympathoadrenal response after trauma or surgery activate the hypothalamic-hypophyseal-adrenal axis by afferent nerve signals which are transmitted from injured tissues by way of C-fibers within the sympathetic nerves. These afferent signals transmitted to the hypothalamus stimulate the hypothalamic-pituitary adrenal axis to secrete corticotropin-releasing factor, which further stimulates adrenocorticotropic hormone (ACTH) secretion from the anterior lobe of the pituitary. ACTH stimulates the adrenals to secrete cortisol, which increases cardiac output and in part mediates the post-traumatic hypermetabolic state [3,16]. The hypermetabolic state, which requires increased blood flow, makes tissues more susceptible to ischemic events [7,8].

Vasopressin, angiotensin II, norepinephrine, endotoxemia and inhalation anesthetics also stimulate release of the corticotropin releasing factor. Beta-endorphin, beta-lipotropin, and alpha-melanocyte-stimulating hormone are also released along with ACTH; these hormones are thought to be cleavage products of the large precursor propiomelanocortin.

The target organ for ACTH is the adrenal cortex. ACTH stimulates the synthesis and release of cortisol in amounts parallel to the degree of injury. For this reason, cortisol has been used as a marker of the degree of the stress response [12–15]. The effects of cortisol and other glucocorticoids, which play a major role in the stress response, include sodium retention, insulin resistance, gluconeogenesis, lipolysis, protein catabolism, demargination of white blood cells and the enhanced catabolic effects of tumor-necrosis factor (TNF) and interleukin-6 (IL-6). Although cortisol is needed for recovery from acute trauma, prolonged extensive cortisol secretion has detrimental effects that lead to critical illness, circulatory dysfunction, organ failure, shock and even death.

Antidiuretic Hormone

Acute blood loss is sensed by atrial receptors, while hypotension is sensed by baroreceptors in the carotid, aortic, and pulmonary arteries and communicated to the hypothalamus. Nerve fibers in the hypothalamus synapse directly with cells in the posterior lobe of the pituitary gland, which then releases antidiuretic hormone into the general circulation. Antidiuretic hormone acts on the renal collecting ducts to actively reabsorb water; thus it causes water retention and is also a powerful vasoconstrictor [17].

Renin-angiotensin

With hypovolemia sensed in the atria and hypotension sensed in the carotid, aortic and pulmonary arteries, there is a signal to the hypothalamus and neurohypophysis to release vasopressin that causes water retention and vasoconstriction. Reduced renal blood flow after trauma activates the aldosterone-renin-angiotensin axis that produces profound vasoconstriction with salt and water retention. The cells are stimulated to secrete renin, which enzymatically cleaves the juxtaglomerular protein, angiotensinogen to yield angiotensin I. This is further cleaved to form angiotensin II. The latter is a very potent vasoconstrictor and vasopressor that acts on the kidney to decrease salt and water excretion. Angiotensin also stimulates the secretion of aldosterone, which further decreases salt and water excretion. These renal physiologic effects last from several hours to several days after injury [3,4,7,17,18].

Opioids

Part of the early stress response is the release of endogenous opioids along with ACTH by the pituitary gland. Also endorphins are released from the adrenal glands by sympathetic stimulation. The opioids are thought to be counter-regulatory inhibitors of the stress response, in that they decrease the sensation of pain and modulate neutrophil and lymphocyte functions, (including T-cell function) thus acting to modulate the immune system. This effectively links the central nervous system responses with immune responses [19,20].

2. Immunochemical Responses after Accidental and Surgical Trauma

A number of complex, inter-related immunochemical responses are initiated by direct injury, surgery, hemorrhage, infection and other acute illnesses. The clinical and immunologic responses occurring after accidental injury are indistinguishable from those after surgical trauma and will be briefly summarized below.

Complement

Tissue injury, local ischemia and tissue hypoxia stimulate the release of mediators including tissue thromboplastin that lead to disruption of the endothelial capillary lining. Subendothelial collagen and basement membrane destruction activate the circulating Hageman factor (Factor XII) that initiates the complement cascade by the intrinsic pathway. Washout coagulation problems occur after large blood volume losses and replacement with banked blood and clear fluids because circulating protein clotting factors are diluted. In addition to initiating the coagulation process, the complex protein clotting system activates the kinin and plasmin systems and initiates multiple inflammatory responses [21].

Arachidonic Acid Cascades: Leukotrienes and Prostaglandins

Injury and ischemia disrupt the endothelial cell membranes. The breakup of these endothelial cell membranes causes the release of arachidonic acid, which produces leukotrienes, or which are converted by cyclooxygenase to produce prostaglandin and thromboxane cascades. Thromboxane tends to aggregate platelets and red cells while a number of the prostaglandins, particularly PGE_1 and PGI_2 dissaggregate red cells. These are also potent mediators of vascular tone and contribute to inflammation, coagulation and cellular activation.

Cytokine Cascades

Endothelial damage triggers multiple cascades that activate T-cells to secrete cytokines, TNF and acute-phase interleukins (IL-1, IL-2, IL-6, and IL-8), which are activated by sepsis, trauma, surgery, adult respiratory distress syndrome (ARDS) and other organ failures. Increased release of these cytokines is associated with an acute-phase reaction and the hypermetabolic state [22,23].

Platelet Activating Factor

Platelet activating factor is produced when arachidonic acid is released from the capillary endothelial cell wall. L-arginine analogues inhibit nitric oxide (NO) and improve blood pressure but they decrease cardiac output and may compromise tissue perfusion [24]. In animal models, the NO donor, SIN-1 increased cardiac output and superior mesenteric artery blood flow and appears to be well tolerated [25]. In experimental preparations, methylene blue, (which inhibits the effects of NO on guanylate cyclase), progressively increases mean arterial blood pressure without decreasing cardiac output, oxygen delivery (DO_2) or oxygen consumption (VO_2) [26].

Nitric Oxide (NO)

The hypotension and myocardial depression of septic shock has been attributed to the action of nitric oxide (NO), which is essential for microcirculatory regulation. NO reduces pulmonary artery (PA) pressure, while NO blockade increases PA pressure. Experimental studies have revealed that inhibition of NO may reduce splanchnic blood flow, increase PA pressure and increase mortality [27,28]. L-arginine analogues inhibit NO and improve blood pressure but they decrease cardiac output and may compromise tissue perfusion [29,30]

Oxygen Free Radicals, Reactive Oxygen Species (ROS)

The reperfusion of ischemic endothelial cells produces bursts of oxygen free radicals or more properly termed, reactive oxygen species (ROS), that are cytotoxic to cells in the immediate environment. When oxygen is restored to hypoxic cells during reperfusion, hypoxanthine accumulated during hypoxia is oxidized by xanthine oxidase. This reaction generates the ROS, superoxide anion radical and hydrogen peroxide, by a series of electron transfers [31]. The ROS damage cells directly by denaturing their proteins, disrupting chromosomes and interfering with the function of various intracellular organelles. Most importantly, these ROS damage cellular membranes by peroxidation of structurally important polyunsaturated fatty acids. The effect of the oxidants on cells is directly related to their quantity and rate of production, which increases with increasing accumulation of toxic unoxidized products as ischemia time is prolonged; i.e., reperfusion injury increases as ischemia time lengthens. Prolonged shock and delayed resuscitation increases the risk of severe damage.

ROS are normally eliminated by the action of endogenous free radical scavengers, such as catalase and superoxide dismutase as well as by antioxidants. With ischemia, activities of these scavengers decrease as they are expended. The ROS activate surface transcription in neutrophils, cytokine transcription in macrophages, and acute phase protein transcription in hepatocytes. The ROS further enhance production of TNF, IL-1 and IL-8, (the proinflammatory cytokines). These newly synthesized cytokines play an important role in amplifying the inflammatory response to ischemia and the reperfusion injury. By activating leukocytes, macrophages and endothelial cells, they further intensify the inflammatory state and initiate the downhill spiral leading to circulatory dysfunction, SIRS and organ failure [31–34].

Antioxidants

Naturally occurring enzymes, such as catalase, superoxide dismutase and glutathione peroxidase play important roles as scavengers of ROS. Ascorbate (Vitamin C), urate, glutathione, tocopherols, flavinoids, carotenoids (beta-carotene, lycopene), and ubiquinol are naturally occurring compounds that are found in a variety of foods and serve as specific therapeutic agents for common dietary deficiencies. More importantly they also function as antioxidants or scavengers of ROS. The antioxidant, N-acetylcysteine (NAC) improves oxygen uptake and cardiac function in experimental animal models of sepsis [35, 36].

3. Ischemia, Poor Tissue Perfusion and Tissue Hypoxia

Ischemia, defined as interruption of blood supply, oxygen and nutrients to localized areas of tissue, produces numerous complex physiologic changes some of which are summarized below.

Reperfusion of Ischemic Capillaries: Washout of Local Mediators

Local injury, reduced flow, ischemia, hypoxia and acidosis in endothelial cells from maldistributed microcirculatory flow and poor tissue perfusion activate several cascades that begin on the endothelial cell surface at the site of injury [22,23]. With ischemia, ATP is broken down to AMP, inosine, adenosine and hypoxanthine. On reperfusion of stagnant capillary networks, endothelial cells generate bursts of oxygen free radicals. (vide supra) Much of this damage does not occur during the original ischemic insult, but later during reperfusion of the ischemic, acidotic capillary networks. The ischemic insult may also be mediated by second messengers such as intracellular calcium, cyclic adenosine monophosphate (cAMP) and phosphatidic acids. Endothelial cells primed by ischemia are more susceptible to subsequent reperfusion and inflammation, but also participate as effectors of inflammatory responses. The gut appears to be particularly susceptible to ischemia, not only as a target organ but also as the source of bacteria and bacterial products that may penetrate the leaky gut mucosal barrier; a phenomenon called bacterial translocation.

Alteration of Membrane Potential

Hypoperfusion during shock results in cell membrane dysfunction [37,38]. Normally, the cell membrane preserves the milieu interior through the maintenance of a negative charge or membrane potential. This potential serves as a semipermeable barrier, preserving the balance of intra and extracellular electrolytes and water. Inappropriate depolarization, as well as prolongation of polarization and repolarization, are early phenomena in low-flow states that occur even before decreases in blood pressure.

Cellular Swelling

Following these changes of membrane potential and due to a relative lack of ATP, the sodium/potassium pump cannot maintain cellular sodium homeostasis [39] and sodium enters the cell causing intracellular swelling. At the same time, potassium leaves through the cellular membrane in an opposite direction. Calcium channels open and extracellular calcium accumulates inside the cell. The increase in intracellular calcium causes cellular contraction by stimulation of the cytoskeleton. Osmotic swelling of the cell occurs with damage to the nuclear and cytoplasmic elements.

Cellular Acidosis

During ischemia, the cell develops an increased redox value associated with an increased ratio of reduced nicotinamide adenine dinucleotide to nicotinamide adenine dinucleotide (NADH/NAD) and intracellular acidosis associated with decreased ATP levels [40]. The increased NADH/NAD ratio occurs because oxygen is absent in the final step of the mitochondrial electron transport chain. This electron transport blockade results in inability to oxidize NADH. Intracellular acidosis occurs secondary to ongoing hydrolysis of ATP to meet the cellular energy requirements.

Unfortunately, clinical indicators of cellular ischemia are not available. Although the characterization of flow dynamics and the estimation of total body oxygen delivery and oxygen consumption provide an estimate of cellular function, precise tissue-specific evaluation of the intracellular environment is at present clinically unavailable. Similarly, estimates of blood lactate and base deficit provide only rough guides of the overall status, changing quite frequently after significant intracellular damage has already occurred.

Alteration in Signal Transduction Pathways

The increased cellular redox state initiates signal transduction pathways associated with nuclear factor κB (NF-κB) [41]. NF-κB is an important transcriptional factor that exists as a heterodimeric complex and controls the inducible expression of a variety of genes that are involved in the immune response. Target genes for NF-κB include cytokines, cytokine receptors, major histocompatability complex (MHC) antigens, acute-phase proteins and several viral enhancers. By activation or blockade of NF-κB according to the cellular redox state, the expression of these secondary proteins may be affected. For example, it has been shown that the generation of reactive oxygen intermediates triggers NF-κB activation. In parallel to NF-κB, other transcriptional factors can be activated through different pathways, often also involving the intracellular redox state and cytokine interaction with membrane receptors. These different transcriptional factors interact to release several immunoregulatory proteins through augmentation or suppression of gene transcription. Modulation of gene transcription by pharmacologic interaction in such transcription pathways is an attractive potential therapeutic option. However, the fine balance between suppression or overproduction and maintenance of necessary levels of such proteins is difficult to achieve with chemical methods. Caution should be exercised in implementing theoretically sound therapies in order to avoid significantly altering responses necessary for appropriate host defense and other important immunoregulatory functions.

Reperfusion of Hypoxic Capillaries

Although cellular priming normally enhances oxygen-dependent killing at sites of infection, shock after trauma may initiate a multitude of priming stimuli that result in the accumulation of toxic intracellular products. These products are not activated or released in the general circulation before reperfusion occurs. Reperfusion stimulates cells to participate in an inflammatory response, as described below.

Production of Inflammatory Mediators

A variety of proteins that are involved in the inflammatory cascade are produced during hypoxic priming and subsequent reperfusion [32–34]. Among them are platelet activating factor (PAF), TNF-α, interleukins (IL-1, -6, -8, -10) and interferons (IFN), to name a few. These mediators are predominantly produced by macrophages. However, by autocrine function they also stimulate macrophages to up-regulate and to achieve a self-sustaining inflammatory phenotype capable of continuous production of inflammatory mediators. TNF-α is secreted in abundance after shock associated with trauma. Its production is stimulated by lipopolysaccharide (LPS) or other macrophage activities such as phagocytosis of particulate material or senescent red blood cells, as typically occurs after trauma. Multiple biochemical pathways exist for its production, which may be independent of priming. IL-1 is capable of up-regulating macrophage production of TNF-α, IL-6, and IL-1 itself. IL-6 is increased after trauma and shock and the degree and persistence of its elevation may be of prognostic significance. Its role in regulating macrophage function is still not clear.

Leukocyte Activation

Leukocyte (neutrophil, monocyte and lymphocyte) function is also affected by reperfusion [7,42]. In particular, polymorphonuclear leukocytes (PMNs) play a central role in the inflammatory cascade. While PMNs are primed during ischemia by increasing their adhesiveness, exposure to abnormal surfaces during reperfusion results in morphologic and biochemical changes defined as activation. At this stage, adhesion is further promoted by a diverse group of surface proteins known as leukocyte adhesion molecules. These mediators include leukotrienes, such as LTB4, platelet-activating factor and other chemoreactants. Activated leukocytes secrete inflammatory proteins which further aggravate the inflammatory response and they may also be a source of ROS. Leukocyte-mediated injury is dependent mainly on leukocyte adherence to the vascular endothelial cell surface and leukocyte-leukocyte aggregation in the microvasculature. Direct injury to the endothelial cells by leukocyte-secreted ROS results in damage of cell-to-cell bridges and formation of intracellular gaps, which allow fluids to diffuse into the extravascular space and edema to develop. Aggregation of leukocytes further compromises the microvascular circulation by occluding capillaries and post-capillary venules, extending the zone of ischemia and tissue necrosis.

Endothelial Cell Changes

The endothelial cell (EC) was once thought to play a passive role in the inflammatory response to shock. It was considered as a barrier only to leukocytes that had the ability to injure it. Now, it is understood that the EC plays an active role in coordinating the response to shock and injury [13]. Its main functions include maintenance of the balance between anticoagulation and procoagulation factors, regulation of smooth muscle tone, control of vascular permeability and receptor-mediated coordination of adhesion and emigration into the extracellular matrix. The EC is capable of producing pro or anticoagulant factors. The normal state of the EC is one of anticoagulation, but when it is subjected to shock, the delicate balance is shifted in favor of procoagulation. The end result is diffuse micro-vascular thrombosis, which can lead to further ischemic organ damage. In addition, this process leads to rapid consumption of clotting factors and can contribute to the consumption coagulopathy sometimes seen in severe trauma.

The control of vasomotor tone by the EC involves a balance between three primary products: prostaglandins, nitric oxide and endothelins. During shock, the balance is tipped in favor of vasoconstriction based on the stimulation of endothelin release and inhibition of nitric oxide, inducing additional damage to poorly perfused structures. The interactions between the EC and the leukocyte that result in leukocyte adhesion and activation are mediated by numerous adhesion molecules, including selectins and integrins. The dynamic role that the EC plays has been increasingly explored, serving as future targets for therapeutic interventions.

4. Acute Clinical Syndromes Produced by Immunologic Disorders

Systemic Immune Response Syndrome (SIRS)

SIRS, a generalized inflammatory state that follows trauma and shock, is responsible for protracted cellular and organ damage or failure in the immediate post-resuscitation period of days or weeks. Activated leukocytes, macrophages, and endothelial cells initiate and amplify the post-ischemic inflammatory state. Although coagulation and inflammation at injury sites are essential for healing, when exaggerated these systems play major roles in the more generalized systemic responses to trauma by stimulating coagulation and inflammation in tissues distant from the initial injury site.

The Inflammatory Cascades

Gradually the SIRS syndrome more actively stimulates inflammatory cascades that initially result from the host responses to blood borne bacterial toxins, including LPS and endotoxin from gram-negative bacteria and cell fragments, exotoxins, and superantigens from gram-positive bacteria [43–45]. Episodes of hypoperfusion and bacterial toxins initiate a common pathway involving TNF-α and IL-1. Like conventional trauma stress responses, the systemic inflammatory response syndrome consists of numerous neurohormonal and immunochemical cascades, changes in the expression and intravascular activity of cytokines, arachidonic acid derivatives, complement pathways, kinin-bradykinin, endothelins, heat-shock proteins, platelet activating factor, macrophage migration inhibitory factor (MIF), and their by-products.

Pathogenesis of ARDS after Trauma and Surgery: Time Course of Events

Next to SIRS, sepsis and septic shock, the most common postoperative and post-traumatic organ failure is adult respiratory distress syndrome (ARDS). The pathogenesis of ARDS should be based on objective physiologic evidence including hypovolemia, low cardiac output, anemia, hypoxemia, adrenomedullary and corticosteroid stress response, the duration of shock or low-flow state, poor tissue perfusion, tissue hypoxia and oxygen debt; all augmented by cascades of mediators.

Oxygen Debt as a Measure of Tissue Hypoxia: Role of the Macrocirculation in Organ Failure

Tissue hypoxia results from inadequate or unevenly distributed microcirculatory blood flow in relation to increased metabolic demands from fever, inflammatory responses, postoperative wound healing, hypovolemia, anesthesia, surgical trauma and failure or delays in replacing blood losses. Progressively increasing tissue hypoxia results in multiple vital organ failure, the major proximate cause of death in ICU patients. We have tested this hypothesis in a consecutive series of 253 high-risk surgical patients, where the amount of oxygen debt was calculated from the difference between serially measured VO_2 and estimated need, $VO_{2(need)}$. This was calculated from the patient's own preoperative VO_2 measurements extrapolated to the intraoperative and to the first 48-hour post-operative periods after corrections for anesthesia and temperature have been made. The net cumulative oxygen debt at any given time was calculated from the integrated area between the actual VO_2 and the estimated $VO_{2(need)}$. Greater oxygen debts were observed in patients with organ failure than in those without organ failure and greater oxygen debts were seen in those who died (all of whom had organ failure) than in those who survived with or without organ failure [46].

Prospective randomized trials have demonstrated that attainment of supranormal values empirically observed in survivors significantly reduced oxygen debt, organ failure and death in high-risk surgical patients. Prior studies indicate that oxygen debts with organ failure were larger than those of patients without organ failures; even larger debts were found in patients who died *with* organ failure. Furthermore, optimal values of cardiac index (CI), DO_2 and VO_2 in prospective trials reduces oxygen debt and thus decreases organ failure and death. The concept that ARDS is caused by antecedent tissue hypoxia is supported by the demonstration of oxygen debt from circulatory deficiencies as the earliest physiologic event associated with high-risk surgical operations, major trauma, and hypovolemia [46]. ARDS does not just materialize as a new entity; rather, it is the end-organ failure of an antecedent circulatory dysfunction in which blood pressure and other superficial signs of shock have been corrected but the underlying tissue perfusion defect is not resolved.

Immunochemical Mediators of ARDS

The early events after hemorrhage, trauma, high-risk surgery and other acute critical illnesses, have been discussed. The uneven microcirculatory flow inevitably leaves some capillary networks predisposed to local hypoxia and acidosis. The endothelial surfaces of these hypoxic, acidotic, vasoconstricted capillary beds in peripheral or visceral circulations activate T-cell lymphocytes and macrophages. With fluid resuscitation, there is reperfusion of poorly perfused capillary networks and in this process, many of these immunochemical mediators are washed out of the microcirculation and into the venous circulation where they go directly to the lungs which is the first capillary network they encounter. Here they play a major role in the development of ARDS and subsequently other organ failures.

It is important to distinguish the initiators, such as high-risk surgery, trauma, hemorrhage, hypovolemia, pre-existing serious cardiac conditions and sepsis from the mediators of immunochemical responses. The initiators may produce low flow states or uneven flow from uneven vasomotion that leaves some capillaries with little or no flow, hypoxia and acidosis. It is obviously easier to prevent immuno-chemical events from occurring than to attempt to treat their consequences, par-ticularly when multi-organ failure is established.

Organ Failures: Relationships of Hemodynamic Patterns to Mediators

Experimentally and clinically the activation of IL-6, IL-8 and tumor necrosis factor, already discussed, have been demonstrated when sepsis or ARDS occurs after trauma. Increased release of these cytokines is associated with an acute-phase reaction and the hypermetabolic state. Meade et al [47] measured plasma levels of complement factors, antitoxins and cytokines in severely traumatized patients on admission to the emergency department and at successive intervals for 48 hours. Those who developed ARDS had initial marked reductions of cardiac index, DO_2, and VO_2 in the first 4 hours after admission, but elevations of plasma interleukin levels which did not reach their maxima until 16 hours after the diagnostic criteria for ARDS had already been met. By contrast, the trauma patients who did not develop ARDS had higher initial cardiac indices, DO_2, and VO_2 values, and lower recorded values for pulmonary shunting as well as lower plasma cytokines. Thus, increased plasma cytokine levels did not precede occurrence of hemodynamic and oxygen transport markers nor the clinical diag-nostic features of ARDS, but they accelerate and augment the disorder as it occurs.

Prevention of ARDS in Severe Trauma and High Risk Surgical Patients

The incidence of postoperative organ failure and death in high-risk trauma and surgical patients was reduced by maintaining adequate tissue perfusion with optimal CI and DO2 to prevent oxygen debt. Moreover, Thangathurai et al [48] further decreased the incidence of ARDS to zero in over 300 high risk cancer patients per year for a three year period by maintaining tissue perfusion intra-operatively with adequate fluids (mostly colloids) and titrated doses of nitro-glycerine to prevent maldistribution of microcirculatory flow as determined by both invasive and noninvasive hemodynamic and oxygen transport monitoring. These data suggest that intraoperative oxygen debt from reduced tissue perfusion is the initiating mechanism that leads to organ failure and that monitoring can facilitate optimization of peripheral tissue oxygenation and prevent postoperative ARDS.

In essence, the physiologic changes that preceded the clinical diagnosis of ARDS include (1) hypovolemia made manifest by reduced blood volume, red blood cell mass and hematocrit; (2) inadequate myocardial performance as indi-cated by a suboptimal increase in CI response to administration of fluids and inotropic agents; (3) inadequate tissue perfusion as indicated by suboptimal DO_2, VO_2, or P_tCO_2/FiO_2 and $PtcCO_2$ and

(4) increased pulmonary vasoconstriction as indicated by increased mean PA pressure and pulmonary vascular resistance (PVR) index. All of these deranged parameters are linked to a primary increase in effective oxygen debt.

5. Immunobiology of Shock in Experimental Models

The considerable progress in shock management during the past 50 years may be attributed to by timely and optimal resuscitation to avoid tissue ischemia. Although cellular ischemia alone is not responsible for tissue damage, the physiologic and immunochemical responses already alluded to produce reperfusion injury from the release of various inflammatory mediators of tissue injury and shock [49].

During low-flow states, cellular changes called "hypoxic priming" occur. The cell readies itself to enter the respiratory burst cycle. Later, when reperfusion is established, the primed cell is activated to participate in an uncontrolled inflammatory process that leads to cellular injury, which is clinically manifested by organ failure or death.

Animal Models of Shock and Their Use to Evaluate Therapy

The understanding of the immunologic response following shock demands extensive experimentation in the animal laboratory. The use of animal models of shock has led to important information on the biology of the normal and pathologic processes and critical insights into the disease. Encouraging messages have been received with regard to the therapeutic modulation of the immune response. However, more often than not the lessons learned in the laboratory do not appear applicable in the clinical setting. Recognition of the differences between conveniently-set animal experiments and the uncontrolled clinical reality is essential for appropriate design and execution of similar studies.

The most commonly used animal models of shock are the following: a) Fixed-pressure and fixed-volume models of hemorrhagic shock have been used and refined for over 60 years. Here, animals are bled to a fixed pressure and maintained at this pressure for a pre-determined time by infusion of fluids or shed blood. b) Fixed-volume models require the removal of a fixed volume of blood over a defined time period and blood pressure is allowed to fluctuate. c) Uncontrolled hemorrhage models; where no surgical control is made during the hemorrhagic period i.e. the animal is allowed to bleed uncontrollably. Variations include models that mimic the pre-hospital stage, where the animal is bleeding uncontrollably without resuscitation, the in-hospital pre-operative stage, (during which the animal continues bleeding but resuscitation to certain end-points is offered) and the operative stage, at which surgical control is achieved and resuscitation is continued to full effect. Usually, hemorrhage in the first two models is produced by allowing a measured amount of blood to flow outside a major artery through a previously placed line. In the third model, an injury is usually created, and the animal is allowed to bleed into a major cavity, (usually the abdomen), in order to simulate the clinical situation.

A number of confounding variables in these classical models need to be considered [43]. First, the sex of the animals can have an effect on the results obtained [44]. Recent work indicates that female mice tolerate sepsis better that male mice due to lack of testosterone. Moreover splenic and macrophage IL-1 production is also suppressed in males. This defective response can be corrected when testosterone secretion is suppressed by castration of the male mice. Second, different strains of the animal species may produce very different results within the same species. Genetic polymorphism within various cytokine loci influence cytokine production and the inflammatory response. Third, the development of shock under controlled laboratory circumstances only remotely simulates the clinical situation. Animals are studied while bleeding without having any additional insults. Human hemorrhagic shock is associated with hypothermia, acidosis, multiple injuries, soft tissue crush and coagulopathy. The fundamental problem with exsanguinating patients is the damage to vascular structures and the gastrointestinal tract with or without spillage of irritant contents rather than just hypotension per se. Additionally, the presence of pre-existing diseases or toxic substances influences the immunologic response, whereas bleeding in healthy laboratory animals is their only pathophysiologic problem. Fourth, the use of heparinization for models of hemorrhagic animal shock is not applicable to clinical conditions (43–45). During experimental hemorrhage, platelet aggregation and diffuse vasoconstriction may alter the bleeding volume. Heparin used to prevent catheter clotting and improve standardization of the model introduces a major confounding variable.

6. Therapy

Therapeutic Strategies

In the last few years there has been an explosion of experimental and clinical work in immunomodulation therapies in trauma, shock and sepsis. Intervention can be performed at various stages of the cascade of the inflammatory response. The cheapest and most effective way of preventing or reducing post-traumatic organ dysfunction and sepsis is most probably the prevention of ischemia/reperfusion which triggers the whole cascade of inflammatory responses in the first instance. The conventional clinical parameters of blood pressure, pulse and urine output are very crude and unreliable markers of adequate tissue perfusion. Early detection and correction of tissue hypoxia is not possible with standard monitoring in the emergency room, the operating room or other areas outside an intensive care unit. A Swan-Ganz catheter which can give adequate information about resuscitation status and oxygen delivery and uptake is not practical outside an intensive care unit environment. Similar limitations apply to other techniques which can measure tissue perfusion, such as intracellular gastric pH monitoring. Base deficit and lactic acid monitoring provide a much more reliable picture of tissue perfusion than the conventional hemodynamic parameters. Base deficit measurements should be part of the usual resuscitation in every significant trauma patient. A more recent development in this field is the improvement and simplication of non-invasive monitoring techniques using bioimpedance principles. These techniques can be applied in the emergency room, operating room or any other place in hospital. The combination of bioimpedance, transcutaneous oxygen and CO_2 monitoring and standard pulse oximetry, provide continuous real-time assessment of cardiac activity, respiratory function and tissue perfusion status [11]. There is clinical evidence that early detection and correction of tissue hypoperfusion reduces the incidence and severity of organ dysfunction.

During the later post-traumatic phase bacterial activators may play an important role in triggering the inflammatory cascade. Appropriate antibiotic treatment or drainage of infected material are then the mainstays of treatment.

Experimental Studies

There are several possible times for intervention during the various stages of the inflammatory process. This section summarizes the effects of some therapeutic interventions evaluated in experimental shock using the approach of Redl et al [50] who analyzed research models targeting factors at four stages: a) the primary induction site, b) the intermediate mediator, c) the final mediator and d) the effector cell.

Primary Induction Site

The importance of prevention and early correction of ischemia and reperfusion has already been discussed. Complement activation peptides are important pro-inflammatory agents and in animal models, it has been shown that blocking this process may be beneficial [51]. Release of endotoxins plays an important role during the early phase of the inflammatory cascade. Numerous therapeutic strategies targeting endotoxins have been developed and tested with variable results. Although animal studies have demonstrated their effectiveness, subsequent human studies have failed to show any significant benefits. The most extensively tested agents reported for clinical use are the E5 murine and HA1A human monoclonal antibodies against endotoxin. Although, all animal and early human studies demonstrated efficacy in Gram-negative sepsis, further large clinical trials failed to show any outcome benefits [52]. Another primary induction site which has been studied very extensively is the gut. with alteration of the effects and extent of bacterial and toxin translocation.

Most animal studies have shown that hemorrhagic shock induces bacteria/endotoxin translocation from the gut [53,54], although others have failed to confirm these findings [55]. Overall, there is experimental evidence that hemorrhagic shock results in translocation and local release of cytokines during the early ischemic phase [53]. In human studies the results are more conflicting, with many studies failing to identify translocation in the portal or the lymphatic system during the early trauma stages [56,57]. In a recent study in trauma patients with hemorrhagic shock, Kale et al [58] identified bacterial translocation in the lymph nodes, portal vein and liver in many hypovolemic trauma patients undergoing emergency laparotomy for trauma. Laboratory work in rats has also shown that, removal of the entire small bowel and colon improves the early survival after prolonged hemorrhagic shock. The authors were unable, however, to show endotoxemia in either the enterectomized group or in the control group. However, in the enterectomized animals, there were higher hepatic ATP levels, suggesting the importance of intestinal participation in hepatic ATP depletion [59]. Selective gut decontamination, (in order to prevent translocation), has been studied extensively in critically ill patients, including trauma victims. Although most studies have reported a lower incidence of pneumonia after such therapy, they have all failed to show any survival benefit [60,61]. This is an area where more and better designed clinical studies are needed.

Therapy at the Intermediate Mediator Level

This phase includes the production and activity of cytokines, adhesion molecules, lipid mediators, and NO. Therapeutic interventions targeting the production or scavenging of cytokines have been extensively tested in laboratory studies with encouraging results. Bahrami et al [62] in a hemorrhagic shock model in rats tested a murine monoclonal antibody to LPS. The 48-hour mortality rate was significantly reduced in the treatment group (mortality 28.6 percent in the treatment group *vs.* 78.6 percent in the control group). Also, lung injury, as assessed by lung wet weight and pulmonary neutrophilic infiltration, was significantly reduced in the treatment group. Abraham and Allbee [63] in a mouse model of resuscitated hemorrhagic shock showed that recombinant interleukin-1 receptor antagonist (IL-1Ra) prevented the post-hemorrhage increases in pulmonary TNF-α levels and diminished the increase in IL-1 and IL-6 mRNA levels normally found after blood loss.

Pellicane et al [64] in a hemorrhagic shock model in mice reported a significantly improved 5-day survival in animals treated with Interleukin-1 receptor antagonist. Their results suggested that IL-1Ra improved the outcome by preventing ATP depletion in vital organs. The timing and dosage of anti-endoxin or anti-cytokine treatment may be critical in the effectiveness and the prevention or treatment of organ dysfunction or sepsis after trauma. O'Riordain et al [65] in a burns animal model showed that administration of anti-TNF antibody on days 0 or 4 when the TNF levels were not elevated did not improve survival. However, anti-TNF therapy on day 7 when the TNF levels were elevated, markedly improved outcome. They also demonstrated that high doses of antibody were not beneficial and may actually be detrimental.

Neutrophil adherence or aggregation play an important role in the inflammatory cascade and organ injury after hemorrhagic shock. The role of blocking of adherence and aggregation of neutrophils in interrupting the inflammatory cascade has been extensively studied in animal studies. Mileski et al (66) in a hemorrhagic shock model in primates showed that inhibition of neutrophil adherence or aggregation with monoclonal antibodies at the time of resuscitation reduced gastric injury and fluid requirements. Pentoxifylline (PTX) has been shown to decrease PMN adhesiveness and to reduce the activated circulating pool of PMNs. Many studies have demonstrated improved outcome with PTX-treated animals in induced hemorrhagic shock [67–70]. Scalia et al [67] in a murine traumatic shock model showed that a recombinant serine protease inhibitor, which reduces neutrophil accumulation in injured tissues, improved survival. Moreover, selectins, which play a major role in the neutrophil-mediated injury after hemorrhagic shock and resuscitation, may be targets for modification, where many animal studies have demonstrated the beneficial effects of selectin blockade. Rivera-Chavez [71] in an uncontrolled hemorrhagic shock and resuscitation model with rats, showed that P-selectin blockade with monoclonal antibodies resulted in increased survival and decreased hepatocellular injury. Winn et al [72] and Ramamoorthy et al [73] using hemorrhagic shock and resuscitation models in rabbits, showed that selectin blockade had a protective effect against ischemia-reperfusion injury.

Lipid mediators (platelet-activating factor, thromboxanes, leukotrienes) play an important role in the inflammatory cascade in traumatic shock [74–77]. Terashita et al [74] showed that the combination of platelet activating factor antagonist and prostaglandin E1 significantly improved survival at 150 minutes and decreased myocardial depressant factor (MDF) in traumatic shock in mice. Many studies showed that treatment with thromboxane synthetase inhibitors improved the survival time and reduced the accumulation of MDF and cathepsin D in experimental traumatic shock [75,76,78]. Leukotriene antagonists have also shown improved survival time and decreased MDF production in traumatic shock [77].

As already stated, NO may be an important player in the pathophysiology of hemorrhagic shock. Although there is controversy about its positive or negative effect in traumatic shock, there has been experimental evidence that NO may have a protective effect resulting in better survival by improving the distribution of capillary blood flow and inhibiting platelet and leukocyte aggregation and adhesion in hemorrhagic shock [79]. However, other conflicting studies have shown that NO inhibition during hypovolemic shock in rats may improve renal function [80].

Final Mediator Level

Oxygen radicals play a critical role as "final" mediators in ischemia-reperfusion organ damage. Numerous pharmacological interventions inhibiting the production of or scavenging oxygen radicals have been studied in experimental shock models. Opposing superoxide generation, inhibiting arachidonic acid oxidation and inhibiting lipid peroxidation are some interventions which have been studied extensively. Fleckenstein et al [81] in a rat hemorrhagic shock model compared the effectiveness of four antioxidants acting at different pathways of oxygen radical generation and reactions. They concluded that inhibition of lipid peroxidation induced by free radicals was more effective than attempting to block specific pathways of oxygen radical production. Superoxide Dismutase (SOD) and allopurinol have been shown to improve survival and protect the gastric mucosa in numerous studies with animal models of hemorrhagic shock [82,83]. Other anti-oxidants, such as Vitamin E have also been shown to improve survival in similar models [84].

Target Level

Membrane stabilization and protection from free radical-induced lipid peroxidation is an attractive therapeutic intervention because all inflammatory pathways end up targeting the cell membrane. The development of non-glucocorticoid 21-aminosteroids (lazaroids) opened new research avenues in the management of hemorrhagic shock and head injuries. Animal work demonstrated significant benefits in treating hemorrhagic shock with lazaroids [85,86]. In experimental cerebral cortical injuries in rats, lazaroids significantly reduced the microvascular permeability at the site of injury and moderately reduced brain swelling [87] with histologically proven reduced axonal injury [88].

Other Modalities

Recombinant bactericidal/permeability-increasing protein (rBPI1) has been shown in numerous studies to have anti-bacterial and anti-endotoxin properties [89]. In vitro studies have shown that rBPI21 inhibits the release of cytokines, free radicals and NO. It also inhibits adhesion of neutrophils and complement activation. In experimental hemorrhagic shock models in rats, rBPI21 was shown to reduce the circulating endotoxin levels, inhibit bacterial translocation, reduce organ damage and improve survival [90,91].

Moderate hypothermia (32–34°C) has been shown to reduce secondary brain injury in animals with traumatic brain damage [92]. Clifton et al [93] showed that rats with traumatic brain injury treated with hypothermia (30°C) demonstrated significantly better beam-walking, beam balance and body weight loss than rats treated with normothermia. One of the suggested mechanisms is the suppression of the post-injury inflammatory response. Hypothermia has been shown to reduce the infiltrations of PMNs into the injured area, inhibit cytokine release and prevent NO synthesis [94, 95].

Clinical Studies

Although a large number of experimental studies showed promising results with immunomodulation in hemorrhagic shock and traumatic brain injury, only a relatively small number of clinical studies have been performed. With very few exceptions, the majority of clinical trials failed to confirm the positive results of the experimental studies. The failure of the murine E5 and human HA1A monoclonal antibodies to improve outcome in large trials in patients with Gram-negative sepsis is one major example with evidence that some patients with Gram-positive sepsis receiving hHA1A were actually harmed by the therapy.

Superoxide Dismutase in Severe Head Injuries, Phase II Trial

A prospective, randomized study of superoxide dismutase has been reported on 104 patients with severe head injuries (i.e. GCS 8 or less). Patients were randomized to receive either placebo or polyethylene glycol-conjugated superoxide dismutase (PEG-SOD), an average of 4 hours after injury. Outcome was assessed using the Glasgow Outcome Scale at 3 and 6 months post-injury. At 3 months, 44 percent of the placebo patients were in a vegetative state or had died as compared with 20 percent in the treatment group which received 10,000 u/Kg of PEG-SOD. At 6 months, these figures were 36 percent and 21 percent respectively (p=0.04). A larger phase III trial has been recommended by this group [96].

Pegorgotein in Severe Head Injuries, Multicenter Trial

A prospective, randomized, multi-center clinical trial has been published with 463 patients with severe closed head injuries (GCS 8 or less after resuscitation and stabilization). The patients received either placebo or pegorgotein (an oxygen free radical scavenger) 10,000 u/Kg or 20,000 u/Kg within 8 hours after injury. The outcome was assessed at 3 months post-injury using the Glasgow Outcome Score. There was no significant difference in neurological outcome or mortality between the study groups [97].

Tirilazad in Head Injury Clinical Trial

A recent prospective, randomized study has been reported including 1,120 patients with head injury. The patients were randomized to receive placebo or the lazaroid (Tirilazad). At 6 months post-injury, 39 percent of patients in the Tirilazad group and 42 percent in the placebo group had good recovery (p=0.461). Mortality was 26 percent and 25 percent respectively. Subgroup analysis has suggested that Tirilazad may be effective in reducing mortality in males with severe head injury and associated subarachnoid hemorrhage (mortality in the Tirilazad group was 34 percent and in the placebo group was 43 percent, p=0.026). [98]

Antithrombin III in Severely Injured Patients Clinical Trial

A further prospective, randomized study has been reported which included patients with severe multiple injuries with injury severity scores (ISS) of 29 or greater. The patients were randomized to receive Antithrombin III (AT III) or placebo within 360 minutes of the injury. There was no difference between the study groups with respect to mortality (AT III group 15 percent, placebo group 5 percent) partial thromboplastin time, prothrombin time, platelets count, plasminogen activator inhibitor I, soluble TNF receptor II, neutrophil elastase, IL-I receptor antagonist, IL-6, or IL-8 levels [99].

rBPI$_{21}$ in Traumatic Hemorrhage, Phase II Clinical Trial

Our group has conducted a prospective, randomized, double-blind, multi-center clinical trial which included trauma patients who required at least two units of blood within 12 hours of injury. 401 patients were randomized to receive rBPI21 (4 mg/Kg) day for two consecutive days) or placebo. The composite end-point rate of mortality or serious complication was 46 percent in the placebo group and 39 percent in the rBPI21 group (p=0.13). The proportion of patients who developed either pneumonia or ARDS was 32 percent in the placebo group and 22 percent in the rBPI21 group (p=0.03). A beneficial trend with rBPI21 which failed to reach statistical significance was observed in both blunt and penetrating trauma and was present across different age groups, ISS and the number of blood units transfused. A large phase III study is currently in progress [100].

Therapy for Macrocirculatory Hemodynamic Patterns: Augmentation of Oxygen Transport

Patients with blunt trauma have hemodynamic patterns of increased cardiac index, hypotension, tachycardia and reduced tissue perfusion/oxygenation. In general, the observed cardiac index and tissue perfusion values are greater in survivors than in nonsurvivors [15, 17, 19, 43, 44]. In high risk surgery and trauma, differences between survivors' and nonsurvivors' hemodynamic patterns have motivated investigators to suggest aggressive fluid therapy titrated to reach optimal physiologic goals, defined by the survivors' patterns, as a strategy to improve patient outcome [32–34]. Fluid therapy is titrated to maintain intravascular volume, improve tissue perfusion and overcome regional circulatory deficiencies caused by uneven, maldistributed vasoconstriction.

The hypothesis is that low flow and poor tissue oxygenation, which lead to organ failure and death, may be documented early in the resuscitation period by non-invasive monitoring. These data may be used to titrate *early* fluid therapy to achieve optimal physiologic criteria in an effort to prevent further deterioration of circulatory function and development of lethal organ failures.

Time Relationships in Therapy of Trauma

Time relationships after severe trauma were studied by Bishop et al [101] where our group has found that optimizing CI, DO$_2$ and VO$_2$ within 24 hours of the injury improves outcome. In prospective randomized studies, we have demonstrated significantly reduced mortality from 39 percent to 18 percent (p < 0.05) and reduced incidence of organ failure from 105 in 65 control patients (1.62 ± 0.28 organ failures/patient) to 37 in 50 protocol patients (0.74 ± 0.28 organ failures/patient; p < 0.01) who were optimized early [101].

Early aggressive therapy to optimize cardiac index, oxygen delivery and oxygen consumption to levels characterizing survivors was demonstrated to improve outcome [101–103]; however, recent studies conducted after organ failure is established, late in the course of illness, have failed to show improvement with this approach. This suggests that therapy should be directed toward improving cardiac output and tissue perfusion as early as possible. Comprehensive non-invasive monitoring for use in the emergency department may be critical to this approach because by the time the patient arrives in the ICU it may already be too late for "early therapy" of this type to prevent lethal organ failure.

7. Summary

After severe injury, high-risk surgery and invasion of the body by pathogens, the body's stress responses subtly progress to what is recognized as the inflammatory response. The interactions of the underlying mechanisms of the stress response are in themselves extraordinarily complex, but when they merge imperceptibly into the larger developing inflammatory process, these interacting mechanisms seem impossible to understand much less ameliorate therapeutically. Faced with this impossible task, recent investigators have singled out several likely candidates as targets, including the H1A1 antibody and anti-cytokine therapies. The results have, however, been frankly disappointing.

Suppression of any one pathway in the multiple inflammatory cascades is likely to be compensated for by the redundancies in the interactions of the other pathways: complement, clotting, corticosteroid, cytokine, eicosanoid, heat shock protein and many other pathways. Many if not most of these mediators of the inflammatory response are interdependent at multiple steps along their progression, making any one factor insignificant in the achievement of the final goal. Immunomodulation although attractive and theoretically compelling, has not yet been shown to be effective; it is not yet "ready for prime time."

It follows from these studies, that for the present, prevention of the many potential insults that cause or augment inflammation is an appropriate therapeutic target. Early recognition by hemodynamic monitoring may be a useful approach to prevent the many minor problems that can rapidly escalate to potentially lethal complications. More importantly, hemodynamic monitoring provides the means to optimize circulatory dynamics to the point where minor problems do not become life threatening and where early non-survivor's hemodynamic patterns can be recognized and reversed with pre-emptive vigorous therapy that attains preset physiologic goals empirically determined for survivors. The onus is on the clinician to provide early therapy targeted to prevent episodes of hypoperfusion or, failing this, to provide adequate salvage therapy after the patient loses control of the inflammatory responses and lapses into lethal organ failures.

References

1. Shoemaker WC. Circulatory mechanisms of shock and their mediators. Crit Care Med 1987; 15:787–93
2. Cunningham DJ. Studies on arterial chemoreceptors in man. J Physiol 1987;385:1–26
3. Waxman K. Physiologic Response to Injury. In: Shoemaker WC, Ayres SM, Grenvik A, Holbrook PR editors. Textbook of Critical Care. Philadelphia: Saunders, 3rd ed, 1995;1395–1402.
4. Gann DS, Lilly MP. The neuroendocrine response to multiple trauma. World J Surg 19983;7:101–18
5. Jaattela A, Ahlo A, Avihainen V, et al. Plasma catecholamines in severely injured patients. Brit J Surg 1975;177:62
6. Maddens M, Sowers J. Catecholamines in critical care. Crit Care Clin 1987;3:871–2.

7. Waxman K. Shock: ischemia, reperfusion and inflammation. New Horiz 1996;4:153–60.
8. Shoemaker WC, Wo CCJ, Demetriades D, Belzberg H, Asensio J, Cornwell E, et al. Early physiologic patterns in acute illness and accidents. New Horiz 1996;4:395–412.
9. Wo CCJ, Shoemaker WC, Appel PL, Bishop MH, Kram HB, Hardin E. Unreliability of blood pressure and heart rate to evaluate cardiac output in emergency resuscitation and critical illness. Crit Care Med 1993;21:218–23
10. Shoemaker WC, Appel PL, Kram HB. Hemodynamic and oxygen transport responses in survivors and nonsurvivors. Crit Care Med 1993; 21: 977–990.
11. Shoemaker WC, Belzberg H, Wo CCJ, Milzman DP, Pasquale MD, Baga L, et al. Multicenter study of noninvasive monitoring as alternatives to invasive monitoring in early management of acutely ill emergency patients. Chest, in press (Oct, 1998).
12. Shoemaker WC, Appel PL, Kram HB. Role of oxygen debt in the development of organ failure, sepsis, and death in high risk surgical patients. Chest 1992;102:208–15.
13. Maier RV, Bulger EM. Endothelial changes after shock and injury. New Horiz 1996;4:211–23.
14. Drexler H. Endothelial dysfunction: clinical implications. Prog Cardiovasc Dis 1997;39:287–324
15. McCuskey RS. The microcirculation during endotoxemia. Cardiovasc Res 1996;32:752–63
16. Harris MJ, Baker RT, McRoberts JW. The adrenal response to trauma, operation, and cosyntropin stimulation. Surg Gynecol Obstet 1990;170:513–16
17. Hilton JG, Marullo DS. Trauma induced increases in plasma vasopressin and angiotensin II. Life Sci 1987;41:2195–3000.
18. Starc TJ, Staluip SA. Time course changes of plasma renin activity and catecholamines during hemorrhage in conscious sheep. Circ Shock 1987;21:129–140.
19. Lloyd DA, Teich S, Rowe NI. Serum endorphin levels in injured children. Surg Gynecol Obstet 1991;172:449–52.
20. Deitch EA, Xu D, Bridges RM. Opioids modulate human neutrophil and lymphocyte function. Surgery 1988;104:41–8.
21. Meakins JL. Host defense mechanisms in surgical patients. Acta Chir Scand 198;55:43–51.
22. Bitterman H, Kinarty A, Lazarovich H, et al. Acute release of cytokines is proportional to tissue injury induced by surgical trauma and shock in rats. J Clin Immunol 1991;11:184–92.
23. Scannell G. Leukocyte responses to hypoxic/ischemic conditions. New Horiz 1996;4:179–83.
24. Yue TI, Farhat M, Rubinovicici R, et al. Protective effect of BN-50739, a new platelet-activating factor antagonistin endotoxin-treated rabbits. J Pharmacol Exp Ther 1990;254:976–81.
25. Chang SW, Feddersen CO, Henson PM, et al. Platelet-activating factor mediates hemodynamic changes and lung injury in endotoxin treated rats. J Clin Invest 1987;79:1498–1509.
26. Dhainaut JF, Tenaillon A, Le Tulzo Y, Schlemmer B, Solet JB, Wolff M, et al.: Platelet activating factor receptor antagonist BN-52021 in the treatment of severe sepsis. Crit Care Med 1994;22:1720–28.
27. Mulder MF, Lambalgen AA, Huisman E, Visser JJ, Van der Bos GC, Thijs LG. Protective role of NO in regional hemodynamic changes during acute endotoxemia in rats. Am J Physiol 1994;266:H1558–64.
28. Petros A, Lamb G, Leone A, Moncada S, Bennett D, Vallanee P. Effects of a nitric oxide synthase inhibitor in humans with septic shock. Cardiovasc Res 1994;28:34–39.
29. Zhang H, Rogiers P, Friedman G, Preiser JC, Spapen H, Buurman WA, et al. Effects of nitric oxide donor SIN-1 on oxygen availability and regional blood flow during endotoxic shock. Arch Surg 1996;131:767–74.
30. Preiser JC, Lejeune P, Roman A, Carlier E, De Backer D, Leeman M, et al. Methylene blue administration in septic shock; a clinical trial. Crit Care Med 1995;23:259–64.
31. Ratych R, Chuknyiska R, Bulkley G. The primary localization of free radical generation after anoxia/reoxygenation in isolated endothelial cells. Surgery 1987;102:122–31.
32. Keel M, Ecknauer E, Stocker R, Ungethum U, Steckholzer U, Kenney J, et al. Different pattern of local and systemic release of pro-inflammatory and anti-inflammatory mediators in severely injured patients with chest trauma. J Trauma 1996;40:907–14.
33. Ghezzi P, Dinarello CA, Bianchi M, Rosandich ME, Repinee JE, White CW. Hypoxia increases production of interleukin-1 and tumor necrosis factor by human mononuclear cells. Cytokine 1991;3:189–94.
34. Hauser CJ. Regional macrophage activation after injury and the compartmentalization of inflammation in trauma. New Horizons 1996;4:235–51.
35. Bakker J, Zhang H, Depierreux M, van Asbeok S, Vinout JL, et al. Effects of N-acetylcysteine in endotoxic shock. J Crit Care 1994;9:236–43.
36. Peake SL, Moran JL, Leppard PI. N-acetyl-L-cysteine depresses cardiac performance in patients with septic shock. Crit Care Med 1996;24:1302–10.

37. Evans JA, Darlington DN, Gann DS. A circulating factor(s) mediates cell depolarization in hemorrhagic shock. Ann Surg 1991;213:549–56.
38. Scannell G, Waxman K, Vaziri ND, Zhang J, Kaupke CJ, Jalali M, et al. Hypoxia-induced alterations of neutrophil membrane receptors. J Surg Res 1995;59:141–5.
39. Miller SE, Miller CL, Trunkey DD. The immune consequences of trauma. Surg Clin N Am 1982;62:167–81.
40. Abraham E. Alterations in transcriptional regulation of proinflammatory and immunoregulatory cytokine expression by hemorrhage, injury, and critical illness. New Horizons 1996;4:184–93.
41. Suzuki YJ, Mizuno M, Packer L. Signal transduction for nuclear factor-kB activation: Proposed licatin of antioxidant-inhibitable step. J Immunol 1994;153:5008–15.
42. Moore FA, Moore EE. Evolving concepts in the pathogenesis of postinjury multiple organ failure. Surg Clin North Am 1995;75:257–77.
43. Redl H, Schlag G, Baharami S, Yao YM. Animal models as the basis of pharmacologic intervention in trauma and sepsis patients. World J Surg 1996;80:519–36.
44. Deitch EA. Animal models of sepsis and shock: a review and lessons learned. Shock 1998;9:1–11.
45. Wichman M, Zellweger R, Ayala A, DeMaso CM, Chaudry IH. Gender differences: improved immune function in females as opposed to decreased immune function in males following hemorrhagic shock. Surg Forum 1995;46:758–9.
46. Shoemaker WC, Appel PL, Kram HB. Role of oxygen debt in the development of organ failure, sepsis, and death in high risk surgical patients. Chest 1992;102:208–15.
47. Meade P, Shoemaker WC, Donnelly TJ, et al. Temporal patterns of hemodynamics, oxygen transport, cytokine, and compliment activity in the development of ARDS after severe injury. J Trauma.
48. Thangathurai D, Charbonnet C, Wo CCJ, Shoemaker WC, Michael MS, Roffey, et al. Intraoperative maintenance of tissue perfusion prevents ARDS. New Horiz 1996;4:453–65.
49. Korthius R, Andeson D, Granger D. Role of neutrophil-endothelial cell adhesion in inflammatory disorders. J Crit Care 1994;9:47–71.
50. Redl H, Schlag G, Bahrams S, Yao YM. Animal models as the basis of pharmacological intervention in trauma and sepsis. World J Surg 1996; 20:487–492.
51. Lindsay TF, Hill J, Fritz F, et al. Blockage of complement activation prevents local and pulmonary albumin leak after lower torso ischemia reperfusion. Ann Surg 1992; 216:677–683.
52. Bone RC, Balk RA, Fein Am, Perl TM, Wenzel RP, Reines HD, et al. A second larger controlled clinical study of E_5, a monoclonal antibody to endotoxin: results of a prospective, multicenter randomized, controlled trial. The E_5 sepsis study group. Crit Care Med 1995; 23:994–1006.
53. Yao YM, Bahrami S, Leichtfried G, Redl H, Schlag G. Pathogenesis of hemorrhage-induced bacteria/endotoxin translocation in rats. Ann Surg 1995;221:398–405.
54. Baker JW, Deitch EA, Li M, Berg R, Specian RD. Hemorrhagic shock promotes bacterial translocation from the gut, J Trauma 1988;28:896–900.
55. Ayala A, Perrin MM, Meldrum DR, Ertel W, Chaudry IH. Hemorrhage induces an increase in serum TNF which is not associated with elevated levels of endotoxin. Cytokine 1990;2:170–4.
56. Peitzman AB, Udekwn AO, Ochoa J, Smith S. Bacterial translocation in trauma patients. J Trauma 1991;31:1086–7.
57. Braithwaite CE, Ross SE, Nagele R, Mure AJ, O'Malley KF, Garcia-Perez FA. Bacterial translocation occurs in humans after traumatic injury: evidence using immunofluorescence. J Trauma 1993;34:586–9.
58. Kale IT, Kuzu MA, Berkaem H, Berkem R, Acar N. The presence of hemorrhage shock increases the rate of bacterial translocation in blunt abdominal trauma. J Trauma 1998;44:171–4.
59. Chang TW. Improvement of survival from hemorrhagic shock by enterectomy in rats: finding to implicate the role of the gut for irreversibility of hemorrhagic shock. J Trauma 1997; 42:223–30.
60. Ramsay G, Van Saene RH. Selective gut decontamination in intensive care and surgical practice: Where are we? World J Surg 1998;22:167–70.
61. Kollef MH. The role of selective digestive tract decontamination on mortality and respiratory tract infections. A meta-analysis. Chest 1994;105:1101–8.
62. Bahrami S, Yao YM, Leichtfried G, Redl H, Schlay G, Di Padora FE. Monoclonal antibody to endotoxin attenuates hemorrhage-reduced lung injury and mortality in rats. Crit Care Med 1997;25:1030–6.
63. Abraham E, Allbee J. Effects of therapy with interleukin-1 receptor antagonist on pulmonary cytokine expression following hemorrhage and resuscitation. Lymphokine Cytokine Res 1994;13:343–7.
64. Pellicane JV, DeMaria EJ, Abd-Elfattah A, Reines HD, Vannice JL, Carson KW. Interleukin-1

receptor antagonist improves survival and preserves organ adenosine-5-triphosphate after hemorrhagic shock. Surgery 1993;114:278–83.

65. O'Riordain MG, O'Riordain DS, Molloy RG, Mannick JA, Radrick ML. Dosage and timing of anti-TNF-alpha antibody treatment determine its effect of resistance to sepsis after injury. J Surg Res 1996;15:95–101.

66. Mileski WJ, Winn RK, Vedder NB, Pohlman TH, Harlan JM, Rice CL. Inhibition of CD18-dependent neutrophil adherence reduces organ injury after hemorrhagic shock in primates. Surgery 1990;108:206–12.

67. Scalia R, Gauthier TW, Lefer AM. Beneficial effects of LEX032, a novel recombinant serine protease inhibitor, in murine traumatic shock. Shock 1995;4:251–6.

68. Barroso-Aranda J, Schmid-Schonbein GW. Pentoxifylline pre-treatment decreases the pool of circulating activated neutrophils, in-vivo adhesion to endothelium, and improves survival from hemorrhagic shock. Biorheology 1990;27:401–18.

69. Flyn WJ, Cryer HG, Garrison RN. Pentoxifylline restores intestinal microvascular boood flow during resuscitated hemorrhagic shock. Surgery 1991;110:350–6.

70. Waxman K, Clark L, Soliman MH, Parazin S. Pentoxifylline in resuscitation of experimental hemorrhagic shock. Crit Care Med 1991;19:728–31.

71 Rivera-Chavez F, Toledo-Pereyra LH, Nora DT, Bachulis B, Ilgenfritz F, Dean RE. P-selectin blockade is beneficial after uncontrolled hemorrhagic shock. J Trauma 1998;45:440–5.

72. Winn RK, Paulson JC, Harlan JM. A monoclonal antibody to P-selectin ameliorates injury associated with hemorrhagic shock in rabbits. Am J Physiol 1994;267:H2391–7.

73. Ramamoorthy C, Sharar SR, Harlan JM, Tedder TF, Winn RK. Blocking L-selectin function attenuates reperfusion injury following hemorrhagic shock in rabbits. Am J Physiol 271:H1871–7.

74. Terashita Z, Stahl GL, Lefer AM. Protective effects of a platelet activating factor (PAF) antagonist and its combined treatment with prostaglandin (PG) E_1 in traumatic shock. J Cardiovasc Pharmacol 1988;12:505–71.

75. Patel JP, Beck LD, Briglia FA, Hock CE. Beneficial effects of combined thromboxane and leukotriene receptor antagonism in hemorrhagic shock. Crit Care Med 1995;23:231–7.

76. Karasawa A, Taylor PA, Lefer AM. Protective effects of KW-3635, a novel thromboxane A_2 antagonist, in murine traumatic shock. Eur J Pharmacol 1990;21:182–8.

77. Bitterman H, Smith BA, Lefer AM. Beneficial actions of antagonism of peptide leukotrienes in hemorrhagic shock. Circ Shock 1988;24:159–68.

78. Hock CE, Lefer AM. Beneficial effect of a thromboxane synthetase inhibitor in traumatic shock. Circ Shock 1984;14:159–68.

79. Daughters K, Waxman K, Nguyen H. Increasing nitric oxide production improves survival in experimental hemorrhagic shock. Resuscitation 1996;31:141–4.

80. Lieberthal W, McGarry AE, Sheils J, Valeri CR. Nitric oxide inhibition in rats improves blood pressure and renal function during hyporolemic shock. Am J Physiol 1991;261:F868–72.

81. Fleckenstein AE, Smith SL, Linseman KL, Beuring LJ, Hall ED. Comparison of the efficacy of mechanistically different anti-oxidants in the rat hemorrhagic shock model. Circ Shock 1991;35:223–30.

82. Tan LR, Waxman K, Clark L, Eloi L, Chieng N, Miller R, et al. Superoxide dismutase and allopurinol improve survival in an animal model of hemorrhagic shock. Am Surg 1993;59:797–800.

83. Tominaga GT, Barley J, Daughters K, Sarfeh IJ, Waxman K. The effect of polyethylene glycol-superoxide dismutase on gastric mucosa and survival in shock with tissue injury. Am Surg 1995;61:925–9.

84. Daughters K, Waxman K, Gassel A, Zommer S. Antioxidant treatment for shock: vitamin E but not vitamin C improves survival. Am Surg 1996;62:789–92.

85. Aoki N, Lefer AM. Protective effects of a novel nonglucocorticoid 21-aminosteroid (UF 74006F) during traumatic shock in rats. J Cardiovasc Pharmacol 1990;15:205–10.

86. Hall ED, Yonkers PA, McCall JM. Attenuation of hemorrhagic shock by the non-glucocorticoid 21-aminosteroid U74006f. Eur J Pharmacol 1988;147:299–303.

87. Mathew P, Bullock R, Teasdale G, McCulloch J. Changes in local microvascular permeability and in the effect of intervention with 21-aminosteroid (Tirilazad) in a new experimental model of focal cortical injury in the rat. J Neurotrauma, 1996;13:465–72.

88. Marion DW, White MJ. Treatment of experimental brain injury with moderate hypothermia and 21-aminosteroids. J Neurotrauma 1996;13:139–47.

89. Horwitz AH, Leigh SD, Abrahamson S, et al. Expression and characterization of cysteine-modified variants of an amino-terminal fragment of bactericidal/ permeability-increasing protein. Protein Expression and Purification 1996;8:28–40.

90. Betz Corradin S, Heumann D, Gallay P, et al. Bactericidal/permeability increasing protein inhibits

induction of macrophage nitric-oxide production by lipopolysaccharide. J Infect Dis 1994;169:105–11.

91. Huang K, Conlon PJ, Fishwild DM. A recombinant amino-terminal fragment of bactericidal/permeability increasing protein (rBPI$_{23}$) inhibits solube CD-14-mediated lipopolysaccharide-induced endothelial adherence for human neutrophils. Shock 1994;1:81–6.

92. Dietrich WD, Alonso D, Busto R, Globus MYT, Ginsberg MD. Post-traumatic brain hypothermia reduces histopathological damage following concussive brain injury in the rat. Neuropathol 1994;87:250–8.

93. Clifton GL, Jiang JY, Lyeth BG, Jenkins LW, Hamm RJ, Hayes RL. Marked protection by moderate hypothermia after experimental traumatic brain injury. J Cereb Blood Flow Metab 1991;11:114–21.

94. Smith JL, Hall ED. Mild pre-and posttraumatic hypothermia attenuates blood-brain barrier damage following controlled cortical impact injury in the rat. J Neurotrauma 1996;13:1–9.

95. Sakamoto KI, Fujisawa H, Koiznmi H, Tsuchida E, Ito H, Sadamitsu D, et al. Effects of mild hypothermia on nitric oxide synthesis following contusion trauma in the rat. J Neurotrauma 1997;14:349–53.

96. Muizelocar JP, Marmarou A, Young HF, Choi SC, Wolf A, Schneider RL, et al. Improving the outcome of severe head injury with oxygen radical scavenger polyethylene glycol-conjuacated superoxide dismutase: a phase II trial. J Neurosurg 1993;78:375–82.

97. Young B, Runge JW, Waxman KS, Harrington T, Wilberger J, Muizelaar JP, et al. Effects of pegorgotein on neurologic outcome of patients with severe head injury. A multicenter, randomized controlled trial. JAMA 1996;276:538–43.

98. Marshall LF, Maas AI, Marshal SB, Bricolo A, Fearnside M, Iannotti F, et al. A multicenter trial on the efficacy of using tirilazad mesylate in cases of head injury. J Neurosurg 1998;89:519–25.

99. Waydhas C, Nast-Kolb D, Gippner-Steppert C, Trupka A, Pfundstein C, Schweiberer L, et al. High-dose antithrombin III treatment of severely injured patients: results of a prospective study. J Trauma 1998;45:931–40.

100. Demetraides D, Smith SJ, Jacobson L, Moncure M, Minei J, Nelson BJ, et al. Bactericidal/permeability increasing protein (rBPI$_{21}$) in patients with hemorrhage due to trauma: results of a multicenter phase II clinical trial. J Trauma (in press).

101. Bishop MW, Shoemaker WC, Appel PL, Wo CJ, Zwich C, Kram HB, et al. Relationship between supranormal values, time delays and outcome in severely traumatized patients. Crit Care Med 1993;21:56–62.

102. Fleming AW, Bishop MH, Shoemaker WC, et al: Prospective trial of supranormal values as goals of resuscitation in severe trauma. Arch Surg 1992;127:1175–81

103. Scalea J, Simon HM, Duncan AO. Geriatric blunt multiple trauma: Improved survival with early invasive monitoring. J Trauma 1990;39:129–36.

3. The Immunology of Sepsis

Stephen J. Parker and Alastair C.J. Windsor

What Are Sepsis and SIRS?

Inflammation is the body's non-specific reaction to tissue injury; the end result of highly amplified yet tightly controlled, humoral and cellular mechanisms aimed principally at limiting the extent of tissue damage. Localised inflammation is an appropriate protective physiological response often resulting in the elimination of the initiating noxious stimulus and the early restoration of homeostasis. Loss of local control or an exaggerated host reaction can, however, result in a progressive immuno-inflammatory process, the systemic inflammatory response syndrome (SIRS), which, in extreme cases, can lead to organ dysfunction and death.

The concept of SIRS encompasses both the clinical and haematological manifestations of an inflammatory process arising from such diverse aetiological triggers as infection, trauma, burns or pancreatitis [1,2]. Sepsis is defined as SIRS arising as a result of infection which can be bacterial, viral, fungal or protozoal in origin (Table 3.1). Bacterial infections are the commonest causes of sepsis but there is no requirement for septic patients to be bacteremic. Bacteremia is a microbiological rather than clinical diagnosis. Severe sepsis represents a more marked homeostatic disturbance, with evidence of tissue hypoperfusion, that remains responsive to intravascular volume replacement. Sepsis that is associated with hypotension and is refractory to fluid resuscitation, requiring inotropic support is termed septic shock. When SIRS is associated with organ dysfunction the multiple organ dysfunction syndrome (MODS) is said to exist, but there is no universally agreed definition of these physiological disturbances. Based on the current definitions, the inter-relationship between infection, sepsis and SIRS is summarised in Figure 3.1.

In this chapter, the roles of endotoxin in gram-negative and exotoxins in gram-positive sepsis will be discussed. The general properties of the pro- and anti-inflammatory cytokines will be outlined and the evidence supporting their roles in the immuno-inflammatory cascade highlighted. The rationale behind immuno-modulatory therapies will be summarised and the reasons why almost all trials of these novel agents have failed will be summised. Pressure of space has meant exclusion of a précis of the roles of the autacoid mediators, the complement and coagulation cascades and the adaptive immune response in sepsis and SIRS. This is in part dealt with in Chapter 2. Regulation of cytokine production at the molecular level will not be discussed.

Table 3.1. The definitions of sepsis, SIRS and MODS. Adapted from Bone [2].

Term	Definition
Bacteraemia	The presence of viable bacteria in the bloodstream.
SIRS	The systemic inflammatory response to a severe clinical insult. The response is manifest by two or more of the following:
	1. Temperature $>38°$ C or $<36°$ C.
	2. Heart rate >90 beats per minute.
	3. Respiratory rate >20 breaths per minute or $P_aCO_2 < 4.3$ kPa.
	4. White cell count $>12,000$ or $<4,000$ per mm^3 or the presence of >10 percent immature forms.
Sepsis	SIRS with documented infection.
Severe sepsis	Sepsis with hypotension, organ hypoperfusion or dysfunction that remains responsive to fluid replacement.
Septic shock	Severe sepsis with hypotension despite adequate fluid resuscitation.
MODS	A state of physiological derangement in which organ function is not capable of maintaining homeostasis.

SIRS = Systemic Inflammatory response syndrome. MODS = Multiple Organ Dysfunction Syndrome.

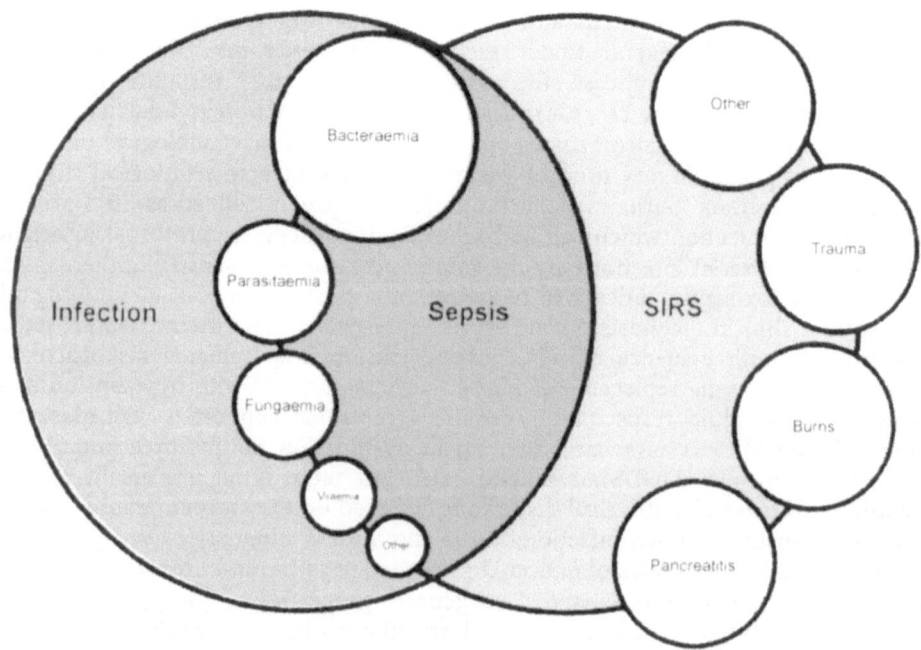

Figure 3.1. The relationship between infection, sepsis and SIRS.

Endotoxin in Gram-negative Sepsis

Bacterial infections are the commonest cause of sepsis with an approximately equal proportion of cases due to gram-positive and gram-negative organisms (Figure 3.2). In those with gram-negative sepsis, *Escherichia coli* and *Pseudomo-*

The Immunology of Sepsis

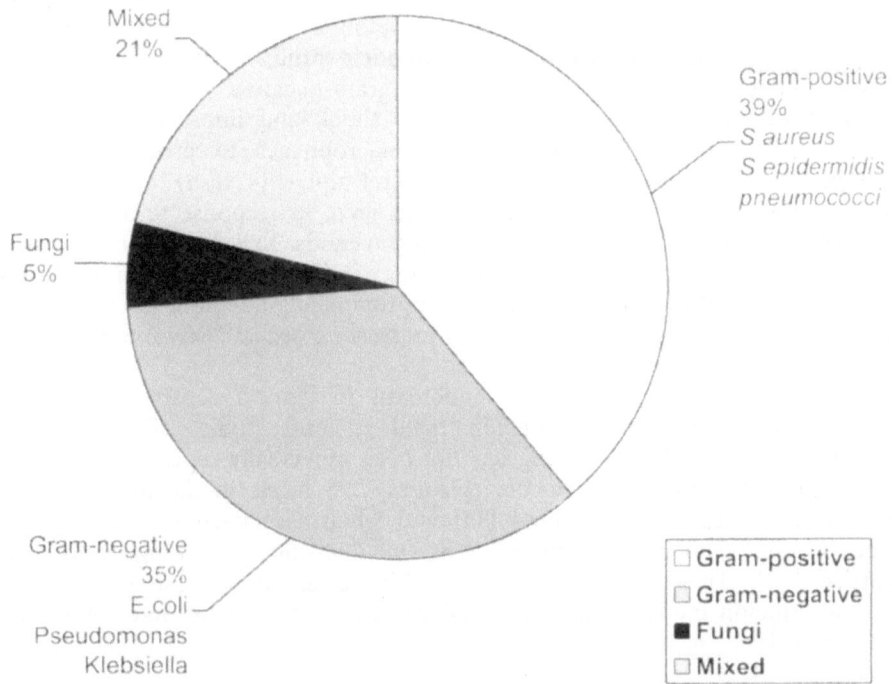

Figure 3.2. Microbiology of positive blood cultures from patients with severe sepsis. Adapted from Brun-Buisson et al [3].

nas aeruginosa are the most frequently identified bacteria with endotoxin believed to play a central role in the underlying pathophysiological disturbances [3,4]. Endotoxin is found within the external membrane of the cell wall of gram-negative bacteria. It was initially isolated as a crude fraction of the bacterial cell wall, containing many molecular components including lipopolysaccharide (LPS). Today, pure LPS preparations are available and the terms LPS and endotoxin are frequently used interchangeably.

LPS has three important molecular components. The highly variable O polysaccharide displays significant variation between bacterial species and confers serotypic specificity. The R region is relatively conserved across all gram-negative species and is not believed to have a specific role in sepsis. The lipid A component appears to be responsible for almost all of the toxicity of LPS and is able to stimulate cytokine release and activate the complement cascade [5]. LPS is released from the cell wall of both growing and damaged bacteria. The host response to LPS is complex and involves interactions between LPS, serum components and specific cell surface receptors. LPS binds to a number of different serum carrier molecules the most important of which is the lipopolysaccharide binding protein (LBP). The LPS-LPB complex then interacts with monocytes via the CD 14 cell surface receptor [6]. Binding of the LPS-LBP complex to cell surface CD14 receptors initiates signal transduction resulting in the transcription and release of pro-inflammatory mediators.

LPS is believed to have a pivotal role in the aetiology of gram-negative sepsis and may also be important in the pathophysiology of other causes of SIRS. Administration of LPS in animal models produces clinical features of sepsis [7] and in both endotoxaemia and gram-negative sepsis models, pre-treatment with anti-LPS antibodies prevents shock and improves survival [8]. In vitro, LPS stimulates monocytes and macrophages to produce the pro-inflammatory cytokine, tumor necrosis factor-alpha (TNF-α) and a similar cytokine response has been demonstrated, in vivo, in response to an LPS challenge [9]. In human volunteer studies, intravenous LPS has been shown to induce physiological and cytokine responses similar to those seen in animal studies [10]. Symptoms of sepsis are seen approximately one hour after endotoxin exposure and occur concurrently with an increase in serum TNF-α concentration [11].

Evidence supporting the role of endotoxin in clinical sepsis is less clear. Elevated LPS levels have been demonstrated in some studies of patients with severe sepsis [12], but, this finding has not been universally repeated [13]. When detected during clinical bacteraemic episodes, LPS levels in the low pico-gram range have usually been measured [14] and when associated with non-meningococcal septic shock, concentrations in the 200–400 pg/ml range have been recorded [15]. These levels are considerably lower than those measured in bacterial infusion models when values greater than 10,000 pg/ml have often been reported [16].

Exotoxins in Gram-positive Sepsis

The cell wall of gram-positive organisms does not possess endotoxin yet these organisms are able to produce a clinically indistinguishable immuno-inflammatory response to that produced by gram-negative bacteria. In severe gram-positive sepsis, due to *Staphylococcus aureus* or *Streptococcus pyogenes*, the response is often the result of the release of superantigenic protein exotoxins [17]. These interact with host T lymphocytes triggering their proliferation and the massive release of proinflammatory cytokines. Gram-positive organisms are also capable of producing proteolytic enzymes that destroy host tissue and augment microbial invasion.

Cytokine Responses in Sepsis

A co-ordinated immuno-inflammatory response requires the regulation of many different cell types. This can be achieved partly by the paracrine actions of soluble protein (cytokine) and lipid or peptide (autacoid) mediators. Many cytokines are generated during the immuno-inflammatory response either as a direct result of activation of macrophages, neutrophils and the endothelium or indirectly via the actions of other inflammatory mediators. Some, including TNF-α, interleukin-1 (IL-1) and Interferon-γ have pro-inflammatory actions whilst others, such as IL-4, IL-10 and Transforming Growth Factor-β have predominantly counter-regulatory activities [18]. "Proximal" cytokines, including TNF-α and IL-1, are released early in the inflammatory process whilst "distal" cytokines, for example IL-2, IL-8 and IL-10, are released later in this pathological continuum.

General Properties of Cytokines

Cytokines regulate both the amplitude and duration of the immuno-inflammatory response. They have multiple effects on cellular growth, differentiation and apoptosis with considerable overlap and redundancy in their actions. There is strong evidence from animal studies to implicate cytokines in the pathophysiology of sepsis because, as discussed above, an endotoxin infusion results in the release of proinflammatory mediators and administration of recombinant cytokines produces a "sepsis-like" illness. Elevated serum cytokine levels are found in the plasma of septic patients and inhibition of cytokine production, at least in animal studies, improves organ dysfunction and survival [19].

Cytokines are not stored within the cell, but, are produced as a result of gene transcription or translation following the initiating stimulus. The specific effects of a particular cytokine depends on its concentration, the cell type on which it is acting, the presence of modulating or regulatory proteins and the density and availability of cell surface receptors. In an attempt to control and localise an inflammatory process, both pro-inflammatory and anti-inflammatory mediators are simultaneously released in response to an aetiological trigger. The balance between these two competing mechanisms is vital if homeostasis is to be maintained. Derangement of either response can result in significant systemic effects. An exaggerated anti-inflammatory response can result in immunosuppression and systemic spread of infection, whereas, an excessive pro-inflammatory response can result in the overflow of cytokines into the systemic circulation resulting in SIRS and MODS [20].

The principal physiological responses to cytokines are the result of their paracrine actions [21]. This localised and often compartmentalised production results in serum concentrations that do not accurately reflect local physiological levels. Support for the importance of paracrine actions of cytokines is given by the lack of correlation between serum cytokine concentrations and the degree of bacteraemia, organ mRNA expression and neutrophil sequestration during experimental sepsis [22]. Quite aptly, serum cytokine levels have been described as being the "Tip of the Iceberg" [23].

Tumor Necrosis Factor-alpha

TNF-α is a 17 kDa polypeptide produced predominantly by cells of the reticuloendothelial system that is believed to have a pivotal role in the evolution of sepsis and SIRS [24]. It has a short half-life with tight control of its expression at both the transcriptional and translational level. It acts directly on cells as well as stimulating the release of other inflammatory mediators. Acting on the endothelium it induces adhesion molecule expression [25] and increases serum procoagulant activity [26]. It releases neutrophils from the bone marrow and, through its chemotactic properties, enhances their migration to the site of tissue damage [27].

In animal models, an intravenous infusion of gram-negative bacteria induces TNF-α expression with serum concentrations rising after 45 minutes, peaking at 90 minutes and returning to baseline levels by six hours [28]. In models of chronic sepsis, such as experimentally-induced peritonitis, serum TNF-α levels often remain low, but, increased mRNA expression has been identified in some organs [29]. Passive immunisation with anti-TNF-α antibodies has been shown to prevent septic shock in animal models of fulminant gram-negative [30] and gram-positive [31] sepsis. In contrast, in bacterial peritonitis models, such a protective effect of anti-TNF-α antibodies has not been consistently demonstrated [32]. The beneficial effects of anti-TNF-α antibodies appear to be maximal when given as prophylaxis, but, delayed administration, in some models, has also been shown to be effective [33]. In those animal models that display a consistent TNF-α response, administration of anti-TNF-α antibodies has been shown to reduce the concentration of other more "distal" pro-inflammatory cytokines [34].

In healthy human volunteers, a TNF-α infusion produces clinical features of sepsis [35]. Elevated serum TNF-α levels have been demonstrated in some patients with sepsis, particularly those with septic shock, and in these studies a correlation has been demonstrated between the serum concentration of TNF-α and the severity of the underlying inflammatory process [36]. However, except for studies in patients with severe meningococcal sepsis, peak serum TNF-α concentrations do not discriminate well between survivors and non-survivors [37]. This may be because serum cytokine responses are often transient and identifying the exact time of the peak concentration can be difficult. Prolonged or persistent elevation of serum TNF-α levels may be a better prognostic indicator [38,39].

The Interleukins

The interleukins are a class of cytokines produced by many different cell types. IL-1 and IL-8 have mainly pro-inflammatory actions whilst IL-4 and IL-10 have predominantly anti-inflammatory effects. IL-1 and IL-6 have been the most extensively studied of this group. The potent immuno-inhibitory actions of IL-10 have attracted recent interest.

IL-1 is a term used to described two closely related mediators—IL-1α and IL-1β. Both activate the IL-1 receptor and have similar biological properties. IL-1β is the predominant form produced by endotoxin-stimulated monocytes and for the purpose of this discussion the term IL-1 refers almost exclusively to this subtype. IL-1 is a key mediator in the immuno-inflammatory cascade, interacting closely with other inflammatory cytokines. In animal models, an LPS infusion induces an increase in serum IL-1 concentration [28] and, as seen with TNF-α, an IL-1 infusion has been shown to produce the clinical features of sepsis [40]. TNF-α also stimulates IL-1 production which in turn, in a positive feedback fashion, enhances the sensitivity of cells to TNF-α [41]. This synergistic effect of IL-1 on TNF-α sensitivity is dependent on the timing of exposure of the effector cells to the two cytokines. Increased IL-1 levels have been demonstrated in patients with severe sepsis [12] and the concentrations recorded correlate well with the severity of the underlying inflammatory process [42]. As with TNF-α, no prognostic value of isolated IL-1 measurements has been demonstrated [40].

IL-6 is a 21 kDa glycoprotein produced by many cell types including lymphocytes, fibroblasts and monocytes. It activates both B and T lymphocytes, induces the production of acute phase proteins, modulates haemopoesis and activates the coagulation cascade. In both animal models and man, an LPS infusion produces a rise in serum IL-6 concentration with a peak seen at approximately four hours [10]. This invariably occurs after an earlier rise in serum TNF-α. IL-6 production appears to be closely linked with that of TNF-α, as anti-TNF-α antibodies have been shown to suppress the IL-6 response to an endotoxin challenge [43]. IL-6 has an important action in attenuating pro-inflammatory cytokine responses and in vitro it has been shown to limit LPS-induced TNF-α and IL-1 production [44].

Of all the cytokines assessed to date, serum IL-6 appears to show the closest correlation with both disease severity and prognosis. In septic patients, the highest levels of IL-6 have been identified in those with septic shock where a correlation with subsequent mortality exists [45,46].

Anti-inflammatory Mediators

In addition to the pro-inflammatory mediators, cytokines with predominantly anti-inflammatory actions have been characterised, of which IL-10 has been the most extensively studied. Treatment of mice with IL-10, prior to an endotoxin challenge, has been shown to reduce plasma TNF-α concentrations and improve survival [47] and neutralisation of IL-10 with anti-IL-10 antibodies has been shown to further increase already elevated TNF-α levels [48]. Increased IL-10 concentrations have been demonstrated in patients with sepsis with the highest levels seen in those with septic shock [49]. IL-10 appears to permit an initial proinflammatory and innate immune response but then limits the magnitude and duration of the process.

Soluble Receptors and Antagonists

The biological activities of cytokines are mediated via cell surface receptors. These often exist in more than one form, each having a different binding affinity for its particular agonist. TNF-α exerts its biological effects through two receptor sub-types with molecular weights of 55 kDa and 75 kDa respectively. Each has distinct functions and a variable affinity for TNF-α [50]. Soluble cytokine receptors have been demonstrated in tissue fluid and plasma in a number of pathological conditions. They are capable of competing with membrane bound receptors for the binding of their respective cytokine and appear to be important in regulating their physiological actions. Receptors reach solution by either being membrane bound molecules that are shed into the circulation or by enzymatic cleavage of cell surface precursor molecules. By whichever mechanisms they are produced, their concentration usually rises in response to the same stimulus that induces the expression of their respective agonist cytokine. Whether they reduce or augment cytokine responses in all situations is unclear. By reducing the number of agonist molecules available to bind to cell surface receptors they could inhibit agonist activity, possibly in an autocrine fashion and thus have potent anti-inflammatory actions. Alternatively, they may augment cytokine responses by stabilising cytokine molecules in solution and retarding metabolism [51].

TNF-α, either in solution or bound to sTNFR, exists in a dynamic equilibrium with the relative balance determining its bioactivity. Administration of LPS to healthy human volunteers results in a large increase in serum TNFR levels with a peak between two and three hours post infusion [10]. The soluble receptor is produced in approximately a ten times concentration excess relative to TNF-α. Elevated levels of sTNFR have been demonstrated in clinical sepsis with good correlations seen between sTNFR levels and APACHE II scores, MOF scores and mortality [52].

Naturally occurring receptor antagonists also exist. These compete with their respective cytokines for receptor binding but do not induce a biological response. IL-1Ra is a 23 kDa protein with an animo acid sequence that is 26 and 19 percent homologous with IL-1β and IL-1α respectively [40]. In animal models, IL-1Ra has been shown to attenuate the responses to endotoxin and gram-negative sepsis [53]. This has been discussed in Chapter 2. Administration of endotoxin to human volunteers results in an increase in IL-1Ra with a peak at approximately three hours post infusion [10]. In clinical sepsis, increased levels of IL-1Ra have been demonstrated far in excess of the IL-1 concentration [54].

Immunomodulatory Therapies

Treatment of sepsis, has until recently, centred around the eradication of established infection with surgery and antibiotics, accompanied by fluid replacement, inotropic support and oxygen therapy. With the realisation that the pathological effects of sepsis and SIRS can result both from the direct actions of micro-organisms and their toxins and indirectly from the hosts' immune response, recent interest has been shown in novel immunomodulatory therapies. In general, these have either inhibited pro-inflammatory or enhanced anti-inflammatory responses. Many of these strategies have been investigated in animal studies, a limited number have progressed to clinical trials and disappointingly few have shown any significant therapeutic effect (Table 3.2).

Sites for Intervention in the Immuno-inflammatory Cascade

The potential therapeutic strategies for modulating the immuno-inflammatory cascade fall into three broad categories: those directed against bacterial components, those aimed at inflammatory mediators and those designed to limit the degree of tissue damage. As sepsis is a dynamic and evolving process, different strategies may be indicated as this pathological continuum advances (Figures 3.3 and 3.4).

The earliest potential site for intervention in the immuno-inflammatory cascade would be to limit the interaction between bacteria, their toxins and host cells. This type of therapy would need to be given early in the pathological process and certainly before significant activation of "proximal" pro-inflammatory cytokines

Table 3.2. Clinical trials of immunomodulatory trials in sepsis and septic shock. Adapted form Zeni et al [95].

Therapy	Agent	Control arm deaths/ Total (%)	Treatment arm deaths/ Total (%)
Anti-TNF-α	Bay x1351 [69]	108/326 (33%)	196/645 (30%)
	Bay x1351 [70]	66/167 (40%)	144/386 (37%)
	Bay x1351 [71]	398/930 (43%)	382/948 (40%)
	MAK 195F [73]	12/29 (41%)	44/93 (47%)
	CDP571 [96]	6/10 (60%)	30/32 (63%)
	CB0006 [72]	6/19 (32%)	27/61 (44%)
IL-Ra	Antril [84]	102/302 (34%)	177/581 (30%)
	Antril [85]	163/456 (36%)	151/450 (34%)
sTNFR	P80 [76]	10/33 (30%)	49/108 (45%)
	P55 [97]	54/140 (39%)	105/304 (34%)

TNF-α = tumor necrosis factor-alpha, IL-Ra = interleukin-1 receptor antagonist, sTNFR = soluble tumor necrosis factor.

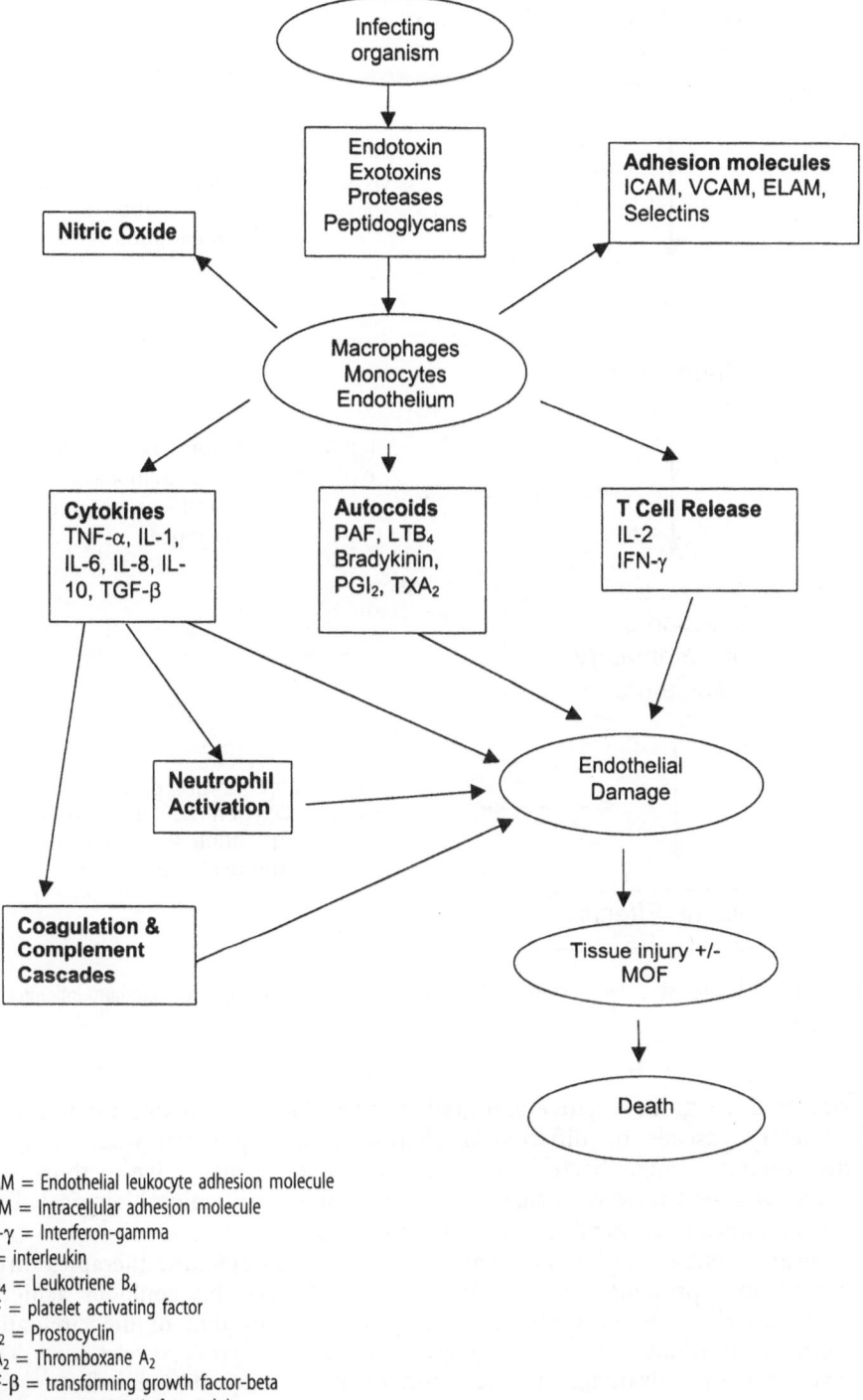

ELAM = Endothelial leukocyte adhesion molecule
ICAM = Intracellular adhesion molecule
IFN-γ = Interferon-gamma
IL = interleukin
LTB$_4$ = Leukotriene B$_4$
PAF = platelet activating factor
PGI$_2$ = Prostocyclin
TXA$_2$ = Thromboxane A$_2$
TGF-β = transforming growth factor-beta
TNF-α = tumor necrosis factor-alpha
VCAM = Vascular cell adhesion molecule

Figure 3.3. An outline of the immuno-inflammatory cascade.

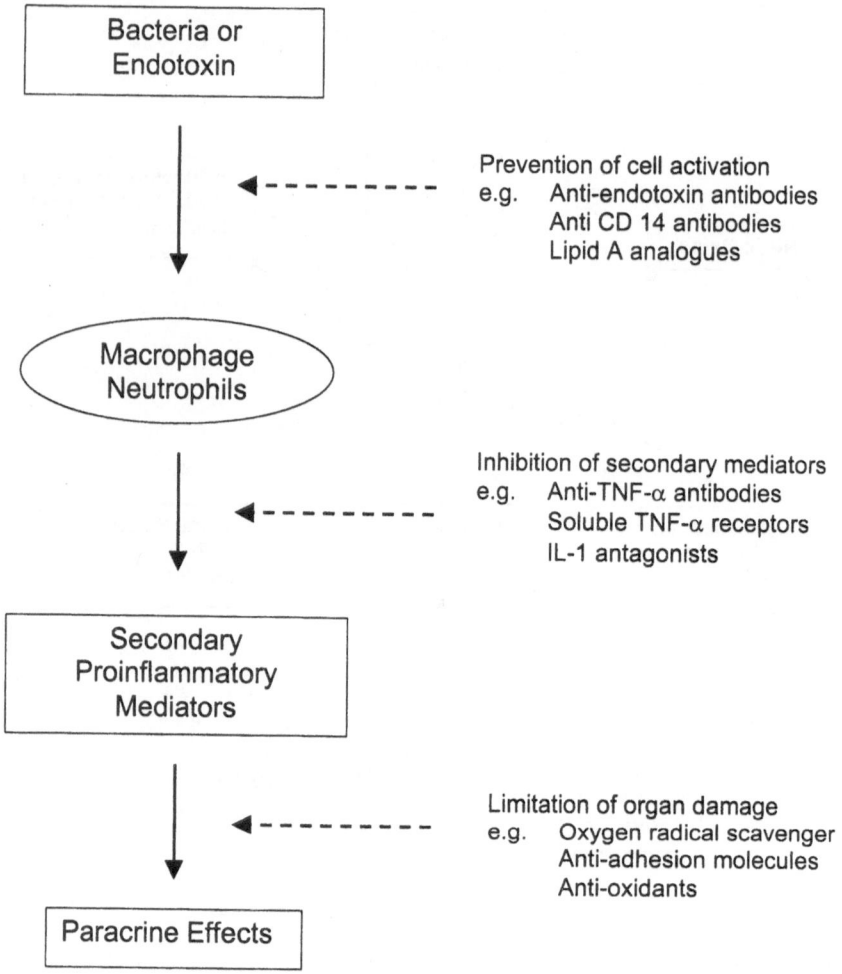

Figure 3.4. Potential sites for immunomodulatory therapies to interrupt the immuno-inflammatory cascade.

has occurred. As gram-negative and gram-positive bacteria activate the immuno-inflammatory cascade by different mechanisms, this approach would only be effective against a single bacterial species and would be ineffective in those with SIRS due to a non-infective cause. Limitations of current microbiological diagnostic techniques often precludes such an approach.

The next potential site for intervention would be anti-cytokine therapies directed against the "proximal" pro-inflammatory cytokines. This could be achieved by inhibition of mediator synthesis or release, neutralisation of the circulating cytokines or blockade or down-regulation of the cell surface receptors. This approach has the advantage that it could be given later in the inflammatory process. Also, as its target is beyond the initial stages of activation, it could be effective in patients with SIRS, irrespective of the underlying aetiology.

Finally, the last potential site for intervention would be to interrupt the pathological processes directly leading to organ dysfunction. Such an approach would require widespread limitation of the actions of the main cellular effectors of the immuno-inflammatory cascade—principally the endothelium, macrophages and neutrophils. Potential approaches include inhibitors of neutrophil migration and activation, free radical scavengers and anti-oxidant agents. Direct inhibition of the secondary messengers involved in signal transduction could also be considered. An attraction of this approach is that it may allow salvage treatment after septic shock is established.

Whilst all of the above approaches have their own advantages and limitations, it should be remembered that immuno-inflammatory responses evolved to protect the host from noxious agents and foreign antigens. Some degree of immune responsiveness is therefore essential and a balance needs to be set between reducing an inappropriately excessive pro-inflammatory response without inducing immuno-deficiency. As multiple mechanisms with considerable redundancy are involved in the immuno-inflammatory cascade combination therapies may be required to ensure the maximal effect [55].

Antiendotoxin Therapies

A number of approaches have been investigated as potential mechanisms for limiting the pathological effects of endotoxin. In animal studies, polyclonal antibodies raised against LPS protected against the effects of endotoxin and lead to the development of polyclonal human anti-sera with high levels of anti-LPS antibodies. In clinical studies, these reduced the mortality associated with gram-negative sepsis [56] and were effective as prophylaxis against gram-negative infection in high risk surgical patients [57].

Following technological advances, anti-LPS monoclonal antibodies (MAb) were developed of which HA-1A and E5 have been the most widely studied. HA-1A is a human anti-Lipid A IgM antibody derived from the spleen of a patient vaccinated with the J5 rough mutant of *E. coli*. E5 is a similar murine anti-Lipid A IgM MAb. Despite the encouraging results seen in animal studies and the enthusiasm generated by the earlier clinical trials of polyclonal antibodies, the results of clinical studies of both of these agents have been disappointing. Three large trials of HA-1A, which enrolled over 3,000 patients with septic shock, failed to show any overall survival benefit [58–60]. A retrospective subgroup analysis of 200 patients with gram-negative bacteremia from the study of Ziegler et al [58], showed improved survival, but, the validity of such a post hoc analysis has been questioned [61]. HA-1A was granted a product licence in Europe in 1992, but, was subsequently withdrawn from the market in 1993. Two large trials of E5, which recruited over 1,500 patients, similarly showed no improvement in overall survival in patients with severe sepsis [62,63].

In addition to anti-endotoxin antibodies, other therapeutic approaches have been used to limit the effects of LPS. Anti-CD14 MAbs has been shown to suppress a wide variety of endothelial, macrophage and neutrophil responses [6] and anti-LBP antibodies have been shown, in animal studies, to protect against potentially lethal endotoxin challenges [64]. LPS neutralising proteins also exist of which bactericidal/permeability-increasing (BPI) protein has been the most extensively studied. BPI is a 55–60 kDa neutrophil primary granule protein with a 45 percent sequence homology to LBP. It has a higher affinity for LPS than LBP and therefore removes LPS from the LPS-LBP complex. A recombinant 23 kDa N-terminal fragment of the BPI protein (rBPI$_{23}$) retains the LPS neutralising capacity and has been demonstrated, in animal studies, to protect against endotox-aemia and gram-negative infection [65]. In human volunteer studies, rBPI$_{23}$ has been shown to abolish the cytokine responses to an endotoxin challenge [66]. LPS analogues, based on the structure of Lipid A, have also been developed and are potent LPS competitive antagonists. A synthetic Lipid A analogue, E5331, has recently been shown to inhibit endotoxin binding to cells, to block LPS-induced TNF-α production and to protect mice from endotoxin and *E. coli*-induced mortality. In human studies, E5331 has been shown to reduce endotoxin-induced cytokine release [67]. To date, there have been no large-scale clinical trials reported of the use anti-CD14 MAbs, anti-LBP MAbs or Lipid A analogues.

Anti-TNF-α Therapies

Anti-TNF-α therapies, in particular the use of anti-TNF-α MAbs, have been extensively investigated in both animal and clinical studies and they have proved to be some of the more promising immunomodulatory treatments of sepsis and SIRS. In animal models of both gram-negative [68] and gram-positive [31] sepsis, anti-TNF-α MAbs have been shown to have several advantageous actions. As expected from the early rise in serum TNF-α following an endotoxin challenge, the maximal benefit of these therapies has usually been seen when given either prophylactically or soon after a septic insult.

Bay x1351 is an IgG$_1$ murine monoclonal anti-TNF-α MAb with a half-life of approximately fifty hours. It has been administered as a single intravenous infusion in three large clinical trials (NORASEPT I, NORASEPT II and INTERSEPT) of patients with sepsis and septic shock of less than twelve hours duration. The NORASEPT I trial randomised 971 patients (478 with septic shock) to receive 7.5 mg/kg, 15 mg/kg anti-TNF-α MAb or placebo [69]. No overall improvement in 28-day mortality was identified. A *post hoc* subgroup analysis showed a significant reduction in mortality at three days in those with septic shock at study entry. The INTERSEPT study randomised 563 patients (420 with septic shock) to receive either 3 mg/kg, 15 mg/kg anti-TNF-α MAb or placebo. It also failed to show an improvement in 28-day mortality, but, more rapid shock reversal and a reduction in organ dysfunction was seen in the antibody-treated groups [70]. As a result of the above two studies, NORASEPT II recruited only patients with septic shock and reported in early 1998. It randomised 1879 patients to receive either 7.5 mg/kg anti-TNF-α MAb or placebo. It demonstrated no difference in 28-day mortality or shock reversal between the two treatment arms [71]. There were no differences in the rate of organ failure except for a significant reduction in the incidence of coagulopathy in the antibody-treated group.

CB0006 is a murine anti-TNF-α MAb which also failed to show any overall survival benefit when used in patients with severe sepsis or septic shock [72]. Subgroup analysis of this study showed, that when compared with historical controls, there was a suggestion of an improvement in survival in those with high serum TNF-α levels at study entry. MAK 195F is a "humanised" F(ab')$_2$ fragment of a murine IgG with a kappa light chain directed against human TNF-α. It too produced no survival benefit in patients with severe sepsis, but, retrospective stratification by serum IL-6 concentration suggested advantageous effects in those with elevated levels of this cytokine at study entry [73]. A similar subgroup analysis of the NORASEPT II data showed no improvement in outcome in those with either elevated TNF-α or IL-6 at study entry.

An alternative therapeutic approach to TNF-α inhibition has been the administration of sTNFRs. To reduce the metabolism of these receptors, increase their affinity for TNF-α and prolong their physiological effects, chimeric molecules have been engineered with dimers of either the p55 or p75 sTNFR attached to the Fc portion of a human IgG. These constructs were effective as TNF-α antagonists in some animal sepsis models, with sTNFR55-IgG being superior to sTNFR75-IgG [74]. In a clinical trial of sTNFR55-IgG, which enrolled almost 500 patients with severe sepsis, there was a trend towards a reduction in 28-day mortality that became significant when predicted mortality and plasma IL-6 levels were included in a logistic regression analysis [75]. In concordance with the results of animal studies, clinical trials of sTNFR75 have been disappointing, with an increased mortality seen in patients treated with higher doses of this receptor construct [76].

Other pharmacological agents also attenuate TNF-α responses. Corticosteroids block TNF-α gene translation and, in animal studies, steroid pre-treatment reduced the mortality from a septic challenge. The encouraging results of animal studies led, in the late 1970s and early 1980s, to the widespread use of steroids in patients with septic shock. A recent meta-analysis showed that the use of steroids in these patients produces no survival benefit and was associated with an increased incidence of secondary nosocomial infection [77]. Phosphodiesterase inhibitors limit TNF-α gene transcription [78]. Pentoxifylline is the most extensively studied of this class of drugs and has been shown to reduce cytokine production [79], reduce neutrophil activation [80] and improve survival in animal models of sepsis [81]. In clinical studies, pentoxifylline reduced cytokine production and improved organ dysfunction scores [82].

Anti-IL-1 Therapies

The most extensively investigated therapy directed against IL-1 has been the use of the IL-1Ra. Since only a few IL-1 receptors need to be activated in order to produce a response, a large excess of IL-1Ra is needed in order to inhibit its actions. In clinical trials of IL-1Ra initially encouraging results were obtained. A phase II study reported a dose-dependent reduction in APACHE II scores and improvement in mortality in 99 patients with severe sepsis [83]. However, two subsequent multicentre placebo-controlled trials, that enrolled over 1,800 patients, failed to confirm these results [84,85].

Why Have Sepsis Trials Failed?

Despite encouraging results in animal studies, no immunomodulatory therapy in clinical sepsis, has, to date, been shown to confer unequivocal benefit in large-scale randomised, double-blind, placebo-controlled trials. Disappointment is especially so in view of the current knowledge of the relative roles of the inflammatory mediators that have been targeted in these studies and the efficacy of these agents in chronic inflammatory states such as rheumatoid arthritis [86]. There are several reasons that appear to account for these divergent results.

Sepsis is an evolving pathological process with the different inflammatory mediators varying in their relative importance throughout the progression of the response. "Proximal" cytokines have predominantly early actions whilst "distal" cytokines are involved later in the pathological process. Therapies targeted against a particular cytokine may be most effective if given during a critical time period and may be of limited benefit, or even cause adverse effects, if given outside a "therapeutic window" [87]. This is especially so for agents directed against the "proximal" cytokines, which in animal studies, have produced the more encouraging results when given either as prophylaxis or immediately after the septic challenge. Profound redundancy exists within the immuno-inflammatory cascade with cytokines displaying many overlapping actions. This, along with the synergistic action of many mediators, suggests that blockade of a single cytokine may not produce a balanced inhibition of the inflammatory response. The complexities of the immuno-inflammatory cascade are such that identifying a "magic bullet" may prove impossible [88]. With the importance of the paracrine actions of cytokines systemic administration of immunomodulatory agents may be ineffective [89].

Most preclinical sepsis studies have been performed using crude animal models that frequently do not mimic well the clinical situation seen in man. In these studies, potential therapeutic agents have often been tested in a limited range of species against a restricted number of bacteria. From animal studies, it is known that both the site and type of infecting organism can influence the response to immunomodulatory therapies. As a result, some authors have expressed concern regarding the rapidity with which potential therapeutic agents progress from simple animal studies to clinical trials without their efficacy being confirmed in a number of animal models [90,91]. Animal studies are usually performed on sex-matched, genetically similar and healthy animals, whereas, patients included in sepsis trials are by their very nature heterogeneous. Age, genetic predisposition, immune status and drug therapy can all alter inflammatory responses. In animal studies, the exact time of onset of a septic insult and its rate of progression can be well controlled, whereas, in clinical studies determining both of these aspects can be very difficult.

Marked variations in physiological and cytokine responses are seen in animals given an identical septic challenge. Also, in healthy human volunteers given an endotoxin infusion or septic patients with similar disease severity, cytokine levels can vary greatly. Innate resistance to infection differs between individuals. In some patients, drugs that augment rather than inhibit the immuno-inflammatory cascade may be the more appropriate form of therapy [92]. Identification of clinical or serological markers that will allow stratification of patients into subgroups who may benefit from a particular form of immunomodulatory therapy is required. There is already some evidence to support this approach as, in many of the anti-TNF-α MAb trials, subgroups of patients were identified, usually in a retrospective post hoc analysis, who by having elevated serum cytokine levels at study entry, appeared to show a survival benefit [73].

A genomic polymorphism has been identified within the TNF-α gene locus that has been shown to influence serum TNF-α levels and subsequent survival in patients with severe sepsis [93,94]. Recognition of such genetic markers may allow identification of high risk patients. With the poor reliability of serum cytokine levels to predict local mediator synthesis, measurement of tissue cytokine expression may provide additional information on the state of the immuno-inflammatory response. At present, new and novel therapeutic agents are being developed at a faster rate than the ability to select who will benefit from them.

The disappointing results of the clinical trials of anti-cytokine therapies has led several authors to question the rationale for this therapeutic approach. In a recent meta-analysis of non-glucocorticoid anti-inflammatory therapies, a marginal benefit from these agents was identified and it was suggested that, at best they accounted for a 10 percent reduction in mortality [95]. It was concluded that many trials of immunomodulatory agents had enrolled insufficient patients to identify a significant difference. In order to reach statistical significance it was estimated that up to 7,000 patients would be needed in some studies, and therefore, the definitive answers regarding the potential benefit of many of these agents may never be known.

References

1. Bone RC. Towards and epidemiology and natural history of SIRS (systemic inflammatory response syndrome). JAMA 1992; 268: 3452–5.
2. Bone RC, Balk RA, Cerra FB, et al. and the ACCP/SCCM Consensus Conference Committee. American College of Chest Physicians/Society of Critical Care Medicine. Definitions of sepsis and organ failure and guidelines for the use of innovative therapies in sepsis. Chest 1992; 101: 1644–55.
3. Sands KE, Bates DW, Lanken PN, et al. for the Academic Medical Center Consortium Sepsis Working Group. Epidemiology of sepsis syndrome in 8 academic medical centres. JAMA 1997; 278: 234–40.
4. Brun-Buisson C, Doyon F, Carlet J, et al. Incidence, risk factors and outcome of severe sepsis and septic shock in adults. JAMA 1995; 274: 968–674.
5. Rietschel ET, Kirikac T, Schade FU, et al. The chemical structure of bacterial endotoxin in relation to bioactivity. Immunobiology 1993; 187: 346–56.
6. Wright SD, Ramos RA, Tobias et al. CD 14, a receptor for complexes of lipopolysaccharide (LPS) and LPS-binding protein. Science 1990; 249: 1431–3.
7. Tracey KJ, Beutler B, Lowry SF, et al. Shock and tissue injury induced by recombinant human cachectin. Science 1986; 234: 470–4.
8. Lynn WA, Golenbeck DT. Lipopolysaccharide antagonists. Immunol Today 1992; 13: 271–6.
9. Feuerstein G, Hallenbeck JM, Vanatta B, et al. Effects of gram negative endotoxin on levels of corticosterone, TNFα, circulating blood cells and the survival of rats. Circ Shock 1990; 30: 265–78.
10. Kuhns DB, Alvord WG, Gallin JI. Increased circulating cytokines, cytokine antagonists and E-selectin after intravenous administration of endotoxin in humans. J Infect Dis 1995; 171: 145–52.
11. Suffredini AF, Fromm RE, Parker MM, et al. The cardiovascular response of normal humans to the administration of endotoxin. N Eng J Med 1989; 321: 280–7.
12. Casey LC, Balk RA, Bone RC. Plasma cytokine and endotoxin levels correlate with survival in patients with the sepsis syndrome. Ann Intern Med 1993; 119: 771–8.
13. Dofferhoff ASM, Bom VJJ, de Vries-Hospers HG, et al. Patterns of cytokines, plasma endotoxin, plasminogen activator inhibitor and acute phase proteins during the treatment of severe sepsis in humans. Crit Car Med 1992; 20: 185–92.
14. Shenep JL, Flynn PM, Barrett FF, et al. Serial quanitation of endotoxemia and bacteremia during therapy for gram-negative bacterial sepsis. J Infect Dis 1988; 157: 565–8.
15. Danner RL, Elin RJ, Hosseini JM, et al. Endotoxemia in human septic shock. Chest 1991; 99: 169–75.
16. Redl H, Schlag G, Bahrami S, Schade U, Ceska M, St_tz P. Plasma neutrophil-activating peptide-1/interleukin-8 and neutrophil elastase in a primate bacteremia model. J Infect Dis 1991; 164: 383–8.
17. Schlievert PM. Role of superantigens in human disease. J Infect Dis 1993; 167: 997–1002.
18. Lynn WA, Cohen J. Adjunctive therapy for septic shock: a review of experimental approaches. Clin Infect Dis 1995; 20: 143–58.
19. Chaudry IH. Sepsis. Lessons learned in the last century and future directions. Arch Surg 1999; 134: 922–9.
20. Bone RC. Towards a theory regarding the pathogenesis of the systemic inflammatory response syndrome: what we do and do not know about cytokine regulation. Crit Care Med 1996; 24: 163–72.
21. Schein M, Wittmann DH, Holzheimer R, et al. Hypothesis: compartmentalization of cytokines in intraabdominal infection. Surgery 1996: 119: 694–700.
22. Mercer-Jones MA, Hadjiminas DJ, Heinzelmann M, et al. Continuous antibiotic treatment for experimental abdominal sepsis: effects on organ inflammatory cytokine expression and neutrophil sequestration. Br J Surg 1998; 85: 385–9.

23. Cavaillon JM, Munoz C, Fitting C, et al. Circulating cytokines: the tip of the iceberg? Circ Shock 1992; 38: 145–52.
24. Tracey KJ, Cerami A. Tumour necrosis factor: an updated review of its biology. Crit Care Med 1993; 21: S415–22.
25. Wyble CW, Hynes KL, Kuchibhotla J, et al. TNF-α and IL-1 upregulate membrane-bound and soluble E-Selectin through a common pathway. J Surg Res 1997; 73: 107–12.
26. Bevilacqua MP, Pober JS, Majeau GR, et al. Recombinant tumor necrosis factor induces procoagulant activity in cultured human vascular endothelium: characterisation and comparison with the actions of interleukin-1. Proc Natl Acad Sci USA 1986; 83: 4533–7.
27. Lukacs NW, Strieter RM, Chensue SW, et al. TNF-alpha mediates recruitment of neutrophils and eosinophils during airway inflammation. J Immunol 1995; 154: 5411–17.
28. Hesse DG, Tracey KJ, Fong Y, et al. Cytokine appearance in human endotoxemia and primate bacteremia. Surg Gynecol Obstet 1988; 166: 147–53.
29. Hadjiminas DJ, McMasters KM, Peyton JC, et al. Tissue tumor necrosis factor mRNA expression following cecal ligation and puncture or intraperitoneal injection of endotoxin. J Surg Res 1994; 56: 549–55.
30. Opal SM, Cross AS, Kelly NM, et al. Efficacy of a monoclonal antibody directed against tumor necrosis factor in protecting neutropenic rats from lethal infection with Pseudomonas aeruginosa. J Infect Dis 1990; 161: 1148–52.
31. Hinshaw LB, Emerson TE, Taylor FB, et al. Lethal staphylococcus aureus-induced shock in primates: prevention of death with anti-TNF antibody. J Trauma 1992; 33: 568–73.
32. Eskandri MK, Bolos G, Miller C, et al. Anti-tumor necrosis factor antibody therapy fails to prevent lethality after cecal ligation and puncture or endotoxemia. J Immunol 1992; 148: 2724–30.
33. Windsor ACJ, Mullen PG, Walsh CJ, et al. Delayed tumor necrosis factor α blockade attenuates pulmonary dysfunction and metabolic acidosis associated with experimental gram-negative sepsis. Ann Surg 1994; 129: 80–9.
34. Fong Y, Tracey KJ, Moldawer LL, et al. ANtibodies to cachectin/tumour necrosis factor reduces interleukin-1α and interleukin 6 appearance during lethal bacteremia. J Exp Med 1989; 170: 1627–33.
35. Michie HR, Manogue KR, Spriggs DR, et al. Detection of circulating tumour necrosis factor after endotoxin administration. N Eng J Med 1988; 318: 1481–6.
36. Damas P, Canivet J-L, de Groote D, et al. Sepsis and serum cytokine concentrations. Crit Care Med 1997; 25: 405–12.
37. Lowry SF, Moldawer LL, Calvano SE. Cytokine markers of the human response to sepsis. In: Vincent J-L ed. Yearbook of intensive care and emergency medicine. Berlin Heidelberg New York: Springer, 1996: 14–23.
38. Martin C, Sauzx P, Mege JL, et al. Prognostic value of serum cytokines in septic shock. Intensive Care Med 1994; 20: 272–7.
39. Pinsky MR, Vincent J-L, Deviere J, et al. Serum cytokine levels in human septic shock. Relation to multiple-system organ failure and mortality. Chest 1993; 103: 565–75.
40. Dinarello CA. Interleukin-1 and interleukin-1 antagonism. Blood 1991; 77: 1627–52.
41. Okusawa S, Gelfand JA, Ikejima T, Connolly RJ, Dinarello CA. Interleukin-1 induces a shock like state in rabbits. Synergism with tumour necrosis factor and the effect of cyclo-oxygenase inhibition. J Clin Invest 1988; 81: 1162–72.
42. Endo S, Inada K, Inoue Y, et al. Two types of septic shock classified by the plasma level of cytokines and endotoxin. Circ Shock 1992; 38: 264–74.
43. Shalaby MR, Waage A, Aarden L, Espevik T. Endotoxin, tumour necrosis factor-α and interleukin-1 induce interleukin-6 production in vivo. Clin Immunol Immunopath 1989; 53: 488–98.
44. Schindler R, Mancilla J, Endres S, et al. Correlations and interactions in the production of interleukin-6 (IL-6), IL-1 and tumour necrosis factor (TNF) in human blood mononuclear cells: IL-6 suppresses IL-1 and TNF. Blood 1990; 75: 40–7.
45. Hack CE, de Groot ER, Felt-Bersma RJF, et al. Increased plasma levels of interleukin-6 in sepsis. Blood 1989; 74: 1704–10.
46. Damas P, Ledoux D, Nys M, et al. Cytokine serum levels during severe sepsis in humans. IL-6 as a marker of severity. Ann Surg 1992; 215: 356–62.
47. Grard C, Bruyns C, Marchant A, et al. Interleukin 10 reduces the release of tumor necrosis factor and prevents lethality in experimental endotoxemia. J Exp Med 1993; 177: 547–50.
48. Marchant A, Bruyns C, Vandenabeele A, et al. Interleukin-10 control interferon- and tumor necrosis factor production during experimental endotoxemia. Eur J Immunol 1994; 24: 1167–71.
49. Van Deuren M, van der Ven-Jongekrijg J, Bertelink AKM, et al. Correlation between proinflammatory cytokines and antiinflammatory mediators and the severity of disease in meningococcal infections. J Infect Dis 1995; 172: 433–9.

50. Tartaglia LA, Goeddel DV. Two TNF receptors. Immunol Today 1992; 13: 151–3.
51. Aderka D, Engelmann H, Maor Y, et al. Stabilisation of the bioactivity of tumor necrosis factor by its soluble receptors. J Exp Med 1992; 175: 323–9.
52. Ertel W, Scholl FA, Gallati H, et al. Increased release of soluble tumor necrosis factor receptors into blood during clinical sepsis. Arch Surg 1994; 129: 1330–7.
53. Fischer E, Marano MA, van Zee KJ, et al. Interleukin-1 receptor blockade improves survival and hemodynamic performance in Escherichia coli septic shock, but fails to alter host responses to sublethal endotoxemia. J Clin Invest 1992; 89: 1551–7.
54. Grdlund B, Sj"lin J, Nilsson A, et al. Plasma levels of cytokines in primary septic shock in humans: correlation with disease severity. J Infect Dis 1995; 172: 296–301.
55. Cross AS, Opal SM, Palardy JE, et al. The efficacy of combination immunotherapy in experimental Pseudomonas sepsis. J Infect Dis 1993; 167: 112–18.
56. Ziegler EJ, McCutchan JA, Fierer J, et al. Treatment of gram-negative bacteraemia and shock with human anti-serum to a mutant Escherichia coli. N Eng J Med 1982; 307: 1225–30.
57. Baumgartner J-D, Glauser MP, McCutchan JA, et al. Prevention of gram-negative shock and death in surgical patients by antibody to endotoxin core glycolipid. Lancet 1985; ii: 59–63.
58. Ziegler EJ, Fisher CJ, Sprung CL, et al. Treatment of gram-negative bacteremia and septic shock with HA-1A human monoclonal antibody against endotoxin. N Eng J Med 1991; 324: 42–436.
59. French National Registry of HA-1A. THe French National Registry of HA-1A (Centoxin) in septic shock. A cohort study of 600 patients. The National Committee for the evaluation of Centoxin. Arch Intern Med 1994; 154: 2484–91.
60. McCloskey RV, Straube RC, Sanders C, et al. for the CHESS Trial Study Group. Treatment of septic shock with human monoclonal antibody HA-1A. A randomised, double-blind, placebo-controlled trial. Ann Intern Med 1994; 121: 1–5.
61. Dellinger RP. Post hoc analyses in sepsis trials: a formula for disappointment? Crit Care Med 1996; 24: 727–9.
62. Greenman RL, Schein RMH, Martin MA, et al. A controlled trial of E5 murine monoclonal IgM antibody to endotoxin in the treatment of gram-negative sepsis. JAMA 1991; 266: 1097–102.
63. Bone RC, Balk RA, Fein AM, et al. and the E5 Sepsis Study Group. A second large controlled clinical study of E5, a monoclonal antibody to endotoxin: results of a prospective, multicenter, randomised controlled trial. Crit Care Med 1995; 23: 994–1005.
64. Gallay P, Heuman D, Le Roy D, et al. Mode of action of anti-lipopolysaccharide-binding protein antibodies for prevention of endotoxemic shock in mice. Proc Natl Acad Sci USA 1994; 91: 7922–6.
65. Evans TJ, Carpenter A, Moyes D, et al. Protective effect of a recombinant amino-terminal fragment of human bactericidal/permeability-increasing protein in an animal model of gram-negative sepsis. J Infect Dis 1995; 171: 153–60.
66. Von der M"hlen MAM, Kimmings AN, Wedel NI, et al. Inhibition of endotoxin-induced cytokine release and neutrophil activation in humans by use of recombinant bactericidal/permeability-increasing protein. J Infect Dis 1995; 172: 144–51.
67. Christ WJ, Asano O, Robidoux ALC, et al. E5331, a pure endotoxin antagonist of high potency. Science 1995; 268: 80–3.
68. Silva AT, Bayston KF, Cohen J. Prophylactic and therapeutic effects of a monoclonal antibody to tumor necrosis factor-α in experimental gram-negative shock. J Infect Dis 1990; 162: 421–7.
69. Abraham E, Wunderink R, Silverman H, et al. and the TNF-α MAb Sepsis Study Group. Efficacy and safety of monoclonal antibody to human tumor necrosis factor α in patients with sepsis syndrome. A randomised, controlled, double-blind, multicenter clinical trial. JAMA 1995; 273: 934–41.
70. Cohen J, Carlet J and the INTERSEPT Study Group. INTERSEPT: an international multicenter placebo-controlled trial of monoclonal antibody to human TNF-α in patients with the sepsis syndrome. Crit Care Med 1996; 24: 1431–9.
71. Abraham E, Anzueto A, Gutierrez G, et al. and the NORASEPT II Study Group. Double-blind randomised controlled trial of monoclonal antibody to human tumour necrosis factor in treatment of septic shock. Lancet 1998; 351: 929–33.
72. Fisher CJ, Opal SM, Dhainaut J-F, et al. Influence of anti-tumor necrosis factor monoclonal antibody of cytokine levels in patients with sepsis. Crit Care Med 1993; 21: 318–27.
73. Reinhart K, Wiegand-L"hnert C, Grimminger F, et al. Assessment of the safety and efficacy of the monoclonal anti-tumor necrosis factor antibody fragment, MAK 195F, in patients with sepsis and septic shock: a multicentre, randomised, placebo-controlled, dose-ranging study. Crit Care Med 1996; 24: 733–42.
74. Evans TJ, Moyes D, Carpenter A, et al. Protective effect of 55- but not 75-kD soluble tumor necrosis factor receptor-immunoglobulin G fusion proteins in an animal model of gram-negative sepsis. J Exp Med 1994; 180: 2173–9.

75. Abraham E, Glauser M, Butler T, et al. p55 Tumour necrosis factor receptor fusion protein in the treatment of patients with severe sepsis and septic shock. JAMA 1997; 277: 1531–8.
76. Fisher CJ, Agosti JM, Opal SM, et al. Treatment of septic shock with the tumor necrosis facto receptor: Fc fusion protein. N Eng J Med 1996; 334: 1697–702.
77. Lefering R, Neugebauer EAM. Steroid controversy in sepsis and septic shock. Crit Care Med 1995; 23: 1294–1303.
78. Doherty GM, Jensen JC, Alexander HR, et al. Pentoxifylline suppression of tumor necrosis factor gene transcription. Surgery 1991; 110: 192–8.
79. Refsum SE, Halliday MI, Campbell G, et al. Modulation of TNF-α and IL-6 in a peritonitis model using pentoxifylline. J Pediatr Surg 1996; 31: 928–30.
80. Hoffmann H. Pentoxifylline in experimental sepsis. In: Faist E, Baue AE, Schildberg FW. The immune consequences of trauma, shock and sepsis—Mechanisms and therapeutic approaches. Volume 2. Legerich: Pabst Science Publisher, 1996: 1245–9.
81. Chalkiadakis GE, Kostakis A, Karayannacos PE, et al. Pentoxifylline in the treatment of experimental peritonitis in rats. Arch Surg 1985; 120: 1141–4.
82. Staubach K-H, Schröder J, Stäber F, et al. Effect of pentoxifylline in severe sepsis. Arch Surg 1998; 133: 94–100.
83. Fisher CJ, Slotman GJ, Opal SM, et al. Initial evaluation of human recombinant interleukin-1 receptor antagonist in the treatment of sepsis syndrome: a randomised, open-label, placebo-controlled multicentre trial. Crit Care Med 1994; 22: 12–21.
84. Fisher CJ, Dhainaut J-F, Opal SM, et al. for the Phase III rhIL-1Ra Sepsis Syndrome Study Group. Recombinant interleukin-1 receptor antagonist in the treatment of patients with sepsis syndrome: results from a randomised double-blind placebo controlled trial. JAMA 1994; 271: 1836–43.
85. Opal SM, Fisher CJ, Dhainaut J-FA, et al. Confirmatory interleukin-1 receptor antagonist trial in severe sepsis. A phase III, randomised, double-blind, placebo-controlled, multicentre trial. Crit Care Med 1997; 25: 1115–24.
86. Moreland LW, Baumgartner SW, Schiff MH, et al. Treatment of rheumatoid arthritis with a recombinant human tumor necrosis factor receptor (p75)-Fc fusion protein. N Eng J Med 1997; 337: 141–7.
87. Ridings PC, Windsor ACJ, Sugerman HJ, et al. Beneficial cardiopulmonary effects of pentoxifylline in experimental sepsis are lost once septic shock is established. Arch Surg 1994; 129: 1144–52.
88. Vincent J-L. Search for effective immunomodulating strategies against sepsis. Lancet 1998; 351: 922–3.
89. Ksontini R, Mackay SLD, Moldawer LL. Revisiting the role of tumour necrosis factor α and the response to surgical injury and inflammation. Arch Surg 1998; 133: 558–67.
90. Piper RD, Cook DJ, Bone RC, et al. Introducing Critical Appraisal to studies of animal models investigating novel therapies in sepsis. Crit Care Med 1996; 24: 2059–70.
91. Deitch EA. Animal models of sepsis and shock: a review and lessons learned. Shock 1998; 9: 1–11.
92. Baue AE. Multiple organ failure, multiple organ dysfunction syndrome and systemic inflammatory response syndrome; why no magic bullets? Arch Surg 1997; 132: 703–7.
93. Stäber F, Petersen M. Bokelmann F, et al. A genomic polymorphism within the tumor necrosis factor locus influences plasma tumor necrosis factor-alpha concentrations and outcome of patients with severe sepsis. Crit Care Med 1996; 24: 381–4.
94. Mira J-P, Cariou A, Grall F, et al. Association of TNF2, a TNF-α promoter polymorphism, with septic shock susceptibility and mortality. JAMA 1999; 282: 561–8.
95. Zeni F, Freeman B, Natanson C. Anti-inflammatory therapies to treat sepsis and septic shock: a reassessment. Crit Care Med 1997; 25: 1095–100.
96. Dhainaut JFA, Vincent JI, Richard C. CDP571, a humanised antibody to human tumor necrosis factor-alpha: safety, pharmacokinetics, immune response and influence of the antibody on cytokine concentrations in patients with septic shock. Crit Care Med 1995; 23: 1461–9.
97. Abraham E, Glauser MP, Butler T, et al. for the Ro 45-2081 Study Group. p55 tumor necrosis factor receptor fusion protein in the treatment of patients with severe sepsis and septic shock. JAMA 1997; 277: 1531–8.

4. Immunodeficiency and the Surgeon

T.G. Allen-Mersh and Andrew Huang

Introduction

Immunodeficiency poses many challenges to the surgeon. The immunodeficient patient, irrespective of age, may present with recurrent infections or infection with an unusual organism and the surgeon has to maintain a high degree of suspicion of the likelihood of underlying significant immune deficiency. On the other hand the surgeon may render a patient immunodeficient with surgery or drugs and therefore need to be proactive in protecting the patient from the consequences.

Classification of Immunodeficiency

Immunodeficiency may be classified into *primary* and *secondary* disorders. Primary immune disorders are due to usually *congenital* intrinsic defects in the immune system whereas secondary or *acquired* immune disorders result from other conditions. Immunodeficiency may be further subdivided into disorders of *specific* and *non-specific* immune mechanisms. Specific deficiencies involve humoral and cell-mediated responses, whereas non-specific deficiencies include defective neutrophil function and specific complement system abnormalities. Many defects are subtle and transient and defy classification.

Causes of Immunodeficiency

Primary Immunodeficiency Disorders

These rare disorders frequently manifest in early childhood with recurrent and severe infections. They may be specific or non-specific immune defects that determine the pattern of infection seen in affected patients.

Defects in Specific Immunity

B-cell deficiency may be qualitative or quantitative; the latter can involve all immunoglobulin classes (panhypogammaglobulinemia) or only one class or sub-class (selective deficiency). In *X-linked hypogammaglobulinemia (Bruton's disease)* infant males present with recurrent pyogenic infections once placentally transferred maternal IgG is lost. There is failure of B-lymphocyte differentiation with negligible IgG, IgM and IgA levels. Patient management consists of lifelong immunoglobulin injections and counseling of female carriers as prenatal diagnosis is possible. *Transient hypogammaglobulinemia* occurs due to a delay in the maturation of the B-cell system and is relatively common in premature infants of both sexes. IgG levels are low but susceptibility to infections is mild and self-limiting. *Common variable deficiency* embraces a combination of defective T-helper cells and B-lymphocytes resulting in late onset immunodeficiency.

T-cell deficiency in isolation is rare and is usually accompanied by variable abnormalities of B-cell function, reflecting the co-operation between the two cell types needed for antibody synthesis. In *DiGeorge syndrome* the thymus and para-thyroid glands fail to develop resulting in decreased levels of T-lymphocytes and hypocalcemic fits from hypoparathyroidism. Resistance to pyogenic bacteria is relatively normal but antibody response to many antigens is impaired because of the need for T-helper cells. Affected children are therefore unable to mount an effective cell-mediated response and are susceptible to infections with fungi, viruses and opportunistic pathogens such as *Pneumocystis carinii* [1]. Thymic grafting paradoxically results in the production of T-lymphocytes which recognize the graft as 'foreign' with frequent subsequent rejection.

Severe combined immunodeficiency (SCID) is an example of a group of disorders where there is defective conjoint humoral and cell-mediated immunity. Death usually occurs in infancy from multiple infections although bone marrow transplantation may effectively restore the immune system.

Defects in Non-specific Immunity

Chronic granulomatous disease is a group of disorders resulting from an enzyme defect of oxygen radical production during neutrophil activation. The classic type is X-linked recessive presenting with severe skin sepsis caused by *Staphylococcus aureus*, Gram-negative bacilli or fungi and complicated by multiple abscesses and non-caseating granulomas. *Chediak-Higashi syndrome* is another example of impaired neutrophil function as a result of defective lysosomes.

Inherited deficiencies of complement components prevent the elimination of immune complexes. C3 deficiencies predispose to recurrent bacterial infections whilst deficiencies in C5, C6, C7, C8 or properdin are associated with systemic infections by encapsulated bacteria such as Neisseria *meningitidis* and *N. gonorrhoea*. *Systemic lupus erythematosus* is an acquired complement deficiency state where the consumption of C1, C4 and C2 components correlates with disease activity [2].

Secondary Immunodeficiency Disorders

Secondary immunodeficiency states are far more common than primary ones but the nature of immune defects and the infection patterns are less well defined. Multiple contributing factors result in varying degrees of immunocompromise and a mixed susceptibility to infections.

Malnutrition and Protein Deficiency

Malnourished populations in the Third World are more susceptible to infections that in turn further hinder their nutrition. There is impaired humoral response after immunization [3] as well as defective cell-mediated immunity, phagocyte function and complement activity [4]. These defects appear to be reversible with adequate protein and calorific diet supplementation [5]. Serious malnutrition however predominantly suppresses cell-mediated immunity as shown by a reduction in CD4+ T-helper cells [6], IL-2 production from lymphocytes and NK activity [7] as well as generalized atrophy of the lymphoid organs.

Malnutrition is prevalent amongst surgical patients to varying degrees [8] predisposing to infections and other complications. This recognition has led to many surgical patients receiving additional nutritional support either enterally [9,10] or parenterally [11]. Immunonutrition enhances host response, induces a switch from acute-phase to constitutive proteins and improves clinical outcome [12].

Protein loss through *nephrotic syndrome* or *protein-losing enteropathy* may be severe enough to cause hypogammaglobulinemia. In nephrotic syndrome the loss of immunoglobulin is selective with a reduction in IgG and relative sparing of IgM levels [13] such that recurrent infections are rarely a significant problem. In *chronic renal failure*, however, patients develop combined T- and B-cell deficiencies that worsen with uremia progression and are often exacerbated by dialysis [14].

Major Trauma, Shock and Burns

Immunodeficiency in these conditions is well recognized and there are defects in cell-mediated, humoral and innate defences. This in part explains the increased incidence of sepsis-related mortality but may also be indirectly related to malnutrition in these patients [15]. Although nutritional support of critically ill patients will not lead to positive nitrogen balance, it can increase protein synthesis, enhance immune function and beneficially modify the body's response to an illness [16].

Malignancy

In disseminated malignancy with cachexia both T and B-cell functions are defective. There is evidence to suggest that cellular immunity in the form of response to cutaneous antigen stimulation [17] and lymphocyte IL-2 production [18] is impaired in patients with advanced colorectal cancer. The degree of immunosuppression, as determined by in vivo and vitro methods, relates to the progression of malignancy [19]. Paradoxically raised levels of circulating soluble cytokines and cytokine receptor levels (immune products) are found in patients with colorectal liver metastases [20]. This raises the possibility that although there is chronic T-lymphocyte stimulation by innate immune responses, the cell-mediated immunity is blocked.

Weight loss, which is prevalent in patients with advanced colorectal malignancy, is not only associated with dietary changes, quality of life or hormones but may also be due to the activation of the innate immune system and the incomplete activation of specific immune responses [21].

Iatrogenic Immunosuppression

Iatrogenic immune suppression may be intentional to prevent transplant rejection or unintentional in the course of disease treatment. *Immunosuppressive drugs* used in transplant surgery affect many aspects of cell function. Lymphocyte and polymorph activities are often impaired, although severe hypogammaglobulinemia is unusual.

Transient *post-operative immunosuppression* in healthy kidney donors is well recognized as demonstrated by depressed B and T cell levels, lymphocyte transformation and delayed hypersensitivity skin testing [22]. The theoretical implication for other surgical patients is that they may be susceptible to opportunistic infections during the peri-operative period and impaired immunological control of disseminated malignant cells during surgery.

Therapeutic radiotherapy targets radiosensitive tissues by ionization and damage to DNA. Most DNA damages are repaired but some are irreparable and when the cell tries to divide it dies in the attempt. In some normal cell lineages (e.g. lymphoid and myeloid cells) the DNA damage triggers immediate programmed cell death (apoptosis). Accidental total body irradiation therefore results in profound neutropenia and thrombocytopenia with severe immunocompromise. Patients with Hodgkin's lymphoma receive lymphoid irradiation but the combination of disease, radiotherapy and chemotherapy all contribute to severe impairment of both humoral and cellular immunity. Patients are therefore susceptible to infections acutely and to secondary malignancies in the long-term [23].

Chemotherapeutic agents are cytotoxic to malignant and any other rapidly dividing normal cells. Therefore both neutrophil and lymphocyte productions are suppressed with subsequent myelotoxicity and immunosuppression. Patients receiving chemotherapy who become septic may therefore require parenteral antibiotics, supplemental Ig and granulocyte-colony stimulating factor (G-CSF).

Splenectomy is another iatrogenic form of secondary immune deficiency and the indications for this procedure have significantly changed over the years with an increased understanding of the immunological importance of the spleen. Splenectomy is now rarely performed as part of staging laparotomy for lymphoma because of less invasive and sensitive radiological techniques such as computed tomography scans. More common indications include idiopathic thrombocytopenic purpura, hemolytic anemias, hypersplenism and traumatic rupture. The spleen is an important immunological organ responsible for antibody production as well as phagocytosis and its removal is associated with a depressed immune response.

This predisposes to potentially lethal infections with opportunistic encapsulated organisms in the syndrome of overwhelming post-splenectomy infection (OPSI). The most common infective organism is *Streptococcus pneumoniae* but *Neisseria meningitidis* and *Hemophilus influenzae* may also be responsible. Most reported episodes of OPSI occur with three years of surgery [24] and children are more susceptible than adults. A review of combined published data showed that 29 (2.5 percent) of 1181 children who underwent trauma splenectomy subsequently developed OPSI, of which 25 per cent were fatal [25]. The growing recognition of this problem has prompted a trend towards splenic salvage rather than splenectomy, especially for children with damaged spleens. In addition to the distinct syndrome of OPSI, splenectomised patients are also susceptible to ordinary post-operative sepsis. Prophylaxis against post-splenectomy infections should be implemented in all patients who undergo total splenectomy. Lifelong penicillins and erythromycin are of proven value in children; pneumococcal and *Hemophilus influenzae* type b immunization are also advised. Influenza immunization may be beneficial but meningococcal vaccination is not routinely recommended at present [26]. Vaccinations should ideally be given two weeks before elective surgery but are not appropriate before the age of two. The value of pneumococcal vaccines in the splenectomized adult is still debated and the long-term benefit in trauma patients remains to be assessed.

There is evidence to suggest that peri-operative *blood transfusions* are associated with immunosuppression in the recipient through the reduction in cell-mediated immunity [27]. This effect was used specifically for the benefit of kidney transplant recipients before more effective immunosuppressive drugs were discovered [28]. However this phenomenon becomes deleterious when managing patients undergoing surgery for colorectal cancers [29]. There is an increased incidence of post-operative infections as well as shortened disease-free interval either from local recurrence or metastases [30,31]. The use of leukocyte-depleted components appears to reduce these risks but others found no significant link between transfusion and prognosis [32]. Nevertheless the use of transfusions in the peri-operative period should be limited to those with significant anemia to avoid other potential complications such as mismatch or infection transmission.

Lymphoproliferative Diseases

These conditions cause severe immunodeficiency because ineffective neoplastic cells replace the normal cells of bone marrow and lymph nodes. *Chronic lymphoid leukemia* results in hypogammaglobulinemia and recurrent chest infections if left untreated. *Non-Hodgkin's lymphoma* is associated with both humoral and cell-mediated defects whereas *Hodgkin's lymphoma* affects cell-mediated immunity predominantly during the late stages. *Multiple myeloma* results in the suppression of polyclonal antibody production and hence the risk of pyogenic bacterial infections is up to ten times that of age-matched controls. During treatment with aggressive chemotherapy combined B and T cell deficiencies will predispose to viral, fungal and bacterial infections.

Infections

Viral infections including cytomegalovirus (CMV), measles, rubella, infectious mononucleosis and viral hepatitis transiently impair cell-mediated immunity. There is a direct cytotoxic effect on the lymphoid cells predisposing to other infections. *Acquired immune deficiency syndrome (AIDS)* due to human immunodeficiency virus (HIV) is an extreme example of secondary immune depression with diverse implications to the surgeon and will be dealt with separately in this chapter. Overwhelming *bacterial infections* may also depress immune function such as the reactivation of Herpes simplex type 1 in the form of cold sores during pneumococcal pneumonia. *Syphilitic infection* results in cell-mediated suppression by blocking lymphocyte transformation whilst *malarial parasites* cause lymphoid and macrophage dysfunction.

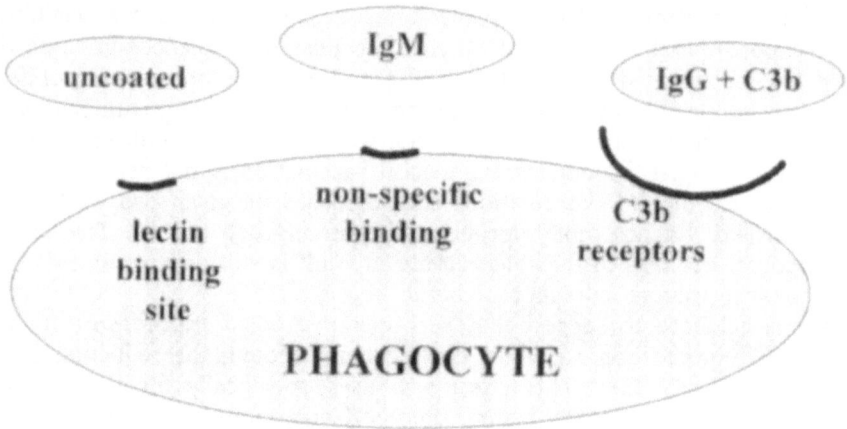

Figure 4.1. Phagocyte, complement and immunoglobulin interactions (Adapted from Roitt [33]).

Pathogenesis of Immunodeficiency

Pyogenic bacteria are opsonized before they become susceptible to phagocytosis by polymorphs and macrophages. Uncoated or IgM-coated bacteria adhere poorly to non-specific sites on the macrophages (innate immunity) with reduced clearance. Conversely specific high affinity receptors for IgG and C3b enable antibody and complement-coated bacteria to be bound strongly and destroyed more easily (acquired immunity) [33]. The complement system augments the effect of antibodies because two adjacent IgG molecules can fix many C3b molecules with an increase in links to the macrophages (Figure 4.1).

Opsonization therefore requires the synergism between complement, antibody and phagocytes and defects in any of the tripartite defence mechanism results in susceptibility to encapsulated organisms. On the other hand T-cell deficiency predisposes to viral and fungal infections which are normally eradicated by cell-mediated immunity. Isolated immune defects as illustrated by primary immunodeficiency disorders predispose to defined infective patterns, but secondary immunosuppression generally results in a mixed susceptibility to bacterial, viral and fungal infections.

Susceptibility in Immunodeficiency

In the clinical setting it is more useful to assess the severity of immunodeficiency rather than its cause [34]. Susceptibility to infections in immunodeficiency can be graded into three groups. The low risk group is more susceptible to organisms that will normally infect healthy individuals. Those in the moderate risk group are in addition at risk from normally harmless commensal organisms. This is commonly seen in surgical practice and includes those who are malnourished, receiving steroids or have advanced malignancies. In contrast patients in the high-risk group such as those receiving chemotherapeutic or immunosuppressive drugs may be severely incapacitated by the same organisms and may require prophylactic antibiotics.

It is generally accepted that immunodeficient patients undergoing surgery should receive selective prophylactic antibiotics. Ethical difficulties in denying immunodeficient patients antibiotics probably explain the lack of controlled evidence to support this general view. Post-operative infective complications are increased despite antibiotic prophylaxis in immunodeficiency but neither infection nor mortality are related to the duration of antibiotic use [35].

In addition to infections, immunocompromised patients also have a higher incidence of cancers due to the impaired surveillance and deletion of any abnormally dividing cells. Transplant recipients are susceptible relatively rapidly to non-Hodgkin's lymphoma (NHL) and non-melanoma skin cancer, whereas HIV patients are affected by Kaposi's sarcoma and NHL more gradually as late phenomena [36]. These cancers are associated to various degrees with oncogenic viruses that are capable of incorporating themselves into the host genome, e.g. Epstein-Barr virus in NHL, human herpes virus type 8 in Kaposi's sarcoma and human papilloma viruses in skin cancer. This issue is discussed more extensively in Chapters 6 and 21.

HIV and the Surgeon

The identification of human immunodeficiency virus (HIV) and acquired immunodeficiency syndrome (AIDS) in the early 1980's made a dramatic impact on surgical practice. Surgeons have long dealt with potentially fatal occupational exposures and indeed hepatitis B has caused more deaths amongst health care workers than any other blood-borne disease. However, HIV differs from hepatitis B in that presently there is no effective immunization as well as its inevitable progression to AIDS. Moreover, there is a greater social stigma associated with HIV than hepatitis despite sharing the same risk factors.

Epidemiology

At the end of 1998 the World Health Organization estimated that 33.4 million people were infected with HIV or had AIDS of whom 32.2 million were adults [37]. Two-thirds of HIV infections are found in sub-Saharan Africa followed by South and South East Asia [38]. HIV has two forms: HIV-1, which causes most disease worldwide and HIV-2 which, is confined mostly to West Africa.

In the UK there were an estimated 25000 adults and children living with HIV or AIDS at the end of 1997. Of the 18000 estimated number of AIDS cases that have occurred since the beginning of the epidemic, approximately 72 percent have died [39] with over two-thirds of AIDS cases have been reported from the Thames regions of London [40].

Viral transmission occurs through sexual contact, parenteral or mucosal exposure to infected blood or body fluids, and from mother to baby in utero, perinatally or via breast milk. In North America and Europe the majority of HIV infections have occurred amongst homosexual/bisexual men and intravenous drug abusers, although the proportion of heterosexually acquired infection has been increasing. Clearly the prevalence of surgical patients with HIV or AIDS depends on geography and subspecialty.

Pathology

HIV is a retrovirus belonging to the sub-family of lentiviruses. The 100–120nm virus particle has a fringed envelope containing two structural glycoproteins gp120 and gp41. The core contains single-stranded ribonucleic acid (RNA), two core structural proteins p24 and p18 as well as the enzyme reverse transcriptase. The core proteins are stable but the part of the envelope gp120 protein is antigenically hypervariable; HIV-1 and 2 also have diverse envelope antigens.

The virus infects particularly the CD4 T-helper lymphocytes by binding via gp120 to the high density CD4 receptors. Other targets for HIV infection are macrophages, neural, renal and perhaps epithelial cells. After binding, RNA is introduced into the cell and the enzyme reverse transcriptase uses this as a template to generate double stranded deoxyribonucleic acid (DNA). This DNA becomes incorporated into the host cell DNA (latent phase) and the provirus eventually transcribes to produce more RNA for viral particles (productive phase). The enzyme viral protease is required to cleave the precursor polyproteins producing essential viral structural proteins and enzymes. Mature viral particles bud from the host CD4 T cell thus destroying it to infect other cells.

HIV infection induces a vigorous immune response that partially clears the virus and decreases the level of HIV-1 genome detectable in plasma. However the infection is not completely cleared, as the proportion of latently infected cells is high in relation to productive cells. A dynamic equilibrium is reached where viral clearance is matched by production and the infection may be asymptomatic for many years. However when viral replication exceeds elimination, the CD4 T-cells eventually become depleted.

The resulting immunodeficiency correlates with the loss of CD4 T-cells but there is also dendritic cell destruction and immune dysregulation with persistent complement activation as well as autoantibody formation. Impairments in antibody formation from B-cells, delayed hypersensitivity and macrophages stem from functionally defective T-cells.

IgA-containing jejunal and rectal plasma cells are also depleted in the gut. These factors render the patient susceptible to opportunistic infections, malignancies and the malnutrition that characterizes AIDS.

Natural History

The US Centers for Disease Control (CDC) has classified HIV infection from its acute infective stage through its progression to AIDS (Table 4.1). After exposure there is a brief seroconversion illness with flu-like symptoms and lymphadenopathy similar to other viral infections. A latent asymptomatic period follows during which the CD4 T-cells fall progressively. The normal CD4 (T cell) count is around 600–1500 cells/μL with the range varying between laboratories. In patients with symptomatic advanced HIV disease, counts below 200 cells/μL are typical [41]. If untreated 25–35 per cent of HIV patients will develop AIDS within two years.

Prognostic indicators are important when assessing HIV patients for surgery and these include CD4 count, viral load (plasma concentration of HIV RNA) and the use of anti-retroviral therapy. A low CD4 count correlates with susceptibility

Table 4.1. CDC classification of HIV disease

Group	Description
I	Acute infection
II	Asymptomatic infection
III	Persistent generalized lymphadenopathy
IV	Other disease
Subgroup A	Constitutional disease
Subgroup B	Neurological disease
Subgroup C	Secondary infectious disease
Category C-1	Specified secondary infectious diseases listed in the CDC surveillance definition for AIDS
Category C-2	Other specific secondary infectious diseases
Subgroup D	Secondary cancers, including those within the CDC surveillance definition for AIDS
Subgroup E	Other conditions

to opportunistic infections and death, whereas the viral load acts a measure of ongoing viral replication. Patients with the highest viral loads are at greatest risk of rapid disease progression; reduction in the load correlates with improved clinical outcome.

Anti-retroviral therapy impairs viral replication thus postponing immunodeficiency and its clinical consequences. Treatment generally consists of two nucleoside analogues (which inhibit reverse transcriptase) plus a protease inhibitor (which prevents viral maturation) or a non-nucleoside inhibitor. Such therapy can reduce viral loads to undetectable levels and increase CD4 count even in patients with advanced AIDS. However viral resistance may decrease the effectiveness of present therapy and where possible, the initial regimen should leave scope for changing to alternative effective combinations if needed.

Presentation to the General Surgeon

HIV patients may have any of the diseases found in normal populations and whilst they are managed the same way precautions are taken to prevent cross-infection. However surgeons may be involved in specific HIV-related conditions such as colorectal and anal disorders as well as providing chronic venous access for chemotherapy (especially for CMV retinitis) or occasionally performing diagnostic lymph node biopsy.

Although lifestyle risk factors are important clues, unusual features of a relatively common surgical condition should raise the suspicion of HIV infection [42].

Anorectal Disease

The most frequent reason for referral to the general surgeon is anorectal disease [43] and approximately half will require surgery [44]. In a cohort of 68 AIDS patients [45], we found the most common conditions were perianal and anal warts (37 percent), anal ulceration (25 percent), perianal sepsis (10 percent), neoplasia (13 percent) and hemorrhoidal disease (15 percent).

Wart Disease

Perianal and anal warts are caused by human papillomaviruses (HPV) which are found in up to 50 percent of male homosexual population [46]. The virus incorporates into the human genome and certain subtypes (16 and 18) have been associated with squamous carcinoma transformation that is about 33 times more common in homosexuals than non-homosexuals. They may have evidence of squamous carcinoma-in-situ before progression to invasive cancer. The objective of anal wart treatment is to control local discomfort or leakage and options include excision or ablation therapy (diathermy, laser or podophyllin). High recurrence rates result from failure to treat internal anal canal warts with subsequent autoinoculation.

Ano-rectal Ulceration

Ano-rectal ulceration ranges from "benign" anal fissures to "idiopathic" AIDS-related ulceration of the anal canal. Benign fissures may be similar to those found in the immunocompetent population but they are unlikely to be secondary to sphincter hypertonicity because prior ano-rectal intercourse decreases the resting pressure of the internal anal sphincter [47]. Trauma secondary to intercourse or HIV-associated diarrhea may be predisposing factors. Treatments are similar to those in seronegative patients but with an emphasis on abstinence from ano-rectal intercourse and careful consideration of sphincterotomy in the presence of diarrhea to avoid incontinence.

Causes of AIDS-related ulcers include specific infections, particularly herpes simplex virus (HSV), CMV or HIV itself and malignancies such as squamous cell carcinoma or non-Hodgkin's lymphoma. These are distinguished from benign fissures in that they are broad-based and deeply erosive, often transgressing sphincter planes with variable number, depth and location [48]. They may therefore be debilitating and painful but only 50 percent of cases will yield a specific causal agent on culture and biopsy. Treatment is directed towards eliminating causative factors and half of the rectal ulcers will respond to acyclovir [45]. Ulcer debridement with removal of pus and stool pockets [49] as well as excision biopsy may be effective especially after failed medical treatment [50].

Perianal Sepsis

HIV patients with perianal sepsis may have simple abscesses, submucosal or high complex fistulae although the latter group is less common than originally thought. Anal intercourse may cause mucosal damage that introduces sepsis beneath that layer with subsequent fistula formation. Early drainage, if the CD4 count is above 100 cells/µL, prevents a synergistic, necrotising gangrene that can occur if sepsis is left unchecked [51]. However wound healing is a significant problem when the CD4 count is less than 50 cells/µL [52] and a conservative approach, for example, with the use of a seton, is probably more appropriate.

Anal Neoplasia

The high incidence of anal intraepithelial neoplasia in HIV patients appears to correlate with the degree of immunosuppression [53]. However there has not been the expected epidemic of invasive squamous anal carcinomas in HIV patients, perhaps being explained by a slower rate of progression of in-situ disease over that of HIV itself. A conservative approach to carcinoma-in-situ is therefore preferred with radiotherapy or surgery reserved for symptomatic or progressive cases. For invasive squamous cell carcinomas chemoradiation is recommended although some are unable to tolerate the diarrhea and skin reactions from radiotherapy [54]. Salvage abdomino-perineal excision of the rectum may be needed for treatment failures although a diverting stoma is more preferable in advanced cases.

Rectal lymphoma presents as an enlarging, painful solid rectal mass and may be mistaken for an abscess or hemorrhoids. Treatment consists of chemotherapy with surgery confined to needle biopsy for diagnosis. This avoids breaching the overlying skin with subsequent ulceration.

Kaposi's sarcoma may present as purple perianal or rectal lesions located in the submucosa. They may cause minor bleeding or present as a fistula; they rarely cause a major problem in the anorectum but act as a marker for the existence of more proximal disease.

Hemorrhoidal Disease

The management of hemorrhoids in HIV patients parallels that seen in non-infected patients and retrospective data suggest that HIV status should not alter the basic indications for surgical management [55]. However many hemorrhoidal 'flare-ups' are actually HSV infections which need to be treated accordingly.

Acute Abdomen

AIDS patients commonly experience abdominal pain but only 2–3% will require an emergency laparotomy [56]. Of the 28 patients who underwent such surgery in our unit, 6 showed features of toxic megacolon, 5 had small bowel obstruction, 6 had localized peritonitis and 3 had a perforated viscus with generalized peritonitis [57]. The most common disease processes encountered were acute CMV colitis, intra-abdominal lymphoma, acute appendicitis and *Mycobacterium avium-intracellulare* (MAI) infection.

Infective Colitis

The commonest organism involved in HIV-related colitis is CMV, which results in vasculitis and subsequent thrombosis of the submucosal blood vessels. As the vasculitis progresses bowel perforation and toxic megacolon can supersede. Patients may be known to have CMV retinitis or are undergoing anti-CMV treatment but pre-operative diagnosis of CMV colitis is often difficult. Segmental bowel resection may be possible for localized perforation but a sub-total colectomy is the operation of choice for toxic megacolon. An anastomosis is avoided in both settings as peritonitis in the immunocompromised patient leads to sepsis and multi-organ failure with a high risk of dehiscence. In addition CMV enteritis may extend to involve other areas of bowel remote from the anastomosis and there is less complication with secondary perforations if the bowel is already defunctioned [58].

Non Hodgkin's Lymphoma

The gastrointestinal tract is the most common extranodal site of AIDS-related lymphoma [59] and its presentation is atypical and aggressive. Emergency laparotomy may be required for bleeding, perforation and obstruction but the results are disappointing. Surgery should therefore be avoided if possible unless there is an acute surgical emergency.

Appendicitis

Appendicitis in HIV patients presents in the same way as the population at large and may in fact be more common [60]. However it may be difficult to distinguish from localized CMV enterocolitis or terminal ileitis with MAI superinfection. CMV may be a cause or co-factor in appendicitis in some HIV patients but larger reviews have identified only normal bacterial flora in most cases [60]. The surgical management is similar to non-HIV patients.

Mycobacterium Avium Intracellulare Infection

MAI affects about 5 percent of severely immunocompromised HIV-infected patients [61]. Vague abdominal pain associated with fever and marrow suppression may be due to hepatosplenomegaly and/or intra-abdominal lymphadenopathy. Diagnosis can be made by CT scan and needle aspirate whilst surgery is reserved for patients with a good functional status and localized disease amenable to minimal intervention.

Outcome of Abdominal Surgery

Laparotomy in the HIV patient carries a perioperative mortality rate of 7–38% [57,62–64] with a higher complication rate for emergencies [62,63]. There is also a significant increase in wound breakdown in HIV patients compared with non-infected groups [65], supported by evidence that scars from HIV/AIDS patients are biomechanically weaker [66].

AIDS patients have more complications with chest problems and sepsis than asymptomatic HIV patients [63] which correlates with the lower overall CD4 count [64,67]. Pragmatically, AIDS patients should undergo anti-retroviral therapy to improve the CD4 count before undergoing elective surgery although presently there is no evidence base to support this. In addition patients with active *Pneumocystis carinii* infection should avoid general anesthesia where possible until treated, whilst regional anesthesia (where possible) has the advantage of less immune suppression [68].

The median survival following abdominal surgery ranges from 7 months in those with AIDS to 40 months in asymptomatic HIV-infected patients [63]. Survival could conceivably lengthen with the more extensive use of effective anti-viral therapy. With careful patient selection, surgery may thus achieve worthwhile palliation in AIDS patients [57]. Therefore surgery should not be withheld due to fear of excessive morbidity or mortality but surgeons should maintain an objective approach when assessing these patients.

References

1. Deerojanawong J, Chang AB, Eng PA, Robertson CF, Kemp AS. Pulmonary diseases in children with severe combined immune deficiency and DiGeorge syndrome. Pediatr Pulmonol 1997;24(5):324–30.
2. Navratil JS, Korb LC, Ahearn JM. Systemic lupus erythematosus and complement deficiency: clues to a novel role for the classical complement pathway in the maintenance of immune tolerance. Immunopharmacology 1999;42(1-3):47–52.
3. Powell GM. Response to live attenuated measles vaccine in children with severe kwashiorkor. Ann Trop Paediatr 1982;2(3):143–5.
4. Rikimaru T, Taniguchi K, Yartey JE, Kennedy DO, Nkrumah FK. Humoral and cell-mediated immunity in malnourished children in Ghana. Eur J Clin Nutr 1998;52(5):344–50.
5. Hulsewe KW, van Acker BA, von Meyenfeldt MF, Soeters PB. Nutritional depletion and dietary manipulation: effects on the immune response. World J Surg 1999;23(6):536–44.
6. Chandra RK. Protein-energy malnutrition and immunological responses. J Nutr 1992;122(3 Suppl):597–600.
7. Villa ML, Ferrario E, Bergamasco E, Bozzetti F, Cozzaglio L, Clerici E. Reduced natural killer cell activity and IL-2 production in malnourished cancer patients. Br J Cancer 1991;63(6):1010–4.
8. McWhirter JP, Pennington CR. Incidence and recognition of malnutrition in hospital [see comments]. Bmj 1994;308(6934):945–8.
9. Keele AM, Bray MJ, Emery PW, Duncan HD, Silk DB. Two phase randomised controlled clinical trial of postoperative oral dietary supplements in surgical patients. Gut 1997;40(3):393–9.
10. Braga M, Vignali A, Gianotti L, Cestari A, Profili M, Carlo VD. Immune and nutritional effects of early enteral nutrition after major abdominal operations. Eur J Surg 1996;162(2):105–12.
11. Bozzetti F, Cozzaglio L, Villa ML, Ferrario E, Trabattoni D. Restorative effect of total parenteral nutrition on natural killer cell activity in malnourished cancer patients. Eur J Cancer 1995;31A(12):2023–7.
12. Gianotti L, Braga M, Vignali A, Balzano G, Zerbi A, Bisagni P, et al. Effect of route of delivery and formulation of postoperative nutritional support in patients undergoing major operations for malignant neoplasms. Arch Surg 1997;132(11):1222–9; discussion 1229–30.
13. Beaman M, Oldfield S, MacLennan IC, Michael J, Adu D. Hypogammaglobulinaemia in nephrotic rats is attributable to hypercatabolism of IgG. Clin Exp Immunol 1988;74(3):425–30.
14. Descamps-Latscha B, Chatenoud L. T cells and B cells in chronic renal failure. Semin Nephrol 1996;16(3):183–91.
15. Saffle JR, Wiebke G, Jennings K, Morris SE, Barton RG. Randomized trial of immune-enhancing enteral nutrition in burn patients. J Trauma 1997;42(5):793–800; discussion 800–2.
16. McMahon MM, Farnell MB, Murray MJ. Nutritional support of critically ill patients. Mayo Clin Proc 1993;68(9):911–20.
17. King J, Caplehorn JR, Ross WB, Morris DL. High serum carcinoembryonic antigen concentration in patients with colorectal liver metastases is associated with poor cell-mediated immunity, which is predictive of survival. Br J Surg 1997;84(10):1382–5.
18. Monson JR, Ramsden C, Guillou PJ. Decreased interleukin-2 production in patients with gastro-intestinal cancer. Br J Surg 1986;73(6):483–6.
19. Kopersztych S, Rezkallah MT, Miki SS, Naspitz CK, Mendes NF. Cell-mediated immunity in patients with carcinoma: correlation between clinical stage and immunocompetence. Cancer 1976;38(3):1149–54.
20. Allen-Mersh TG, Glover C, Fordy C, Henderson DC, Davies M. Relation between depression and circulating immune products in patients with advanced colorectal cancer. J R Soc Med 1998;91(8):408–13.
21. Fordy C, Glover C, Henderson DC, Summerbell C, Wharton R, Allen-Mersh TG. Contribution of diet, tumour volume and patient-related factors to weight loss in patients with colorectal liver metastases. Br J Surg 1999;86(5):639–44.
22. Slade MS, Simmons RL, Yunis E, Greenberg LJ. Immunodepression after major surgery in normal patients. Surgery 1975;78(3):363–72.
23. Swerdlow AJ, Douglas AJ, Hudson GV, Hudson BV, Bennett MH, MacLennan KA. Risk of second primary cancers after Hodgkin's disease by type of treatment: analysis of 2846 patients in the British National Lymphoma Investigation. BMJ 1992;304(6835):1137–43.
24. Francke EL, Neu HC. Postsplenectomy infection. Surg Clin North Am 1981;61(1):135–55.
25. Sherman R. Perspectives in management of trauma to the spleen: 1979 presidential address, American Association for the Surgery of Trauma. J Trauma 1980;20(1):1–13.

26. Guidelines for the prevention and treatment of infection in patients with an absent or dysfunctional spleen. Working Party of the British Committee for Standards in Haematology Clinical Haematology Task Force [see comments]. BMJ 1996;312(7028):430–4.

27. Quintiliani L, Pescini A, Di Girolamo M, Iudicone P, Martini F, Guglielmetti M, et al. Relationship of blood transfusion, post-operative infections and immunoreactivity in patients undergoing surgery for gastrointestinal cancer. Haematologica 1997;82(3):318–23.

28. Chavers BM, Sullivan EK, Tejani A, Harmon WE. Pre-transplant blood transfusion and renal allograft outcome: a report of the North American Pediatric Renal Transplant Cooperative Study. Pediatr Transplant 1997;1(1):22–8.

29. Stephenson KR, Steinberg SM, Hughes KS, Vetto JT, Sugarbaker PH, Chang AE. Perioperative blood transfusions are associated with decreased time to recurrence and decreased survival after resection of colorectal liver metastases. Ann Surg 1988;208(6):679–87.

30. Beynon J, Davies PW, Billings PJ, Channer JL, Protheroe D, Umpleby HC, et al. Perioperative blood transfusion increases the risk of recurrence in colorectal cancer. Dis Colon Rectum 1989;32(11):975–9.

31. Parrott NR, Lennard TW, Taylor RM, Proud G, Shenton BK, Johnston ID. Effect of perioperative blood transfusion on recurrence of colorectal cancer. Br J Surg 1986;73(12):970–3.

32. Weiden PL, Bean MA, Schultz P. Perioperative blood transfusion does not increase the risk of colorectal cancer recurrence. Cancer 1987;60(4):870–4.

33. Roitt I. Roitt's essential immunology. 9th ed. Oxford: Blackwell; 1997.

34. Primrose J, Giles G. Surgical immunology and organ transplantation. In: Cuschieri A, Giles G, Moossa A, editors. Essential Surgical Practice. 3rd ed. Oxford: Butterworth-Heinemann; 1995. p. 132–4.

35. Moesgaard F, Lykkegaard-Nielsen M. Preoperative cell-mediated immunity and duration of antibiotic prophylaxis in relation to postopertive infectious complications. A controlled trial in biliary, gastroduodenal and colorectal surgery. Acta Chir Scand 1989;155(4–5):281–6.

36. Mueller N. Overview of the epidemiology of malignancy in immune deficiency. J Acquir Immune Defic Syndr 1999;21 Suppl 1:S5–10.

37. WHO. Global AIDS surveillance–Part I. Wkly Epidemiol Rec 1998;73(48):373–6.

38. Burton AH, Mertens TE. Provisional country estimates of prevalent adult human immunodeficiency virus infections as of end 1994: a description of the methods. Int J Epidemiol 1998;27(1):101–7.

39. UNAIDS/WHO. Epidemiological fact sheet on HIVS/AIDS and sexually transmitted diseases. UK. 1998:1–12.

40. Anon. AIDS and HIV infection in the United Kingdom: monthly report. Communicable Disease Report. CDR Weekly 1998;8(9):83.

41. Anon. Major advances in the treatment of HIV-1 infection. DTB 1997;35:25–9.

42. Truskett PG. HIV infection in surgical practice. Med J Aust 1993;158(4):264–5.

43. Miles AJ, Mellor CH, Gazzard B, Allen-Mersh TG, Wastell C. Surgical management of anorectal disease in HIV-positive homosexuals. Br J Surg 1990;77(8):869–71.

44. Wexner SD, Smithy WB, Milsom JW, Dailey TH. The surgical management of anorectal diseases in AIDS and pre-AIDS patients. Dis Colon Rectum 1986;29(11):719–23.

45. Allen-Mersh T. Anorectal problems in AIDS patients. In: Cochrane J, Wastell C, editors. The impact of HIV on surgical practice. London: The Royal College of Surgeons of England; 1992. p. 48–50.

46. Sohn N, Robilotti JG, Jr. The gay bowel syndrome. A review of colonic and rectal conditions in 200 male homosexuals. Am J Gastroenterol 1977;67(5):478–84.

47. Miles AJ, Allen-Mersh TG, Wastell C. Effect of anoreceptive intercourse on anorectal function. J R Soc Med 1993;86(3):144–7.

48. Schmitt SL, Wexner SD, Nogueras JJ, Jagelman DG. Is aggressive management of perianal ulcers in homosexual HIV- seropositive men justified? Dis Colon Rectum 1993;36(3):240–6.

49. Viamonte M, Dailey TH, Gottesman L. Ulcerative disease of the anorectum in the HIV+ patient [published erratum appears in Dis Colon Rectum 1993 Nov;36(11):990]. Dis Colon Rectum 1993;36(9):801–5.

50. Miles AJ, Connolly GM, Barton SE, Allen-Mersh TG, Hawkins DA, Gazzard BG, et al. Persistent ulceration of the anal margin in homosexuals with HIV infection. J R Soc Med 1991;84(2):87–8.

51. Consten EC, Slors JF, Danner SA, Offerhaus GJ, Bartelsman JF, Van Lanschot JJ. Local excision and mucosal advancement for anorectal ulceration in patients infected with human immunodeficiency virus. Br J Surg 1995;82(7):891–4.

52. Lord RV. Anorectal surgery in patients infected with human immunodeficiency virus: factors associated with delayed wound healing. Ann Surg 1997;226(1):92–9.

53. Metcalf AM, Dean T. Risk of dysplasia in anal condyloma. Surgery 1995;118(4):724-6.
54. Chadha M, Rosenblatt EA, Malamud S, Pisch J, Berson A. Squamous-cell carcinoma of the anus in HIV-positive patients. Dis Colon Rectum 1994;37(9):861-5.
55. Hewitt WR, Sokol TP, Fleshner PR. Should HIV status alter indications for hemorrhoidectomy? Dis Colon Rectum 1996;39(6):615-8.
56. Ferguson CM. Surgical complications of human immunodeficiency virus infection. Am Surg 1988;54(1):4-9.
57. Davidson T, Allen-Mersh TG, Miles AJ, Gazzard B, Wastell C, Vipond M, et al. Emergency laparotomy in patients with AIDS [see comments]. Br J Surg 1991;78(8):924-6.
58. Lowy AM, Barie PS. Laparotomy in patients infected with human immunodeficiency virus: indications and outcome [see comments]. Br J Surg 1994;81(7):942-5.
59. Raphael BG, Knowles DM. Acquired immunodeficiency syndrome-associated non-Hodgkin's lymphoma. Semin Oncol 1990;17(3):361-6.
60. Flum DR, Steinberg SD, Sarkis AY, Wallack MK. Appendicitis in patients with acquired immunodeficiency syndrome. J Am Coll Surg 1997;184(5):481-6.
61. Dryden MS, Shanson DC. The microbial causes of diarrhoea in patients infected with the human immunodeficiency virus. J Infect 1988;17(2):107-14.
62. Deziel DJ, Hyser MJ, Doolas A, Bines SD, Blaauw BB, Kessler HA. Major abdominal operations in acquired immunodeficiency syndrome. Am Surg 1990;56(7):445-50.
63. Yii MK, Saunder A, Scott DF. Abdominal surgery in HIV/AIDS patients: indications, operative management, pathology and outcome. Aust N Z J Surg 1995;65(5):320-6.
64. Albaran RG, Webber J, Steffes CP. CD4 cell counts as a prognostic factor of major abdominal surgery in patients infected with the human immunodeficiency virus. Arch Surg 1998;133(6):626-31.
65. Davis PA, Corless DJ, Gazzard BG, Wastell C. Increased risk of wound complications and poor healing following laparotomy in HIV-seropositive and AIDS patients. Dig Surg 1999;16(1):60-7.
66. Davis P, Corless D, Appleton S, Wastell C. Weakness of healed wounds in patients with HIV and AIDS. Br J Surg 1999;86 (Suppl 1):28-9.
67. Emparan C, Iturburu IM, Ortiz J, Mendez JJ. Infective complications after abdominal surgery in patients infected with human immunodeficiency virus: role of CD4+ lymphocytes in prognosis. World J Surg 1998;22(8):778-82.
68. Balabaud-Pichon V, Steib A. [Anesthesia in the HIV positive or AIDS patient]. Ann Fr Anesth Reanim 1999;18(5):509-29.

Commentary on Section I

Andrew P. Zbar

The aims of the first section of this book are to lay down general principles of immunology and to define broad immunologic responses in surgery, stress and sepsis as well as the surgeon's interaction with the immunosuppressed patient.

In Chapter 1, Plunkett and colleagues make the assumption that the reader is conversant with the basic ontology of the immune system. In their treatise, they allude to the theoretical paradigm of immunology as proposed by Matzinger and Fuchs. [1] What is unique about this view is its change of the overall concept of the origins of inherent danger to the organism and the purpose of immunologic defence. Broadly, the original ideas as outlined by Burnet in the middle of the 20th century revolved around the suggestion that the host's immune response was principally towards exogenous, "non-self" stimuli [2] and the implications of this view which was the backbone of immunology as taught to all medical students, were that immunocytes functioned as specialized surveillance cells for non-self haptens and immunogens and that the T cell repertoire in particular was developed against foreign antigens very early in development. This view cannot be sustained in the current era of transgenic immunology, with knowledge regarding immunoglobulin switching in the periphery of mature B cells, the new understanding of T cell receptor co-stimulation to newly exposed foreign peptides and the poor clinical responses towards tumors which express tumor-associated antigens.

What Matzinger proposed was a change in this self/non-self paradigm where the immune system will only respond to dangerous signals (essentially derived from dying or damaged cells not undergoing programmed cell death) and potentially linked to genetic polymorphisms. These signals must effectively be carried to immunocompetent lymphocytes by activated dendritic (and other) antigen-presenting cells, which incorporate the second-signal models for T cell stimulation already shown by Bretscher and Cohn [3] and Janeway [4]. In this way, any immunologic "theory of everything" has to account for the observed facts of immunology and the Matzinger theory goes some considerable way to explaining why there is limited maternal/foetal immunologic interaction, why circulating auto-antibodies after apoptotic or infarctive cell death can be short-lived and relatively harmless, why spontaneous tumor regression occurs (particularly during acute systemic infection or following partial extirpative surgery) and why there is a necessity for repeated vaccination strategies with the use of adjuvants in anti-tumor immunotherapies [5]. The theory is, however, just that and there is little at present to explain the on/off switch between tolerance and auto-activation, why circulating auto-antibodies are not more destructive and the mechanisms involved in B cell sequence variation following their activation [6]. Moreover, it accounts for normal thymic apoptosis, B cell apoptosis within germinal centers, "natural" cell death during breast/uterine and ovarian involution and the immunologic responses towards hematopoietic and gastrointestinal cell turnover. These non-dangerous events all represent constitutive signals for cells that are dying physiologically. The system permits immune responsiveness without receptor specificity or self/non-self discrimination, but it does not fully explain the persistent need for immunosuppression following allografts or the nature of immunoprivelege in sites such as the CNS or the eye.

The ontogeny of the immune system is further covered in Chapter 9. In theory, it should have some basic evolutionary advantage, although it is unclear why endogenous and exogenous foreign antigens should be initially processed differentially as peptide epitopes combined with MHC molecules for cell surface expression. This is of considerable importance since the aberrant presentation and processing of antigen is a significant mechanism whereby many solid tumors escape immunologic detection and elimination.

References

1. Fuchs EJ, Matzinger P. Is cancer dangerous to the immune system? Seminars Immunol 1996;8:271–80
2. Burnet FM. The concept of immunologic surveillance. Prog Exp Tumor Res 1970;13:1–27
3. Bretscher P, Cohn M. A theory of self-nonself discrimination: paralysis and induction involve the recognition of one and two determinants on an antigen, respectively. Science 1970;169:1042–9
4. Janeway CA Jr. The immune system evolved to discriminate infectious nonself from noninfectious self. Immunol Today 1992;13:11–6
5. Matzinger P. Tolerance, danger and the extended family. Ann Rev Immunol 1994;12:991–1045
6. Lafferty KJ, Cunningham AJ. A new analysis of allogeneic interactions. Aust J Exp Biol Med Sci 1975;53:27–42

In Chapter 2 Demetriades and colleagues discuss the subcellular and immunological responses to shock, ischaemia and reperfusion. Many of these studies have been conducted in animal models. It is uncertain whether much of this work actively translates into clinical studies, particularly since strain differences have been shown in resistance to standardized ischaemia [1]. For example, reactive oxygen species are implicated in the pathogenesis of many surgical disorders such as adult respiratory distress syndrome (ARDS), atherosclerosis and cancer and genetically-engineered animal models as well as syngeneic strains which eliminate genetic polymorphism have recently been used as tools for understanding the functional aspects of antioxidant enzymes in cellular defences against different forms of oxidant injury [2]. Transgenic rodents, which overexpress different isoforms of superoxide dismutase (SOD), catalase and glutathione peroxidase, appear to show increased tolerance to standardized ischaemia-reperfusion in myocardial, CNS and drug-induced toxicity. The reverse results have been noted in knockout models for these enzymes and similar experiments have been found with knockout transgenics specific for the different forms of NO synthase (neuronal nNOS; endothelial eNOS or inducible iNOS) in experimental head injury. eNOS is critically involved in maintaining cerebral blood flow and reducing infarct size, whereas both iNOS and nNOS play key roles in local neurodegeneration; showing an important bias in ischaemia-reperfusion response with genetic variation [3].

The immunology of CNS trauma in particular is still poorly understood. Recent experimental models of neurotrauma have shown that adoptive transfer of reactive T cells or active immunization with myelin basic protein promotes recovery from spinal cord injury, where there is already impaired lymphocyte and early hematopoietic progenitor cell activity [4,5]. The authors refer to the effects of lazaroids (in particular tirilazad mesylate) which are inhibitors of lipid membrane peroxidation and which have been shown to be beneficial in spinal cord trauma [6] The action of these agents is complex increasing membrane stability, scavenging lipid peroxyl radicals and reducing lipid peroxidation-induced arachidonic acid release. They localize in the cerebrovascular endothelium acting primarily on the blood-brain barrier and attenuating subarachnoid hemorrhage injury and ischaemia-induced blood-brain barrier permeability. Phase III trials of these agents in spinal cord and head injury, ischaemic stroke and spontaneous subarachnoid hemorrhage are underway in Europe and Australasia [7].

In the immune reaction to trauma (including deliberate surgical trauma), one of the recent areas of excitement has been in the attenuated immunosuppression which appears to occur after minimally invasive surgery when compared with conventional open surgery. These studies have shown variations in T cell proliferation in vitro to standard mitogens and expression of cell surface monocyte receptor molecules (HLA-DR, CD80 and L-Selectin). These effects have been noted in patients undergoing cholecystectomy (laparoscopy vs. open), [8] Nissen fundoplication [9] and colorectal resection for cancer [10] These findings have been accompanied by reductions in the traditional IL-6 rise seen following open surgery, conversion of peripheral lymphocyte cytokine profiles from a Th1 to a relatively suppressed Th2 pattern [11] and variations in the number of detectable CD3 and CD4:CD8 ratios, NK subsets, intra-peritoneal macrophages and B cells in the peripheral blood of laparoscopic compared with open cases [12–14].

The relevance of such immunosuppression following conventional surgery lies in many recent clinical case reports as well as many experimental studies which have suggested that laparoscopic cancer surgery is associated with an increased risk of tumor spread to abdominal wall wounds (port-site metastases). There seems little evidence that this is caused by mechanical wound contamination, but rather disturbance of peritoneal anti-tumor immunity perhaps compounded by the effects of CO_2 pneumo-peritoneum [15,16].

The other area of importance to the immunity of the post-surgical patient with cancer is the use of peri-operative allogeneic blood and blood product transfusion. There is considerable debate concerning the effect of peri-operative blood transfusion on cancer-specific outcome particularly in colorectal cancer, with some papers suggesting that the presence of post-operative infection in combination with blood transfusion is deleterious [17]. This effect has been confirmed for patients with a range of other solid cancers including gastric cancer, (with less of an effect for packed red blood cells), breast cancer and esophageal carcinoma, although not in hepatocellular carcinoma [18–21].

The final view on blood transfusions and their effect on cancer outcome is not fixed as yet. At present active policies regarding leukocyte depletion of perioperative transfused blood don't seem to exert an effect and differences in survival rather than locoregional cancer recurrence may be due to a complicated post-operative course rather than the effects of immunosuppression induced by allogeneic cell exposure [22]. The issue is not obviated by the use of autologous blood transfusion in patients with malignancy.

References

1. Baker JE, Konorev EA, Gross GJ, Chilian WM, Jacob HJ. Resistance to myocardial ischaemia in five rat strains: is there a genetic component of cardioprotection? Am J Physiol Heart Circ Physiol 2000;278:H1395–400
2. Ho YS, Magnent JL, Gargano M, Cao J. The nature of antioxidant defense mechanisms: a lesson from transgenic studies. Environ Health Perspect 1998;106 Suppl 5:1219–28
3. Samdani AF, Dawson TM, Dawson VL. Nitric oxide synthase in models of focal iscahemia. Stroke 1997;28:1283–8
4. Hauben E, Butovsky O, Nevo U, Yoles E, Moalem G, Agranov E, et al. Passive or active immunization with myelin basic protein promotes recovery from spinal cord contusion. J Neurosci 2000;1:6421–30
5. Iversen PO, Hjeltnes N, Holm B, Flatebo T, Strom-Gundersen I, Ronning W, et al. Depressed immunity and impaired proliferation of hematopoietic progenitor cells in patients with complete spinal cord injury. Blood 2000;96:2081–3
6. Clark WM, Hazel JS, Coull BM. Lazaroids. CNS pharmacology and current research. Drugs 1995;50:971–83
7. Taylor BM, Fleming WE, Benjamin CW, Wu Y, Mathews WR, Sun FF. The mechanism of cytoprotective action of lazaroids 1:Inhibition of reactive oxygen species formation and lethal cell injury during periods of energy depletion. J Pharmacol Exp Ther 1996;276:1224–31
8. Brune IB, Wilke W, Hensler T, Feussner H, Holzmann B, Siewert JR. Normal T lymphocyte and monocyte function after minimally invasive surgery. Surg Endosc 1998;12:1020–4
9. Pertilla J, Salo M, Ovaska J, Gronroos J, Lavonius M, Katila A, et al. Immune response after laparoscopic and conventional Nissen fundoplication. Eur J Surg 1999;165:21–8
10. Schwenk W, Jacobi C, Mansmann U, Bohm B, Muller JM. Inflammatory response after laparoscopic and conventional colorectal resections — results of a prospective randomized trial. Langenbecks Arch Surg 2000;385:2–9
11. Brune IB, Wilke W, Hensler T, Holzmann B, Siewert JR. Downregulation of T helper type 1 immune response and altered pre-inflammatory and anti-inflammatory T cell cytokine balance following conventional but not laparoscopic surgery. Am J Surg 1999;177:55–60
12. Berguer R, Bravo N, Bowyer M, Ferrick D. Measurement of intracellular gamma-interferon, interleukin-4 and interleukin-10 levels in patients following laparoscopic cholecystectomy. J Invest Surg 2000;13:161–7
13. Walker CB, Bruce DM, Heys SD, Gough DB, Binnie NR, Eremin O. Minimal modulation of lymphocyte and natural killer cell subsets following minimal access surgery. Am J Surg 1999;177:48–54
14. Jackson PG, Evans SR. Intraperitoneal macrophages and tumor immunity: a review. J Surg Oncol 2000;75:146–54
15. Neuhaus SJ, Watson DI, Ellis T, Rofe AM, Jamieson GG. The effect of immune enhancement and suppression on the development of laparoscopic port site metastases. Surg Endosc 2000;14:439–43
16. Neuhaus SJ, Watson DI, Ellis T, Rofe AM, Mathew G, Jamieson GG. Influence of gases on intraperitoneal immunity during laparoscopy in tumor-bearing rats. World J Surg 2000;24:1227–31
17. Mynster T, Christensen IJ, Moesgaard F, Nielsen HJ. Effects of combination of blood transfusion and postoperative infectious complications on prognosis after surgery for colorectal cancer: Danish RANX05 Colorectal Cancer Study Group. Br J Surg 2000;87:1553–62
18. Dhar DK, Kubota H, Tachibana M, Kotoh T, Kinugasa S, Shibakita M, Kohno H, Nagasue N. A tailored perioperative blood transfusion might avoid undue recurrences in gastric carcinoma patients. Dig Dis Sci 2000;45:1737–42.
19. Pysz M. Blood transfusions in breast cancer patients undergoing mastectomy: possible importance of timing. J Surg Oncol 2000;75:258–63
20. Dresner SM, Lamb PJ, Shenfine J, Hayes N, Griffin SM. Prognostic significance of peri-operative blood transfusion following radical resection for oesophageal carcinoma. Eur J Surg Oncol 2000;26:492–7
21. Kwon AH, Matsui Y, Kamiyama Y. Perioperative blood transfusion in hepatocellular carcinomas: influence of immunologic profile and recurrence free survival. Cancer 2001;91:771–8

22. Van de Watering LM, Brand A, Houbiers JG, Klein Kranenbarg WM, Hermans J, van de Velde C, Cancer Recurrence and Blood Transfusion Study Group. Perioperative blood transfusions, with or without allogeneic leucocytes, relate to survival, not to cancer recurrence. Br J Surg 2001;88:267–72

In Chapter 3, Parker and Windsor outline the importance of the cytokine cascade and attempts to attenuate it in human sepsis, septic models and in the systemic inflammatory response syndrome (SIRS). Anti-endotoxin strategies are fully discussed in the chapter. Endotoxin is a potent stimulator of the inflammatory response and probably initiates most Gram-negative sepsis. A range of anti-endotoxins have been tried in clinical studies including anti-LPS antibodies, LPS-binding proteins and lipoproteins, polymyxin B conjugates, lipid A analogues and extracorporeal techniques for endotoxin removal [1]. The latest phase II trials utilizing the monoclonal IgM anti-endotoxin antibody E5 in life-threatening Gram-negative sepsis have proved disappointing although there is some improvement in mortality for those patients treated with E5 who initially present with shock and who display anti-endotoxin antibodies directed against lipid A and lipid X [2,3].

These confirm the doubtful effects of earlier studies assessing the role of HA-1A (a human IgM monoclonal antibody raised against the *E. coli* J5 (Rc) endotoxin) or recombinant bactericidal/permeability increasing protein. The latter has been shown to impair LPS-mediated TNF production in human blood in vitro and to protect against an LD60 dose of endotoxin in mice, although human studies are awaited [4]. Newer approaches specifically designed to attenuate endotoxin will include endotoxin analogues, new antibodies directed against novel endotoxin epitopes, subunit vaccines, binding columns and recombinant human proteins and small molecule inhibitors of endotoxin synthesis and intracellular signaling.

The immunologic concepts of sepsis and SIRS are changing. Whether or not the monitoring of septic patients with pro-inflammatory blood markers (TNF, IL-1, IL-6, IL-8 and C-reactive protein), markers of invasive infection (procalcitonin), inherent immunosuppressive functions (TGF-β1L-10 and PGE2) or monocytic function and phenotype (HLA DR, CD14 levels or ex vivo TNF secretion capacity) will be clinically important in the future is at present unknown [5]. Recent work has shown that the glycosyl-phosphatidylinositol-linked glycoprotein CD14 is expressed as a pattern recognition receptor on myeloid cells, binding to gram-negative and gram-positive bacterial cell walls affecting the signaling of Toll-like receptors and the NF-κB kinase, implying a central role in responses to microbial pathogens. This has been coupled to work showing that CD14 antisense oligonucleotide therapy prevents lethal LPS-induced shock in animals and that CD14 expression by monocytes in humans is impaired in severe sepsis, suggesting a potential new modality of therapy [6]. The poor results also alluded to by Parker and Windsor regarding therapy with platelet activating factor and bradykinin antagonists, IL-1r therapy, monoclonal anti-TNF antibodies and soluble dimeric TNF receptor fusion proteins, means that new strategies against sepsis must be developed.

As mentioned in the last part of the chapter, genetic polymorphisms will affect the overall immunological response against microbial invasion. These may be represented in heat shock protein variations or altered expression of MHC class II molecules in response to LPS exposure [7]. Given that it is estimated that more than 50,000 people die each year in the United States from septic shock or

SIRS-related illnesses [8] our future understanding of individual genetic variation in cytokine production and release, NO synthase expression and coagulation factor polymorphism will provide relevant information to identify which patients are more or less likely to develop potentially fatal sepsis or multi-organ dysfunction. Moreover, it may assist in defining those capable of responding to anti-mediator strategies [9].

References

1. Hellman J, Warren HS. Antiendotoxin strategies. Infect Dis Clin Nth Am 1999;13:371–86.
2. Angus DC, Birmingham MC, Balk RA, Scannon PJ, Collins D, Kruse JA, et al. E5 murine monoclonal antiendotoxin antibody in gram-negative sepsis: a randomized controlled trial. E5 Study Investigators. JAMA 2000;282:1723–30.
3. Pape HC, Remmers D, Grotz M, Schedel I, von Glinski S, Oberbeck R, er al. Levels of antibodies to endotoxin and cytokine release in patients with severe trauma: does posttraumatic dysergy contribute to organ failure? J Trauma 1999;46:907–13.
4. Marra MN, Thornton MB, Snable JL, Wilde CG, Scott RW. Endotoxin-binding and neutralizing properties of recombinant bactericidal/permeability-increasing protein and monoclonal antibodies HA-1A and E5. Crit Care Med 1994;22:559–65.
5. Volk HD, Reinke P, Docke WD. Immunological monitoring of the inflammatory process: which variables? When to assess? Eur J Surg Suppl 1999;584:70–2.
6. Furusako S, Takahashi T, Mori S, Takahashi Y, Tsuda T, Namba M, et al. Protection of mice from LPS-induced shock by CD14 antisense oligonucelotide. Acta Med Okayama 2001;55:105–15.
7. Piani A, Hossle JP, Birchler T, Siegrist CA, Heumann D, Davies G, et al. Expression of MHC class II molecules contributes to lipoplysaccharide responsiveness. Eur J Immunol 2000;30:3140–6.
8. Tobias PS, Lee H, Orr S, Soldau K, Tapping R. Innate immune system recognition of microbial pathogens. Immunol Res 2000;21(2–3):341–3.
9. Stuber F. Effects of genetic polymorphisms on the course of sepsis: is there a concept for gene therapy? J Am Soc Nephrol 2001;12 Suppl 17:S60–4.

In Chapter 4, Allen-Mersh and Huang discuss the role the surgeon plays in the immunosuppressed patient. These days this may involve vascular access surgery or occasionally the treatment of such patients with complicated lymphoproliferative disease or Kaposi's sarcoma which presents as a surgical emergency. In the 1980's there was a vogue for lymph node biopsy in patients with HIV disease. The commonest histologic finding is follicular hyperplasia in patients with AIDS-related complex (ARC) or persistent generalized lymphadenopathy, although other features, most notably epithelioid histiocyte accumulation, follicle mantle zone effacement, burnt-out follicles and plasmacytosis are often seen.

Although these biopsies can be performed without significant morbidity, their value is doubtful with secondary infections and neoplastic disease being identified in only 10% of cases. Moreover, this avoids the small potential risk (between 1 per 200,000 to 1 per 2,000,000) to the surgeon [1]. Formal lymph node biopsy is still indicated in patients with unexplained generalized symptoms, atypical enlargement of lymph nodes or the exclusion of concomitant disease in patients with previously defined infectious or neoplastic processes [2–4]. Many of these biopsies have been supplanted by fine needle aspiration (FNA) where B cells fail to show light chain restriction in follicular hyperplasia [5] and where in-situ hybridization on frozen section specimens or microfragments will detect viral RNA with considerable accuracy or can be used for the detection of gag DNA by polymerase chain reaction (PCR). Lymph node aspiration may also be used to follow response to therapy. There is evidence that undetectable plasma viraemia using ultrasensitive PCR technology does not always reflect complete HIV suppression within lymph nodes since it appears that protease inhibitors target HIV reservoirs in lymphoid tissue better than nucleoside analogues [6]. There is further evidence that Gallium-67 scanning may avoid lymph node biopsy or FNA in some patients with follicular hyperplasia [7].

General surgeons may encounter these patients in their practice presenting with complicated CMV infections of the intestinal tract, appendicitis, spontaneous bacterial peritonitis, cholecystitis, obstructive jaundice or with protean manifestations of coincident Tuberculosis [8,9]. There may also be a place for increased laparoscopy in these patients with less attendant disturbed post-operative immunity.

References

1. Goldberg D, Johnston J, Cameron S, Fletcher C, Stewart M, McMenamin J, et al. Risk of HIV transmission from patients to surgeons in the era of post-exposure prophylaxis. J Hosp Infect 2000;44:99–105.
2. Wong R, Rappaport W, Gorman S, Darragh M, Hunter G, Witzke D. Value of lymph node biopsy in the treatment of patients with the human immunodeficiency virus. Am J Surg 1991;162:590–2.
3. Gerstoft J, Pallesen G, Mathiesen LR, Pedersen C, Gaub J, Lindhardt BO. The value of lymph node histology in human immunodeficiency virus related persistent generalized lymphadenopathy. APMIS Suppl 1989;8:24–7.
4. Burton F, Patete ML, Goodwin WJ Jr. Indications for open cervical node biopsy in HIV-positive patients. Otolaryngol Head Neck Surg 1992;107:367–9.
5. Oertel J, Oertel B, Lobeck H, Huhn D. Immunocytochemical analysis of lymph node aspirates in patients with human immunodeficiency virus infection. J Clin Pathol 1990;43:844–6; J Aquir Immune Defic Syndr Hum Retrovirol 1995;10 Suppl 2:S57–S61.
6. Ruiz L, van Lunzen J, Arno A, Stellbrink HJ, Schneider C, Rull M, et al. Protease inhibitor-containing regimens compared with nucleoside analogues in the suppression of persistent HIV-1 replication in lymphoid tissue. AIDS 1999;13:F1–8.
7. Podzamczer D, Ricart I, Bolao F, Romagosa V, Bonnin D, Guionnet N, et al. Gallium-67 scan for distinguishing follicular hyperplasia from other AIDS-associated diseases in lymph nodes. AIDS 1990;4:683–5.
8. Mueller GP, Williams RA. Surgical infections in AIDS patients. Am J Surg 1995;169 (5A Suppl):34S–38S.
9. Hudson CP, Wood R, Maartens G. Diagnosing HIV-associated tuberculosis: reducing costs and diagnostic delay. Int J Tuberc Lung Dis 2000;4:240–5.

SECTION II

TRANSPLANT IMMUNOLOGY

5. Allorecognition and Tissue Typing in Organ Transplantation

Paul E. Morrissey, Reginald Y. Gohh and Anthony P. Monaco

Chapters 5 through 8 should be read together. Although some areas are covered by different authors, the chapters have been designated separately for the assessment of factors involved in allorecognition and tissue matching (Chapter 5), immuno-suppressant pharmacology (Chapter 6), clinical transplantation and strategies to deal with patterns of rejection (Chapter 7) and immunologic aspects specific for xenotransplantation (Chapter 8).

Introduction

The beginning of solid-organ transplantation can be traced back to the technical achievement of Alexis Carrel. In 1902, he described the techniques of vascular anastomosis, thus ushering in accounts of autograft and homograft transplantation. Although a number of animal-to-human kidney transplants were reported in the ensuing three decades, a human donor organ was not used until 1933, by the Russian surgeon Voronoy. This and other attempts at using human kidneys for transplantation failed owing to acute tubular necrosis and rejection.

The history of transplantation unfolds over the 20th century, beginning with futile attempts at experimental allotransplantation and human xenotransplantation at the turn of the century. The next 50 years were fraught with failure. During this period, the recognition of self in the context of histocompatibility antigens [1] and the central role of the lymphocyte [2] in allorecognition were discovered. Allograft rejection, particularly of allogeneic skin, mediated by a cellular response, (lymphocytes) was a sentinel observation arising from controlled experiments in a rabbit model and histologic studies in the Royal Air Force burn clinics during World War II [3]. These two discoveries represent the beginnings of transplantation immunology and both were the basis later for the awarding of the Nobel Prize in Physiology and Medicine (Table 5.1). Midway through the 20th century, the transplant community was invigorated with new enthusiasm by two important discoveries. The first was the creation of acquired neonatal tolerance in mice by Peter Medawar and colleagues. The second was the first successful renal transplant, performed between identical twins at the Peter Bent Brigham Hospital

Table 5.1. Nobel Prize awards in physiology or medicine relevant to transplantation

1908	Paul Erlich	Antibody secretion and phagocytosis as cellular defenses
	Elie Metchnikoff	
1912	Alexis Carrel	Suturing of vessels and transplantation of organs termed "the boldest and most difficult of operations"
1960	Sir Peter Medawar	Immunologic basis of failed transplants
	Sir Frank Macfarlane Burnet	Concept of self and non-self, clonal deletion
1980	Baruj Benaceraf	HLA and histocompatibility
	Jean Dausset	Genetic control of immune responses (HLA)
	George D. Snell	Resistance to transplanted tumors genetically determined
1988	George Hitchings	Important principles in drug therapy (azathioprine)
	Gertrude Elion	
1990	Joseph E. Murray	Successful kidney transplantation in man
	E. Donnall Thomas	Bone marrow transplantation
1996	Robert Zinkernagel	Discovery of how immune system recognizes virus-infected cells (T-cell receptor)
	Paul Doherty	

in Boston on December 23, 1954, and was performed by the team of Moore, Murray, Merrill and Harrison.

These events took place in an era where multiple, previous attempts at renal transplantation had produced few short-term (weeks to months) survivals, but no long-term survivors. End-stage renal disease meant certain death. Perhaps the greatest achievement in transplantation medicine, however, was the first successful organ transplant accomplished under immunosuppression six years following the twin transplant [4]. Present strategies in all solid organ transplantation involve the use of potent immunosuppressive agents, the mechanisms of which are intricately understood. The development of these agents, (azathioprine, prednisone, cyclosporine, mycophenolate mofetil, tacrolimus and sirolimus, to date), in addition to advances in immunologic understanding, have contributed to the high success rates in kidney, liver, heart, pancreas and lung transplantation.

Advances in transplantation immunology have played a significant role in prolonging allograft survival, leading to the development of novel immunosuppressive agents (including antilymphocyte antibodies) and to our understanding of allograft rejection and the means by which our pharmacological interventions thwart the process. Furthermore, newer advances in immunotherapy offer hope for an era where donor-specific unresponsiveness or tolerance to solid organ transplants may become a reality. The New York Academy of Sciences sponsored the first international transplant conference in 1954. The meeting was titled "The Relation of Immunology to Tissue Homotransplantation" [5]. In this chapter, the role of immunology in transplant allorecognition, in acute and chronic rejection and in clinical applications over the past 45 years is discussed. Particular attention is given to key concepts that have been successfully applied to the current practice of transplant medicine, with lesser emphasis on the theoretical constructs that serve as the basis for continued research and progress toward tolerance. Achieving this goal will represent the ultimate application of transplantation immunology in clinical solid organ transplantation.

Major Histocompatibility Complex

First defined by Snell and Benaceraf in the mouse, it is now clear that specific genes encode for cell surface proteins that are unique to each individual. These self-determining antigens are expressed on all nucleated cells and collectively contribute to the recognition of allografted material as foreign and initiate rejection. While transplantation of foreign tissues represents a 20th century phenomenon, the ability to recognize foreign proteins is of profound biologic importance, primarily in the fight against infectious diseases and tumor antigens.

The principle immunologic function of the major histocompatibility complex (MHC) is the production of proteins that present foreign peptide fragments (antigen) to T lymphocytes. The foreign antigenic fragments derived from processing of viral, tumor, or allogeneic cells become attached to MHC molecules and are then recognized by T cells as "non-self". This recognition initiates an immunologic cascade intent on destruction of "foreign" tissue with preservation of the host. While immunoglobulin B-cell receptors recognize parts of whole antigens (epitopes), the T-cell receptor complex (TCR) recognizes processed fragments of peptide antigens, often only 11–20 amino acids in length, presented in the context of the MHC [6]. (See Chapters 1 and 9)

The T-cell receptor complex specifically recognizes non-self proteins expressed on the membrane-bound MHC complex. This cell-cell interaction is critical for allorecognition by T lymphocytes which otherwise are unresponsive to invading organisms or foreign tissue.

Structure of the MHC/HLA

The determination of self is defined by a single genetic locus in all mammalian species so far studied. In man, these are defined on a short sequence of chromosome 6 and are inherited in Mendelian fashion. Two distinct classes of MHC antigens, class I (HLA-A, -B, -C) and class II (HLA-DR, -DP, -DQ), are located on adjacent sequences of DNA and are separated on chromosome 6 by a third class of antigens which comprise the complement system. Human MHC molecules are termed human leukocyte antigens (HLA). There is extensive allelic polymorphism (multiple forms of the genes are present in the population) for HLA.

HLA molecules are transmembrane glycoprotein heterodimers (composed of two differing amino acid chains). The class I molecule is comprised of a 45 kDa heavy chain encoded by the MHC and an associated invariant β2-microglobulin molecule which is encoded outside the MHC. Class II molecules are composed of a 32 kDa α chain and a 28 kDa β chain, both of which are encoded by the MHC (Table 5.2). Despite the distinct proteins that comprise class I and class II HLA, the three-dimensional structures of the molecules are remarkably similar and this fact is reflected in their functionality. The molecules extend approximately 70Å from the cell surface and at their distal extent express a groove that serves as a holder for amino acid fragments. The peptide-binding groove lies between parallel α helices supported on a structure of β-pleated sheets. The ends of the groove are open in class II molecules, consistent with the finding that amino acid sequences expressed by class II molecules are longer than those associated with class I molecules and vary from between 12–30 amino acids. [7, 8] (Figure 5.1).

Individuality results from genetically encoded amino acid substitutions in MHC molecules, the majority of which occur in the region of the peptide-binding

Table 5.2. Features of human leukocyte antigens

Class I	Class II
Two chains:	Two chains:
Alpha chain — α1,α2,α3	Alpha chain — α1,α2
β2-microglobulin	Beta chain — β1,β2
Polymorphisms arise from α1,α2	Variant HLA-DR arise from β1,β2
Found on most nucleated cells	Found on antigen presenting cells
Class II HLA Expression	
Constitutive expression on antigen presenting cells	
B-cells, monocytes, dendritic cells	
Induced expression:	
Activated T-cells, allograft epithelial cells and capillary endothelium	

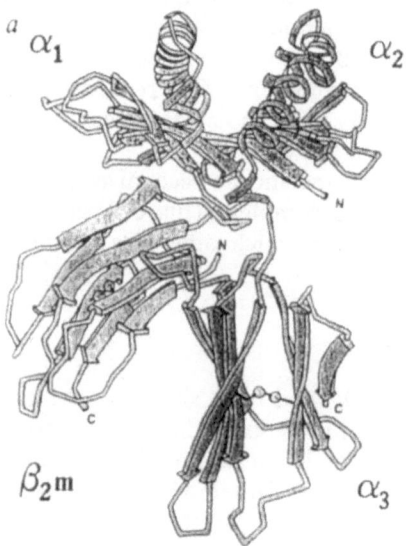

Figure 5.1. Schematic representation of the structure of HLA-A2. The β-strands are shown as thick arrows and the α-helices are represented as helical ribbons. The antigen presentation site is between the polymorphic α1 and α2 domains at the top [8].

groove. Substitution at this "business" end of the molecule enables varying presentations of amino acid sequences and interactions with the TCR [9]. As T lymphocytes recognize foreign antigen fragments in the context of MHC presentation, it is likely that the conformation of the HLA molecules as well as the specific amino acid sequence of the bound peptide are relevant to the cell-cell interactions and ultimately to T-cell activation

HLA in Allorecognition and Rejection

Host recognition of foreign tissue is complex, having evolved over millions of years as a defence mechanism against infection. When the host is invaded, (or transplanted), foreign tissue is present. Functional aspects of transplanted organs are the same between individuals of the same species, yet each cell is unique in the expression of MHC molecules, prohibiting the interchange of organs between individuals. HLA are the most polymorphic genes known and hypervariable regions define specific HLA subtypes. Individual HLA combinations contribute to self-recognition, represent foreign antigen after transplantation and participate in antigen binding by the TCR complex. Class I and class II HLA vary in their cellular expression where Class I molecules are expressed on most nucleated cells. Class II molecules are associated with specialized antigen presenting cells (APC), most notably, B-lymphocytes, monocytes, macrophages and dendritic cells.

Allograft endothelial cells express class I MHC. Since the allograft itself does not express class II MHC or costimulatory molecules, (such as B7 or CD40 for example), these cells do not stimulate helper T-cells and initiate acute rejection. Ultimately, the allograft becomes the target for cytotoxic T-cells such as CD8+ cells that recognize foreign antigen in the context of class I MHC and destroy the allograft (vide infra). The events culminating in acute rejection include processing of the antigen, presentation of antigen in the context of MHC (HLA), recognition by the T-cell, T-cell activation with proliferation of cytotoxic effector cells and eventual cell death.

Minor Histocompatibility Antigens

The β-microglobulin chain and male-female differentiation antigens (male H-Y antigen) serve as minor antigens for transplant immune responses. Minor antigen differences are unlikely to influence the fate of an HLA mismatched allograft in the setting of sufficient immunosuppression, but can precipitate alloimmune responses if immunosuppression is limited. Minor histocompatibility antigens are presented as peptides in the antigen-binding groove of MHC class I or class II molecules and can precipitate acute rejection [10, 11] and they may also contribute to chronic rejection in liver allografts [12].

These concepts have been studied extensively by the expression of minor histocompatibility antigens in an MHC-identical mouse, transfecting donor mice with β-galactosidase prior to skin transplantation. Recipient mice rejected grafts with associated rises in circulating IFN-γ and IL-2. These cytokines predominate in acute rejection and are not detectable in a well functioning allograft [13]. Although the strength of the reaction was decreased 30-fold compared with MHC mismatched grafts, the qualitative effect was identical [14]. This work, transplants across H-Y (male minor antigen) and autosomally encoded minor antigen differences, demonstrating that cytokine-mediated acute rejection occurs between minor and major MHC differences via indirect or direct pathways [15].

Inheritance of HLA

HLA antigens are inherited in Mendelian fashion with half of the genetic material from each parent. Each set of MHC genes on a single chromosome is defined as a haplotype and therefore children are 1-haplotype matches with each parent and may or may not match other HLA antigens on the second haplotype in a random fashion. Siblings have a 25 percent chance of inheriting the same alleles from each parent (a 2-haplotype match), a 50 percent likelihood of sharing one-haplotype and a 25 percent chance of inheriting separate alleles from each parent (0-haplotype match). Unrelated individuals may share common HLA antigens by random selection (coincidence). HLA antigens are variably immunogenic. HLA-DR, HLA-B and HLA-A antigens are respectively less alloreactive. In practical terms, six antigens, two alleles each for HLA-A, -B and -DR are identified in the process of tissue typing (identifying the HLA antigens expressed by an individual or their phenotype). A 2-haplotype matched sibling carries a significant immunologic advantage over all other nonidentical transplant pairs [16]. The estimated half-life of such a kidney is 22 years, more than double the average survival of a cadaver kidney transplant. Even better, identical twins match each other at all major and minor histocompatibility sites and the resultant transplant is the equivalent of an autograft (i.e. requires no immunosuppression).

HLA Matching in Transplantation

Despite the importance of HLA antigens in initiating the alloimmune response the importance of matching HLA antigens between donor and recipient is modest. Improvements in allograft function attributable to HLA matching vary by individual organ and in fact by percentages small enough that controversy exists regarding the true benefit derived by delays in organ transplantation brought about by the time-consuming practice of HLA matching [17]. Benefits to HLA matching have been shown for pancreas, kidney and heart transplantation with the benefit being greatest for the pancreas, somewhat less for kidneys and of even lesser value for heart transplantation.

The greatest amount of research has been in cadaver kidney transplantation where HLA matching is always performed [18]. HLA-A, -B, -DR matching plays some role in the assignment of kidney and pancreas allografts. In the United States, zero-mismatched allografts are shared by mandate with phenotypically matched recipients on a national rather than regional basis.

Practical issues influence the application of HLA matching in solid organ transplantation. ABO compatibility and medical necessity determine the allocation of livers, hearts and lungs. Allowable cold ischemic times, (the period from procurement until transplantation), are less than 12 hours and optimally 3–6 hours for these allografts. Preoperative cross-match testing is only performed in cardiothoracic transplantation when the recipient is highly sensitized (i.e. there are high levels of circulating antibody to HLA antigens). Typically, prior to organ procurement, the heart and lung recipients have been identified, notified and in fact, are often undergoing surgery in preparation for removal of the diseased organ and the anticipated transplant. Poorly matched cardiac and pulmonary allografts are associated with a higher frequency of acute rejection episodes and decreased graft survival at one year. However, heart transplants are performed on the basis of medical urgency, thereby obviating any attempts at HLA matching. The benefit of HLA matching is clearer in pancreas transplantation, particularly pancreas after kidney and pancreas transplantation alone. In this setting, acute rejection is common, immune events within the allograft are difficult to monitor and the prompt diagnosis of acute rejection is relatively problematic.

The likelihood of acute rejection is proportional to the degree of HLA-B, HLA-DR mismatch, [19] with current immunosuppression. Therefore, well-matched allografts experience less acute rejection and show improved survival. However, this advantage has already begun to diminish in the era of improved immunosuppression (mycophenolate mofetil, tacrolimus, etc.). That HLA matching is less crucial in simultaneous kidney-pancreas transplantation and illustrates a fundamental point in modern transplantation. Detecting acute rejection is problematic in pancreas transplantation in the absence of a kidney from the same donor. Late detection of acute rejection is costly in terms of allograft function and long-term survival. Therefore, avoiding acute rejection by HLA matching is presumably of greater importance in pancreas transplantation alone or pancreas after kidney transplantation where acute rejection is more difficult to identify. In simultaneous kidney-pancreas transplantation and kidney transplantation and liver transplantation alone, serologic markers of injury readily detect acute rejection and pharmacologic intervention can salvage the allograft in 95 percent of cases, somewhat less for kidneys and hearts and least for livers.

Zero-mismatched Kidneys (Phenotypic Matches)

One-year allograft survival following cadaver renal transplantation continues to improve. Currently, 88 percent of first cadaver renal allografts are functioning after one year [20]. Attempts to diminish immune responses by minimizing donor and recipient HLA incompatibilities have contributed to this success [18]. In the United States, cadaver kidneys for transplantation are assigned based on some combination of patient waiting time, HLA match and geography. Modest improvements in transplantation outcomes can be demonstrated for each degree of HLA matching. Allograft survival at one year for completely mismatched kidneys is 87 percent, increasing to 90 percent for five antigen-matches and 92 percent for 0-mismatched kidneys [20]. Kidney donors and recipients are typed for class I (HLA-A, -B) antigens and class II (HLA -DR) antigens. Thus, HLA typing is incomplete as HLA-C, -DP and -DQ antigens are not typed and no matching is predicated on minor histocompatibility differences.

However, the typed antigens seem to play the greatest role in alloimmune recognition, possibly because they show the greatest polymorphism. Zero-mismatched kidneys, (all typed antigens in the recipient are present in the donor), are shared nationally and benefit from an improved graft survival, which is almost equivalent to a live donor kidney. Zero-mismatched allografts are considered phenotypically identical between donor and recipient. Differences often exist due to "blanks" (HLA antigens in the donor or recipient that cannot be identified) in the typing process. This arises when both HLA alleles in the donor or recipient express the same antigen (HLA-A2 for example is inherited from each parent). Genotypically-matched allografts share identical gene sequences for HLA as arises by chance for some cadaver donor-recipient pairs and would be the case for all HLA 2-haplotype identical siblings.

Tissue Typing

Immunology plays a role in the day-to-day affairs of clinical transplantation. Some of the testing is of academic interest only while other pre-transplant testing is integral to the success of the transplant procedure. Specific assays have been developed to determine HLA antigens of the donor and recipient (tissue typing), testing for donor-specific antibodies (cross-match) and determining the recipient's reactivity to alloantigens in the general population (panel reactive antibody, PRA).

The applications of these tests to transplantation and their relative value for various allografts are discussed below.

Tissue typing is performed on lymphocytes recovered from cadaver donor lymph nodes or peripheral blood. Tests for class I antigens are performed on peripheral blood lymphocytes or T-cells and those for class II on B-lymphocytes. Class I antigens are determined serologically, whilst class II antigens may be determined serologically or by PCR methodologies.

Lymphocytes are separated from other leukocytes in a blood sample by running the sample over immunomagnetic beads coated with monoclonal antibodies for lymphocytes and then eluting the trapped cells for analysis or by eliminating non-lymphocytic cells in a sample by the addition of specific antibodies and complement to effect cell lysis of all but the lymphocytes. Recovered lymphocytes are added to microtiter trays loaded with monoclonal antibodies to known HLA types. These monoclonal antibodies are produced commercially in hybridoma lines after recovering the serum antibodies generated by pregnant women exposed to paternal HLA by the fetus. After the tray is incubated, allowing the antibody to bind to specific antigen, complement is added, resulting in lysis of cells with bound antibody. A fluorescent dye demonstrates lysed versus intact (viable) cells.

Molecular Tissue Typing

Specific oligonucleotide probes that can identify individual DNA for determining class II HLA (and class I in some laboratories) have replaced the conventional serologic methods described above [21]. This technology involves amplifying a specific locus using the polymerase chain reaction (PCR), then adding specific known probes and detecting their binding by radioactive or enzymatic markers. DNA-based typing was first accomplished with high resolution using restriction fragment-length polymorphism (RFLP) typing and later by sequence-specific oligonucleotide probes (PCR-SSOP) or by PCR with sequence-specific primers (PCR-SSP). Commonly, combinations of serologic and DNA-based techniques are performed. RFLP analysis is based on restriction endonuclease cleavage at polymorphic restriction sites. The technology relies on linkage disequilibrium between polymorphic restriction sites.

In part due to poor specificity, RFLP has been replaced by newer methodologies. The cloning and sequencing of HLA antigens has enabled precise identification by PCR primers. Polymorphic regions of HLA molecules can be amplified through PCR methodologies. The amplified DNA sequences can then be identified with selected oligonucleotide probes (SSOP). Alternatively, the sequence can be amplified by a series of known primers. A completely matched primer (SSP-sequence specific primer) will produce a more efficient PCR reaction than a primer with mismatches. The alleles undergoing the greatest amplification are identified by agarose gel electrophoresis. Currently, this represents the most versatile, quick and inexpensive technique for testing all of the class II loci.

With the introduction of DNA-based technologies, genetic polymorphisms involving HLA have become ever more numerous. The known specificities now number 95 HLA-A loci, over 200 HLA-B loci, 50 HLA-C loci and greater than 118 HLA-DR loci [22]. It is known that many of these distinct specificities share common epitopes (antigen-binding sites). These cross-reacting groups (CREGs) represent common amino acid sequences shared across a group of HLA molecules ("public" antigens) and usually do not differ in their ability to induce an immune response. A patient may be exposed to the HLA-B7 molecule by blood transfusion and develop a specific antibody to –B7 (private antigen) or an antibody to a public antigen on the –B7 molecule which is shared by HLA-B7, B27, B42, B54, B55 and B56. A highly sensitized patient (PRA > 60%) may have a few antibodies formed against public antigens rather than multiple antibodies to specific HLA "private" antigens. Matching of CREGs rather than HLA has been proposed as a means of achieving better allograft matching within smaller population groups [23].

Panel Reactive Antibodies (PRA)

Patients develop anti-HLA antibodies through prior exposure to HLA antigens. This occurs with (1) pregnancy, (2) blood transfusion or (3) prior organ transplantation, particularly when an allograft is lost to acute rejection. These preformed cytotoxic antibodies can be screened for by the microlymphocytotoxicity test. On a regular basis, the serum of all wait-listed patients is added to T and B-cells from a wide pool of donors with known HLA specificities. Complement is added and cell lysis is monitored by the ability of viable (intact) cells to exclude vital red dye. The methodologies are identical to those applied to cross-match testing with the exception that the assay utilizes a panel of cells which express a wide variety of known HLA antigens, rather than lymphocytes from an individual donor. The panel reactive antibody (PRA) is expressed as a percent of positive reactions against the entire pool of tested HLA. A 0 percent PRA implies an absence of pre-formed antibodies. In contrast, potential recipients with greater than 80 percent PRA have pre-formed antibodies to most HLA antigens and often have to wait years or even decades for a potential allograft. These patients are referred to as highly sensitized. For many of these patients, receipt of a 0-mismatched allograft represents their only hope of successful transplantation. Recipients with PRA >30 percent are at an increased risk of acute rejection compared with unsensitized recipients and in general, are treated with increased immunosuppression at the time of transplantation.

Blood Transfusion

The generation of memory B-cells to HLA molecules leads to high titers of anti-HLA antibodies in a potential transplant recipient and increases the waiting time for transplantation and the risk of acute rejection. Because of this, pre-transplant blood transfusions are avoided. In the past, this was challenging, but the advent of recombinant human erythropoietin (rhEpo) has enabled most dialysis patients to maintain adequate hemoglobin without transfusion. It came as somewhat of a surprise, when it was revealed that patients transplanted in the 1970s who received multiple blood transfusions had better outcomes than those who did not [24].

Numerous studies in the 1980s confirmed the beneficial effect, which was hypothesized to result from an immunosuppressive effect of blood transfusion or by eliminating a population of "high-responders" to HLA. This latter group would become sensitized by the blood transfusions, making it more difficult to find cross-match negative donors, delaying the time to transplantation and increasing the risk of acute rejection. Alternatively, experimental studies with blood transfusions in animals, (mostly rodents), showed that transfusions induced so-called suppressor lymphocytes which possessed an immunoregulatory function to depress the allograft immune response, thus prolonging graft survival. Whatever the etiology of the effect, it was lost when subsequent improvements in standard immunosuppression, particularly the advent of cyclosporine, negated the minor beneficial effect of pre-transplant blood transfusions [25]. Subsequent research efforts were directed towards donor-specific blood transfusions (DST). DST is given in small quantities under immunosuppression to lessen the risk of sensitization. Only a salutary effect of decreased donor-specific hyporesponsiveness (18 percent versus 3 percent of controls), was produced but with no detectable difference in the allograft [26].

Pre-transplant Cross-match

Recipients of renal allografts are at varying risk for antibody-mediated hyperacute rejection. This threat has been reduced to a rare occurrence (<0.1 percent) by the routine performance of a pre-transplant cross-match. The purpose of the test is to identify pre-formed antibodies in the recipient's serum against donor HLA, a situation immunologically analogous to an ABO incompatible blood transfusion. A sufficient titer of pre-formed antibody could result in immediate loss of a renal allograft. Interestingly, due to the short preservation times allowed for heart, lung and liver allografts, these organs are usually transplanted without cross-match testing. Furthermore, a positive cross-match in liver or combined liver-kidney transplantations has minor consequences [27]. The vulnerability of renal allografts to pre-formed recipient anti-HLA antibody in contrast to heart, liver or lung allografts is probably due to the unusual susceptibility of the renal endothelium to damage by antigen-antibody reactions. In contrast, more than 80 percent of renal allografts are lost within minutes to hours of transplantation when placed in the setting of a positive cross-match [28]. Since this early observation a cross-match test performed with donor lymphocytes has been the standard prior to renal transplantation. Donor lymphocytes serve as a target for recipient antibodies.

Cross-match testing may be performed similarly to the serologic determination of HLA antigens. Patients awaiting a renal transplant send a serum sample to the tissue-typing laboratory each month. The recipient's serum is incubated with donor lymphocytes and complement is added. A positive cross-match is confirmed by cell lysis. Modifications of the standard "NIH Cross-match" have improved the sensitivity of the test. The original microlymphocytotoxicity reaction lacks sensitivity by today's standards. Applying the Amos (wash) technique or adding anti-human globulin (AHG) to the standard procedure improves the sensitivity of the test (Figure 5.2). The wash eliminates anti-complement elements in the serum. After the reaction of lymphocytes and serum antibody, excess serum is washed off to eliminate unbound IgG. AHG binds to recipient antibodies (IgG) ensures that a complement-fixing isotype is present on the lymphocyte and increases the sensitivity of the test. Finally, the application of flow cytometry to the cross-match has produced the most sensitive technique yet available. The recipient's serum is mixed with donor lymphocytes and incubated with mouse anti-T or anti-B antibody conjugated with phycoerythrin and an anti-human IgG conjugated with flourescein. The cells are separated by the flow cytometer. Very

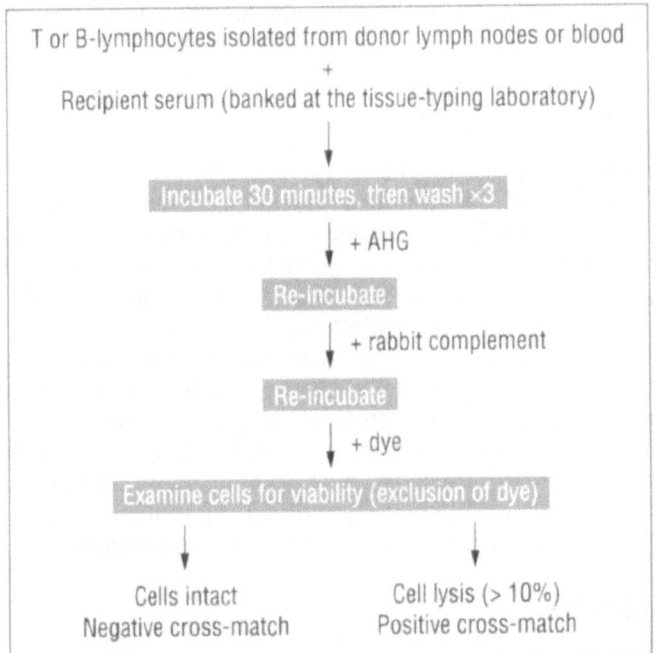

T or B-lymphocytes isolated from donor lymph nodes or blood
+
Recipient serum (banked at the tissue-typing laboratory)

Incubate 30 minutes, then wash ×3

+ AHG

Re-incubate

+ rabbit complement

Re-incubate

+ dye

Examine cells for viability (exclusion of dye)

Cells intact   Cell lysis (> 10%)
Negative cross-match   Positive cross-match

Figure 5.2. Cross-match testing is performed uniformly prior to renal transplantation and in many centers in a retrospective fashion after liver and heart transplantation. The original "NIH test" has been made more sensitive by the addition of the antihuman globulin step. T cells and B cells are separated by antibody coated beads or nylon wool columns. Anti-class I is identified by the lysis of donor T cells and anti-class II is identified by the lysis of B cells.

low levels of antibody are detectable. Positive results for T and to a lesser extent B-cell cross-matches are associated with an increased frequency of acute rejection and poorer one-year graft survival.

Mixed Lymphocyte Reaction

Alloreactivity against a specific donor can be assessed through the mixed lymphocyte culture/reaction (MLR). This test serves as a useful tool in research and can be applied as a measure of donor-specific hyporesponsiveness or hyporeactivity [29]. In brief, responder lymphocytes (from spleen, lymph nodes or peripheral blood) are incubated with irradiated stimulator cells in triplicate wells for 3–4 days. The cells are then pulsed with [^{3}H] thymidine and harvested 18 hours later. Thymidine incorporation is quantified by liquid scintillation as counts per minute and serves as a measure of responder cell proliferation (responsiveness to alloantigen). Unfortunately, the in vitro MLR fails to accurately predict in vivo responses and acute rejection can occur despite marked reductions in MLR response [30]. As a result, application of the MLR to predict the adequacy of immunosuppression, immune reactivity against the allograft or the ability to wean immunosuppression, has not proved reliable.

The assigned immunosuppressive regimen for each patient is currently relegated to the art of medicine. A laboratory assay which predicts the adequacy of immunosuppression, would serve as an invaluable contribution to clinical transplantation.

Acute Rejection

The recognition of allograft antigens by the immune system leads to a sequence of events that, unchecked by immunosuppression, results in the elimination of the foreign material. Generally these events include both a non-specific inflammatory component and an antigen-specific immune response, both of which are driven by marrow-derived leukocytes. T-cells and antibody-producing B-cells mediate the specific response. In particular, the T lymphocyte is critical to the immune response and it has been demonstrated that rejection will not occur in hosts absent of these cells (congenitally athymic "nude" mice) [31]. Once awoken from a dormant state by the recognition of antigen, activated T-cells induce the recruitment, differentiation and activation of many other cells. The inflammatory response is mediated by macrophages, polymorphonuclear cells and natural killer (NK) cells, which can be non-specifically activated by ischemia, reperfusion injury and the trauma associated with the transplant surgical procedure.

Antigen Recognition

The first step in the initiation of the immune response is the recognition of antigen. It is the difference in histocompatibility antigens between allograft donor and recipient that leads to an immune response against an allograft. The very high degree of polymorphism in the class I and II antigens that comprise the MHC is the one distinguishing feature that makes it unique compared with other regions of the genome and it is this feature that creates serious problems for transplantation purposes. This polymorphism presumably evolved as an immune defence mechanism against infections, since species with a limited array of MHC antigens are easily overwhelmed by infections. From a practical standpoint, the consequences of MHC polymorphism are that combinations of MHC-identical donors and recipients are extremely uncommon among unrelated individuals.

The discovery of the MHC was based on its ability to induce allograft rejection. Indeed, the most frequent and aggressive rejection occurs when the MHC disparities between the donor and the recipient are the greatest [32]. However, normally the principle function of the MHC gene products is to present antigens in the form of fragments of foreign proteins (peptides), forming non-covalently bound complexes that can be recognized by T-cells through specific receptors [33]. During the ontogeny of the immune system, T lymphocytes were selected whose receptors could specifically recognize foreign antigens in the context of MHC molecules. Simultaneously, self-reactive T-cells were removed by a variety of mechanisms, resulting in a state of self-tolerance [34].

Antigen Processing

Foreign antigens (viral proteins, transplanted MHC molecules) are first present in the host as functionally intact proteins. However, they are recognized immunologically as short antigenic sequences in the peptide-binding groove of the MHC. Protein molecules must be "processed" for MHC expression [34]. Class I molecules bind cytoplasmic peptides in the endoplasmic reticulum (Figure 5.3). The

The MHC Class I Processing and Presentation Pathway

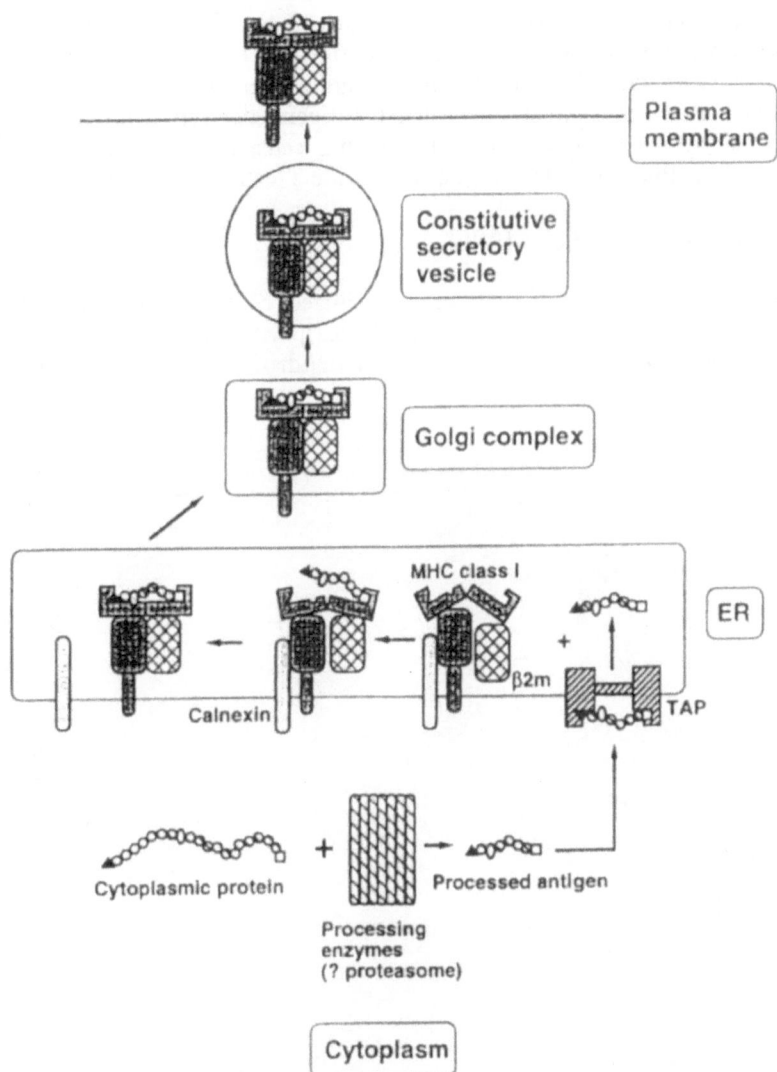

Figure 5.3. Schematic representation of class I antigen processing and presentation. Class I molecules bind peptides derived from cytosolic proteins. Proteins are processed to small peptide fragments by proteasome complexes, which are multicatalytic protease assemblies. The "transporter associated with antigen processing" (TAP) heterodimer then transports peptide fragments to the endoplasmic reticulum (ER) where they are packaged with the class I MHC. Release of calnexin allows protein movement out of the ER to the Golgi complex and eventual expression on the cell surface [9].

peptide sequences are cleaved by enzymes attached to proteasome complexes, transported to the endoplasmic reticulum and then bundled with class I MHC. The amino acid sequences, (only 8–11 residues in length), are recognized by T-cells as foreign antigen. Class II molecules are loaded with peptide fragments in the endosomes and lysosomes. Cell membrane bound proteins are endocytosed by the presenting cell and cleaved into small fragments. These fragments are incorporated into the groove of the class II molecule and the entire complex is then presented on the cell surface (Figure 5.4). In short, viral-infected cells provide an abundant source of foreign antigen in the cytoplasm, which becomes associated with class I MHC. T-cells recognize these cells as foreign and initiate cytotoxic reactions against them. Inert antigens derived from the cell wall are processed by specialized antigen processing cells, bound to class II molecules, expressed on the cell surface and also activate T-cells. (See Chapter 9)

Antigen Presenting Cells (APC)

Antigen presenting cells (APC) are specialized cells that initiate and modulate immunity. APC take many forms (Table 5.2), with dendritic cells initiating the most powerful immune responses. Mature dendritic cells express high concentra-

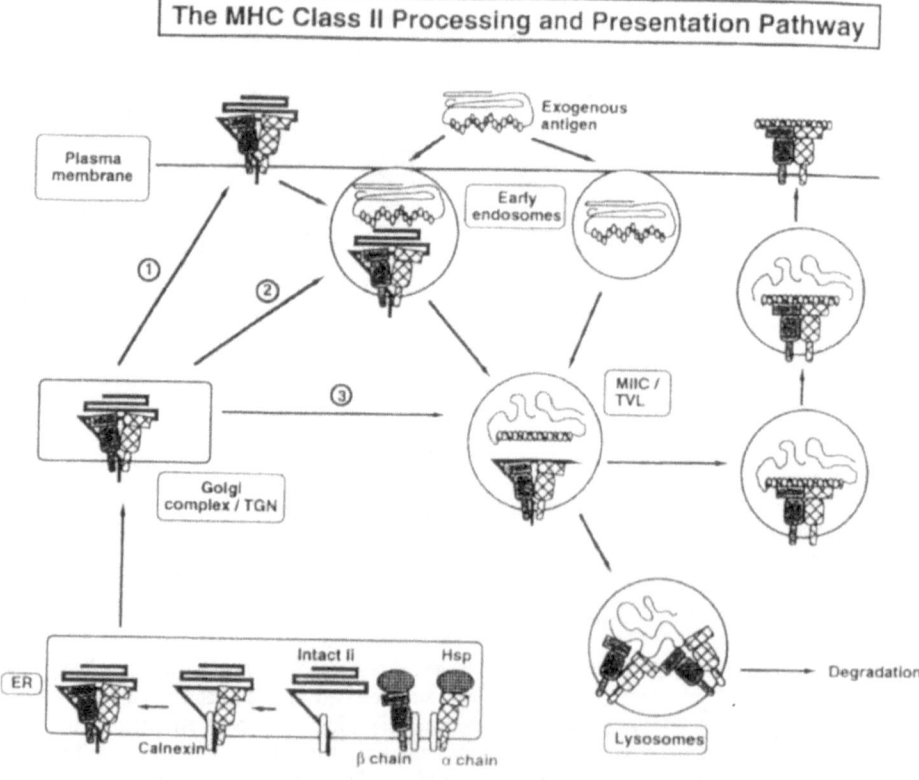

Figure 5.4. Schematic representation of class II antigen processing and presentation. Foreign proteins contained in endosomes are processed for expression with class II MHC molecules. Class II MHC molecules assemble in the ER. The dissociation of Ii from the class II molecule makes the antigen-binding site available for peptide molecules. Lysosomes contain antigen, particularly resident pathogens. Tubulovesicular lysosomes in macrophages and MIIC in B-lymphocytes are major sites of class II MHC accumulation and possibly of peptide loading. Intact, peptide-loaded class II MHC molecules are then transported to the cell surface for expression [9].

Table 5.3. Interactions between T lymphocytes and antigen presenting cells (APC)

T-CELL	APC	Role
TCR / CD3	MHC – Ag	Recognition of foreign antigen (signal 1)
CD2 (LFA-2)	CD58 (LFA-3)	Cell-cell binding
CD 11a / 18 (LFA-1)	CD54 (ICAM-1)	Cell-cell binding
ICAM-3	CD 11a / 18(LFA-1)	Cell-cell binding
CD154 (gp 39)	CD40	Costimulation (signal 2)
CD28	$B7_1$, $B7_2$ (CD80, CD86)	Costimulation
IL-2 Receptor	- - -	Activation (signal 3)

Abbreviations: TCR= T-cell receptor, MHC= major histocompatibility complex, Ag= antigen, CD= clusters of differentiation, LFA= lymphocyte function associated antigen (CD11a = α-subunit, CD18 = β-subunit), ICAM= intercellular adhesion molecule, IL= interleukin.

tions of both class I and class II MHC antigens and thus are able to stimulate both CD4+ and CD8+ cells. These cells capture antigens, process foreign peptides for presentation with the MHC and travel to secondary lymphoid organs to recruit host immune responses against the allograft [35]. Also, expression of class II MHC can be induced on endothelium and some allograft epithelial cells, which can subsequently be recognized by host T-cells. Dendritic cells, B-cells and macrophages are referred to as "professional" antigen presenting cells and provoke vigorous T-cell activation, while "amateur" antigen presenting cells require priming by cytokines (e.g. INF-γ) to express class II MHC and provoke weaker T-cell responses. Full activation of T-cells requires a co-stimulatory signal from the APC to specific T-cell receptors. These signals result from binding of CD40, CD80 (B7-1) or CD86 (B7-2) to their respective T-cell receptors CD154 (CD40 ligand) and CD28 (Table 5.3). Blockade of the co-stimulatory signal prevents acute rejection and leads to long-term allograft survival in animal models [36,37].

Direct and Indirect Allorecognition

T-cells recognize foreign antigen by two distinct "direct" and "indirect" pathways. Direct recognition occurs when T-cells recognize intact allogeneic MHC molecules on the surface of donor cells (Figure 5.5). These molecules may be class II MHC expressed on passenger leukocytes that accompany the allograft (donor APC recognized by recipient lymphocytes). The indirect pathway is a more physiologic mechanism accounting for T-cell responsiveness to viral infection [38]. Indirect recognition occurs when T-cells recognize peptide antigens in the context of self-MHC [39,40]. Viral antigens, for example, are presented by host APC to host lymphocytes. In organ transplantation, foreign proteins may be derived from donor MHC molecules as these proteins confer uniqueness or individuality.

Both direct and indirect mechanisms play a role in transplant rejection. Direct recognition of donor antigens expressed on donor APC provides a powerful stimulus for T-cell alloactivation. It is possible that early responses to the allograft result from direct recognition of antigen presenting cells within the graft (so-called "passenger leukocytes"). Over time, the graft becomes populated with recipient, bone marrow-derived APCs and indirect recognition predominates. In this construct, early acute rejections are the result of T-cell subpopulations stimulated

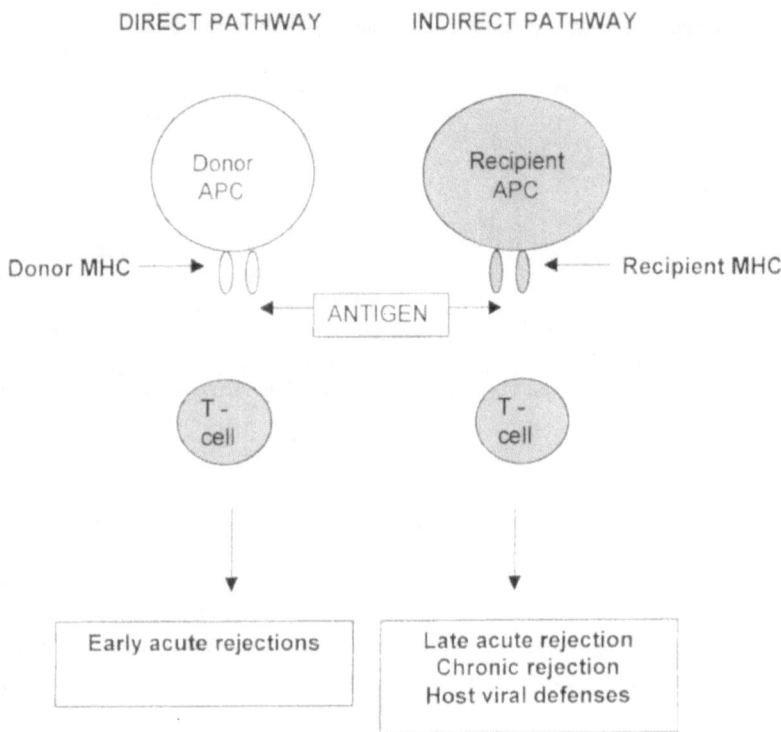

DIRECT PATHWAY   INDIRECT PATHWAY

Figure 5.5. Direct and indirect allorecognition. Alloantigen may be presented to T-cells for recognition by either of two distinct pathways. The direct pathway is unique to transplantation and requires the presence of foreign (donor) cells expressing their intact MHC molecules. Donor antigen is presented in this context and recognized by host T-cells. The indirect pathway arose as a mechanism for the recognition of viruses, tumor antigens and other foreign proteins. Allopeptides processed by recipient antigen presenting cells (APC) and minor histocompatibility antigens are recognized via the indirect pathway.

through the direct pathway of recognition and later alloimmune events (late acute rejection, chronic rejection and allograft accommodation or acceptance) which predominantly involve indirect T-cell-APC interactions.

Experimental evidence supports the hypothesis that acute and chronic rejection may be largely the respective consequences of both direct and indirect allorecognition. Foreign peptides in the context of donor APC (non-self MHC) induce a vigorous response by T-cells, which unchecked by immunosuppression initiates acute rejection. That direct recognition contributes primarily to the development of acute rejection is supported by efforts to eliminate donor-derived APC prior to transplantation [41]. These allografts rarely suffer early acute rejection, but suffer the indolent immune consequences of chronic rejection. Similarly, acute rejection occurs when donor-recipient recognition is boosted by adoptive transfer of T-cells specific for direct recognition of allogeneic MHC molecules [42]. In short, experiments limiting donor APC lessen the chances of acute rejection, while stimulation of host T-cells via the direct pathway leads to acute rejection. However, there are no absolutes in this scheme. In an elegant study using donor cells from class II MHC knock out mice, it was demonstrated that indirect alloresponses were capable of mediating acute rejection in the absence of direct allorecognition [43].

Chronic rejection, alternatively, may be a consequence of indirect recognition. Alloantibodies may play a significant role in the development of chronic rejection. These antibodies are derived from B-cells serving as APC and stimulating T-cells via the indirect pathway [44]. This is supported by experimental evidence that allografts depleted of APC remain susceptible to chronic rejection after the infiltration of host APC into the graft [41]. Moreover, rat cardiac allografts, transplanted across minor MHC differences recognized via the indirect pathway, are lost to chronic rejection [45]. In some models, indirect allorecognition results in preferential activation of Type 2 (suppressor) cytokines, production of alloantibody by B-cells and growth factor production by endothelial and smooth muscle cells. Together these responses contribute to chronic allograft rejection. That indirect allorecognition can initiate acute or chronic rejection in transplant organs demonstrates the redundant and highly complex nature of the immune system.

T-Cell Activation

The T-cell receptor (TCR) is a heterodimer comprised of two polypeptide chains, α and β, which are associated with several proteins of the CD3 complex [46]. Although the T-cell antigen receptor is responsible for the exquisite specificity of a T-cell clone for a specific antigen sequence, it is the CD3 complex that transduces the signal of activation to the T-cell. Once the antigen-specific T-cell receptor on the surface of the T-cell is triggered, a series of intracellular events ensues, resulting in de novo expression of a range of genes, including those encoding various cytokines and cell-surface proteins [47].

One of the unique features of the immune response is that recognition of antigen is not sufficient to trigger the full activation of the T-cell. The activation of the T-cell cannot occur without the participation of additional signaling mechanisms. A second or co-stimulatory signal must be delivered in collaboration with successful antigen engagement. Without such signals, a T-cell may become anergic or unresponsive [48]. Since such a state would be highly desirable in transplantation, enormous interest has been directed at studying these mechanisms. There are a number of cell surface proteins on T-cells that could function as co-stimulatory molecules and potentially contribute to their activation. One interaction that has garnered significant attention is that between the CD28 molecule on the CD4+ T lymphocyte and its ligand B7 on the surface of the APC [49]. This interaction initiates a signaling process distinct from that delivered through the TCR and which results in an increased rate of cytokine gene activation. The production of IL-2 and other stimulatory cytokines (signal 3) leads to activation and proliferation of T-cells, thereby amplifying their response (Figure 5.6).

T-cells also receive important signals from cytokines. Activation begins with binding to specific cytokine receptors, with the downstream effect being the amplification of both immune and inflammatory processes following transplantation. Cytokines have been demonstrated to increase MHC expression and enhance target cell injury and inflammation involving neutrophils and platelets. They have also been shown to increase the expression of cellular adhesion molecules on endothelial and epithelial cells, thus facilitating the migration of leukocytes across the vascular endothelium of the transplanted organ. Alternatively, some cytokines inhibit the immune response. Therefore, it is the balance between stimulatory and inhibitory cytokines that determines the strength of any given immune response to antigenic stimuli [12].

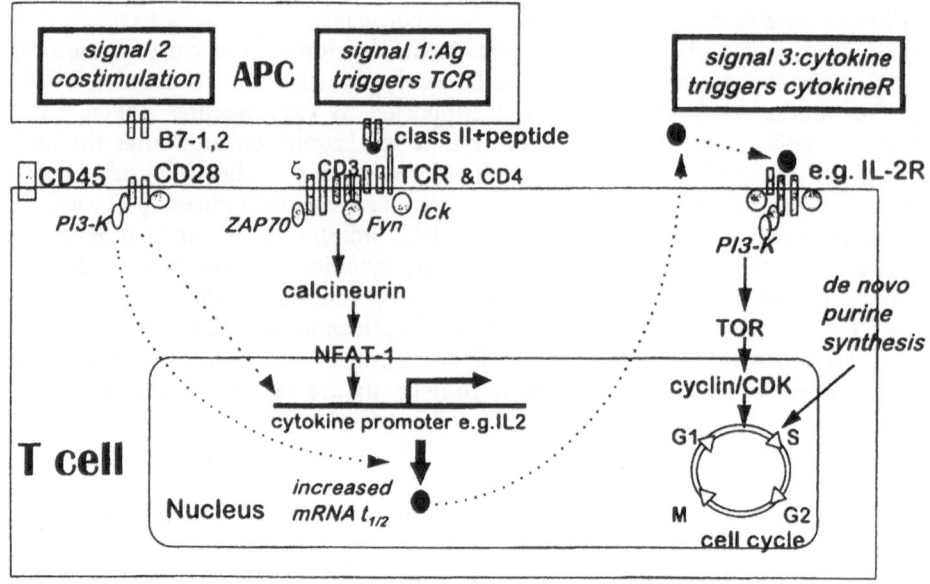

Figure 5.6. The three-signal model of T cell activation. Signal I involves recognition of foreign antigen in the context of MHC by the T cell receptor complex. This initiates signal transduction pathways that lead to the production of cytokines (IL-2). Full activation requires a costimulatory signal (signal 2). Released cytokines then stimulate nascent cells (signal 3) to proliferate by binding to specific receptors (IL-2 receptor, e.g.). Cell division is effected by intracellular pathways such as the one involving the "target of Rapamycin" (TOR) molecule (Halloran PF, Lui SL. Approved Immunosuppressants. In: Norman DJ, Suki WN. editors. Primer on Transplantation, Thorofare, NJ: ASTP, 1998; 93–102).

Th1 and Th2 Paradigm

Helper T-cell progenitors can be channeled in at least two different directions during the development of an immune response. Following stimulation of the immune system, a pattern of response emerges in which one set of cytokines appears to favor the development of an antibody response to an antigen (Th2 response) while simultaneously down-regulating the cellular response; conversely, the generation of another milieu of cytokines favors the development of a cellular immune response (Th1 response) [50]. This is known as the Th1/Th2 paradigm. Exactly how a Th1- or Th2-dominant response is determined is uncertain but it is postulated that the local cytokine milieu plays a significant regulatory role in determining which type of T helper cells are expanded after antigen stimulation. Current thinking suggests that Th1 cells produce primarily IL-2, INF-γ, and TNF-α, favoring the development of cell-mediated immunity. Conversely, Th2 cells produce primarily IL-4, IL-5, IL-6, IL-10 and IL-13 that promote humoral immune responses. It is postulated that administration of cytokine signals favoring an immune response driven by the Th2 pathway may be less damaging than the Th1-driven system since acute rejection is dominated by cell-mediated mechanisms. To assess the validity of this theory, several groups have tried to assess the role of key cytokines by performing experiments in which the over-expression or absence of these cytokines is evaluated in an attempt to push the immune system toward either a Th1 or Th2 response. Although the injection of

IL-2 or IFN-γ can prevent the induction of tolerance, the injection of IL-4 does not induce tolerance [51–53]. Other experiments have also shown that rejection can occur in both IL-2 and IFN-γ knockout mice [54,55]. Therefore, the Th1/Th2 model represents an oversimplification of the alloimmune response. However, the model emphasizes the important role that cytokines play in the determination of allograft rejection versus acceptance.

Forms of Allograft Rejection

Hyperacute rejection occurs within minutes of reestablishing blood flow to the donor organ. The allograft becomes mottled, cyanotic and swollen, resulting in immediate destruction of the organ. Histologically, the reaction is characterized by antibody deposition, endothelial cell damage, fibrinoid necrosis and infiltration of polymorphonuclear infiltrates, platelet thrombi and relatively minimal lymphocytic infiltrate [56]. Hyperacute rejection is caused by pre-formed antibodies binding to donor alloantigens on the vascular endothelium, resulting in the local fixation of complement (vide supra). Patients with a history of prior exposure to MHC antigens through previous transplant procedures, blood transfusions, or pregnancies are at risk for developing antibodies reactive with alloantigens. Fortunately, due to the widespread application of pre-transplant cross-match testing, this form of rejection is now a rare event, occurring in less than 0.1 percent of kidney transplants.

Of interest is the fact that liver transplants are performed with little regard to existing anti-donor recipient activity. Thus, they are frequently performed despite a positive cross-match and with no attempt to match HLA antigens between the donor and recipient. Acute rejection occurs in over 60 percent of liver transplant recipients within 90 days of surgery, but typically has no or little long-term consequences. Liver allografts are resilient or resistant to immune events for unclear reasons. In part, this may be due to the enormous regenerative capacity displayed by the liver, but it is also apparent that the immune response to liver allografts is different from other allografts, with examples of spontaneous tolerance occurring in several rodent models [57].

Antibody may also mediate tissue damage through the activity of NK cells in antibody-dependent cellular cytotoxicity (ADCC). In this case, the alloantibody acts as a bridge between the target tissue and both the effector cell and the killer cell. The latter has an IgG Fc receptor capable of affixing cytophilic antibody [58]. In human transplant recipients, specific donor-directed ADCC has been associated with rejection in a number of studies. For instance, Tilney and colleagues have demonstrated high levels of anti-donor ADCC activity within the infiltrating cell population of rejecting rat heart allografts [59]. In contrast, several laboratories, using a variety of different experimental models, have found that allografts can survive for extended periods of time in the presence of high levels of NK effector activity [60]. Therefore, the role of ADCC activity in allograft rejection has not been firmly established.

Acute Cellular Rejection

Acute rejection continues to be a major problem in clinical transplantation, occurring in 15-40% of renal transplant recipients. Fortunately, the majority of acute rejection episodes are reversible with use of high doses of corticosteroids, anti-lymphocyte globulin or the monoclonal murine antibody OKT3. In 1952, Woodruff made the observation that acute rejection occurred far more frequently in the initial six weeks after engraftment and decreased both in incidence and severity after this period [61]. This phenomenon, termed "immune adaptation" does not have a well-established immunologic explanation but is a consistent observation in human solid organ transplantation.

Histopathologically, acute rejection is characterized by an acute mononuclear cell infiltrate with associated endarteritis and perivascular cuffing of mononuclear cells. Immunohistochemical studies demonstrate that the mononuclear cells consist of a mixture of T lymphocytes, macrophages, B-cells and large granular lymphocytes, with occasional polymorphonuclear leukocytes, eosinophils, and basophils [62]. It is important to note that the pattern of cellular infiltrate varies from one organ to another and also considerably within a single organ itself. As has been suggested previously, the T lymphocytes play an essential role in the initiation of allograft rejection because congenitally athymic, nude mice or T lymphocyte deprived animals are incapable of rejecting either xeno- or allografts. The helper T lymphocyte appears to be the most important cell in the induction of acute rejection. T-helper (CD4+) cells are critical in initiating rejection, whilst CD8+ cells are not required and only contribute to the speed of the actual rejection [60]. Following the initiating event, elaboration of cytokines results in activation and recruitment of specific (CD8+ cytotoxic T lymphocytes) and non-specific (macrophage, NK cells) effector cells within the allograft. Delayed-type hypersensitivity, analogous to acute rejection, involves a non-specific effector phase that is characterized by an infiltrate of lymphocytes and macrophages. More recent studies have suggested that the cytotoxic T lymphocyte (CTL) responses dominate the acute rejection process early. CTLs kill their targets through the elaboration of perforins or granzymes, through the activation of the Fas death pathway in the target cell or through the secretion of TNF-α [63]. Apoptosis, (or programmed cell death), is the final common pathway for each of these effector cell mechanisms.

It should also be mentioned that antibody is frequently associated with acute rejection episodes. The target of these antibodies is the endothelium of arterioles, the microcirculation and glomeruli. Hence, many of the histopathologic changes observed with acute rejection, such as arteriolar thrombosis, interstitial hemorrhage and fibrinoid necrosis of the arteriolar walls, may well be the result of the deposition of antibody and the consequent activation of complement [64]. However, the presence of donor-specific antibody does not necessarily correlate with the presence of acute allograft rejection and its presence may be entirely compatible with normal allograft function.

Chronic Rejection

Since the inception of solid organ transplant programs, the short-term patient and allograft survival have progressively improved due to advancements in organ preservation, the development of a powerful array of immunosuppressive agents and improved management of post-transplant complications. Kidney, liver and heart allograft survival rates approach 80–85% at one year. Despite these early successes, the allograft attrition rate after the first year has not changed significantly. For instance, the half-life of cadaver donor renal allografts remains at 8 to 9 years, despite more than 80 percent functioning at the end of the first year

[65]. The rate of decline of other organs is similarly disappointing. The incidence of coronary arteriosclerosis in heart allografts reaches 50 percent by 5 years, leading to a 25 percent mortality rate. Half of all lung transplants have failed within a similar period, primarily due to an entity known as bronchiolitis obliterans [66]. Interestingly, liver allografts appear to enjoy a relatively improved survival, presumably due to the lower immunogenicity and regenerative properties of this organ [67].

Although multiple factors including recurrent disease and drug toxicity contribute to the allograft loss after the first year, an entity known as chronic rejection accounts for the majority of allograft losses when death with function is censored from the analysis. Chronic rejection is defined as a progressive decline in allograft function which occurs months or years after transplantation and is manifested histologically by the presence of gradual vascular obliteration that occurs universally in all types of allografts, eventually leading to fibrotic changes and a decline in allograft function [68]. The term "chronic rejection" may actually be misleading, since it implies an exclusively immune pathogenesis. However, it is clear that both immune (alloantigen dependent) and non-immune (alloantigen-independent) factors are important and perhaps a better term to describe this entity would be "chronic allograft dysfunction". The relative contribution of either of these mechanisms is difficult to ascertain, since both immune and non-immune mechanisms can result in very similar patterns of tissue injury. Unfortunately, this entity has been resistant to current rejection therapies and results in the gradual loss of the allograft.

Undoubtedly the immune system plays a major role in the pathogenesis of chronic rejection. Immunologic parameters such as histocompatibility difference, acute rejection episodes and pre-sensitization have all been noted to have an adverse effect on allograft survival [69]. Recurrent episodes of acute cellular rejection, particularly if severe or late, have been clearly demonstrated to be a risk factor for the development of acute rejection. In contrast, freedom from acute rejections has been shown to be protective from the development of chronic allograft dysfunction [70]. In this setting, it is felt that although the numbers of allograft-infiltrating T lymphocytes diminish after an acute event, they and the cytokine products that they elaborate may continue to provide a smoldering low-grade immunologic response and subsequent indolent injury. Thus, chronic rejection may result from inadequately treated acute rejection episodes. The fact that protocol biopsies in patients with no allograft dysfunction often show focal inflammatory lesions is suggestive proof of such a process [71].

An alternative hypothesis suggests that immune regulatory mechanisms that actually have been induced to prevent acute rejection may paradoxically promote the chronic process. In this theory, the cytotoxic Th1-like response is inhibited, resulting in a predominant Th2 type immune reaction. Although this tends to down-regulate the cytotoxic response, it does support the production of immunoglobulin resulting in antibody-mediated allograft response [72]. Lending support to this theory is the fact that IgG deposits may be seen in vessel walls during chronic rejection and that donor-specific antibody may be found in the circulation of such individuals. However, it is not clear whether the presence of such antibodies is causally related to allograft dysfunction.

In recent years, increasing attention has been paid to the influence of alloantigen-independent factors in the etiology of chronic rejection. It has been clearly demonstrated that syngeneic kidney transplants may develop histopathological lesions that resemble those of chronic rejection, although the time period over which such lesions develop is usually longer than in allogeneic models [73]. This suggests that these lesions may develop independently of allogeneic immune reactions. Non-immune parameters such as delayed renal allograft function, donor age and even brain death due to stroke have been demonstrated to have a powerful influence on allograft survival [74]. In fact, it has been estimated that these factors may have as powerful effect on allograft survival as HLA mismatch. What is particularly interesting is that many of these factors have also been shown to influence the progression of chronic renal disease in native kidneys. The common denominator of all these factors is the induction of injury and subsequent inflammation. Since chronic rejection has been predominantly studied in renal allografts, the following comments will pertain primarily to this model.

Subjecting a kidney to ischemia produces both morphologic and immuno-histochemical changes that are comparable to those found in allografts with chronic rejection. Similarly, prolonged cold ischemia (preservation) and warm ischemia (re-anastomosis) in a renal allograft are risk factors for long-term survival, particularly in the setting of delayed allograft function [75]. The early lesions of ischemic renal injury consist not only of acute tubular necrosis but also of inflammatory changes that result in the increased expression of MHC Class I and II molecules in tubular and interstitial cells respectively. Injury could therefore increase the probability of rejection and subsequent rejection could further induce inflammation, perpetuating the so-called "injury triangle" [76]. Another key factor that may influence early allograft function is injury due to brain death itself. Although little is known about the systemic effects of brain death, recent work by Tilney et al. suggests that a massive release of inflammatory mediators, cytokines and adhesion molecules into the circulation of such individuals could occur, potentially altering the phenotype of the donor vascular endothelium [77].

Effect of Nephron Mass

Aside from injuries in the donor at the time of transplantation, certain pre-existing chronic conditions in the donor may also have a significant influence on the long-term function of the allograft. Donor age itself is a strong predictor of poor long-term allograft outcome and lesions of chronic rejection appear to be more common in donors of older age. In renal transplantation, the effects of donor aging appears to be due to decreased "nephron dose", in which an inadequate nephron mass is postulated to be a risk factor for progression to chronic rejection [78]. The percentage of sclerosed glomeruli increases from 5 percent in the fourth decade to 10–30% in the eight decade. Therefore, the use of the older and "marginal" donor may affect the input quality of the transplanted tissue where it has been suggested that the effects of donor age may explain about 30 percent of the variance in kidney transplant outcomes beyond one year. The nephron-dosing hypothesis may also be applied to scenarios in which there is a significant size disparity between donor and recipient or to explain the improved survival of female recipients of gender-mismatched cadaveric renal allografts. Although these observations do highlight the importance of nephron number on transplant survival, the effects are small compared with the effects of donor age and delayed allograft function.

Other Factors in Chronic Rejection

Hyperlipidemia, toxicity from immunosuppressive drugs and infectious complications, particularly cytomegalovirus (CMV) infections, also contribute to chronic rejection. The prominence of vascular lesions in chronic rejection and some pathologic similarities to atherosclerosis has led to the suggestion that lipid abnormalities may contribute to the process of chronic rejection [79,80]. Immunosuppressive drugs may affect the long-term function of renal allografts by either inadequately suppressing the alloimmune response or by producing side-effects which histologically resemble chronic rejection [81]. The nephrotoxic effects of the calcineurin inhibitors (cyclosporine and tacrolimus) have been well described. Both drugs enhance the transcription and secretion of transforming growth factor-β (TGF-β) in a variety of cell types including T-cells, proximal tubular cells and fibroblasts. TGF-β promotes the accumulation of extracellular matrix and the production of type IV collagen, thus contributing to the interstitial fibrosis seen in allografts experiencing chronic rejection [82].

Clinical transplant data in both liver and heart transplantation supports a link between CMV infection and the development of chronic rejection [83,84]. CMV infection is associated with coronary re-stenosis [85] and in heart transplant patients and allograft atherosclerosis appears to develop earlier and with greater frequency in patients who have had associated CMV infection. A causal connection is not clear, since patients often develop CMV infection following an episode of acute rejection and therefore, are more likely to have experienced severe rejection.

Strategies to Prevent Chronic Rejection

Chronic rejection remains the most important cause of allograft loss in long-term studies with a prevalence rate ranging from 10 to 80 percent in renal transplant patients, depending on the duration of follow-up. It remains one of the major challenges facing transplant physicians today. Immunosuppressive therapy is generally ineffective, except perhaps in those patients who have been inadequately immunosuppressed due to overzealous tapering of drug therapy or non-compliance. Fortunately, there appears to be room for optimism. Using data obtained through the United Network for Organ Sharing, Hariharan et al. have recently demonstrated that since 1988, there has been a substantial increase in both short- and long-term survival of kidney allografts from both living and cadaveric donors [86]. Between 1988 and 1996, the one-year survival rate for both living donors (88.8–93.9%) and cadaver allografts (75.5–87.7%) improved significantly. Subsequently, the estimated half-life for allografts from living donors increased steadily from 12.7 to 21.6 years and that for cadaveric allografts increased from 7.9 to 13.8 years. The improvement is not attributable to any of the newer immunosuppressive drugs, since it took place in an era where maintenance immunosuppressive medications consisted of cyclosporine, azathioprine and prednisone. Rather, it reflects a reduction in the rate of acute rejection that has resulted in lower rates of allograft failure due to chronic rejection. Interestingly, Hariharan and colleagues also found that the cold-ischemia time and the titer of serum panel reactive antibodies in recipients have decreased overtime, which may have contributed to the lower rates of acute rejection in this cohort of patients. What is perhaps overlooked in this study is the contribution of better clinical care of non-immunologic risk factors, including perhaps better treatment of hypertension and hyperlipidemia and more effective prophylaxis or treatment of serious infectious complications.

Tolerance

The ultimate goal of transplantation research would be the creation of an environment where the recipient would accept an allograft without immunosuppression and remain immunocompetent so as not to become susceptible to infection and cancer. Additionally, achieving tolerance would solve the problem of chronic allograft rejection that affects the majority of transplanted organs. Several animal models have been developed, particularly in the past five years, where limited exposure to immunosuppression at the time of engraftment results in donor-specific hyporesponsiveness (tolerance). These models vary in their methodologies and in the robustness of the "tolerance" achieved. Some of the experimental mechanisms are discussed below along with the potential mechanisms through which tolerance might be achieved (Table 5.4).

For many years tolerance models were based on the creation of a state of hematopoietic chimerism [87]. Indeed, the tolerance observed to skin allografts in cattle by Sir Peter Medawar was the result of blood group and presumably bone marrow-derived blood elements shared between freemartin cattle. These cows share a common placenta in utero, allowing prenatal exposure to non-self antigens during the period of thymic selection of T lymphocyte clones. Fraternal twins become blood group chimeras and as adults can accept skin grafts from one another. Medawar and colleagues subsequently published a model of acquired neonatal tolerance in which experimental, in utero exposure to alloantigen (splenocytes) produced animals that were tolerant to skin allografts after birth [88]. Tolerance has only been achieved in humans in rare case reports of patients who underwent bone marrow transplantation for hematologic disorders and subsequent renal engraftment from the bone marrow donor [89].

However, the transplanted organ may itself produce a form of microchimerism where small numbers of donor and recipient leukocytes become intermingled

Table 5.4.   Mechanisms of tolerance induction*

Deletion (Apoptosis)
Thymic deletion — Neonatal tolerance induction, intrathymic injection of allogeneic cells, whole alloantigen or donor MHC peptides.
Peripheral deletion — Bone marrow chimeras, mixed hematopoietic chimerism (with or without myeloablation, lymphoid irradiation).
Suppression (Immune deviation)
Th1 → Th2 shift (favoring IL-4, IL-10, IL-13)
T suppressor cells
Veto cells — inactivate/delete alloreactive T-cells
Anergy (Inactivation)
Costimulatory blockade (CD28, CD154)
Donor-specific blood transfusions
Bone marrow infusion with or without ALG

*Although individual hypotheses have been proposed to explain tolerance, the mechanism of experimental tolerance is usually multifactorial and may, in fact, involve some or all of these events.

Two-Way Paradigm (Organ)

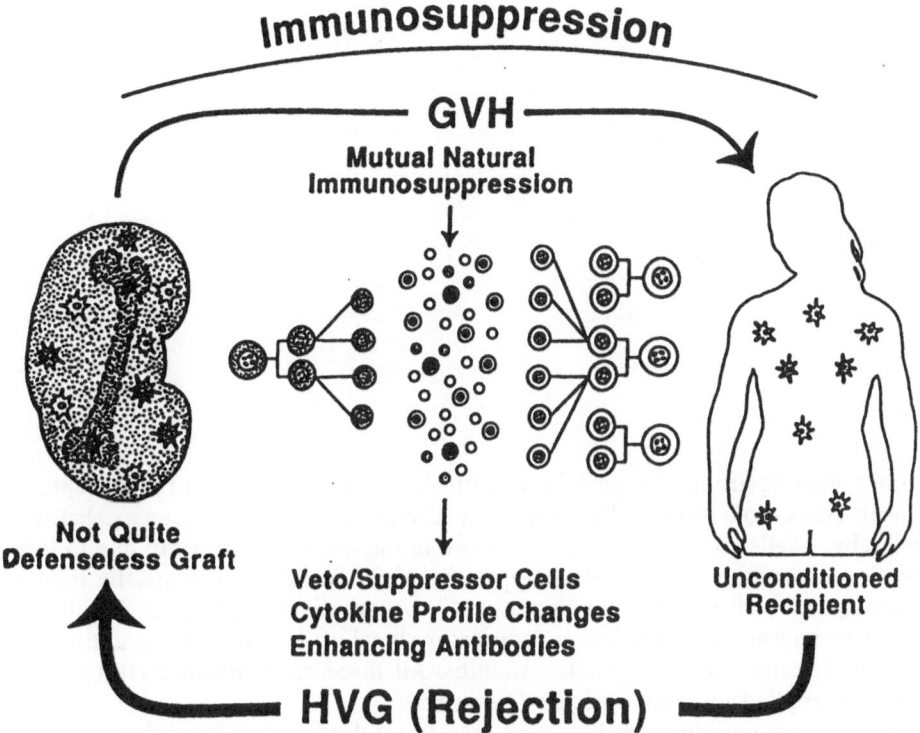

Figure 5.7. Microchimerism, establishing a microscopic (cellular) presence of the donor in host lymphoid compartments, has been postulated as a mechanism for allograft acceptance, accommodation and possibly tolerance. Bone marrow-derived donor leukocytes in the allograft infiltrate the host and can be identified by sensitive staining methodologies even many years following organ transplantation. These cells may contribute to overall immunosuppression through as yet poorly defined immunologic mechanisms possibly involving suppressor cell activity or alterations in the cytokine milieu that promote anergy. Along with the recipient immune system these cells participate in bidirectional "cross-talk", which on one axis leads to a host-versus-graft (HVG) reaction while simultaneously donor cells participate in graft-versus host (GVH) reaction (Starzl TE, Rao AS, Trucco M, et al. Explanation for loss of the HLA matching effect. Transplant Proc 1995;27:57–60).

throughout the allograft and the lymph compartments. This exchange of donor and recipient APCs, particularly of the dendritic type, may play a role in acceptance or accommodation toward the allograft [90] (Figure 5.7). Although, this is a weak form of allograft acceptance, microchimerism may play a role in the long-term survival of allografts, in the ability to reduce immunosuppression and in the absence of chronic rejection noted in some transplant recipients. Nonetheless, at this time, tolerance to an allograft cannot be routinely achieved in humans.

Tolerance to self arises in utero and occurs mainly through deletion of T-cell clones in the thymus. The presentation of self-antigen to developing thymocytes capable of responding results in their destruction (apoptosis). The remaining T-cell repertoire, (approximately 10 billion cells), is capable of recognizing and becoming activated by non-self antigens. Experimentally, deletion of reactive T-cell

Table 5.5. Progression toward tolerance

Allograft environment	Immunosuppression	Current status
New allograft	High	All transplants
Accommodation	Moderate	Humans
HLA matched	Low	6-Ag match kidneys
Microchimerism	Low	Some allograft recipients
		Liver > kidney, heart
Mixed hematopoietic chimerism	Low	Animal models
Donor-specific unresponsiveness	Low	Animal models
		Multiple experimental mechanisms
Tolerance	None	Rodent and primate models
Robust tolerance	None	Rodents; no response to repeat challenge with donor antigen (skin graft, e.g.)

clones may occur in the periphery (outside the thymus) and produce antigen-specific unresponsiveness. Tolerance may also arise from suppressor mechanisms, whereby T-cells encounter antigen, but are not activated presumably due to intervention of immunomodulatory (suppressor) cells that downregulate the immune response (so-called "immune ignorance"). Alternatively, activated T-cells may either be anergized or produce a suppressor signal after encountering antigen and become tolerized to that specific stimulus. All three mechanisms have been successfully applied in animal models (Table 5.5).

The early experiments of Medawar created a tolerance based on the deletion of specific alloreactive clones. In utero exposure to antigen in the form of bone marrow-derived cells results in the thymic deletion of reactive T-cell clones. In rodents, exposure to donor antigen by thymic injection of mature animals, with a short course of immunosuppression, has led to donor-specific tolerance. Even islet cells, whose transplantation remains an elusive goal in clinical transplantation, can be successfully engrafted with these protocols [91]. Unfortunately, thymic injection is not practical in human transplantation where end-organ disease presents in adulthood after the thymus has involuted and reactive clones of T-cells have already been selected.

All strategies for tolerance in humans must eliminate or make unresponsive a set of T-cell clones in the periphery that are already programmed to respond to a specific foreign antigen as well as prevent their reappearance from bone marrow-derived stem cells. T-cell-APC interactions offer several strategies for tolerance induction. Blocking cytokine production or cytokine-induced T-cell activation or T-cell proliferation are the mechanisms of our present maintenance immunosuppressive armamentarium. However, mechanisms that abrogate immune responsiveness or promote suppressor responses may lead to donor-specific tolerance. The requirements for immunosuppression are highest when an allograft is initially placed. Acute rejection rates are lower in the period 3–6 months after transplantation and are less than 5 percent thereafter. The current practice of immunotherapy reflects this process of host accommodation to the allograft.

Induction with antibodies directed against TCRs offer some protection against acute rejection early after transplantation. In time, doses of maintenance immunosuppression are reduced as the host becomes accommodated to the allo-grafted tissue. HLA matched or 2-haplotype matched kidneys are another way of weakening the immune reaction with attendant decreases in immunosuppressive requirements. The recognition of microchimerism after solid organ transplanta-tion in humans has also suggested a mechanism for the accommodation of allo-grafts. Starzl has proposed that leukocytes became interchanged between the allograft and the host compartments (bloodstream, lymph nodes, liver, spleen). This provides an environment for immunologic "cross-talk" and results in some measure of graft acceptance. This is supported by the demonstration of micro-chimerism in some individuals greater than 20 years following organ transplanta-tion and the excellent function of some of these allografts even in the absence of immunosuppression. Furthermore, the concept fits well with clinical observation regarding liver transplantation. Immunosuppressive requirements, in general, are lower for liver allografts than other solid organ transplants. Many patients can be maintained successfully on one immunosuppressive drug after liver transplanta-tion. The liver is transplanted with a large source of allogeneic leukocytes (lym-phoid cells, antigen presenting cells, Kupffer cells) that can interact with host immune cells and promote allograft acceptance. Whether this involves suppressor mechanisms, apoptosis of reactive lymphoid clones or immunologic fatigue is not known. In contrast, skin allografts are more immunogenic than solid organ trans-plants. Skin allografts are commonly rejected in animal models treated with immunosuppressive regimens that are adequate for solid organ transplantation. However, donor-specific skin grafts can be accepted in some animals that have been "tolerized" by a previous solid organ transplant [92]. While skin allografts are difficult to maintain, possibly owing to the high numbers of dendritic (Lan-gerhan's) cells, liver allografts are tolerogenic in animal models [93] and possibly in multi-organ transplantation in humans [27].

Tolerance remains an elusive goal in human transplantation. However, true tol-erance has been achieved in rodent models of hematopoietic chimerism and donor-specific unresponsiveness based on T-cell anergy (from oral, intravenous or intrathymic injection of donor MHC antigens). Interestingly, the development of tolerance by co-stimulatory blockade also requires T-cell activation by IL-2 [94] and INF-γ [95] and stimulated T-cells are more susceptible to apoptosis. T-cells activated in the setting of co-stimulatory blockade, progress to activation-induced cell death (AICD), which results in the depletion of reactive T-cell clones and anergy [96]. An intriguing observation has been that preventing early T-cell activation with standard immunosuppressive agents abrogates tolerance by inter-fering with the MHC-TCR response (signal 1). This experimental observation has not been noted with sirolimus (rapamycin) which functions downstream from signal 1 events [97,98].

Hale et al. have recently described an attractive model of allograft tolerance [98]. These investigators added a brief course of sirolimus to the anti-lymphocyte globulin donor-specific bone marrow protocol of Monaco and colleagues [99] to produce tolerance to strongly immunogenic skin allografts across a complete his-tocompatibility mismatch. The advantage of this protocol was that tolerance was achieved without the use of irradiation for cytoablation. Cytoreduction induced by anti-lymphocyte globulin, reconstitution with donor bone marrow and a short course of sirolimus produced multilineage chimerism. Skin grafts on animals administered an adequate dose of donor bone marrow survived indefinitely and the complete absence of an immune response to repeat challenge with donor skin indicated a robust form of tolerance. This protocol could easily and safely be applied to human solid organ transplantation. Live donor renal transplantation offers an ideal opportunity for recipient conditioning with donor hematopoietic cells proximate to the transplant event.

Recent experimental models have achieved long-term allograft acceptance in primates even after discontinuing immunosuppression. While earlier primate experiments applied successful strategies from rodent models, (bone marrow ablation followed by reconstitution), newer models have invoked lymphoid depletion by antibodies or co-stimulatory blockade at the time of alloantigen presentation, with encouraging results [100,101]. Prolonged co-stimulatory blockade with anti-CD154 (monthly injection for 5 months) in nine MHC-mismatched monkeys resulted in well functioning kidneys with no evidence of acute rejection after more than one year [102]. Interestingly, standard immunosuppression interfered with the response to anti-CD154 and 5/11 monkeys treated with immunosuppressive drugs developed acute rejection. These studies provide some optimism for eventually achieving tolerogenic immunosuppressive regimens in humans without the toxicity associated with myeloablation and immune reconstitution. However, anti-donor antibodies have developed in all of these models, often resulting in chronic rejection. Furthermore, few of the researchers have placed donor skin grafts on "tolerant" animals or challenged them by administering pro-inflammatory cytokines to test the strength of the tolerance achieved.

References

1. Snell GD. Methods for the study of histocompatibility genes. J Genetics 1948;49:87–108.
2. Brent L. A history of transplantation immunology. San Diego: Academic Press, 1997.
3. Medawar P. Memoir of a thinking radish. New York: Oxford University Press, 1986.
4. Merrill JP, Murray JE, Harrison JH, et al. Successful homotransplantation of the kidney between nonidentical twins. N Engl J Med 1960;262:1251–60.
5. Rogers BO. The relation of immunology to tissue homotransplantation. Ann N Y Acad Sci, 1955; 59:277–466.
6. Doherty PC, Zinkernagel RM. A biological role for the histocompatibility antigens. Lancet 1975;1:1406–9.
7. Chicz RM, Urban RG, Lane Ws et al. Predominant naturally processed peptides bound to HLA-DR1 derived from MHC-related molecules are heterogenous in size. Nature 1992;358:764–768.
8. Bjorkman PJ, Saper MA, Samraoui B et al. Structure of the human class I histocompatibility antigen, HLA-A2. Nature 1987;329:506–12.
9. Germain RN. MHC-dependent antigen processing and peptide presentation: providing ligands for T lymphocyte activation. Cell 1994, 76: 287–99.
10. Nicholls SM, Bradley BB, Easty DL. Effects of mismatches for MHC and minor antigens on corneal graft rejection. Invest Ophthalmol Vis Sci 1991;32:2729–34.
11. Sano Y, Streilein JW, Ksander BR. Detection of minor alloantigen-specific cytotoxic T-cells after rejection of murine orthotopic corneal allografts. Tx 1999;68:963–70.
12. Candinas D, Gunson BK, Nightingale P, et al. Sex mismatch as a risk factor for chronic rejection of liver allografts. Lancet 1995;346:1117–21.
13. Dallman MJ. Cytokines as mediators of organ graft rejection and tolerance. Curr Opinion in Immunol 1993;5:788–93.
14. Valujskikh A, Matesis D, Heeger PS. Characterization and manipulation of T-cell immunity to skin grafts expressing a transgenic minor antigen. Transplantation 1999;68:1029–36.
15. Roopenian DC, Davis AP, Christianson GJ, et al. The functional basis of minor histocompatibility loci. J Immunol 1993;151:4595–4605.
16. Terasaki PI, Cecka JM, Gjertson DW, et al. High survival rates of kidney transplants from spousal and living unrelated donors. N Engl J Med 1995;333:333–6.
17. Helderman JH, Goral S. The allocation of cadaver kidneys. N Engl J Med 1999;341:1468–9.

18. Opelz G, Wujciak T. Cadaveric kidneys should be allocated according to the HLA match. Transplant Proc 1995;27:93-7.
19. Gruessner A, Sutherland DER. Pancreas transplantation in the US and non-US as reported to the UNOS and International Pancreas Transplant Registry (IPTR). In: Cecka JM, Terasaki PI, editors. Clinical Transplants. Los Angeles: UCLA Tissue Typing Laboratory, 1996; 47-68.
20. U.S. Scientific Registry of Transplant Recipients and the Organ Procurement and Transplantation Network. 1999 Annual report, Washington, DC: Department of Health and Human Services, 1999.
21. Bunce M, Young NT, Welsh KI. Molecular HLA typing — the brave new world. Transplantation 1997;64:1505-13.
22. Prasad VK, Heller G, Kernan NA, et al. The probability of HLA-C matching between patient and unrelated donor at the molecular level. Transplantation 1999;68:1044-50.
23. Thompson JS, Thacker LR. CREG matching for first kidney transplants performed by the SEOPO. Clinical Transplantation 1996;10:586-93.
24. Opelz G, Terasaki PI. Dominant effect of transfusion on kidney graft survival. Transplantation 1980;29:153-5.
25. Opelz G. Improved kidney graft survival in nontransfused recipients. Trans Proc 1987;19:149-52.
26. Alexander JW, Light JA, Donaldson LA, et al. Evaluation of pre- and post-transplant donor-specific transfusion/cyclosporine A in non-HLA identical living donor kidney transplant recipients. Transplantation 1999;68:1117-24.
27. Morrissey PE, Gordon F, Shaffer D, et al. Combined liver-kidney transplantation in patients with cirrhosis and renal failure. Liver Transplant Surg 1998;4:363-9.
28. Patel R, Terasaki PI. Significance of the positive cross-match test in kidney transplantation. N Engl J Med 1969;280:735-9.
29. Reinsmoen NL, Kaufman D, Matas A, et al. A new in vitro approach to determine acquired tolerance in long-term kidney allograft recipients. Transplantation 1990;50:783-90.
30. Steilein JW, Strome P, Wood PJ. Failure of in vitro assays to predict accurately the existence of neonatally induced H-2 tolerance. Transplantation 1989;48:630-4.
31. Rygaard J. Skin allografts in nude mice. Acta Path Microbiol Scand 1974;82:93-104.
32. Gorer PA. The antigenic basis of tumor transplantation. J Pathol Bacteriol 1938;47: 231-52.
33. Von Boehmer H, Swat W, Kisielow P. Positive selection of immature ab T cells. Annu Rev Immunol 1993;135: 67-80.
34. Gorman RN, Margulies DH. The biochemistry and cell biology of antigen processing and presentation. Annu Rev Immunol 1993;11:403-50.
35. Lotze MT, Thomson AW, editors. Dendritic cells: biology and clinical applications. San Diego: Academic Press, 1999;1-733.
36. Steptoe RJ, Thomson AW. Dendritic cells and tolerance induction. Clin Exp Immunol 1996;105:397-402.
37. Sayegh M, Turka L. The effect of T-cell costimulatory activation pathways in transplant rejection. N Engl J Med 1998;338:1813-21.
38. Sherman AL, Chattopadhyay S. The molecular basis of allorecognition. Annu Rev Immunol 1993;11:385-402.
39. Shoskes DA, Wood KJ. Indirect presentation of MHC antigens in transplantation. Immunology Today 1994;15:38.
40. Gould DS, Auchincloss HJ. Direct and indirect recognition: the role of MHC antigens in graft rejection. Immunol Today 1999;20:77-82.
41. Lechler RI, Batchelor JR. Restoration of immunogenicity to passenger cell-depleted kidney allografts by the addition of donor strain dendritic cells. J Exp Med 1982;155:31-41.
42. Shirwan H. Chronic allograft rejection. Do the Th2 cells preferentially induced by indirect alloantigen recognition play a dominant role? Transplantation 1999;68:715-26.
43. Auchincloss HJ, Lee R, Shea S et al. The role of "indirect" recognition in initiating rejection from skin grafts from MHC class II-deficient mice. Proc Natl Acad Sci USA 1993;90:3373-7.
44. Bradley JA, Mowat AM, Bolton EM. Processed MHC class I alloantigen as the stimulus for CD4+ T cell-dependent antibody-mediated graft rejection. Immunol Today 1992;13:434-8.
45. Cramer DV, Qian S, Harnaha J, et al. Cardiac transplantation in the rat. I. The effect of histocompatibility differences on graft atherosclerosis. Transplantation 1989;47:414-9.
46. Garboczi DN, Ghosh P, Utz U, et al. Structure of the complex between human T-cell receptor, viral peptide and HLA-A2. Nature 1996;384:134-41.
47. Cantrell D. T cell antigen signal transduction pathways. Annu Rev Immunol 1996;14:259-74.
48. Schwartz RH. A cell culture model for T lymphocyte clonal anergy. Science 1990;248:1346-56.
49. Lenschow DJ, Walinus TL, Bluestone JA. CD28/B7 system of T cell costimulation. Annu Rev Immunol 1996;14:233-58.

50. Mosmann TR, Coffman RL. Th1 and Th2 cells: different patterns of lymphokine secretion lead to different functional properties. Annu Rev Immunol 1989;7:145–73.
51. Dallman MJ, Shiho O, Page TH, et al. Peripheral tolerance to Alloantigen results from altered regulation of the interleukin 2 pathway. J Exp Med 1991;173:79–87.
52. Bugeon L, Cuturi M-C, Hallet M-M, et al. Peripheral tolerance of an allograft in adult rats-characterization by low interleukin -2 and interferon-g mRNA levels and by strong accumulation of major histocompatibility complex transcripts in the allograft. Transplantation 1992;54:219–25.
53. Mueller R, Davies JD, Krahl T, Sarvetnick N. IL-4 expression by allografts from transgenic mice fails to prevent allograft rejection. J Immunol 1997;159:1599–603.
54. Strom TB, Roy-Chaudhury Pm, Manfro R, et al. The Th1/Th2 paradigm and the allograft response. Curr Opin Immunol 1996;8:688–93.
55. Steiger J, Nickerson PW, Seurer W, et al. IL-2 knockout recipient mice reject islet cell allografts. J Immunol 1995;155:489–98.
56. Williams GM, Hume DM, Hudson RPJ, et al. "Hyperacute" renal allograft rejection in man. New Engl J Med 1969;280:735–9.
57. Furges O, Morris RJ, Dallman MJ. Spontaneous acceptance of liver allografts in the rat: analysis of the immune response. Transplantation 1994;57:171–7.
58. Perlmann P, Holm G. Cytotoxic effects of lymphoid cells in vitro. Adv Immunol 1969;11:117–93.
59. Tilney NL, Strom TB, MacPherson SG, et al. Surface properties and functional characteristics of infiltrating cells harvested from acutely rejection cardiac allografts in inbred rats. Transplantation 1975;20:323–30.
60. Mason DW, Dallman MJ, Arthur RP, et al. Mechanisms of allograft rejection: the roles of cytotoxic T cells and delayed-type sensitivity. Immunol Rev 1984;77:167–84.
61. Woodruff M. The transplantation of homologous tissue and its surgical applications. Ann R Coll Surg Eng 1952;11:173–95.
62. Bishop GA, Hall BM, Duggin GG, et al. Immunopathology of renal allograft rejection analyzed with monoclonal antibodies to mononuclear cell markers. Kidney Int 1986;29:708–17.
63. Wever PC, Buonstra JC, Laterveer JC, et al. Mechanisms of lymphocyte-mediated cytotoxicity in acute renal allograft rejection. Transplantation 1998; 66:259–64.
64. Dunnill MS. Histopathology of rejection in renal transplantation. In: Morris PJ editor. Kidney transplantation: principles and practice. 2nd ed. New York:Grace and Stratton 1984;355–82.
65. Cecka JM, Terasaki PI. The UNOS scientific renal transplant registry. In: Terasaki PI, Cecka JM, editors. Clinical transplants. Los Angeles: UCLA Tissue, Typing Laboratory; 1994:1–18.
66. Hosenpud JD, Novick PT, Breen TJ, et al. The registry of the International Society for Heart and Lung Transplantation: eleventh official report, 1994. J Heart Lung Transplant 1994;13:561–70.
67. Ludwig J, Wiesner RH, Batts KP, et al. The acute vanishing bile duct syndrome (acute irreversible rejection) after orthotopic liver transplantation. Hepatology 1987;7:476–83.
68. Paul LC, Hayry P, Foegh M, Dennis MJ, et al. Diagnostic criteria for chronic rejection/accelerated allograft atherosclerosis in heart and kidney transplants: joint proposal from the fourth Alexis Carrel Conference on Chronic Rejection and Accelerated Arteriosclerosis in Transplanted Organs. Transplant Proc 1993;25:2022–23.
69. Halloran PF, Melk A, Barth C. Rethinking chronic allograft nephropathy: The concept of accelerated senescence. J Am Soc Nephrol 1999;10:167–81.
70. Kahan BD. Toward a rational design of clinical trends in immunosuppressive agents in transplantation. Immunol Rev 1993;136:29–49
71. Shoshes DA, Wood KJ. Indirect presentation of MHC antigens in transplantation. Immunol Today 1994;15:32–8.
72. Hutchinson IV. Immunological mechanisms of long-term allograft acceptance. In: Paul LC, Solez K, editors. Organ transplantation: Long-term Results. New York: Marcel, Dekker, 1992; 1–31.
73. Tullius SG, Heemann U, Hancock WW, et al. Long-term kidney isografts develop functional and morphologic changes which mimic those of chronic allograft rejection. Ann Surg 1994;220:425–32.
74. Ojo AO, Wolfe RA, Held PF, Port FK et al. Delayed allograft function: Risk factors and implications for renal allograft survival. Transplantation 1997;63:968–74.
75. Cecka JM, Cho YW, Terasaki PI. Analyses of the UNOS Scientific Renal Transplant Registry at three years — early events effecting transplant success. Transplantation 1992;53:59–64.
76. Goes N, Urmson J, Ramassen V, Halloran PF. Ischemic acute tubular necrosis induces an extensive local cytokine release. Transplantation 1995;59:565–72.
77. Terasaki PI, Cecka JM, Gjertson DW, et al. High survival rate of kidney transplants from spousal and living unrelated donors. N Engl J Med 1995;333:333–6.

78. Gjertson DW. A multifactor analysis of kidney allograft outcomes at one and five years post-transplantation: 1996 UNOS update. In: Clinical Transplants 1996. editors. Cecka JM, Terasaki PI. Los Angeles: ULCA Tissue Typing Laboratory, 1997; 343–60.
79. Massy ZA, Kasiske BL. Post-transplant hyperlipidemia: mechanisms and management [review]. J Am Soc Nephrol 1996;7:971–7.
80. Guijarro L, Massy ZA, Kasiske BL. Clinical correlation between renal allograft failure and hyperlipidemia. Kidney Int 1995;48:S56–9.
81. Massy ZA, Guijarro C. Wiederkehr MR. Chronic renal allograft rejection: Immunologic and non-immunologic risk factors. Kidney Int 1996;49:518–24.
82. Skuda C, Longuino LR, Ruoslahti E, et al. Elevated expression of transforming growth factor β and prostacyclin expression in experimental glomerulonephritis. J Clin Invest 1996;86:453–62.
83. O'Grady JC, Sutherland S, Harvey F, et al. Cytomegalovirus infection and donor/recipient HLA antigens: Interdependent cofactors in pathogenesis of vanishing bile duct syndrome after liver transplantation. Lancet 1988;2:302–5.
84. Gao SZ, Hunt SA, Schroeder JS, et al. Early development of accelerated allograft coronary artery disease: Risk factors and course. J Am Coll Cardiol 1996;28:673–9.
85. Zhou YF, Leon MB, Waclawiw MA, et al. Association between prior CMV infection and the risk of restenosis after coronary atherectomy. N Engl J Med 1996;335:624–30.
86. Hariharan S, Johnson CP, Bresnahan BA, et al. Improved allograft survival after renal transplantation in the United States, 1988–1996. N Engl J Med 2000;342:605–12.
87. Jankowski RA, Ildstad ST. Chimerism and tolerance: from freemartin cattle and neonatal mice to humans. Hum Immunol 1997;52:155–61.
88. Billingham R, Brent L, Medawar P. Actively acquired tolerance of foreign cells. Nature 1953;172:603–6.
89. Sayagh MH, Fine NA, Smith JL et al. Immunologic tolerance to renal allografts after bone marrow transplants from the same donor. Ann Int Med 1991;114:954–5.
90. Starzl TE, Demetris AJ, Murase AJ, et al. Cell migration, chimerism and graft acceptance. Lancet 1992;339:1579–82.
91. Posselt AM, Odonco JS, Barker CF, et al. Promotion of pancreatic islet allograft survival by intra-thymic transplantation of bone marrow. Diabetes 1992;41:771–5.
92. Bishop GA, Sun J, DeCruz DJ, Rokahr KL, et al. Tolerance to rat liver allografts III. Donor cell migration and tolerance-associated cytokine production in peripheral lymphoid tissues. Immunol 1996;156:4925–31.
93. Kamada N, Davies HS, Roser B. Reversal of transplantation immunity by liver grafting. Nature 1981;292:840–2.
94. Lenardo MJ. Interleukin-2 programs mouse alpha-beta T lymphocytes for apoptosis. Nature 1991;353:858–61
95. Konieczny BT, Dai Z, Elwood ET, et al. IFN-gamma is critical for long-term allograft survival induced by blocking the CD28 and CD40 ligand T cell costimulation pathways. Immunol 1998;160:2059–64.
96. Larson C, Pearson T. The CD40 pathway in allograft rejection, acceptance and tolerance. Curr Opin Immunol 1997;9:641–7.
97. Li Y, Zheg XX, Li XC et al. Combined costimulation blockade and rapamycin but not cyclosporine produces permanent engraftment. Transplantation 1998;66:387–8.
98. Hale DA, Gottschalk R, Umemura A et al. Establishment of stable multilineage hematopoietic chimerism and donor-specific tolerance without irradiation. Transplantation 2000;69:1242–51.
99. Wood ML, Orosz CG, Gottschalk R, Monaco AP. The effect of injection of donor bone marrow on the frequency of donor reactive CTL in antilymphocyte serum-treated, grafted mice. Transplantation 1992;54:665–9.
100. Armstrong N, Buckley P, Oberley T et al. Analysis of primate renal allografts after T-cell depletion with anti-CD3-CRM9. Transplantation 1998;66:5–13.
101. Kirk AD, Harlan DM, Armstrong NN et al. CTLA4-Ig and anti-CD40 ligand prevent renal allograft rejection in primates. Proc Natl Acad Sci USA 1997;94:8789–94.
102. Kirk AD, Burkly LC, Batty DS et al. Treatment with humanized monoclonal antibody against CD154 prevents acute renal allograft rejection in nonhuman primates. Nature Med 1999;5:686–93.

6. Immunosuppressive Therapy in Solid Organ Transplantation

Nick Torpey, J. Andrew Bradley and John J. Fung

Introduction

In the early days of transplantation, no effective immunosuppressive agents were available and early attempts to perform kidney transplantation between individuals who were not genetically identical failed because of acute rejection. The breakthrough came in 1959 when Schwartz and Dameshek discovered the immunosuppressive properties of 6-mercaptopurine and Calne went on to show that azathioprine (AZA), one of its derivatives, was able to prevent rejection of canine kidney allografts. Azathioprine alone was not sufficient to prevent human kidney allografts from rejecting but when combined with corticosteroids it was possible to achieve 50 percent 1-year graft survival. This was a remarkable achievement and for the next twenty years AZA plus steroids, (sometimes supplemented with polyclonal anti-lymphocyte antibodies), remained the standard immunosuppressive therapy after renal transplantation.

The next major advance came in the late 1970s with the discovery of the novel immunosuppressive agent Cyclosporin A (CyA) by Borel at the Sandoz (now Novartis) laboratories. The potent immunosuppressive properties of CyA in organ transplantation were demonstrated by Calne and White in Cambridge England and it quickly became the mainstay of immunosuppressive regimens for the next two decades. The combination of CyA, AZA and steroids not only resulted in 80 percent 1-year graft survival after renal transplantation, but for the first time allowed cardiac and hepatic transplantation to be undertaken with good clinical results.

During the 1990s tacrolimus became available and challenged the place of CyA as the principal immunosuppressive agent for preventing graft rejection. Mycophenolate mofetil (MMF), sirolimus and monoclonal antibodies to the interleukin-2 receptor have also recently been licensed for clinical use. These newer agents have all been subjected to randomized controlled trials to determine their efficacy in organ transplantation and the transplant surgeon and physician no longer have to rely on a single immunosuppressive regimen for all patients. It is now possible to tailor immunosuppression to suit the clinical needs of the recipient, although this approach is still at a relatively early stage of development.

In this chapter we describe those immunosuppressive drugs currently used in human organ transplantation, outline their mode of action, pharmacology and adverse effects, and discuss the consequences of long-term immunosuppression. Chapter 7 should be read along with this chapter for a suggested rationale of combination therapy during rejection episodes of solid organ transplants.

Immunosuppressive Agents

Allograft rejection is mediated by T-lymphocyte dependent effector mechanisms. After activation CD4 and CD8 T cells undergo proliferation and clonal expansion. This is dependent on the availability of IL-2 and other T cell growth factors released by T helper cells. Such cells play a central role in allograft rejection and are able, through the release of cytokines, to orchestrate the immunological effector mechanisms responsible for rejection. Key cytokines include T cell growth factors such as IL-2, IL-4 IL-7 and IL-15 together with pro-inflammatory cytokines such as interferon-γ (IFN-γ) and tumor necrosis factor-α (TNF-α). Cytotoxic T cells, delayed type hypersensitivity responses (DTH) and alloantibody responses may all contribute to acute rejection.

Immunosuppressive agents can be classified according to the point at which they act in the process of T cell activation and clonal expansion (Figure 6.1). Most

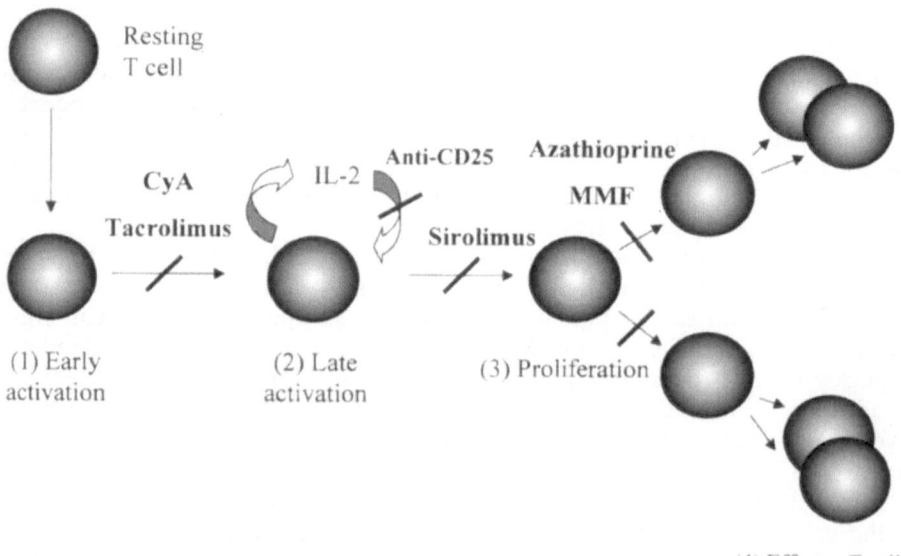

Fig. 6.1. Site of action of immunosuppressive agents (1) Resting T cells respond to donor MHC, either directly on graft antigen presenting cells (APC) or indirectly as peptides presented by recipient APC. (2) Antigen-activated T cells secrete IL-2 and express the IL-2 receptor. (3) T cell growth factors promote clonal expansion of activated T cells (4). These cells develop effector functions (for example as cytotoxic T lymphocytes), secrete pro-inflammatory cytokines that recruit other immune cells, and promote B cell production of alloantibody (4). The sites of action of CyA, tacrolimus, anti-CD25 antibodies, sirolimus, azathioprine and MMF are shown. Steroids and polyclonal anti-lymphocyte antibodies act at multiple sites.

contemporary immunosuppressive regimens use a combination of agents with different modes of action. The risk of acute rejection is highest in the first few weeks after transplantation and accordingly the number and dose of immunosuppressive agents is highest at the time of transplantation ("induction therapy"). As the risk of acute rejection declines immunosuppressive therapy is reduced so as to minimize side-effects ("maintenance therapy"). Immunosuppressive therapy cannot, however, be withdrawn completely without risking graft loss from rejection and maintenance therapy is therefore continued indefinitely.

Calcineurin Inhibitors: (Cytokine Suppressive Agents)

When a T lymphocyte is activated by antigen, a coordinated program of multiple gene activations is set in motion; this program eventually leads to the proliferation of the activated T cell. CyA and tacrolimus block the transcription of 10 genes of at least 60 that are activated in the T cell. Some of these include IL-2, IL-3 and IL-4, granulocyte-macrophage colony-stimulating factor and interferon-gamma. The inhibition of the production of IL-2 is their key effect and has been extensively studied [1-3]. These drugs are known to block the activation of the IL-2 gene by interfering with the binding of specific transcription factors to the promoter (control region) of IL-2, preventing RNA synthesis.

Cyclosporin

Pharmacology

CyA is a lipid soluble cyclic peptide produced by the fungus *Tolyplocadium inflatum* (Figure 6.2(a)). The drug is insoluble in water and the oral bioavailability is about 30 percent, with considerable variability (range = 10–60%) [4]. Hepatic metabolism is the only significant elimination mechanism and drug alteration is via the cytochrome P450 IIIA enzymes [5]. At least 17 metabolites are identifiable and at least a few are immunosuppressive although of considerably less potency than the parent compound. CyA, in common with tacrolimus and sirolimus, has many clinically important interactions with drugs sharing cytochrome p450 (CYP 3A4) metabolism (Table 6.1).

Co-administration of a large list of interactive drugs can cause unexpected increased or decreased serum levels by induction, or by competitive inhibition of P450. For these reasons, it is essential that levels be monitored regularly and that dosage is adjusted accordingly [6]. Bioavailability has been a particular problem with the original formulation of CyA (Sandimmun®), which was dependent on bile salts for absorption. Cyclosporin microemulsion (Neoral®) has more predictable pharmacokinetics and has replaced Sandimmun worldwide in both adult and pediatric transpantation. Neoral® does not require bile excretion for its bioavailability and is better dispersed and absorbed when compared with CyA. The relative bioavailability of Neoral, compared with Sandimmune is increased between 74 percent and 139 percent [7] and the total AUC is increased by 30 percent [8]. Once absorbed, CyA is extensively bound to red blood cells and plasma proteins with only 5 percent of the drug free in plasma. The metabolites of CyA are excreted in the urine.

Both the immunosuppressive action and side-effects of CyA are dependent on its blood concentration. Unpredictable absorption, metabolism, distribution and

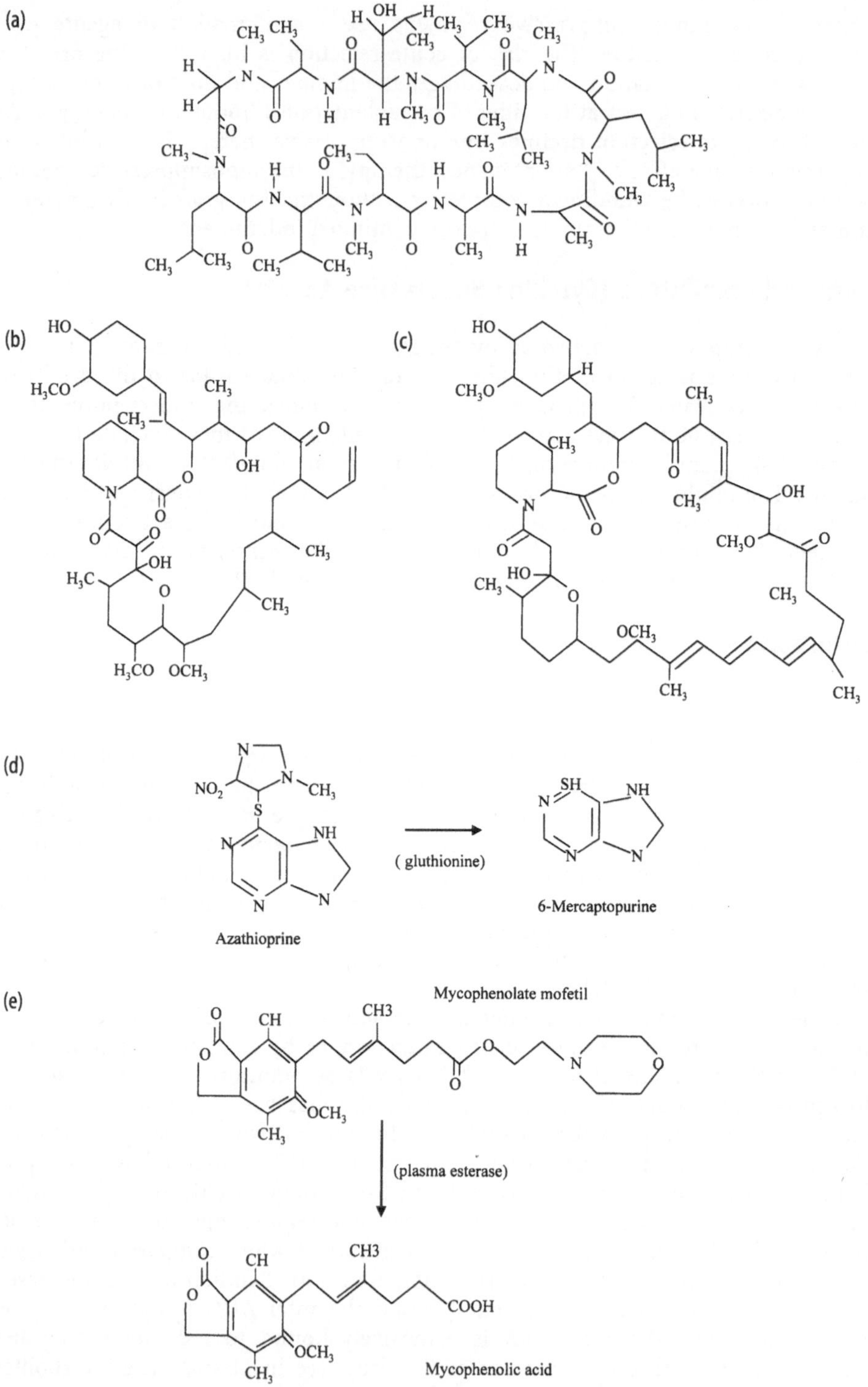

Figure 6.2. Structure of chemical immunosuppressive agents. (a) Cyclosporin A. (b) Tacrolimus. (c) Sirolimus. (d) Azathioprine and 6-Mercaptopurine. (e) MMF.

Table 6.1. Drugs that induce or inhibit CYP3A4. Drugs that induce activity of CYP3A4 reduce the bioabailability of cyclosporin, tacrolimus and sirolimus, whereas inhibition of CYP3A4 reduces their metabolism and increases bioavailability

Inducers of CYP3A4
Carbamazepine
Phenytoin
Phenobarbitone
Rifampicin
Sulphonamides (if given IV)
Inhibitors of CYP3A4
Macrolide antibiotics
Ketoconazole and other — azole antifungals
Diltiazem and Verapamil
Progestogens
Cimetidine
St Johns Wort
Grapefruit juice

excretion mean that monitoring CyA levels in whole blood is essential. This is most precisely achieved by calculating the area under the blood concentration-time curve (AUC, Figure 6.3), which measures total CyA exposure following an oral dose. Such measurements have been shown to predict doses that prevent acute rejection without causing acute drug toxicity, [9,10] but require multiple carefully timed blood samples making this method impractical for routine clinical use. Most units rely on trough CyA levels, which for Sandimmun correlate poorly with AUC measurements. In patients taking Neoral, trough levels may be more representative of the AUC levels, [11] and there is evidence that 2 hour post-dose levels (C_2), which may be more predictive of AUC could be more reliable in predicting efficacy in both heart [12] and liver [13] transplant recipients.

Mode of Action

The immunosuppressive action of CyA is to prevent antigen-specific T cell activation and the molecular basis of this effect is well understood [14,15] (Figure 6.4). CyA enters T cells and binds to the cytoplasmic protein cyclophilin — a member of the immunophilin family. The resulting CyA/cyclophilin complex inhibits the activity of the calcium/calmodulin dependent phosphatase calcineurin, (PP2B-protein phosphatase 2B), thus preventing the de-phosphorylation of the cytoplasmic subunit of the transcription factor NF-AT (nuclear factor of activated T cells). NFAT increases the affinity of other transcription factors for binding to the enhancer domains of T cell-specific genes which encode for T cell cytokines such as IL-2, IL-3 and IL-4, IFN-γ and TNF-α. By preventing NF-AT translocation, CyA inhibits the expression of these cytokines and exerts a potent immunosuppressive effect on T ymphocytes. In contrast to IL-2, the expression of TGFβ is enhanced in the presence of CyA. TGFβ inhibits T cell activation but may also promote renal fibrosis, one of the consequences of long term CyA treatment [16].

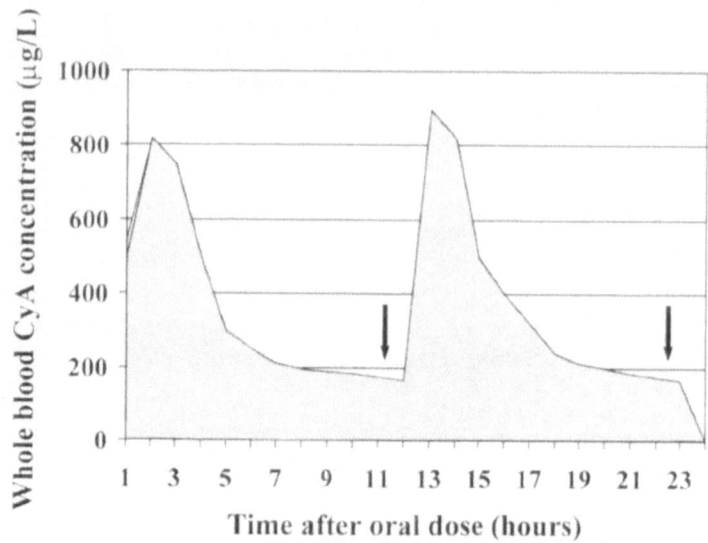

Figure 6.3. Whole blood CyA concentration following oral administration. Total CyA exposure is derived by calculating the area under the concentration-time curve (AUC — shaded area). Arrows indicate "trough" CyA levels.

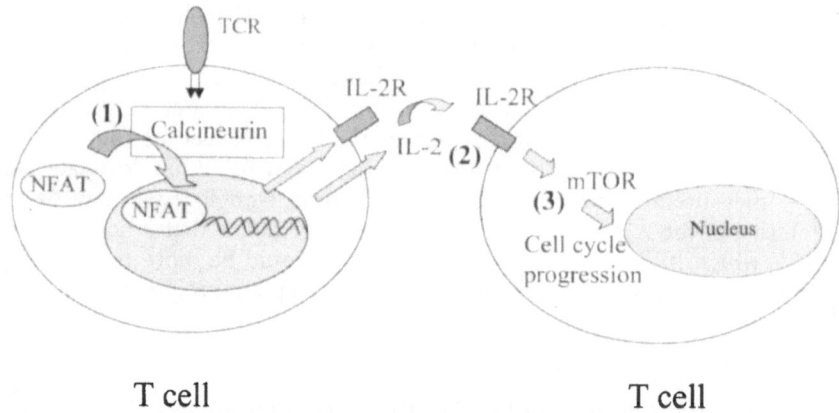

Figure 6.4. T-cell activation. Ligation of the T-cell receptor (TCR), accompanied by ligation of T-cell costimulatory molecules by ligands on APC, leads to Ca^{++}-dependent activation of the phosphatase calcineurin, dephosphorylation of NF-AT and upregulation of IL-2 and IL-2Rα gene expression (and the genes for many other cytokines). 1–2, acting in either autocrine or paracrine fashion, stimulates protein synthesis and T cell proliferation at least in part by activation of the phosphatase mTOR. (1) Calcineurin inhibition by cyclosporin and tacrolimus. (2) Blockade of IL-2 receptor by anti-CD25 antibodies (3) mTOR inhibition by sirolimus.

Adverse Effects

All drugs that non-specifically suppress the immune system increase the risk of infection and malignancy (vide infra). Table 6.2 lists other adverse effects of CyA. Nephrotoxicity is the most important, particularly in renal transplantation and is probably the result of renal ischaemia caused by CyA-induced vasoconstriction of

Table 6.2. Side effects of pharmacological immunosuppressive agents

	Cyclosporin	Tacrolimus	Rapamycin	Azathioprine	MMF	Steroids
Hypertension	+++	++	+	−	−	++
Dyslipidaemia	++	+		−	−	++
Diabetes	+		−	−	−	+++
Nephrotoxic	+++		−	−	−	−
Neurotoxic	Tremor Fits Neuropathy (all +)	Tremor Fits Neuropathy (all +++)	Headache	−	−	Psychiatric symptoms
Blood	HUS (rare)	HUS (rare)	Anaemia Leucopenia ↓↓ platelets	Anaemia Leucopenia ↓ platelets	Anaemia Leucopenia ↓ platelets	
Cosmetic	Hirsuitism Gingival hyperplasia	Alopecia (rare)	−	−	−	Obesity Bruising
Other	↑K$^+$	↑K$^+$	↓ wound healing Rashes GI upset	GI upset Pancreatitis	GI upset Diarrhoea Teratogenic	Cataract Pancreatitis Osteoporosis

the afferent arterioles with progressive renal fibrosis in between 15–40% of patients. [17–19] CyA levels are usually high in acute nephrotoxicity but may not be so in chronic CyA nephrotoxicity.

Hypertension, which frequently develops within weeks of commencing therapy, [20] hyperkalaemia and fluid overload often accompany both acute and chronic nephrotoxicity and each may mimic renal allograft rejection. For this reason a renal biopsy is often necessary to confirm the diagnosis of CyA nephrotoxicity. Native kidneys are also adversely affected by CyA with up to 10 percent of other organ recipients treated with CyA (or tacrolimus) developing dialysis-dependent renal failure [21,22].

Minor neurotoxicity (tremor) is common (10–55%) and many patients improve over time without a change in therapy. More severe symptoms such as seizures have also been associated with CyA [23] and hypomagnesemia and hypocholes-terolemia are believed to be risk factors for CyA neurotoxicity. CyA is diabeto-genic, although analysis of this effect is confounded by the frequent concomitant use of steroids. Hepatotoxicity, manifested by an increased cholestatic tendency, may be quite common, but a reduction in dosage often improves this effect and it does not appear to be a major clinical problem.

Rarely, CyA may cause haemolytic-uraemic syndrome, leading to acute renal failure. In addition to hypertension, CyA also promotes an atherogenic lipid profile, leading to increased cardiovascular risk. Cosmetic connective tissue side-effects of CyA are common and can be distressing to the patient. These include hirsutism, gingival hyperplasia and coarsening of the facial features [24].

Tacrolimus

Pharmacology

Tacrolimus (FK 506, Prograf) is a macrolide antibiotic isolated from the bacterium *Streptomyces tsukubaenis* (Figure 6.2b). Although structurally distinct from CyA its immunosuppressive properties are very similar and mediated through calcineurin inhibition. In terms of the suppression of alloimmunity, tacrolimus appears to have more immunosuppressive efficacy than CyA. Clearly, tacrolimus is a highly effective immunosuppressant; clinical trials have validated less rejection in tacrolimus-based immunosuppressive regimens when compared with CyA-based immunosuppressive regimens [25–36]. One reason for the greater efficacy of tacrolimus over CyA may lie in the relative resistance of tacrolimus to p-glycoprotein counter-transport, which lowers intracellular levels of such drugs.

Tacrolimus is well absorbed, but like CyA, bioavailability is very variable (5–60%) because of extensive cytochrome p450 metabolism. Unlike CyA, however, trough levels of tacrolimus correlate well with AUC measurements and a high trough level predicts toxicity, particularly in patients with hepatic dysfunction [37–39]. Surprisingly, however, there is no evidence that monitoring tacrolimus levels leads to reduced rates of acute rejection. Both CyA and tacrolimus have a plasma half-life of about 12 hours and are administered in two daily doses 12 hours apart. Both can be given intravenously at 30 percent of the oral dose.

Mode of Action

Tacrolimus, like CyA, binds to immunophilins in the cell cytoplasm. These are known as FK binding proteins (FKBPs), of which there are several isoforms; FKBP12 being the most important. Like CyA/cyclophilin, tacrolimus/FKBP12 inhibits calcineurin activity (Figure 6.4). In addition, tacrolimus exhibits additional immunosuppressive effects independent of NF-AT inhibition, at least in vitro [14,15].

Adverse Effects

The common adverse effects of tacrolimus are shown in Table 6.2. Nephrotoxicity is comparable to CyA [40–42]. The incidence of long-term renal injury, as seen with CyA, is at present unknown. Tacrolimus is more likely than CyA to cause neurotoxicity [43], particularly tremor, parasthesia and occasionally fits, but is largely free of cosmetic side-effects. Although hypertension and hyperlipidaemia may occur less frequently with tacrolimus than CyA, there is a significant incidence of diabetes mellitus following treatment with tacrolimus. In two trials comparing CyA and tacrolimus in renal transplantation, diabetes occurred in 12 percent and 20 percent of the tacrolimus-treated patients compared with 2 percent and 4 percent of those receiving CyA [33,44]. Black patients treated with tacrolimus seem to be particularly at risk of developing diabetes [44]. Gastrointestinal side-effects include diarrhea and anorexia, which is similar to that seen with other macrolide antibiotics, such as erythromycin.

Which Calcineurin Inhibitor?

The introduction of tacrolimus into clinical practice provided the first real alternative to CyA as the principal immunosuppressive agent in organ transplantation.

Many studies have compared the two medications. Two large prospective randomized trials have compared tacrolimus with CyA (Sandimmun) as part of combination therapy in renal transplantation [33,44]. Both followed patients for one year following transplantation and both showed a reduction in biopsy-proven acute rejection from 45 percent in the CyA group to 25–30% with tacrolimus and a significant reduction in the incidence of severe rejection requiring anti-lymphocyte antibody treatment. There was no difference in patient or graft survival or in serum creatinine at the end of the study. Long-term follow up is awaited. Neither study compared tacrolimus with Neoral, which is more effective than Sandimmun in preventing both single and multiple episodes of acute rejection [45]. Nevertheless it seems likely that tacrolimus is slightly more potent than Neoral, based on trials in recipients of other organ transplants (vide infra) and the effect of tacrolimus to "rescue" severe rejection in patients already taking CyA [46].

Tacrolimus and CyA (Sandimmun) have been compared in two large trials in liver transplantation [29,30]. Tacrolimus resulted in a significant reduction in acute rejection and reduced the number of episodes of severe or refractory rejection. An as yet unpublished study comparing tacrolimus with Neoral (the TMC study) confirms the benefit of tacrolimus and importantly demonstrates a survival advantage in tacrolimus-treated patients at 6 months post-transplantation. Studies in heart and lung transplantation also suggest reduced rates of acute rejection with tacrolimus [47]. After lung transplantation, tacrolimus may improve both 1 and 3 year survival when compared with CyA [48] and may be more effective in preventing the development of obliterative bronchiolitis [49].

Sirolimus (Rapamycin, Rapamune®)

Pharmacology

The use of Sirolimus has been approved for use in kidney transplantation as an adjunct to CyA-based immunosuppression [50,51]. Sirolimus is a macrolide isolated from the bacterium *Streptomyces hygroscopicus*. The organism was first recovered from a soil sample from Easter Island (Rapa Nui, hence Rapamycin). Sirolimus is structurally related to tacrolimus (Figure 6.2(c)) and also binds to FKBP12, but has a distinct immunosuppressive action. Sirolimus is well absorbed and is a substrate for p-glycoprotein counter-transport and it is extensively metabolised by the same cytochrome p450 enzyme responsible for CyA and tacrolimus metabolism, resulting in bioavailability of only 15 percent. It is sequestered in erythrocytes and has a half-life of about 65 hours, allowing once-daily dosing but making a loading dose necessary. Trough sirolimus levels and AUC measurements correlate well with low and high levels, predicting rejection and toxicity respectively [52]. In a large US study sirolimus was successfully given at two fixed doses in combination with CyA without routine monitoring of sirolimus levels [53]. Care should be taken when sirolimus and CyA are used in combination because each drug increases blood concentration of the other. To avoid toxicity, the two agents can be administered four hours apart or be given together with careful monitoring of blood levels. Sirolimus, like tacrolimus and CyA, has many important drug interactions (Table 6.1).

Mode of Action

Sirolimus inhibits DTH and both B and T cell responses to alloantigen. It binds to FKBP12 without inhibiting calcineurin activity. Instead the sirolimus/FKBP complex inhibits the activity of the protein kinase mTOR (mammalian target of rapamycin). mTOR is an important part of the signaling pathways activated by IL-2 and other cytokines and controls the activity of at least three regulatory molecules important for protein synthesis [15] (Figure 6.4). mTOR inhibition prevents the initiation of protein synthesis (by blocking the activity of the 5 cap-binding protein eIF-4E) and by blocking ribosomal activity (preventing phosphorylation of riboso-mal S6 protein via p70S6 kinase). Sirolimus inhibits the activity of both D and E-type cyclins. This has the net effect of blocking T cell proliferation in response to IL-2 and other T cell growth factors. The immunosuppressive effects of calcineurin inhibitors and sirolimus are complimentary. CyA and tacrolimus inhibit the first phase of T cell activation, preventing progression of the cell cycle from G0 to G1. Sirolimus acts immediately down stream, blocking progression from the G1 to the S phase. Although tacrolimus and sirolimus both bind to the same immunophilin, they may still be used together, because FKBP12 is present to excess in T cells [54].

Adverse Effects

Sirolimus causes dose-dependent hypercholesterolaemia, hypertriglyceridaemia and thrombocytopenia (Table 6.2). Leukopenia and anaemia are less common as is anorexia, vomiting, diarrhea, diabetes mellitus and testicular atrophy. In vitro, sirolimus inhibits the proliferation of fibroblasts and smooth muscle cells, which may explain the impaired wound healing and excess of lymphoceles observed in clinical trials (52). Sirolimus has been implicated in rare cases of interstitial pneumonitis. It is not nephrotoxic, but may exacerbate the nephrotoxic effects of CyA (vide infra).

Hypertension, nephrotoxicity and hepatotoxicity have not been reported[1] [55].

Sirolimus or Calcineurin Inhibitors?

Two prospective, randomized studies have compared sirolimus and CyA (Neoral), each given as part of triple therapy regimens in combination with prednisolone and azathioprine/MMF [57,58]. Patient and graft survival was equivalent after 1 year of follow up. Although acute rejection rates were not significantly different between the sirolimus and CyA groups, there was a trend for greater use of bolus steroids to treat acute rejection in those patients on sirolimus. Despite this, graft function (as measured by serum creatinine levels and estimated creatinine clear-ance) was better in the sirolimus groups.

An alternative approach is to take advantage of the synergistic immunosuppres-sive effects of sirolimus and CyA and to use both agents together. A recent large US study randomised renal transplant recipients to receive 2mg sirolimus, 5mg sir-olimus or AZA in combination with CyA (Neoral) and prednisolone [53]. Results at six months showed an impressive reduction in acute rejection to 17 percent and 12 percent in the two sirolimus groups compared to 30 percent with AZA. Patient and graft survival was similar in all groups, but surprisingly those patients on sirolimus had significantly higher serum creatinine levels, (possibly because sirolimus

---

1 SDZ RAD, 40-0-(2-hydroxyethyl)-rapamycin, is a rapamycin analog which acts by inhibiting growth factor-driven cell proliferation [56]. Although it has less in vitro activity compared with sirolimus, it has similar immunosuppressive properties when given orally.

enhances CyA nephrotoxicity). The full results of several studies in which sirolimus and CyA are initially given in combination, but where the CyA dose is subsequently reduced or eliminated, are awaited. Preliminary data suggest that this strategy results in low rates of rejection and improved renal function. There is little data on the use of sirolimus with tacrolimus [54], although this combination was used in a recent successful series of pancreatic islet transplants [59].

Anti-proliferative Drugs

Agents commonly used for immunosuppression in this class include the anti-metabolites, such as azathioprine (AZA) [60] and mycophenolate mofetil (MMF). Interference with purine metabolism is known to cause immunosuppression, thus, not surprisingly, these agents are most toxic to proliferating cells that are making new DNA. In the past and on occasion in present times, the use of alkylating agents, such as cyclophosphamide and methotrexate have also been used as immunosuppressants. These agents differ from AZA and MMF in that they non-specifically damage cellular macromolecules by alkylating them, particularly DNA; being toxic to all actively dividing cells.

Azathioprine (AZA)

AZA has been used as an immunosuppressive agent both in organ transplantation and many inflammatory and autoimmune diseases for almost forty years. It has also been used in numerous maintenance immunosuppressive regimens. Prior to the advent of cyclosporine-CyA, AZA was used in conjunction with corticosteroids as the mainstay of immunosuppression, however, it has no usefulness in the treatment of acute rejection episodes. Since the advent of CyA and tacrolimus, AZA has been relegated to an adjunctive role, generally in combination with either agent. The addition of AZA to either tacrolimus or CyA-based regimens may allow for reduction of dosages of these agents with resultant decreased side effects due to CyA or tacrolimus.

AZA is an inactive pro-drug (Figure 6.2(d)). It is well absorbed after oral administration and converted in the liver to 6-mercaptopurine, which is further metabolized by most cell types (Figure 6.5(a)). It is an imidazole derivative of 6-mercaptopurine which is the active metabolite following hepatic and erythrocyte metabolism.

The principal immunosuppressive activity of AZA depends on metabolism to thioguanine nucleotides [15]. Thioguanine nucleotides are incorporated into and damage DNA and RNA, thus causing inhibition of transcription and arrest of cell proliferation [61]. Alternatively, 6-mercaptopurine can be metabolised by thio-purine methyltransferase (TPMT) to thio-inosinic acid. This is an important route of drug elimination, although methyl-thioinosine monophosphate inhibits the enzyme PRPP synthase, thus inhibiting de novo purine synthesis (Figure 6.5(a) and 6.5(b)). The 6-thioguanine nucleotides (TGN) are known to incorporate into DNA, although the altered molecule is not stable allowing strand breaks in the chromosomes. The final inactive end metabolite is 6-thiouric acid, which is excreted by the kidneys.

TPMT activity is determined by a genetic polymorphism. About 1:300 patients are homozygous for a low activity allele and are at risk for severe myelosuppression. Tests to determine TPMT genotype are available but not used widely in routine clinical practice [62].

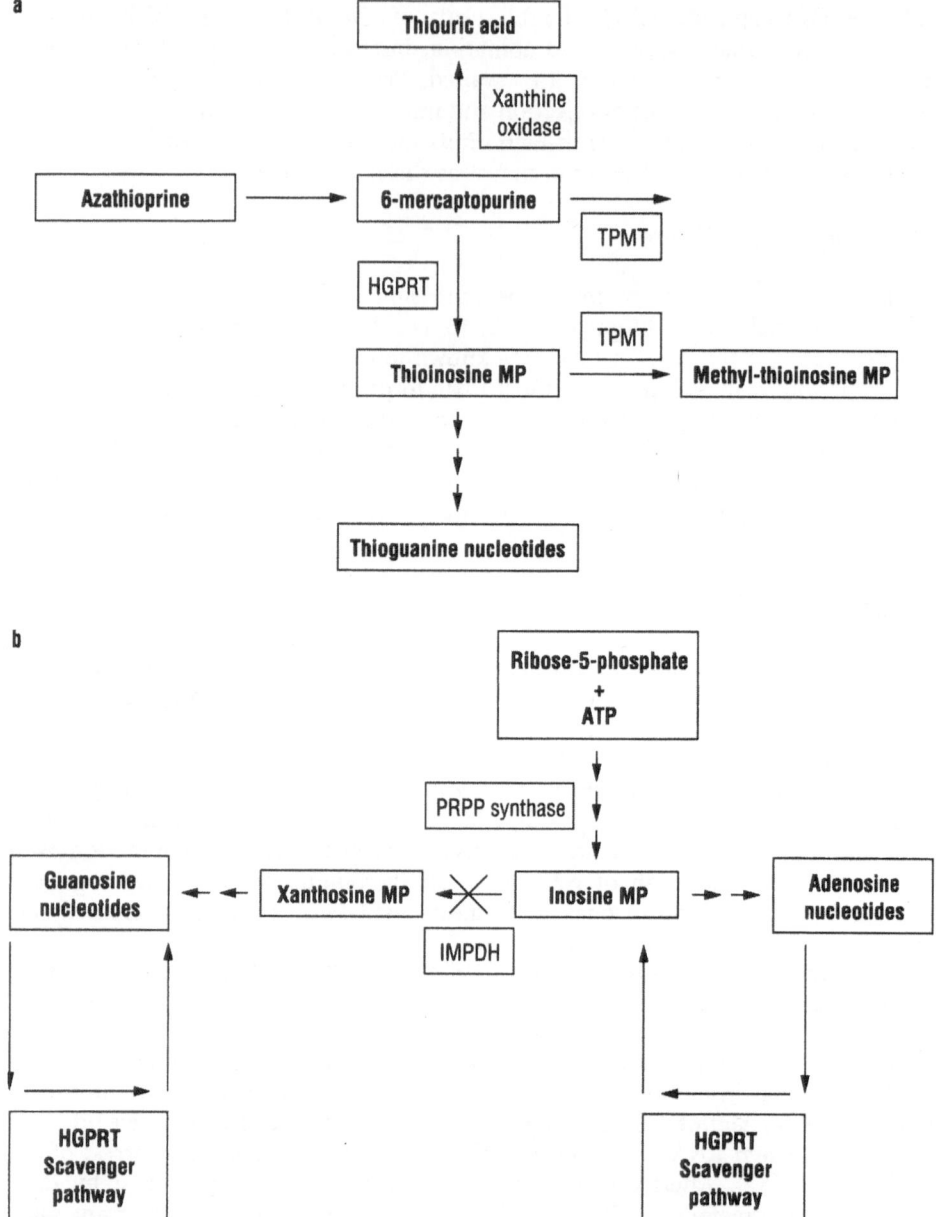

Figure 6.5(a) Metabolism of Azathioprine. Metabolism via xanthine oxidase and thiopurine methyl-transferase (TPMT) leads to inactivation of azathioprine and excretion of mostly inactive metabolites in urine. Metabolism via HGPRT to thioinosinc monophosphate (TIMP) leads to the generation of thioguanine nucleotides, the active metabolites of azathioprine. **(b)**. Action of mycophenolic acid (MPA). De novo purine synthesis is from ribose-5-phosphate and ATP via the enzyme 5-phosphoribosyl-1-pyrophosphate (PRPP) synthase, ultimately giving inosine monophosphate (IMP). IMP is metabolised to adenosine (ATP, dATP) and guanosine (GTP, dGTP) nucleotides. The rate-limiting enzyme in GTP/dGTP synthesis is inosine monophosphate dehydrogenase (IMPDH), which is inhibited by MFA. Rapidly proliferating T and B lymphocytes are unable to generate sufficient purine nucleotides via scavenger pathways and rely on de novo purine synthesis.

The main side effect of AZA is dose-limiting bone marrow suppression, which may be severe. For this reason it is important to monitor the full blood count closely, particularly for the first few weeks of treatment. Pancytopenia and thrombocytopenia with megaloblastic anemia is the pattern usually seen and deaths from bone marrow suppression have been reported. As with other anti-proliferative drugs, nausea, vomiting and hair loss may occur. AZA may also cause reversible acute cholestasis and rarely results in a severe veno-occlusive liver disease [63] and an interstitial pneumonitis. AZA therapy has also been associated with an increased risk of pancreatitis believed to be due to a hypersensitivity reaction [64]. Its use seems safe in pregnancy; as although it is mutagenic, fetal cells do not express the enzyme HGPRT (Figure 6.5(a)) and thus cannot produce potentially toxic thioguanine nucleotides.

The most important drug interaction is that between AZA and allopurinol. Metabolism of AZA via xanthine oxidase is an important route of drug elimination (Figure 6.5(a)). Because allopurinol inhibits xanthine oxidase it significantly increases the immunosuppressive and toxic effects of AZA, necessitating a 75 percent dose reduction. A safer approach in patients who need concurrent allopurinol treatment is to replace azathioprine with MMF. The usual starting dose of azathioprine is 1–2mg/kg.

Mycophenoloc Acid (MPA) and Mycophenolate Mofetil (MMF)

Mycophenolic acid (MPA) inhibits inosine monophosphate dehydrogenase, which is involved in the de novo synthesis of guanosine monophosphate. Mycophenolated motefil (MMF) is a relatively new immunosuppressive agent, but is already in widespread use [65–70]. It would be logical to use the drug in a fashion similar to AZA and the anti-proliferative effect may be more specific than AZA with less toxicity. The ability to block humoral responses effectively may make the drug specifically useful in antibody-mediated processes. MMF, like AZA, is a pro-drug form of MPA which was synthesized in an attempt to provide more stability and better bioavailability. (Figure 6.2(e)) It is well absorbed and rapidly hydrolyzed to the active compound MPA.

MPA is 90 percent bound to plasma proteins and is metabolised to inactive MPA glucuronide in the liver. MPA glucuronide is secreted into the bile and either reabsorbed and excreted in the urine or converted back to MPA by glucuronidases from gut flora. The result is increased exposure of the intestinal epithelia to MPA, accounting for the gastrointestinal side effects that are a common feature of MMF treatment. Most trials of MMF have used fixed dosing regimens, however, measurements of trough MPA levels and particularly MPA AUC values have shown a significant correlation between MPA exposure and acute rejection after kidney and possibly cardiac transplantation [71].

MPA is a non-competitive inhibitor of the enzyme inosine monophosphate dehydrogenase (IMPDH), which catalyses the rate-limiting step in the de novo synthesis of guanosine nucleotides (Figure 6.7(b)). Activated lymphocytes rely on de novo purine synthesis and upregulate the expression of the type II isoform of IMPDH, for which MPA has a high binding affinity. Hence MPA selectively inhibits the proliferation of activated lymphocytes. Unlike AZA, MPA is not mutagenic and spares other cell types that are able to utilise salvage pathways of purine synthesis. At a cellular level IMPDH inhibition has two effects. First, de novo production of guanosine nucleotides is blocked, preventing DNA and RNA

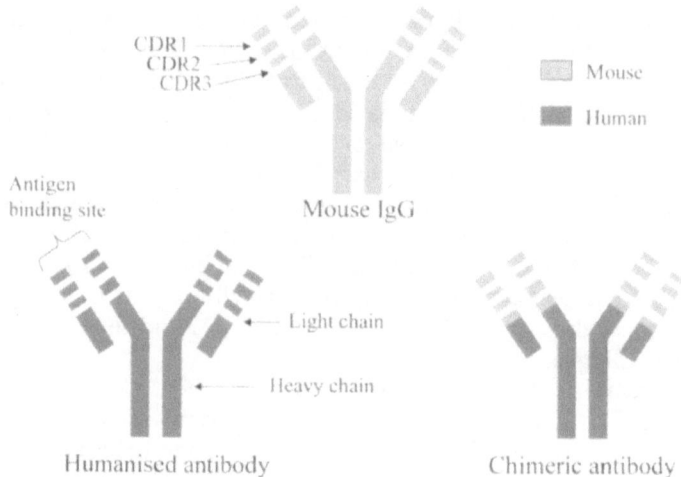

Figure 6.6. Engineered monoclonal antibodies. Murine antibodies can be engineered to make them less immunogenic. Humanized antibodies retain only murine complementarity determining regions (CDR) responsible for antibody specificity on a human Ig framework, whereas chimeric antibodies have murine variable regions and human constant regions.

synthesis. Second, there is a relative excess of adenosine nucleotides, which inhibit PRPP synthase and which further shuts down de novo purine synthesis (Figure 6.5(b)). In addition to T cell inhibition, MMF blocks antibody production by B-cells and inhibits smooth muscle cell proliferation.

Adverse effects of MMF are shown in Table 6.2. Gastrointestinal symptoms including nausea, vomiting and diarrhoea are common and generally resolve if the dose of MMF is reduced. MMF causes bone marrow suppression to a similar degree as AZA and patients treated with MMF are probably more likely to develop invasive CMV disease [72]. MMF is neither nephrotoxic nor hepatotoxic, but in animal studies, it may be teratogenic and should not be used in patients wishing to become pregnant.

Azathioprine or Mycophenolate?

Four important randomised trials have established MMF as a potent immunosuppressive agent in organ transplantation. Three trials in renal transplantation have used immunosuppression with Neoral and prednisolone and added either MMF or AZA [73,74], or MMF or placebo [67]. At six months, biopsy-proven acute rejection occurred in 38 percent, 35 percent and 46 percent of patients in the AZA/placebo groups respectively and in 20 percent, 20 percent and 17 percent of patients receiving MMF 2g daily. Patients in the MMF groups were significantly less likely to have severe or steroid-resistant rejection. MMF at a dose of 3g produced a similar reduction in the rate of rejection but with significantly more side-effects. 3 year follow-up of the Tricontinental MMF Renal Transplantation Study [74,76] and the European MMF Cooperative Study [67,77] suggest a trend towards improved graft survival in MMF-treated patients. Review of US renal registry data similarly demonstrates a trend to improved 4-year graft survival in MMF compared with AZA-treated patients (86% vs 82%)[78].

The fourth important study of MMF was in heart transplant patients [79]. A modest reduction in both the incidence and severity of acute rejection was associated with a reduced number of patient deaths at 1 year in MMF-treated patients (6%) compared with AZA-treated patients (11%). Similar results have been obtained in smaller trials of liver and lung transplant recipients [70].

Many other trials involving MMF have been published, particularly in renal transplantation. These include the use of MMF in combination with sirolimus [58], as a calcineurin inhibitor-sparing agent, in protocols to allow steroid withdrawal and as rescue therapy for refractory rejection [70]. Some of these trials are discussed in more detail.

Cyclophosphamide (CPM)

CPM has been used in place of AZA, particularly when there is suspected AZA-associated hepatitis. CPM is also the most widely used preparatory treatment for bone marrow transplantation. It is useful in high doses, both to incapacitate the recipient's immune system, (preventing rejection of grafted marrow) and in neoplastic diseases requiring marrow transplantation with effective chemotherapy.

Side-effects are considerably more common and serious with the high-dose therapy used for bone marrow transplantation. Virtually all patients experience nausea, vomiting and hair loss and as many as 15 percent of patients experience clinically significant cardiac dysfunction. Infertility has also been associated with these doses. Hemorrhagic cystitis is a well-known side effect of CPM, but the reported incidence is very variable (0.5–40%).

Corticosteroids

Synthetic glucocorticoids have been used as immunosuppressive agents in both induction and during maintenance therapy for more than 40 years. There are four principal glucocorticosteroid compounds used in transplantation: hydrocortisone, prednisone, prednisolone and methylprednisolone. Because hydrocortisone can only be given intravenously and possesses the greatest mineralocorticoid properties per unit of glucocorticoid activity, its routine application in transplantation has been relatively limited. The latter three agents have more glucocorticoid activity in proportion to their mineralocorticoid activity.

Most transplant units use oral prednisolone (or prednisone) and intravenous methylprednisolone, which are bio-equivalent and have little mineralocorticoid activity. Oral absorption is excellent and once in the circulation, glucocrticoids are 90 percent bound to plasma proteins. Free glucocorticoid readily diffuses across cell membranes. Metabolism is by hepatic p450 enzymes and although drugs that either induce or inhibit these enzymes influence clearance of glucocorticoids, the need for tailored dose-adjustment is uncommon.

Steroids have many effects on inflammation and the immune response [80]. Corticosteroids have broad effects including: 1) antagonism of inflammatory mechanisms by stabilization of lysosomal membranes and suppression of prostaglandin synthesis; decreasing capillary permeability and inhibiting histamine and bradykinin release; 2) decreasing lymphocyte and macrophage traffic and reducing absolute numbers of neutrophils and eosinophils and 3) inhibiting leukocyte adhesion to endothelium. They interfere with the production of IL-1 and IL-6, thus blocking the early steps of T cell activation. At high doses glucocorticoids are also inherently lympholytic. At therapeutic doses, glucocorticoids act through the cytosolic glucocorticoid receptor. The drug/receptor complex is translocated to the cell nucleus, where it activates the transcription of certain genes and inhibits others. Among those activated is the gene for I-κβ, which inhibits the activity of NF-κβ, an important transcriptional activator of the genes for many pro-inflammatory cytokines. Numerous other genomic effects of glucocorticoids have been described.

The overall effect is to down-regulate the expression of cytokines, chemokines and adhesion molecules, including IL-1, IL-2, IL-4, IL-6, IFN-γ, TNF-α, the IL-2 receptor, ICAM-1 and selectins. By this mechanism glucocorticoids inhibit T cell activation and proliferation at multiple levels, as well as interfere with macrophage and monocyte function. Very high doses of glucocorticoids (for example 250–1,000 mg methylprednisolone) have receptor-independent, non-genomic immunosuppressive effects. These effects occur rapidly and include the sequestration and lysis of circulating leucocytes and cytotoxic T lymphocytes. Used in this way, high dose intravenous methylprednisolone is the standard treatment for acute rejection and successfully reverses up to 75 percent of rejection episodes. (See Chapter 7).

As with all corticosteroids used in transplantation, the side-effects are numerous and well known, causing considerable morbidity (Table 6.2) [81,82]. Some are related to the total dose and duration of administration. An increased incidence of serious infections has been well documented in patients receiving corticosteroids. Impaired fibroblast growth and collagen synthesis contributes to poor wound healing; hence, surgical wounds and anastomoses are at increased risk for breakdown. Long-term use of steroids is of particular concern in transplant recipients, with increased risk of cardiovascular disease (hypertension, hyperlipidaemia and hyperglycaemia), bone disease (osteoporosis, avascular necrosis and growth retardation in children, secondary to suppression of the pituitary-adrenal axis) and cataracts or glaucoma. The use of high dose glucocorticoids, for example to treat acute rejection, may be associated with peptic ulceration, (in approximately 2%), pancreatitis and psychiatric disorders.

Hypertension may relate to the fluid retention properties of the synthetic corticosteroids. Soft-tissue and dermatologic changes such as fat redistribution, skin atrophy and striae produce the characteristic "Cushingoid" appearance. Although rare, acute adrenal insufficiency can develop unexpectedly if the patient is stressed, even up to 12 months after stopping steroids. Current immunosuppressive protocols aim to minimise steroid use and if possible to withdraw steroids in stable patients (See Chapter 7).

Immunosuppressive Antibodies

Polyclonal Anti-lymphocyte Antibodies [83]

The first immunosuppressive antibodies to enter clinical use were polyclonal anti-lymphocyte antibodies, produced by immunising animals (rabbits, goats and horses) with either purified thymocytes or lymphocytes. Antibodies cross-reacting with other cellular molecules in blood are generated but removed by extensive absorption to blood components. Several commercial preparations are currently

Table 6.3. Cambridge Protocol for Immunosuppression in Renal Transplantation

	Definition	Induction	Maintenance	FKI/CyA levels
High Risk	PRA > 85% and 1 or 2 DR mismatch	IL2R Antibody FK 0.1mg/kg po	FK 0.1mg/kg bd MMF Ig bd Pred 20mg	10–15 μg/L FK reducing to 5–10 μg/L at 1 yr
Medium Risk	PRA > 10% or 2 DR mismatch	IL2R Antibody FK 0.1mg/kg po	FK 0.1mg/kg bd Aza 1.5mg/kg Pred 20mg	10–15 μg/L FK reducing to 5–10 μg/L at 1 yr
Low Risk	All others	CyA 5mg/kg po	CyA 4mg/kg bd Aza 1.5mg/kg Pred 20mg	250–300 μg/L CyA reducing to 200–250 at 3 mo 150–200 at 6 mo 100–150 after 1 yr
Delayed Graft Function	Need for dialysis post operatively (except for ↑K⁺)	Half-dose FK/CyA and double-dose prednisolone Substitute MMF for azathioprine for 3 months In high risk group, consider course of ATG/OKT3		
Steroids		Aim for 5mg/day by 3 months. Possible reduction to 0mg in stable patients by 1 year		

PRA, panel reactivity; pred. prednisolone; rno, month; yr, year.

available and although known collectively as anti-thymocyte globulin (ATG), the potency and specificity to various T cell antigens differs between preparations.

ATG is administered as purified γ globulin, which contains a mixture of antibodies directed against many cell surface molecules on T and B cells, macrophages and natural killer (NK) cells. Binding of these antibodies to their cell surface antigens has a number of effects. Most importantly, antibody opsonisation leads to cell lysis and rapid depletion of both memory and activated T lymphocytes within 24 hours. In addition, antibody-mediated cross-linking of T cell receptors may cause partial activation and block the proliferative response to alloantigen [84].

The place of immunoglobulin therapy in immunosuppressive regimens is in a state of flux [85]. These agents were originally shown to be effective in the reversal of acute rejection. More recently, they have been introduced immediately after transplantation with this practice referred to as "prophylactic" or "induction" therapy. This use is based on the concept that early incapacitation of the immune system may theoretically reduce the propensity for subsequent rejection although this early intensification of immunosuppression is not universally accepted.

Apart from their use in induction therapy, they may be reserved for the treatment of severe or steroid-resistant acute rejection. Routine use of ATG in renal transplantation has not significantly improved long-term patient or graft survival, although there may be some benefit in patients considered at high risk for acute rejection [86–88]. Moreover, the potentially severe side effects of ATG and the impressive reduction in acute rejection episodes achievable with tacrolimus, MMF, sirolimus and anti-CD25 antibodies has made ATG induction therapy a less attractive option.

ATG is usually given as a 7–10 day course at a dose determined by the patients body weight. Monitoring the level of CD3⁺ lymphocytes in peripheral blood, which should be reduced to 50–100 cells/μl, allows for a significant reduction in dose, thus minimizing side-effects. ATG must be administered via a central vein to avoid thrombophlebitis. A very small number of patients may become sensitized to heterologous proteins from earlier exposure (e.g. equine hyperimmune tetanus immune globulin), although anaphylaxis occurs in fewer than 1 percent of patients. Nonetheless, a skin test prior to use is recommended. Polyclonal preparations cause a high incidence of reactions and the side-effects are related to the limitations of its heterologous nature and contaminating antibody specificities. There is often a "first-dose effect" of fever, rigors, headache, myalgias, arthralgias, serum sickness, thrombocytopenia and diarrhoea, probably related to cytokine release. Skin rash is also a fairly frequent occurrence (10–30%). ATG can cause neutropenia and thrombocytopenia, and increases the risk of early cytomegalovirus (CMV) infection. There is a 2–3 fold increase in the incidence of post-transplant lymphoproliferative disease (PTLD) in ATG-treated patients (vide infra).

Monoclonal Anti-lymphocyte Antibodies OKT3 (Orthoclone®, Muromonab-CD3)

Hybridoma technology has allowed the development of single-specificity monoclonal antibodies such as OKT3. These drugs are much more uniform, standardized and potent as immunosuppressants. For this use, OKT3 has been shown to be more effective than high doses of steroids. OKT3 is a murine IgG2a monoclonal antibody directed against CD3, a non-polymorphic component of the T cell receptor complex. OKT3 binding results in rapid activation and depletion of circulating T cells within minutes. Those cells that persist either have no surface expression of CD3 or have CD3 blocked by OKT3 binding with co-capping and internalization of the complex. In either case, the cells are non-functional. Like ATG, OKT3 is a powerful immunosuppressant when used for induction therapy and to treat acute rejection and has a similar side effect-profile. OKT3 is by far the most extensively studied of the monoclonal antibodies [89] and its current use is described below.

OKT3 is administered as a peripheral IV bolus. There is a profound first-dose effect necessitating pre-treatment with IV methylprednisolone, despite which fevers, rigors, headache, tachycardia, bronchospasm, elevation or depression of blood pressure and diarrhoea are common. In addition, there is a significant risk of pulmonary oedema (especially in fluid over-loaded patients), aseptic meningitis and encephalitis. Cytokine release is thought to be responsible for these effects and may also contribute to a significant incidence of delayed graft function in renal transplant recipients treated with OKT3. Other side-effects are shared with ATG.

Because OKT3 is a murine antibody it may induce the formation of neutralising anti-murine antibodies, thus limiting the effectiveness of repeated treatment. Individuals vary in the amount and type of antibody they form directed against the mouse antibody, a phenomenon known as the human anti-murine antibody (HAMA) response. (See Chapter 9) The nature of the specificity of HAMA is dependent upon the type of antibody infused. If the entire murine antibody is infused, then HAMA are anti-heterophilic (i.e. species un-specific), anti-isotypic (against the mouse heavy chain), or anti-idiotypic (against the antigen binding site). These antibodies tend to either block the function of the monoclonal antibody or accelerate its clearance.

The use of OKT3 has declined sharply in recent years as newer immunosuppressive agents have become available. The potent suppression of T lymphocyte populations is known to be associated with an increased incidence of viral infection and lymphoproliferative disorders [90]. It is not clear whether antibody therapy is any worse than other immunosuppression in producing these disorders. Some evidence suggests that problems arise because antibodies are used for too long a time or too late in the course of resistant rejection when the immunosuppression burden is already high.

IL-2 Receptor Antibodies (Anti-CD25, Anti-Tac Antibodies)

Molecular mechanisms elaborating IL-2 and IL-2 receptor (IL-2R) gene transcription have led to IL-2 receptor-targeted therapy [91]. For example, whilst constitutive IL-2R is present as a heterodimer with a beta chain and a common hematopoietin gamma chain, the affinity for IL-2 is markedly up-regulated by the expression of CD25, a T-cell activation antigen, (or Tac also known as IL-2R alpha chain), normally expressed on activated T cells. [92,93].

Basiliximab (Simulect®) and daclizumab (Zenapax®) are both monoclonal antibodies directed against the α-subunit of the high affinity IL-2 receptor (IL-2Rα, or CD25). These antibodies represent a significant advance in the development of immunosuppressive agents. First, they were specifically chosen because they inhibit a crucial step of T cell activation. Second, both antibodies are genetically engineered to prevent the development of a human anti-mouse neutralising antibody response. Dacluzimab is a chimeric antibody, consisting of human constant and murine variable regions, whilst basiliximab is a humanised antibody, where only the antigen binding (complementarity-determining, CDR) regions are murine in origin (Figure 6.6). Only 10 percent of the dacluzimab antibody is of murine origin, resulting in a lower immune response to the foreign protein and an increased half-life. It has a long serum half-life (about 20 days). In contrast basiliximab is a hybrid monoclonal antibody produced in vitro from a murine myeloma cell line transfected with plasmid-borne recombinant gene constructs coding for murine variable chains binding human constant-regions. The resulting monoclonal antibody has even less murine amino acid sequences than daclizumab. Both agents appear to be almost free from the side-effects of non-specific depression of the immune system.

After antigen-specific activation, T cells produce IL-2 and express the high affinity IL-2R. Subsequent T cell proliferation is dependent on IL-2 signaling through IL-2R (Figure 6.4). The IL-2R is composed of α (CD25), β (CD122) and γ (CD132) subunits. The IL-2Rα subunit is expressed only after initial antigen specific T cell activation and is required for IL-2 signaling. Both basiliximab and daclizumab bind to IL-2Rα and block IL-2R function preventing T cell proliferation. In contrast to ATG and OKT3, the anti-CD25 antibodies cause neither antigen-independent T cell activation nor cytokine release. Anti-CD25 antibodies are used in combination with a calcineurin inhibitor as prophylaxis against rejection. Inclusion of CyA/tacrolimus is desirable since high levels of IL-2 may cause T cell proliferation through interaction with the low affinity IL-2R. Anti-CD25 antibodies have little effect on cytotoxic effector cells and are not effective in treating acute rejection episodes.

Two important randomised placebo-controlled trials using anti-CD25 antibodies in renal transplantation have been published. The addition of basiliximab to baseline immunosuppression with Neoral and prednisolone reduced biopsy-proven acute rejection in the first six months following transplantation from 44 percent to 30 percent [94]. A similar reduction (35 percent to 22 percent) was obtained with the addition of daclizumab to triple therapy comprising Neoral, AZA and prednisolone [95]. Episodes of severe rejection needing ATG treatment were significantly fewer in the anti-CD25 antibody-treated patients. After one year of follow-up, however, patient and graft survival were similar in all treatment groups. Notably, no side-effects were associated with anti-CD25 antibody administration and there was no increase in either infection or malignancy when compared with placebo. In clinical trials, basiliximab was well tolerated without evidence of cytokine-release syndrome, hypersensitivity reactions, or anti-idiotype antibody response in transplant recipients given concomitant steroids, AZA and CyA immunosuppression. Similar trials are currently underway in heart, lung, liver and pancreas transplantation.

New Agents Under Development

A large number of new immunosuppressive agents are currently being assessed to determine their value in organ transplantation. Pharmacological agents in this category include the malonitrilamides (e.g.leflunomide), brequinar sodium, 15-deoxyspergualin and FTY720. Of these, FTY720 is of particular interest because it causes immunosuppression by interfering with lymphocyte homing, a mechanism distinct from all other agents. FTY720 is currently undergoing phase 2 clinical evaluation in renal transplantation with promising results.

15-Deoxyspergualin (DSG) was discovered by a drug development program investigating anti-tumor agents in Japan. The drug was shown to be very active against lymphoid tumors only and later was shown to be immunosuppressive. The molecular basis for the action of DSG is unknown but appears to be different to that of all previously known immunosuppressant drugs. DSG appears to bind to a constitutive member of the heat shock protein 70 (Hsp70) and may inhibit the translocation of NF-kB to the nucleus during T and B cell activation. In human studies in kidney and pancreas transplantation, the incidence of acute rejection was significantly decreased when DSG was combined with CyA [96–99]. The toxic effects seen in transplanted patients have been gastrointestinal in nature, (anorexia and nausea), reversible bone marrow suppression (to lymphocytes and thrombocytes) and reversible hypotension. The bone marrow suppression appears to be the most significant side-effect.

A wide variety of biologic agents are also undergoing assessment in pre-clinical or clinical transplant settings. These include monoclonal antibodies to CD4, CD2, CD52 and intercellular adhesion molecule-1 (ICAM-1). There is also intense interest in the concept of using monoclonal antibodies and fusion proteins which block the CD40-CD154 and the B7-CD28 co-stimulatory pathways. In animal models, co-stimulatory blockade has been shown to promote long-term allograft survival in the absence of conventional immunosuppressive drugs. Although initial attempts to use this approach in the clinic have so far proved disappointing, further studies are proposed. CTLA4-Ig is one such chimeric fusion protein that blocks the B7-CD28/CTLA4 (cytotoxic T lymphocyte antigen-4) pathway. It has recently been used in clinical trials for the prevention of infection in kidney transplantation [100].

Long Term Complications of Immunosuppression

Modern immunosuppressive treatment accompanied by improvements in patient selection, tissue typing, surgical techniques and post-operative care, has substantially improved the outcome following solid organ transplantion. More than 50 percent of heart, liver and kidney transplant patients survive for 10 years following transplantation and many recipients of living-donor renal transplants can be expected to have adequate graft function even after 20 years [101]. The price of this success is prolonged exposure to immunosuppressive agents and the consequences of non-specific suppression of the immune system, particularly infection and malignancy. Moreover, several commonly used immunosuppressive drugs increase cardiovascular risk and as discussed already, may lead to irreversible renal failure.

Infection

In the early days of transplantation, infection was responsible for up to 50 percent of patient deaths, particularly amongst those treated with very high doses of corticosteroids. Improved diagnosis, treatment and prophylaxis have dramatically decreased this figure. In one recent study 12 percent of liver transplant recipients followed for 6 years died from infection [22] and a retrospective analysis of stable renal transplant recipients in the USA reported a mortality of only 2.2 patients per 1,000 per year from infection [102]. Nevertheless, infections of the type commonly encountered in the general population and opportunistic infections remain a significant cause of morbidity in transplant recipients [103], particularly during periods of intense immunosuppression. Many patients are at risk of infection even before transplantation. Uraemia, diabetes and advanced liver disease non-specifically depress the immune system and patients with inflammatory lung, liver or kidney disease may have already received considerable immunosuppressive therapy. Some patients on transplant waiting lists have recurrent or persistent infections relating to their underlying cause of organ failure, for example bronchiectasis, cystic fibrosis, viral hepatitis or reflux nephropathy and a few are critically ill on intensive care units.

Infections following transplantation can be divided into those occurring peri-operatively, those occurring at the time of peak immunosuppression (typically opportunistic infections presenting during the first six months) and those that may persist for many years. Peri-operative infection is related to pre-existing risk factors in the recipient (vide supra), major surgery involving the chest, vasculature, biliary tree or urinary tract and indwelling venous and urinary catheters. These infections are almost always bacterial and caused by the same nosocomial pathogens responsible for infection in general surgical practice. It is uncommon for active infection of this sort to be transmitted with the graft. Most units give broad-spectrum antibiotic prophylaxis determined by the local pattern of antibiotic resistance.

There are many opportunistic infections that may occur following transplantation. The most important include *Pneumocystis carinii* pneumonia (PCP), toxoplasmosis, herpesvirus infections (especially cytomegalovirus (CMV) and Epstein Barr virus; EBV), tuberculosis and particularly in critically ill patients, disseminated fungal infections. Human herpesvirus 8 (HHV8), which causes Kaposi's sarcoma (KS), and BK virus, (which may cause a progressive nephropathy in renal transplant recipients), are two more recently described opportunistic pathogens [104,105]. Some opportunistic infections, notably CMV, EBV, HHV8 and toxoplasmosis can be conveyed with the graft and transplantation of an organ from a sero-positive donor to a sero-negative recipient is associated with an increased risk of infection. Serological testing for CMV and toxoplasmosis is routinely used to identify such high-risk patients and to guide prophylactic treatment.

CMV is the most important opportunistic infection affecting transplant recipients, affecting between 20–50% of transplant recipients [103, 106]. The syndrome of leucopenia, thrombocytopenia, atypical lymphocytosis and fever, with positive identification of CMV virus or by the presence of acute-response CMV IgM antibodies, has been termed the "CMV syndrome". Progression of disease to invasive CMV entails positive identification of the CMV virus or viral antigens within tissue. Reduction of immunosuppression allows for recovery of immunity and subsequent sero-conversion, which provides protection against CMV re-activation.

It is common practice to use prophylactic anti-microbial therapy for the first six months following transplantation. Trimethoprim-sulfamethoxazole (co-trimoxazole, Septrin®) is by far the most successful agent used and has almost eliminated PCP as well as significantly reduced the number of urinary tract infections in renal transplant recipients. Septrin is also effective prophylaxis for toxoplasmosis. Patients at high risk for CMV may be given either oral aciclovir or ganciclovir. Patients with a history of TB or who have lived in an endemic area, may be given one year's treatment with isoniazid as the incidence of TB is 100 times more frequent in the immunosuppressed population when compared with the general population. Prophylaxis against oral candidiasis with either amphotericin lozenges or nystatin is usually necessary only for the first month following transplantation.

Malignancy

The long-term risk of malignant disease in immunosuppressed transplant recipients is considerable and the incidence of certain cancers is over 100 times that observed in the general population. Occasionally, undiagnosed malignancy in the donor is transmitted in an organ graft to the recipient, or undiagnosed malignancy in the recipient declares itself following transplantation. However, the majority of cancers following transplantation arise as a consequence of immunosuppressive therapy. The overall exposure to immunosuppression, rather than to particular agents, is the most important risk factor although there is probably a specific association between ATG/OKT3 treatment and post-transplant lymphoproliferative disease (PTLD) and between the use of AZA and skin cancer. Perhaps more importantly, immunosuppression is associated with infection by or re-activation of oncogenic viruses, particularly EBV, HHV8, papillomavirsuses (which may cause skin, uterine cervical and anal cancers and pre-malignant anal intra-epithelial neoplasia [107]) and hepatitis B and C.

Analysis of post transplant malignancy registries has demonstrated that the type of cancers developing in transplant recipients differs significantly from the general population [108,109]. Skin cancer, particularly squamous carcinomas (SCC), KS, PTLD and cervical, vulval, anoperineal and renal carcinoma account for most of the excess risk. There does not seem to be a significant increase in the incidence of lung, prostate, colon and breast cancers, with some evidence suggesting a surprising reduction in breast cancer in immunosuppressed patients

[110]. Skin cancer and lymphoma are the two most important malignancies that develop following transplantation.

Skin tumours, particularly SCC, account for between 30 and 80 percent of post-transplant malignancies. Most occur in sun-exposed areas and patients should be advised to take appropriate precautions to protect against excessive exposure to sunlight. The spectrum of PTLD can range from a benign lymphoid proliferation such as a mononucleosis syndrome to a frankly malignant lymphoid tumor. PTLD has been associated with all types of immunosuppressive therapy but the incidence is higher with the use of T cell specific immunosuppressive agents, such as CyA and tacrolimus.

PTLD occurs in 1–3% of patients, representing a 30-fold increase in the risk of lymphoma over the general population. The majority are B-cell lymphomas containing the EBV genome and they occur within the first few years following transplantation [111] (See Chapter 21). Risk factors for the development of PTLD include grafting an organ from an EBV sero-positive donor to an EBV sero-negative recipient (which is a common occurrence in paediatric transplantation), concurrent CMV infection and the use of ATG/OKT3. Treatment is by drastic reduction in immunosuppression to allow the recipient cytotoxic T cell response against EBV to recover. Should this fail to control the disease the outcome is usually very poor.

Cardiovascular Disease

Many patients on transplant waiting lists either have established vascular disease or are at high risk of its development. This particularly applies to chronic dialysis patients, most of whom are hypertensive and an increasing number of whom are diabetic. Transplantation effectively reduces the risk of death from cardiovascular disease in these patients [112], yet their cardiovascular mortality following transplantation is still 10 times that of the general population. In some studies "death with a functioning graft" is the leading cause of renal allograft failure and cardiovascular disease the leading cause of death [102]. Cardiac transplant recipients are also at high risk of coronary artery disease because chronic rejection of heart allografts is manifest as progressive, immunologically-mediated graft arteriosclerosis. Consequently, effective treatment of cardiovascular risk factors is essential to prolong both patient and graft survival.

Cardiovascular risk in transplant recipients is compounded by the adverse effects of immunosuppression. CyA, tacrolimus and steroids all contribute to hypertension, hyperlipidaemia and diabetes and sirolimus is a potent cause of hyperlcholesterolaemia. Strategies to reduce exposure to both steroids and calcineurin inhibitors have been described above and all transplant recipients should receive advice on smoking, diet and exercise. Aspirin is routinely prescribed as prophylaxis to prevent cardiovascular events. Many patients will require treatment with lipid-lowering agents and anti-hypertensive medications. Data from the Collaborative Transplant Study clearly demonstrates that systolic blood pressure below 140mmHg is associated with prolonged survival of renal allografts [113].

Conclusions and Future Prospects

Currently available immunosuppressive therapy is now very effective at preventing acute allograft rejection and one year graft survival rates of around 85 percent are now common following solid organ transplantation. The wide selection of immunosuppressive agents now in use makes for a more flexible approach when prescribing immunosuppressive regimens, with the possibility of tailoring therapy according to donor and recipient risk factors, so as to maximise graft survival and minimise side-effects. Unfortunately, none of the available agents have yet been shown to prevent the development of graft loss from chronic rejection, which remains a major cause of allograft failure. The long-term goal in transplantation is to develop clinically applicable strategies for inducing specific immunological tolerance to the graft, thereby avoiding the need for long-term use of nonspecific immunosuppressive agents. Recent progress in the laboratory suggests that transplant tolerance is a realistic proposition in due course, although a number of obstacles remain to be overcome. In the meantime, the introduction into clinical practice of new pharmacological agents may further refine immunosuppressive protocols and reduce the incidence of nephrotoxicity and other agent-specific complications.

References

1. Henderson DJ, Naya I, Bundick RV, et al. Comparison of the effects of FK-506, cyclosporin A and rapamycin on IL-2 production. Immunology 1991;73:316.
2. Siekierka JJ, Hung SHY, Poe M, et al. A cytosolic binding protein for the immunosuppressant FK506 has peptidyl-prolyl isomerase activity but is distinct from cyclophillin. Nature 1989;341:755.
3. Harding MW, Galat A, Uehling DE, et al. A receptor for the immunosuppressant FK506 is cis-trans peptidyl-prolyl isomerase. Nature 1989;341:758.
4. Freeman DJ. Pharmacology and pharmacokinetics of cyclosporine. Clin Biochem 1991;24:9.
5. Watkins PB. The role of cytochromes P-450 in cyclosporine metabolism. J Am Acad Dermatol 1990;23:1301.
6. Keown PA:.Optimizing cyclosporine therapy: Dose, levels, and monitoring. Transplant Proc 1988;20:382.
7. Levy G, Grant D. Potential for CsA-Neoral in organ transplantation. Transplant Proc 1994;26:2932.
8. Kovarik JM, Mueller EA, van Bree JB, et al. Cyclosporine pharmacokinetics and variability from a microemulsion formulation — a multicenter investigation in kidney transplant patients. Transplantation 1994;58:658.
9. Senel MF, Van Buren CT, Welsh M, et al. Impact of early cyclosporin average blood concentration on early kidney transplant failure. Transplant Int 1998;11:46–52.
10. Mahalati K, Belitsky P, Sketris I, et al. Neoral monitoring by simplified sparse sampling area under the concentration-time curve: its relationship to acute rejection and cyclosporin nephrotoxicity early after kidney transplantation. Transplantation 1999;68:55–62.
11. Kahan BD, Dunn J, Fitts C et al. Reduced inter- and intrasubject variability in cyclosporin pharmacokinetics in renal transplant recipients treated with a microemulsion formulation in conjunction with fasting, low fat meals or high fat meals. Transplantation 1995;59:505–11.
12. Cantarovich M, Elstein E, De Vaarennes B, et al. Clinical benefit of Neoral dose monitoring with cyclosporin 2-hour post-dose levels compared with trough levels in stable heart transplant patients. Transplantation 1999;68:1839–42.
13. Levy G. Relationship of pharmacokinetics to clinical outcomes. Transplant Proc 1999;31: 1654–58.
14. Screiber SL, Crabtree GR. The mechanism of action of cyclosporin A and FK506. Immunology Today 1992;13:136–42.
15. Kung L, Gourishankar S, Halloran PF. Molecular pharmacology of immunosuppressive agents in relation to their clinical use. Curr Opin Organ Transplant 2000;5:268–75.
16. Pankewycz OG. Transforming growth factor-β and renal graft fibrosis. Curr Opin Organ Transplant 2000;5:336–42.
17. Keown PA, Stiller CR, Wallace AC: Effect of cyclosporine on the kidney. J Pediatr, 1987;111:1029.
18. Remuzzi G, Bertani T. Renal vascular and thrombotic effects of cyclosporine. Am J Kidney Dis 1989;13:261.
19. Rush DN: Cyclosporine toxicity to organs other than the kidney. Clin Biochem 1991;24:101.

20. Luke RG. Mechanism of cyclosporine-induced hypertension. Am J Hypertens 1991;4:468.
21. Hornberger J, Best J, Geppert J, et al. Risks and costs of end stage renal disease after heart transplantation. Transplantation 1998;66:1763–70.
22. Jain A, Reyes J, Kashyap R, et al. What have we learned about primary liver transplantation under tacrolimus immunosuppression? Long-term follow up of the first 1000 patients. Annals of Surgery 1999;230:441–9.
23. Scott JP, Higenbottam TW. Adverse reactions and interactions of cyclosporin. Med Toxicol Adverse Drug Exp 1988;3:107.
24. Reznick VM, Lyons Jones K, Durham BL, et al. Changes in facial appearance during cyclosporine treatment. Lancet 1987;1:1405.
25. Fung JJ, Todo S, Jain A, et al. Conversion from cyclosporin to FK506 in liver allograft recipients with cyclosporine related complications. Transplant Proc 1990;22:6–12
26. Fung JJ, Jain A, Hamad I, et al. Long term effects of FK506 following conversion from cyclosporine to FK506 for chronic rejection in liver transplant recipients. Hepatology 1993;18:74A
27. Sher LS, Cosenza CA, Michel J, et al. Efficacy of tacrolimus as rescue therapy for chronic rejection in orthotopic liver transplantation: a report of the U.S. Multicenter Liver Study Group. Transplantation 1997;64:258.
28. Fung J, Eliasziw M, Todo S, et al. The Pittsburgh randomized trial of tacrolimus compared to cyclosporine for hepatic transplantation. J Am Coll Surg 1996;183:117.
29. The European FK506 Multicenter Liver Study Group. Randomized trial comparing tacrolimus and cyclosporin in prevention of liver allograft rejection. Lancet 1994;334: 423.
30. The United States Multicenter FK506 Liver Study Group. A comparison of tacrolimus (FK506) and cyclosporine for immunosuppression in liver transplantation. N Engl J Med 1994;331:1110.
31. Jordan ML, Naraghi R, Shapiro R, et al. Tacrolimus rescue therapy for renal allograft rejection — five year experience. Transplantation 1997;63:223.
32. FK506 Kidney Transplant Study Group. A comparision of tacrolimus (FK506) and cyclosporine for immunosuppression after cadaveric kidney transplantation. Transplantation 1997;63:977–83
33. Mayer AD, Dmitrewski J, Squifflet JP et al . Multicenter randomized trial comparing tacrolimus and cyclosporine in the prevention of renal allograft rejection. A report of the European tacrolimus multicenter renal study group. Transplantation 1997;64:436.
34. Mentzer RM, Jahania MS, and Lasley RD. Tacrolimus as a rescue immunosuppressant after heart and lung transplantation. The U.S. Multicenter FK506 Study Group. Transplantation 1998;65:109.
35. Corry RJ, Egidi MF, Shapiro R et al. Tacrolimus without antilymphocyte induction therapy prevents pancreas loss from rejection in 123 consecutive patients. Transplant Proc 1998;30:521
36. Gruessner RWG for the Tacrolimus Pancreas Transplant Study Group. Tacrolimus in pancreas transplantation: a multicenter analysis. Clin Transplantation 1997;11:299.
37. Regazzi MB, Rinaldi M, Molinaro M, et al. Clinical pharmocokinetics of tacrolimus in heart transplant recipients. Ther Drug Monit 1999;21:2–7.
38. Venkataramanan R, Jain A, Warty VS, et al. Pharmacokinetics of FK506 in transplant patients. Transplant Proc 1992;23:2736–40.
39. Warty VS, Venkataramanan R, Zendehrouh P, et al. Practical aspects of FK506 analysis (Pittsburgh experience). Transplant Proc 1992;23:2730–1.
40. Cillo U, Alessiani M, Fung JJ, et al. Major adverse effects of FK506 used as an immunosuppressive agent after liver transplantation. Transplant Proc 1993;25:628–34
41. Fung JJ, Alessiani M, Abu-Elmagd K, et al. Adverse effects associated with the use of FK506. Transplant Proc 1991;23:3105–8
42. Moutabarrik A, Ishibashi M, Kameoka H, et al. FK506 mechanism of nephrotoxicity: Stimulatory effect on endothelin secretion by cultured kidney cells. Transplant Proc 1992;23:3133–6.
43. Eidelman BH, Abu-Elmagd K, Wilson J, et al. Neurologic complications of FK-506. Transplant Proc 1991;23:3175–8.
44. Pirsch JD, Miller J, Deierhoi MH, et al. A comparison of tacrolimus (FK506) and cyclosporin for immunosuppression after cadaveric renal transplantation. Transplantation 1997;63:977–83.
45. Keown P, Niese D. Cyclosporin microemulsion increases drug exposure and reduces acute rejection without incremental toxicity in de novo renal transplantation. Kidney Int 1998;54:938–44.
46. Woodle ES, Thistlethwaite R, Gordon JH, et al. A multicentre trial of FK506 therapy in refractory acute renal allograft rejection. Transplantation 1996;62:594–9.
47. Meiser BM, Uberfuhr P, Martin S, et al. Single-centre randomised trial comparing tacrolimus (FK506) and cyclosporin in the prevention of acute myocardial rejection. J Heart Lung Transplant 1998;17:782–7.
48. Reichenspurner H, Kur F, Treede H, et al. Optimisation of the immunosuppressive protocol after lung transplantation. Transplantation 1999;68:67–71.

49. Keenan RJ, Dauber JH, Iacono AT, et al. Long-term follow-up clinical trial of tacrolimus versus cyclosporin for lung transplantation. J Heart Lung Transplant 1998;17:58–63.
50. Morris RE. Rapamycins: Antifungal, antitumor, antiproliferative and immunosuppressive macrolides. Transplant Rev 1992;6:39–87.
51. Morris RE, Meiser BM, Wu J, et al. Use of rapamycin for the suppression of alloimmune reactions in vivo: Schedule dependence, tolerance induction, synergy with cyclosporine and FK 506, and effect on host-versus-graft and graft-versus-host reactions. Transplant Proc 1991;23:521–4.
52. Kahan BD, Napoli KL, Kelly PA, et al. Therapeutic drug monitoring of sirolimus: correlations with efficacy and toxicity. Clin Transplant 2000;14:97–109.
53. Kahan BD. Efficacy of sirolimus compared with azathioprine for reduction of acute renal allograft rejection: a randomised multicentre study. Lancet 2000;356:194–202.
54. McAlister VC, Gao Z, Peltekian K, et al. Sirolimus-tacrolimus combination immunosuppression. Lancet 2000;355:376–7.
55. Murgia MG, Jordan S, Kahad BD. The side effect profile of sirolimus: A phase I study in quiescent cyclosporine-prednisone-treated renal transplant recipient. Kidney Int 1996;49:209–16
56. Schuurman HJ, Cottens S, Fuchs S et al. SDZ, a new rapamycin derivative. transplantation 1997;64:32–5.
57. Groth CG, Backman L, Morales J-M, et al. Sirolimus (Rapamycin)-based therapy in human renal transplantation. Transplantation 1999;67:1036–42.
58. Kreis H, Cisterne JM, Land W, et al. Sirolimus in association with mycophenolate mofetil induction for the prevention of acute graft rejection in renal allograft recipients. Transplantation 2000;69:1252–60.
59. Shapiro AM, Lakey JR, Ryan EA, et al. Islet transplantation in seven patients with type 1 diabetes mellitus using a glucocorticoid-free immunosuppressive regimen. N Engl J Med 2000;343:230–8.
60. Schwartz R, and Dameshek W. The effects of 6-mercaptopurine on homograft reactions. J Clin Invest 1960;39:952.
61. Chan GL, Erdmann GR, Gruber SA, et al. Azathioprine metabolism: Pharmacokinetics of 6-mercaptopurine, 6-thiouric acid and 6-thioguanine nucleotides in renal transplant patients. J Clin Pharmacol 1990;30:358.
62. Coulthard SA, Rabello C, Robson J, et al. A comparison of molecular and enzyme-based assays for the detection of thiopurine methyltransferase mutations. Br J Haematology 2000;110:599–604.
63. Lia-no F, Moreno A, Matesanz R, et al. Veno-occlusive hepatic disease of the liver in renal transplantation: Is azathioprine the cause? (see comments). Nephron 1989;51:509.
64. Frick TW, Fryd DS, Goodale RL, et al. Lack of association between azathioprine and acute pancreatitis in renal. Lancet, 1991;337:251.
65. Sollinger HW, Deierhoi MH, Belzer FO, et al. RS-61433: A phase I clinical trial and pilot rescue study. Transplantation 1992;53:428–32.
66. Sollinger HW, for the US Renal Transplant Mycophenolate Mofetil study group. Mycophenolate mofetil for the prevention of acute rejection in primary cadaveric renal allograft recipients. Transplantation 1995;60:225–32.
67. European Mycophenolate Mofetil cooperative study group. Placebo-controlled study of mycophenolate mofetil combined with cyclosporin and corticosteroids for prevention of acute rejection. Lancet 1995;345:1321–5
68. McDiarmid SV. Mycophenolate mofetil in liver transplantation. Clin Transplantation 1996;10:140–5
69. Pescovitz MA, for the Mycophenolate mofetil acute renal rejection study group. Mycophenolate mofetil for the treatment of a first acute renal allograft rejection. Transplantation 1998;65:235–41
70. Mele TS, Halloran PF. The use of mycophenolate mofetil in transplant recipients. Immunopharmacology 2000;47:215–45.
71. Van Gelder T, Hilbrands LB, Vanrenterghem Y, et al. A randomised, double-blind multicentre plasma concentration controlled study of the safety and efficacy of oral mycophenolate mofetil for the prevention of acute rejection after kidney transplantation. Transplantation 1999;68:261–6.
72. Meulen CG, Wetzels FM, Hilbrands LB. The influence of mycophenolate mofetil on the incidence and severity of primary cytomegalovirus infections and disease after renal transplantation. Nephrol Dial Transplant 2000;15:711–4.
73. Sollinger HW and the US Renal Transplant Mycophenolate Mofetil Study Group. Mycophenolate mofetil for the prevention of acute rejection in primary cadaveric renal allograft recipients. Transplantation 1995;60:225–32.
74. Tricontinental Mycophenolate Mofetil Renal Transplantation Study Group. A blinded, randomised clinical trial of mycophenolate mofetil for the prevention of acute rejection in cadaveric renal transplantation. Transplantation 1996;61:1029–37.

75. European Mycophenolate Mofetil Study Group. Placebo controlled study of mycophenolate mofetil combined with cyclosporin and corticosteroids for prevention of acute rejection. Lancet 1995;345:1321–5.
76. Mathew TH and the Tricontinental Mycophenolate Mofetil Renal Transplantation Study Group, A blinded, long-term, randomised multicentre study of mycophenolate mofetil in cadaveric renal transplantation. Results at three years. Transplantation 1998;65:1450–4.
77. European Mycophenolate Mofetil Cooperative Study Group. Mycophenolate mofetil in renal transplantation: 3-year results from the placebo-controlled trial. Transplantation 1999;68:391–6.
78. Ojo AO, Meier-Kriesche HU, Hanson JA, et al. Mycophenolate mofetil reduces late renal allograft loss independent of acute rejection. Transplantation 2000;69:2405–09.
79. Kobashigawa JA, Miller L, Renlund DG, et al. A randomised active-controlled trial of mycophenolate mofetil in heart transplant recipients. Transplantation 1998;66:507–15.
80. Adcock IM. Molecular mechanisms of glucocorticoid actions. Pulmonary Pharm Therapeutics 2000;13:115–26.
81. Tornatore KM, Reed KA, Venuto RC. Methylprednisolone and cortisol metabolism during the early post-renal transplant period. Clin Transplant 1995;9:427.
82. Boitard C, Bach JF. Long-term complications of conventional immunosuppressive treatment. Adv Nephrol 1989;18:335.
83. Maes BD, Vanrenterghem YF. Induction with polyclonal antibodies. Curr Opin Organ Transplant 1999;4:305–11.
84. Merion R, Howell T, Bromberg J. Partial T cell activation and anergy induction by polyclonal antilymphocyte globulin. Transplantation 1998;65:1481–9.
85. Taylor RM. Monoclonal and polyclonal antibodies: Clinical aspects. Immunol Lett 1991;29:113–6.
86. Szczech L, Berlin J, Aradhye S, et al. Effect of anti-lymphocyte induction therapy on renal allograft survival: a meta-analysis. J Am Soc Nephrol 1997;8:1771–7.
87. Szczech L, Berlin J, Feldman HI, et al. The effect of anti-lymphocyte induction therapy on renal allograft survival. Ann Intern Med 1998;128:817–26.
88. Katznelson S, Cecka J. Immunosuppressive regimens and their effects on renal allograft outcome. In: Cecka J, Terasaki P, editor. Clinical Transplants 1996. Los Angeles, CA: UCLA Tissue Typing Laboratory, 1996; 361–71.
89. Kreis H, Legendre C, Chatenoud L. OKT3 in organ transplantation. Transplant Rev 1991;5:181–99.
90. Cockfield SM, Preiksaitis J, Harvey E, et al. Is sequential use of ALG and OKT3 in renal transplants associated with an increased incidence of fulminant posttransplant lymphoproliferative disorder? Transplant Proc 1991;23:1106–7.
91. Kirkman RI, Barrett LV, Gaulton GN et al. Administration of an anti-interleukin-2 receptor monoclonal antibody prolongs cardiac allograft survival in mice. J.Exp.Med 1985;162:358.
92. Kirkman RL, Shapiro ME, Carpenter CB et al. A randomized prospective trial of anti-Tac monoclonal antibody in human renal transplantation. Transplantation 1991;51:107.
93. Kovarik J, Wolf P, Cisterine JM, Mourad G, et al. Disposition of basiliximab, an interleukin-2 receptor monoclonal antibody, in recipients of mismatched cadaver renal allografts. Transplantation 1997;64:1701–5.
94. Nashan B, Moore R, Amlot P, et al. Randomised trial of basiliximab versus placebo for control of acute cellular rejection in renal allograft recipients. Lancet 1997;350:1193–8.
95. Vincenti F, Kirkman R, Light S, et al. Interleukin-2 receptor blockade with daclizumab to prevent acute rejection in renal transplantation. N Engl J Med 1998;338:161–5.
96. Katoh H, Ohkohchi N, Orii T, et al. Effectiveness of 15-DSG on steroid resistant acute rejection in living related transplantation.Transplant Proc 1997;29:533–4.
97. Takahashi K, Ota K, Tanabe K, et al. Effect of a novel immunosuppressive agent, deoxyspergualin, on rejection in kidney transplant recipients. Transplant Proc 1990;22:1606–12.
98. Okazaki H, Sato T, Jimbo M, et al. Prophylactic use of deoxyspergualin in living related renal transplantation. Transplant Proc 1991;23:1094–5.
99. Okubo M, Tamura K, Kamata K, et al. 15-Deoxyspergualin "rescue therapy" for methylprednisolone-resistant rejection of renal transplants as compared with anti-T cell monoclonal antibody (OKT3). Transplantation 1993;55:505.
100. Kirk AD, Harlan DM, Armstrong NN, et al. CTLA4-Ig and anti-CD40 ligand prevent allograft rejection in primates. Proc Natl Acad Sci 1997;94:8789–94.
101. Hariharan S, Johnson CP, Bresnahan BA, et al. Improved graft survival after renal transplantation in the United States, 1988–1996. N Eng J Med 2000;342:605–12.
102. Ojo AO, Hanson JA, Wolfe RA, et al. Long-term survival in renal transplant recipients with graft function. Kidney Int 2000;57:307–13.
103. Fishman JA, Rubin RH. Infection in organ transplant recipients. N Engl J Med 1988;338:1741–51

104. Regamey N, Tamm M, Wernli M, et al. Transmission of human herpesvirus 8 infection from renal transplant donors to recipients. N Engl J Med 1998;339:1358–63.
105. Nickeleit V, Hirsch HH, Binet IF, et al. Polyomavirus infection of renal allograft recipients: from latent infection to manifest disease. J Am Soc Nephrol 1999;10:1080–9.
106. Abu-Nader R, and Patel R. Current management strategies for the treatment and prevention of cytomegalovirus infection in solid organ transplant recipients. Bio Drugs 2000;13:159–75.
107. Zbar AP, Fenger C, Efron J, BeerGabel M, Wexner SD. The pathology and molecular biology of anal intra-epithelial neoplasia (AIN): comparisons with cervical and vulvar intra-epithelial carcinoma. Int J Colorect Dis 2002(in press)
108. Shiel AG, Flavel S, Disney AP, et al. Cancer incidence in renal transplant patients treated with azathioprine or cyclosporin. Transplant Proc 1987, 19:2214–2216.
109. Penn I. Cancers complicating organ transplantation. N Engl J Med 1990;323:1767–9.
110. Stewart T, Tsai SC, Grayson H, et al. Incidence of de-novo breast cancer in women chronically immunosuppressed after organ transplantation. Lancet 1995;346:796–800.
111. Paya CV, Fung JJ, Nalesnik MA, et al. Epstein-Barr virus-induced post-transplant lymphoproliferative disorders. ASTS/ASTP EBV-PTLD task force and the Mayo clinic organised international consensus development meeting. Transplantation 1999;68:1517–25.
112. Wolfe RA, Ashby VB, Milford EL, et al. Comparison of mortality in all patients on dialysis, patients on dialysis awaiting transplantation, and recipients of a first cadaveric transplant. N Engl J Med 1999;341:1725–30.
113. Opelz G, Wujciak T, Ritz E. Association of chronic kidney graft failure with recipient blood pressure. Kidney Int 1998;53:217–22.

7. Clinical Transplantation and the Immunology of Organ Rejection

John J. Fung and J. Andrew Bradley

Immunologic Considerations

Transplantation of tissue between areas of the same individual is termed autografting and is not subject to rejection. Tissues transplanted between genetically identical individuals (syngeneic grafting) is termed isografting. Allografts (also known as homografts) are tissues transplanted between genetically disparate individuals within the same species. Xenografts (also known as heterografts) are tissues transplanted between disparate species.

Recognition of genetic disparity is directed towards antigens on the cell surface of the transplanted tissues. These antigens are generally classified as "transplantation antigens". The best defined group of antigens and those most thoroughly studied are the major histocompatibility complex (MHC) antigens. (See Chapter 5) However, other less well characterized transplant antigens have also been identified, such as the rejection by female recipients to antigens found on the Y chromosome in syngeneic male donors. In humans, the MHC antigens are also called human leucocyte antigens (HLA). This group of genes is located on the short arm of chromosome 6 and the segment of this chromosome is termed a haplotype. Each individual possess two chromosomes 6 and therefore there are two haplotypes.

Each haplotype consists of a group of three classes of genes, encoding three classes of antigens, termed Class I, Class II and Class III antigens. Class I antigens can be subdivided into HLA-A, HLA-B, and HLA-C antigens and are composed of two polypeptide chains, an alpha heavy chain (which is trans-membranous) and β_2-microglobulin. The normal biologic function of Class I antigens is for surveillance of T cells to recognize self — thus virally infected cells or tumor cells expressing foreign peptides in conjunction with Class I MHC antigens will be destroyed by cytotoxic T cells. The distribution of these antigens is such that most nucleated cells posses them on the cell surface as do platelets. Class II antigens are more restricted in their distribution, being present on those cells involved in the development of an immune response. These cells, include antigen processing cells, B cells, activated T cells and cells which are involved in an inflammatory process. Like Class I antigens, they are heterodimers (two distinct polypeptide chains, termed alpha and beta chains), but both chains are trans-membranous. Three major allelic loci have been identified and have been sub-divided into HLA-DR, HLA-DQ, and HLA-DP antigens. These antigens are thought to play an important role in the signaling process for antigen presenta-tion between antigen processing cells and effector lymphocytes. Other proteins coded within the Class II MHC region include proteins involved in assembly of MHC molecules.

Class III antigens are composed of a number of complement components. The entire HLA complex is inherited by simple Mendelian laws and the expression of the two haplotypes is co-dominant. Each parent contributes one HLA haplotype to each offspring. The probability of one offspring sharing either two or zero haplotypes with another sibling is 25 percent, whilst the probability of sharing one haplotype with another sibling is 50 percent.

There are numerous allelic forms of each subgroup of Class I antigens. This polymorphism is thought to confer various degrees of resistance to epidemic infections and thus preserve species survival. Currently there are over 95 alleles of HLA-A, 207 alleles of HLA-B and 50 alleles of HLA-C. There are varying fre-quencies of any given allele amongst different ethnic groups and many alleles have not been defined. Previous studies have suggested that HLA-A and HLA-B antigens are more involved in allograft recognition, whilst HLA-C antigens are less involved.

Class II antigens are currently detected by serologic, cellular typing, or DNA identification methods. Numerous alleles for HLA-DR, HLA-DQ and HLA-DP have been identified. Previously, only the HLA-DR antigen system could be easily typed by serologic methods and as a result, it is the only locus which is routinely determined in clinical solid organ transplantation. With the advent of molecular typing, HLA-DQ and HLA-DP can be easily typed, however, little is known about the impact of matching these alleles in solid organ transplant outcomes (although this is critical in bone marrow transplantation). In allogeneic bone marrow transplantation, the mixed lymphocyte reaction can be utilized to detect subtle differences in HLA Class II antigens between recipient and donor.

Clinical tissue typing includes the determination of histocompatibility between the donor and recipient, by comparing the HLA phenotypes of both the donor and recipient, by determining the degree of previous sensitization (often expres-sed as panel reactive antibody — PRA) and finally the determination of cross-match compatibility as already described in Chapter 5. Sensitization to HLA antigens occurs following pregnancy (females may develop HLA antibodies to paternal antigens found in the fetus), blood transfusions (from contaminating white cells and platelets) and from previous organ transplants. The PRA gives an indication of the degree of reactivity of serum from an individual towards a selec-ted group of HLA allelic specificities. The higher the PRA, the more likely a subsequent cross-match will be positive. The cross-match determination is simply a complement-mediated cytotoxicity assay of recipient serum towards HLA antigens found on the donor cells (lymphocytes). A positive cross-match suggests that anti-donor HLA antibodies exist in the recipient and may impact on subsequent allograft function. More recently, flow cytometry has been used to determine whether anti-donor HLA antibodies exist in the recipient.

There are no effective methods of reducing these pre-formed antibodies, however, preventing sensitization is the most effective method of maintaining low PRA values. This is accomplished by minimizing blood transfusions and by the use of recombinant erythropoietin, indicated for anemia in renal failure. Cross-matches are done at the time that a potential ABO compatible organ is identified. With the data on histocompatibility in hand, a number of clinical strategies can be formulated based on the impact of these parameters on patient and graft survival. Data from both European and American centers, when analyzed in large numbers, suggest a long-term benefit of HLA matching between the donor and recipient in kidney transplantation. The probability of achieving full HLA match is in the order of 1:1 million if all the Class I and Class II loci of HLA are considered. This probability of "perfect matching" is enhanced if HLA-C, HLA-DQ and HLA-DP antigens are not included and six antigen matches can be found in 1:10,000. This is the rationale for developing a national policy that preferentially transplants "perfectly" matched organs (6 antigen matched HLA-A, -B, -DR).

Understanding Allograft Recognition

The initial host response to the donor organ is through recognition of HLA antigens on the surface of the endothelium or by shedding of soluble alloantigens or cells which are then processed in regional lymph nodes or in the spleen. The afferent limb is responsible for sensitization of recipient cells against donor antigens. Either the donor cells themselves (such as passenger leucocytes), or recipient antigen processing cells, present the alloantigen to recipient T lymphocytes in lymphoid tissues.

Lymphocytes are pre-programmed to recognize foreign antigen during their development in the thymus. Antigen specificity is determined by an antigen-binding unit on the T cell surface, the T cell receptor (TCR; see Chapter 1). The specificity and diversity of the binding site of the TCR results from its amino acid composition and the variation in this composition from T cell to T cell. The gene sequence coding for the TCR rearranges during early thymocyte development, such that each T cell ends up with a different TCR binding specificity. Because the gene rearrangements are completely random, a huge library of binding sites capable of recognizing both "self" and "foreign" molecules is generated. Thymocytes with TCRs that bind strongly to "self" molecules (and thus potentiate the development of autoimmunity), are subsequently destroyed by negative selection, whereas some interaction between TCRs and "self" molecules is necessary in order to assure appropriate T cell–antigen presenting cell interactions, i.e. positive selection.

Lymphocytes re-circulate at a rate of 1 percent to 2 percent per hour, migrating through all tissues of the body. Re-circulation routes are not random and specialized cell-surface "homing" molecules on T lymphocytes mediate attachment to specific endothelial molecules in targeted tissues. Once inside tissue, antigen presenting cells such as dendritic cells and macrophages make intimate contact with the lymphocytes and present foreign antigen that has already been processed intra-cellularly by the antigen presenting cell. The antigen presenting cell phagocytoses foreign protein and enzymatically cleaves it to the size of small peptides 8 to 12 amino acids in length which are loaded onto MHC molecules. The MHC molecule carries the peptide fragment to the cell surface where it is displayed to T cells.

The TCR is a cell surface molecule. The TCR associates with "accessory" molecules, including CD3 and either CD4 or CD8. The TCR/CD3 complex interacts with the peptide fragment in the binding grove of the MHC molecule of the antigen presenting cell and this complex is stabilized by the CD4 or CD8 molecule of the T cell. This interaction initiates intracellular signaling pathways which result in the activation and subsequent proliferation of that T cell clone recognizing the particular antigen fragments of foreign protein. It is the requirement for antigen presentation by antigen presenting cells bearing an MHC molecule specific to the host that is the basis for MHC-restricted antigen recognition.

Antigen-directed proliferation of T cell clones is absolutely required for an effective immune response. It is driven by a positive feedback loop between T cells and soluble autocrine and paracrine cytokines. Cells recognizing antigen make the potent T cell growth factor (interleukin-2 (IL-2)) and simultaneously become responsive to IL-2 by expressing the IL-2 receptor. This dual synthesis allows the cells to stimulate clonal expansion. During an ongoing immune response, proliferating T cells recruit many other cell types and immune mechanisms into action. T cells also produce other cytokines, IL-1 through 6, IL-9 and IL-10 as well as interferon-gamma, tumor necrosis factor (TNF)-alpha and TNF-beta, granulocyte colony-stimulating factor (G-CSF) and granulocyte-monocyte colony-stimulating factor (GM-CSF). These substances have at least three important functions. First, cytokines can attract and activate other leukocytes. For example, CD4 helper T cell cytokines attract macrophages and CD8-bearing cytotoxic lymphocytes into rejecting allografts. They also trigger macrophage activation and CD8 lymphocyte cell maturation. The resulting multi-cellular tissue infiltration has traditionally been referred to as the delayed-type hypersensitivity (DTH; Type IV) response. CD4 helper T cell cytokines are also responsible for the activation of B cells and thus indirectly for the majority of antibody production. Second, cytokines up-regulate both MHC molecules on tissues and adhesion molecules on endothelium. This aids in the entry and accumulation of leukocytes in the tissue and an accelerated recognition of "foreign" molecules. Third, cytokines activate distant organ responses such as the hepatic acute-phase response, bone marrow phagocyte synthesis and the hypothalamic-pituitary axis, producing the systemic signs of inflammation. (See Chapter 2)

Once the antigen is consumed or removed, the process down-regulates. A number of sensitized memory T cells remain and contribute to a stronger secondary response on re-challenge with the same antigen. Other mechanisms of T cell regulation which relate the expression of regulatory molecules (such as Fas ligand), may also play an important role in T cell mediated responses. T cell responses also diminish with the removal of IL-2, a phenomenon known as "activation-induced cell death" or AICD which is an apoptotic phenomenon. (See Chapter 12) Apoptosis, also termed "programmed cell death" or "physiological cell death", is a mechanism of cell death which is an energy-dependent process mediated by specific receptor-ligand interactions leading to endonuclease activation with extensive chromosomal DNA degradation.

In the case of transplanted solid organs, recipient T lymphocytes enter the graft rapidly. Conversely, donor antigen presenting cells also exit the graft immediately after reperfusion. Thus, recipient lymphocytes potentially become sensitized to donor (foreign) antigens both inside and outside of the transplanted organ. The first wave of donor antigen presenting cells that exit the allograft present antigen via direct antigen presentation, in that recipient T cells that respond do not require antigen processing by recipient antigen presenting cells.

Normally, the frequency of reactive T cells that respond to a foreign peptide in context with "self" MHC is of the order of 1:1,000, however, in the "direct" pathway of allorecognition, up to 10 percent of recipient T cells will respond. It has been suggested that the ferocity of acute rejection is due to the large number of T cells that respond to direct antigen presentation, while chronic rejection may be due to delayed type hypersensitivity reactions from "indirect" antigen presentation.

The migration of donor cells out of transplanted organs has often been suggested to play a role in initiation of organ rejection. However, in some circumstances, donor-derived immunocompetent lymphocytes recognize recipient HLA as foreign and initiate a process called graft-versus-host disease (GVHD). While GVHD is the major immune reaction occurring after allogeneic bone marrow transplantation, it can also occur after solid organ transplantation. Patients receive allogeneic bone marrow as treatment for a variety of hematologic malignancies. Donor cells which are activated to recipient MHC infiltrate recipient tissues and create a DTH response, primarily in the skin, gastrointestinal tract, liver and lung.

Non-immunologic Considerations

The widespread application of solid organ transplantation has necessitated the use of donors that were traditionally considered sub-optimal. The liberalization of donor criteria such as age and stability has increased the potential donor pool. The impact of such cadaveric donors is now being appreciated where lower short and long-term function of these organs has been identified. A number of donor factors have been identified which increase the likelihood of short-term and long-term allograft failure. Prolonged cardiac massage, severe hypoxemia, high levels of inotropic drug support, prolonged and severe hypotension and possibly endocrine factors, may play a role in initial organ dysfunction. The microvasculature of the allograft is the primary site affected by ischemia and reperfusion injury. In addition, several non-immunologic factors, such as hyperlipidemia, degree of initial allograft damage due to preservation, hypertension, drug toxicity, the presence of cytomegalovirus (CMV) infection and donor factors (such as age) may accelerate graft loss for primarily immunologic reasons, i.e. development of chronic rejection. Reperfusion of ischemic organs leads to disturbance in microvascular blood flow, increased leucocyte adhesion, up-regulation of adhesion molecule and MHC expression, often masking the development of acute rejection.

This has led to a greater utilization of organs from living donors, mostly from related sources. In kidney transplantation, HLA identical (2 haplotype matched, sibling) transplants have the advantage of early allograft function, decreased rejection episodes and prolonged allograft survival. HLA non-identical (1 haplotype matched, either sibling or parent and 0 haplotype matched, either non-related or sibling) transplants, have decreased survival when compared with HLA identical grafts, however, the outcomes in these patients are as good as with perfectly HLA-matched cadaveric kidney allografts. This suggests that non-immunologic conditions can override the impact of HLA matching and other immunologic factors.

Clinical Transplant Outcomes

The icons of significance in clinical transplantation vary according to the type of transplant. For solid organ transplantation, these have traditionally been patient and allograft survival. However, these outcomes are crude measures of success, since immunologic factors contribute significantly to the end results. In solid organ transplantation, the development of rejection is a significant clinical event.

In kidney transplantation, hyperacute rejection occurs in over 80 percent of transplants where positive cross-matches occur and histocompatibility testing is important in preventing this antibody-mediated event. Even with careful selection of cross-match negative donor-recipient combinations, patients with a PRA exceeding 40–60% have a decreased graft survival. The losses are generally due to rejection. Hyperacute rejection has also been seen in heart transplant patients, but hyperacute rejection of the liver is not seen to the same extent, even in the face of a positive cross-match. Liver allografts are thought to be relatively resistant to antibody mediated injury, perhaps because of their unique dual blood flow and its role in removing antigen-antibody complexes, as well as because of the secretion of soluble Class I HLA antigens from the liver which neutralize alloantibodies.

Clinical Patterns of Rejection

Transplantation of an organ among genetically non-identical individuals can lead to its destruction by a process called rejection. There are various types of rejection.

1. Hyperacute rejection occurs soon after reperfusion of the organ and is characterized by rapid thrombotic occlusion of the graft microvasculature. This process is mediated by pre-existing antibodies in the recipient which bind to the endothelium of the microvasculature of the donor organ. This binding activates the complement cascade, which in turn promotes intra-vascular thrombosis. Hyperacute rejection was first described in cases of ABO incompatible organs. Subsequently, hyperacute rejection has been recognized in cases where IgM and/or IgG antibodies were directed against human leucocyte antigens (HLA) found on the donor organ.
2. Acute rejection can entail humoral and/or cellular mechanisms. In humoral rejection, endothelial cells of the donor microvasculature show changes of vasculitis without thrombi. With cell-mediated acute rejection, there is an inflammatory change in the allograft due to a mononuclear infiltrate, usually in the perivascular regions, which may result in distal ischemia if advanced.
3. Chronic rejection is a slow process leading to fibrosis and obliterative arteriopathy and ischemia of the functional elements of the graft. This phenomenon is not yet clearly understood, however, recurrent bouts of acute cellular rejection can lead to rapid development of chronic rejection as soon as 6–12 weeks after transplantation.

Rejections can be minimized by different approaches: 1) using ABO compatible and lymphocytotoxic cross-match negative allografts; 2) minimizing allogeneic differences between donor and recipient, e.g. HLA-matched kidney transplantation; and 3) ensuring adequate induction immunosuppression.

Prevention of Rejection Using Specific Agents

The foundation of transplantation has been the necessity of utilizing drug therapy to suppress the recipient immune response. Failure of achieving sufficient immunosuppression is associated with high incidences of graft loss from rejection. The present goal of immunosuppressive regimens is to suppress responses to the allograft whilst preserving sufficient immunity to prevent infection or the development of malignancies. The ultimate goal of immunomodulation is to achieve donor-specific tolerance without alterations in immunity to other antigens. As knowledge of the molecular mechanisms of rejection have advanced, a greater understanding of how many immunosuppressants work has evolved. More importantly, new strategies are guided by this knowledge, resulting in site-directed immunosuppression. Virtually every known step of the immune process can be targeted and many new drugs are now in various stages of development. This topic has been extensively covered in the preceding chapter.

Current Anti-rejection Protocols

For nearly 20 years following the introduction of cyclosporin A, (CyA) most transplant programs have adopted very similar immunosuppressive regimens using a combination of CyA/azathioprine/prednisolone (often known as triple therapy), with or without anti-thymocyte globulin (ATG)/OKT3 antibody treatment (quadruple therapy). In some European units, dual therapy, (CyA/Azathioprine or CyA/prednisolone) or even CyA monotherapy has been successfully used in low-risk renal transplants [1]. The development of tacrolimus, mycophenolate mofetil (MMF), sirolimus and anti-CD25 antibodies has given rise to many alternative and potentially more effective immunosuppressive protocols, some of which have been tested in clinical trials. (See Chapter 6) Moreover, increasing awareness of the long-term side effects of immunosuppression, particularly malignancy, cardiovascular disease and calcineurin inhibitor nephrotoxicity, is beginning to influence the choice of immunosuppressive agent. As a result there are many different protocols currently in use. What follows is an attempt to present a modern approach to the immunosuppression used for induction therapy, maintenance therapy and the treatment of acute rejection.

Induction Therapy

The incidence of acute rejection is highest in the first weeks and months following transplantation. Accordingly, more intense immunosuppressive treatment, (often known as "induction therapy"), is used to cover this period. Implicit in this approach is the assumption that the benefits of preventing acute rejection in terms of graft and patient survival outweigh the additional side effects of increased immunosuppression. Surprisingly, such benefits have been hard to demonstrate. For example, initial experience with CyA in renal transplantation demonstrated a significant reduction in acute rejection without noticeable improvement in long-term graft survival [2]. Tacrolimus, MMF or anti-CD25 antibodies reduce acute rejection at 6 months by 30–50% without any improvement in either patient or graft survival at one year. Similar reductions in acute rejection can be achieved using ATG/OKT3 induction therapy but with questionable benefit after follow-up at two years [3–5].

Longer follow-up of two recent trials suggests that patients experiencing acute rejection in the first 6 months following renal transplantation are significantly more likely to have lost their graft by 3 years (26 and 35%) than those patients who remained free of rejection (6 and 7%) [6,7]. Retrospective studies also demonstrate a detrimental effect of early rejection on long-term renal allograft survival [8,9] and a recent analysis of all US renal transplants performed between 1988–1996 suggests that projected graft half-life is doubled in patients who remain free of rejection [10]. Consequently attempts to reduce early acute rejection appear justified, at least in renal transplantation.

Although the details of induction immunosuppression protocols vary between transplant centers, most are broadly similar irrespective of the organ transplanted. Immediately before or during the transplant operation high-dose glucocorticoid, typically 500–1,000mg methylprednisolone, is given [11]. In some units the first dose of calcineurin inhibitor is also given pre-operatively. Triple immunosuppressive therapy with CyA/tacrolimus, azathioprine/MMF and steroids is started post-operatively. The choice between Neoral and tacrolimus is often determined by local experience and by their individual side-effect profiles. Thus tacrolimus might be avoided in black patients because of the significant risk of diabetes, whereas the cosmetic side-effects of CyA may be unacceptable to some patients. The potential benefits of tacrolimus in renal, liver and lung transplantation have already been discussed in Chapter 6.

MMF has replaced azathioprine in many renal transplant units, particularly in the USA because of its superior protection against acute rejection [12–14] and potential long-term benefits [6,7,15]. However, the substantial cost of MMF has limited its use in some UK and European centers. Most units now use low-dose steroids, for example 20mg prednisolone, which are as effective in reducing acute graft rejection as the high dose regimens used in the 1980s [16].

The use of antibodies in induction therapy is controversial. ATG/OKT3 induction with CyA or tacrolimus-based triple therapy is commonly used in heart, lung and intestinal transplantation. In renal transplantation the lack of proven long-term benefit and significant side-effects of ATG/OKT3 have considerably reduced their use, especially since comparable reductions in acute rejection rates are now obtained with anti-CD25 antibodies, tacrolimus or MMF-containing regimens. Indeed, comparison of the US trials of tacrolimus [17] or MMF [12] (which used ATG) with similar European trials [13,18], (which did not), shows almost identical acute rejection rates irrespective of whether ATG was used. One rationale for the use of ATG/OKT3 as induction therapy in renal transplantation was that it could allow the introduction of calcineurin inhibitors to be delayed until the onset of reasonable graft function, thus eliminating CyA/tacrolimus nephrotoxicity in the immediate post-operative period. Although delayed graft function (DGF) is a risk factor for early graft failure [19], recent studies do not support a contributory role for CyA [20] and most renal transplant units now reserve ATG for the treatment of steroid resistant rejection or for induction therapy in very high risk patients. Trials comparing ATG and anti-CD25 antibodies in cardiothoracic and high-risk renal transplants are in progress.

Some groups of patients seem to be at particular risk for early acute rejection of renal allografts. These include children, black patients, recipients who receive grafts poorly-matched for HLA antigens, recipients highly sensitised against HLA antigens and recipients who have previously rejected a graft. There is some evidence that ATG induction may benefit these patients [5]. More importantly, knowledge of the recipient's immunological risk might allow immunosuppressive treatment to be tailored to each individual patient. In the same way, immunosuppressive regimens can be tailored to take account of risks attributable to the donor kidney. In particular, the shortage of suitable donor organs has resulted in many units using kidneys from increasingly elderly, often hypertensive donors (so-called "marginal" donors). These kidneys seem especially sensitive to ischemic and nephrotoxic injury and several groups have reported preliminary results using sirolimus, MMF or anti-CD25 antibody/ATG-based therapy in these types of transplants without the use of potentially nephrotoxic calcineurin inhibitors [21,22].

Maintenance Therapy

Following 3–6 months of stable graft function, it is common practice to gradually reduce the intensity of immunosuppression. The aim is to provide continuing prophylaxis against acute rejection whilst minimizing both the cumulative dose of immunosuppression and the adverse effects of specific drugs. No particular maintenance regimen has been shown to be clearly superior and there are few trials providing prospective data on long-term graft survival using different protocols. Nevertheless there is general agreement that dose reduction and in some circumstances, complete withdrawal of calcineurin inhibitors and steroids is appropriate.

CyA and tacrolimus both have significant long-term side effects. Most importantly, they increase the risk of cardiovascular disease through adverse effects on lipids, blood pressure and diabetes, and both are nephrotoxic. Nephrotoxicity is of particular concern in renal transplantation, but up to 6 percent of liver transplant [23,24] and 10 percent of heart transplant recipients [25] will develop end-stage renal failure, largely as a result of CyA/tacrolimus treatment. Three strategies are available to minimise CyA/tacrolimus exposure. First, almost all units reduce the dose of CyA/tacrolimus over time according to trough whole-blood levels. Typical target CyA levels are 250–350 μg/L at the time of transplantation, falling to 100–150 μg/L at one year (10–15 and 5–10 μg/L for tacrolimus). The difficulties in interpreting trough CyA/tacrolimus levels have been discussed in the preceding chapter.

The second approach is to withdraw CyA/tacrolimus altogether. Two trials in stable renal transplant recipients receiving CyA/MMF/steroids have shown that gradual CyA withdrawal improves renal function and lipid profiles at the expense of a 10–20% incidence of acute rejection [26,27]. Similar studies in which CyA is replaced with sirolimus are underway. The final approach is to eliminate CyA/tacrolimus from both induction and maintenance therapy by using sirolimus, MMF or anti-CD25 antibodies [21,28,29]. Unfortunately, long-term follow up information on this approach is not yet available.

Similar approaches have been used to reduce steroid exposure. Most induction regimens use only low dose steroids [16] and in those patients free of rejection, the dose is reduced rapidly. Liver transplant recipients for example, are often weaned from steroids within 3 months of transplantation. Trials in renal transplant recipients suggest that it is safe to withdraw steroids between 3 and 6 months post-transplant but, as with CyA/tacrolimus withdrawal, there is an excess of acute rejection episodes [30]. Late withdrawal of steroids, up to 6 years post-transplant is also possible but in some patients it may precipitate a deterioration in renal function and consequently requires close monitoring [31]. It is not clear if increased use of newer immunosuppressive agents will allow a more rapid reduction of steroid dose with fewer rejection episodes, although preliminary data with MMF suggest that this may be the case. Use of these drugs may also permit steroid-free immunosuppression.

Treatment of Acute Rejection

Depending on the organ transplanted, some 20–50% of transplant recipients will experience at least one episode of acute rejection despite modern induction therapy. Acute rejection is the leading cause of graft loss in the first year after transplantation and in renal allografts the severity of rejection may have a negative impact on long-term graft survival, particularly if there is persistent loss of graft function despite treatment [9]. Consequently, prompt diagnosis and effective treatment of acute rejection are essential. Three treatments are in current use.

First line treatment of acute rejection in most units is high dose intravenous steroids, usually 500-1,000mg of methylprednisolone given on three consecutive days, which is effective in 60–80% of cases. Patients with severe rejection or those who do not respond to steroids, are treated with a 10–14 day course of OKT3/ATG. Both antibody preparations are superior to steroids and are effective in 90 percent of rejection episodes. However, their significant side-effects (and cost) mean that most transplant programs do not use either ATG or OKT3 as first line treatment for rejection, thus minimizing the development of neutralizing antibodies and reserving ATG/OKT3 for steroid-resistant rejection. An important additional consideration is that multiple courses of antibody treatment considerably increase the risk of lymphoma, (up to 11% in one report) [32], justifying cautious use of ATG/OKT3 both as part of induction therapy and in the treatment of rejection. Finally, both tacrolimus [33] and MMF [34,35] can be used as "rescue therapy" either in patients who have recurrent episodes of acute rejection or who have rejection resistant to steroids and antibody. Tacrolimus is substituted for CyA and/or MMF for azathioprine. Clearly this is only an option if the patient is not already taking tacrolimus and MMF, making it reasonable to avoid one or the other in induction regimens.

Conclusions

Organ transplantation is undergoing rapid changes as immune mechanisms of allograft rejection are dissected and biotechnology yields molecules which can inhibit immune responses at various steps in the rejection cascade. Advances in therapeutic drug monitoring are helping the clinician to "fine tune" immunosuppressive therapy and commence early weaning, however, the importance of immunosuppressive drug therapy based on clinical judgment cannot be overemphasized.

References

1. Ponticelli C, Tarantino A, Segoloni G, et al. A randomised study comparing three cyclosporin-based regimens in cadaveric renal transplantation. J Am Soc Nephrol 1997;8:638–45.
2. Thiel G, Bock A, Spondlin M, et al. Long-term benefits and risks of cyclosporin-A (Sandimmun): an analysis at 10 years. Transplant Proc 1994;26:2493–8.
3. Szczech L, Berlin J, Aradhye S, et al. Effect of anti-lymphocyte induction therapy on renal allograft survival: a meta-analysis. J Am Soc Nephrol 1997; 8:1771–7.
4. Szczech L, Berlin J, Feldman HI, et al. The effect of anti-lymphocyte induction therapy on renal allograft survival. Ann Intern Med 1998;128:817–26.
5. Katznelson S, Cecka J. Immunosuppressive regimens and their effects on renal allograft outcome. In: Cecka J, Terasaki P. Editors. Clinical Transplants Los Angeles, CA: UCLA Tissue Typing Laboratory, 1996;361–71.
6. Mathew TH and the Tricontinental Mycophenolate Mofetil Renal Transplantation Study Group. A blinded, long-term, randomised multicentre study of mycophenolate mofetil in cadaveric renal transplantation. Results at three years. Transplantation 1998;65:1450–4.
7. European Mycophenolate Mofetil Cooperative Study Group. Mycophenolate mofetil in renal transplantation: 3-year results from the placebo-controlled trial. Transplantation 1999;68:391–6.
8. Humar A, Hassoun A, Kandaswamy R. Immunologic factors: the major risk for decreased renal allograft survival. Transplantation 1999;68:1842–6.
9. Vereerstraeten P, Abramowicz D, De Pauw L et al. Absence of a deleterious effect on long-term kidney graft survival of rejection episodes with complete functional recovery. Transplantation 1997;63:1739–43.
10. Hariharan S, Johnson CP, Bresnahan BA, et al. Improved graft survival after renal transplantation in the United States, 1988-1996. N Eng J Med 2000;342:605–12.
11. Fricke L, Klutter H, Feddersen A, et al. Pre-operative application of glucocorticoids efficaciously reduces the primary immunological response in kidney transplantation. Clin Transplant 1996;10:432–6.
12. US Renal Transplant Mycophenolate Mofetil Study Group, Sollinger HW. Mycophenolate mofetil for the prevention of acute rejection in primary cadaveric renal allograft recipients. Transplantation 1995;60:225–32.
13. Tricontinental Mycophenolate Mofetil Renal Transplantation Study Group. A blinded, randomised clinical trial of mycophenolate mofetil for the prevention of acute rejection in cadaveric renal transplantation. Transplantation 1996;61:1029–37.
14. European Mycophenolate Mofetil Study Group. Placebo controlled study of mycophenolate mofetil combined with cyclosporin and corticosteroids for prevention of acute rejection. Lancet 1995;345:1321–5.
15. Ojo AO, Meier-Kriesche HU, Hanson JA, et al. Mycophenolate mofetil reduces late renal allograft loss independent of acute rejection. Transplantation 2000;69:2405–9.
16. Gore SM, Oldham JA. Randomised trials of high- and low-dose steroids in renal transplantation. Transplantation 1986;41:319.
17. Pirsch JD, Miller J, Deierhoi MH, et al. A comparison of tacrolimus (FK506) and cyclosporin for immunosuppression after cadaveric renal transplantation. Transplantation 1997;63:977–83.
18. Mayer AD, Dmitrewski J, Squifflet JP et al. Multicenter randomized trial comparing tacrolimus and cyclosporine in the prevention of renal allograft rejection. A report of the European tacrolimus multicenter renal study group. Transplantation;1997,64:436.
19. Ojo AO, Wolfe RA, Held PJ, et al. Delayed graft function: risk factors and implications for renal graft survival. Transplantation 1997;63:968.
20. Kasiske B, Johnson H, Goerdt P, et al. A randomised trial comparing cyclosporin induction with sequential therapy in renal transplant recipients. Am J Kidney Dis 1997;30:639–45.
21. Hong JC, Kahan BD. Use of anti-CD25 monoclonal antibody in combination with rapamycin to eliminate cyclosporin treatment during the induction phase of immunosuppression. Transplantation 1999;68:701–4
22. Land W. Mycophenolate mofetil-based immunosuppressive therapy: induction, maintenance and conversion protocols in renal transplantation. Transplant Proc 1999;31:27–32.
23. Hornberger J, Best J, Geppert J, et al. Risks and costs of end stage renal disease after heart transplantation. Transplantation 1998;66:1763–70.
24. Jain A, Reyes J, Kashyap R, et al. What have we learned about primary liver transplantation under tacrolimus immunosuppression? Long-term follow up of the first 1,000 patients. Ann Surg 1999;230:441–9.

25. Abramowicz D, Manas D, Lao M, et al. Preliminary results of a randomised controlled study investigating the withdrawal of Neoral in stable renal transplants receiving mycophenolate mofetil in addition to Neoral and steroids. Transplantation 1999;67(suppl):240.
26. De Sevaux RG, Smak-Gregor PJ, Hene RJ et al. Withdrawal of cyclosporine or prednisolone in renal transplant recipients treated with mycophenolate mofetil, cyclosporine and prednisolone: a randomised study. Transplantation 1999;67(suppl):240.
27. Groth CG, Backman L, Morales J-M, et al. Sirolimus (Rapamycin)-based therapy in human renal transplantation. Transplantation 1999;67:1036–42.
28. Kreis H, Cisterne JM, Land W, et al. Sirolimus in association with mycophenolate mofetil induction for the prevention of acute graft rejection in renal allograft recipients. Transplantation 2000;69:1252–60.
29. Hricik DE, O'Toole M, Schulak JA, et al. Steroid-free, cyclosporin-based immunosuppression after renal transplantation: a meta-analysis of controlled trials. J Am Soc Nephrol 1993;4:1300–5.
30. Ratcliffe PJ, Dudley CR, Higgins RM, et al. Randomised controlled trial of steroid withdrawal in renal transplant recipients receiving triple immunosuppression. Lancet 1996;348:643–8.
31. Vanrenterghem Y. Strategies to reduce or replace steroid dosing. Transplant Proc 1999;31 (suppl):7–10.
32. Swinnen LJ, Constanzo-Nordin MR, Fisher SG, et al. Increased incidence of lymphoproliferative disorder after immunosuppression with the monoclonal antibody OKT3 in cardiac transplant recipients. N Engl J Med 1990;323:1723–8.
33. Woodle ES, Thistlethwaite R, Gordon JH, et al. A multicentre trial of FK506 therapy in refractory acute renal allograft rejection. Transplantation 1996;62:594–9.
34. Mycophenolate Mofetil Acute Renal Rejection Study Group. Mycophenolate mofetil for the treatment of a first acute renal allograft rejection. Transplantation 1998;65:235–41.
35. Mycophenolate Mofetil Renal Refractory Rejection Study Group. Mycophenolate mofetil for the treatment of refractory, acute cellular renal transplant rejection. Transplantation 1996;61:722–9.

8. The Immunology of Xenotransplantation

Christoph Knosalla and David K.C. Cooper

Introduction

Today, the shortage of organ donors is a major limiting factor to organ transplantation. In 1999 in the USA, 72,110 patients were waiting for an organ transplant, while only 21,516 (16,862 cadaveric and 4,714 living) donor organs became available in the same year [1]. This shortage results in increasing waiting times for patients requiring kidney transplantation and a mortality of greater than 10 percent per year in patients waiting for heart or liver transplantation. For children, the shortage in organ availability is even more marked. These limitations, which show no immediate signs of being resolved, have increased the interest in the use of xenogeneic organs. Xenotransplantation offers an unlimited source of organs and cells, the opportunity for the surgical procedure to be performed on an elective basis and the ability to extend the indications for organ transplantation.

Definitions

Xenotransplantation (XTx) refers to the transplantation of tissues or organs between different species. When the human is considered as the potential organ recipient, XTx includes non-human primate-to-human or non-primate mammal-to-human transplantation. There have been clinical attempts using both of these models, where both non-human primates and pigs have been used as sources of organs [2]. In experimental settings, many different models have been described.

Some years ago it was proposed by Calne that XTx should be classified as either *concordant* or *discordant*. When *hyperacute rejection* (HAR, occurring within minutes or hours) results, the donor-recipient pair is considered *discordant*. If rejection is delayed longer than 24 hours and follows a pattern similar, but possibly accelerated, to allograft rejection, he has suggested that the pair be considered *concordant*.

The major differences between these two groups is that in discordant pairs, HAR results from the existence of pre-formed natural antibodies in the recipient directed against antigens in the donor species. These antibodies bind to the antigens on the donor organ vascular endothelium and activate complement, resulting in HAR. Because these antibodies are produced in the host without the need for prior immunization by a specific organ transplant, they are referred to as natural xeno-reactive antibodies. When transplantation is carried out between concordant species, there is no or a very low level of natural xeno-reactive antibody in the recipient directed at donor antigens. However, a rapid induced response develops, leading to rejection more rapidly than would normally be observed in allograft models.

Choice of Source Animal

Although the non-human primates offer the advantage of phylogenetic proximity, their limited availability and limited breeding capacity, together with other factors such as the cost of maintenance, the potential risk of transferring viral infection, (xenozoonosis) and ethical concerns relating to their use in large numbers for the purposes of transplantation, have led to limited enthusiasm for their use in this respect. In contrast to these logistic and ethical objections, the pig is widely viewed as the most suitable source of organs for humans for a number of reasons as outlined in Table 8.1, [3] however, it creates specific immunological problems that must be resolved if it is to be utilized in this capacity.

Immunological Barriers

Hyperacute Rejection (HAR)

From the immunological perspective, the pig is *discordant* to humans. Transplantation of a pig organ into a human or non-human primate is frequently rapidly rejected within minutes or hours, although longer survival has been documented. Work in the 1960s by several groups, in particular by Perper and Najarian [4], demonstrated the mechanism of discordant xenograft rejection to be that of antibody-mediated complement activation. More recent studies, particularly by Good et al [5] have indicated that the major determinant on the pig vascular endothelium to which human antibodies are directed is a galactose oligosaccharide. The major difference between the carbohydrate structures exposed on the vascular endothelium of the pig when compared with the human is the presence of Galα1-3Gal (Gal) epitopes on the pig vascular endothelium, which can be considered as the equivalent of the human ABO blood type antigens.

All placental mammals, (except humans, apes and Old World monkeys), express a functional gene (α1,3 galactosyltransferase) that produces the enzyme that synthesizes Gal epitopes [6]. Glycoproteins and glycolipids containing Gal epitopes are found on many pig tissues, including the entire vascular endothelium [7]. Because animals that express a functional gene are immunologically tolerant to Gal, they do not, of course, produce antibodies that bind to the Gal epitope. In contrast, in humans, apes and Old World monkeys, the functional gene appears to have been lost during evolution [6] and these species therefore produce antibodies to Gal epitopes. The transplantation of a pig organ into a human is therefore initially rejected by anti-Gal antibody with binding to Gal antigens and the activation of complement.

It is believed that anti-Gal antibodies develop in humans and other non-human primates during the early weeks of neonatal life as a response to colonization of the gastrointestinal tract by various microorganisms (bacteria, viruses and fungi) which express Gal structures on their cell surfaces [8]. There is evidence to suggest that anti-Gal antibodies account for approximately 80–90% of the natural anti-pig antibody in humans, although this varies considerably between individuals. The exact character of natural antibodies that are directed to other porcine determinants remains uncertain, but Zhu [9] has provided evidence that antibodies other than anti-Gal can lead to porcine cell destruction although with significantly diminished cytotoxicity when compared with anti-Gal antibodies.

The presence of pre-formed natural anti-Gal antibody leads to immediate destruction of a transplanted pig organ. Macroscopically, the transplanted organ swells (sometimes to twice its normal size and weight), becomes black from a combination of interstitial hemorrhage and ischemia and rapidly ceases to function. Histopathologically, HAR is characterized by thrombus formation, which is more accentuated initially in the venous system than in the arterial, with disruption of the vascular endothelium, interstitial hemorrhage, and edema [10]. Infiltration of polymorphonuclear leukocytes may then follow. Immunohistologically, HAR is characterized by the deposition of IgM, IgG, IgA and complement on the vascular endothelium. The underlying mechanism, and the macroscopic and microscopic appearances are similar to the HAR that can develop following transplantation of an ABO-incompatible organ allograft as discussed in Chapters 5 and 7.

Prevention of HAR

If anti-pig antibodies are depleted from the recipient serum, then HAR can be avoided. This can either be achieved through a course of plasmapheresis or through the passage of plasma through immunoaffinity columns of synthetic Gal oligosaccharides that deplete the plasma only of anti-Gal antibody [11]. The latter technique has some advantages over plasma exchange because of its specificity, since beneficial antibodies are not removed in the process. Although it has been demonstrated that such immunoadsorption is efficient in preventing HAR, anti-Gal antibody continues to be produced, however, resulting in a delayed form of rejection over several days (vide infra).

An alternative approach is to deplete or inhibit the complement that is the ultimate destructive agent in xenorejection and this can be achieved through the use of purified cobra venom factor [12] or the administration of soluble complement receptor type 1 (sCR1) [13]. These agents work in different ways, with Cobra venom factor activating the alternate pathway of complement and leading to rapid complement depletion at the C3 point of the pathway. sCR1 inhibits both the classical and alternate pathways of complement by binding to proteins at the C3 and C5 level, thus preventing development of subsequent activated complement factors, with both agents protecting a xenograft from HAR for several days. However, long-term administration of any agent that depletes or inhibits complement is associated with a potential risk of infection and therefore this form of therapy cannot be continued indefinitely, hence complicating the design of clinical studies.

A third approach has been the development of genetically engineered pigs which express one or more human complement-regulatory proteins (CRPs) [14,15]. Such CRPs can protect human cells from autologous complement activation under most circumstances. Pigs express pig CRPs for the same purposes, but there is evidence that pig CRPs do not protect successfully against human complement. Therefore, the introduction of one or more human CRPs by transgenic technology has been shown to be beneficial in protecting pig organs. There is some evidence, however, that it is the *quantity* of CRPs rather than the *quality* that is important and that an increase in the expression of pig CRPs might be as effective as the introduction of a human CRP [16].

The human complement regulatory system includes several different proteins for manipulation, such as decay accelerating factor (CD55, DAF), membrane cofactor protein (CD46, MCP) and membrane inhibitor of reactive lysis (CD59). Organs from pigs expressing one or more of these CRPs have been demonstrated to successfully block human (or non-human primate) complement activation in vitro and to prevent HAR when a pig organ is transplanted into a primate. However, as with antibody depletion and/or complement inhibition, such transgenic organs remain susceptible to a subsequent rejection phenomenon that develops in the pig-to-primate model over time, known as *acute humoral xenograft rejection* (AHXR).

Acute Humoral Xenograft Rejection (AHXR)

This form of rejection develops after some days or weeks and at present remains the major immunological barrier to successful XTx. Macroscopically, AHXR appears as a patchy discoloration on the graft, which reflects small areas of focal ischemia and/or congestion. Hemorrhagic spots may develop, indicating interstitial blood extravasation. There are as yet no clinical laboratory data that are diagnostic of the development of AHXR, although it can be associated with a progressive thrombocytopenia, due to consumption of platelets in the graft combined with a disturbance of coagulation parameters; (in particular a fall in fibrinogen to below detectable levels and a dramatic increase in prothrombin time), both of which are believed to be markers of endothelial cell activation.

Table 8.1. Relative advantages and disadvantages of baboons and pigs as sources of organs and tissues for transplantation into humans

	Baboon	Pig
Availability	Limited	Unlimited
Breeding potential	Poor	Good
Size of adult organs	Inadequate[a]	Adequate (in selected herds)[a]
Similarity to humans		
Anatomy	Close	Close
Physiology	Close	Moderately close
Cost of maintenance	High	Low
Immunologic compatibility	Concordant	Discordant
Necessity for blood-type compatibility with humans	Important	Probably unimportant
Experience with genetic engineering	None	Considerable
Risk of infection transfer (xenozoonosis)	High	Low
Public opinion about use	Mixed	Favorable

[a] The size of certain baboon organs, e.g. the heart, is inadequate for transplantation into adult humans. Breeds of miniature swine are approximately 50 percent of the weight of domestic pigs at birth and sexual maturity and reach a maximum 200–300lb (< 130 kg)

SECTION III

PRINCIPLES OF TUMOR IMMUNOLOGY

combination pharmacologic therapy. For example, Zaidi et al [23] demonstrated that survival of an hDAF transgenic pig kidney could be maintained for over two months with immunosuppression provided by a cocktail of cyclophosphamide, cyclosporine and corticosteroids. There is little evidence, however, that even this therapy prevents the induced antibody response to the pig organ. At our own center, Bühler et al [20] have demonstrated that co-stimulatory blockade using an anti-CD154 monoclonal antibody does successfully prevent the induced antibody response. This certainly reduces the antibody load on the transplanted organ, but has not been entirely successful in preventing AHXR.

There is considerable evidence that endothelial cell activation plays a central role in the development of AHXR, especially for the activation of the coagulation system and agents which reduce such activation have been demonstrated to be beneficial. Once again, cyclophosphamide appears to be capable of inhibiting endothelial cell activation, but its long-term use is limited due to its significant immunosuppressive effect and side-effects. There have been several studies in rodent models of changes in gene expression in the endothelial cells after XTx, demonstrating up-regulation of "beneficial" genes which promote a state of *accommodation* in which the endothelium develops resistance to the effect of antibody [24]. Although accommodation has not yet been documented conclusively in any pig-to-primate model. Approaches incorporating gene therapy or further transgenic technology, therefore, remain future possibilities to stimulate clinical endothelial accommodation.

As intravascular disseminated coagulation appears to be a significant feature of AHXR, approaches have been undertaken to inhibit platelet aggregation and/or coagulation by treatment of xenograft recipients with various agents. To date, these attempts have failed to prevent AHXR. Indeed, one of the major effects of cyclophosphamide, in addition to its immunosuppressive effect, may be the fact that it reduces platelet numbers and, in particular, platelet aggregation.

As both HAR and AHXR appear to result largely from the presence of anti-Gal antibodies, it would clearly seem beneficial to develop a pig that did not synthesize and express this epitope. "Knockout" (KO) of the α1,3galactosyltransferase gene has been achieved in mouse embryonic stem cells by homologous recombination [25]. However, pluripotent embryonic stem cells are not available in pigs and so Gal-knockout has not yet been achieved in pigs. The technique of nuclear transfer holds some promise of overcoming this technical problem and several groups are currently attempting to develop Gal-knockout pigs using this new technology. Although it is unlikely a Gal-knockout pig would resolve all of the immunological problems inherent in xenotransplantation, we can be optimistic that it will lead to significant progress in the field of pig-primate transplantation.

A final strategy to diminish humoral responsiveness might be to decrease the expression of Gal on donor pig organs by increasing expression of another oligosaccharide, an approach that has been named *competitive glycosylation* [26]. For example, the introduction of the gene for the H(O) blood group saccharide (α1,2fucosyltransferase), that competes with 1,3-galactosyltransferase for its substrate (a sugar known as N-acetyllactosamine), has been demonstrated in in vitro models to lead to the replacement of Gal in up to 80–90% of its distribution. However, this low expression of Gal is still sufficient to lead to ultimate cell destruction by anti-Gal antibody and it would seem necessary to replace *all* Gal epitopes if this approach is to be successful.

Cellular Xenograft Rejection

In vitro evidence suggests that the cellular response to a pig xenograft will be at least as strong, if not stronger, than that towards an allograft [27]. The cellular response in vivo, however, remains poorly defined, largely because AHXR has not yet been successfully overcome. Pino-Chavez [18] has described the microscopic features of a cell-mediated response that develops even in the presence of intensive immunosuppressive therapy. However, conclusions regarding the pure cell-mediated response (in the absence of AHXR) must be interpreted with great caution, as data are currently extremely limited. It would seem likely, however, that if AHXR could be overcome, a cell-mediated response may then subsequently develop.

Chronic Xenograft Rejection

It would also seem likely that chronic rejection, e.g. graft atherosclerosis, will develop in transplanted pig organs and will possibly develop more rapidly than in allo-transplants. Because of the need for prolonged intensive immunosuppressive therapy in order to suppress the cell-mediated response and the possible development of early chronic rejection, there are those working in this field who believe that only techniques to allow the development of immunological tolerance will be successful in xenotransplantation. Our own center has been investigating this possibility for several years.

Immunological Tolerance

Some scientists involved in this field of research believe that it is unlikely the immunological barriers to xenotransplantation will be overcome unless immunological tolerance (unresponsiveness) to the transplanted organ can be induced [28]. Approaches towards this goal in our own laboratory have included efforts to induce both B and T cell tolerance by induction of mixed hematopoietic chimerism using pig bone marrow cells or peripheral blood mobilized progenitor cells [22, 29]. This approach has not yet been successful due largely to the continuing presence of anti-Gal antibody and the rapid removal of pig cells from the blood of non-human primates by macrophages.

More recently, based on successful experiments in mice, in which the transplantation of pig thymic tissue has induced a state of tolerance to pig skin grafts [30] and in pigs, (in which tolerance to allografts was achieved by the transplantation of a composite "thymokidney"), we have investigated co-incident thymic transplantation in the pig-to-baboon model [31]. The transplantation of vascularized pig thymic tissue in the form of a pig thymokidney (autologous thymic tissue placed under the pig's renal capsule and allowed to revascularize before transplantation into a baboon) has been only partially successful in this respect due, once again, to the persistence of natural anti-Gal antibodies which have prevented long-term graft survival and have hindered the development of T-cell tolerance by this approach.

Finally, the introduction into the non-human primate's own bone marrow cells of the gene for α1,3galactosyltransferase might allow for the deletion of the B cells responsible for anti-Gal antibody production as the primate's autologous bone marrow cells would then express this epitope [32]. Although this approach (along with the mixed hematopoietic chimerism strategy), have been successful in rodent models (using Gal-knockout mice which produce anti-Gal antibody), neither has yet been successful in the pig-to-primate model.

Comment

If XTx using the pig as the source of organs could be developed successfully, its potential in clinical medicine is immense [33]. Not only would organs be available for transplantation electively and in unlimited numbers, but conditions such as diabetes mellitus might be cured by the transplantation of large numbers of pig pancreatic islets. Indeed, in almost any condition where there is inadequate cell function, e.g. inadequate dopamine production in patients with Parkinson's disease, the XTx of cells may potentially offer a cure. With the current rate of advance in biotechnology, it seems likely that the remaining barriers to successful XTx can be overcome within the foreseeable future.

Acknowledgements

The authors thank their many colleagues at the Transplantation Biology Research Center and at Immerge BioTherapeutics who have contributed to the studies summarized in this review, and David H. Sachs, MD, and Leo Bühler, MD, for their critical reviews of the manuscript. Christoph Knosalla, MD was supported by a research grant of the Deutsche Forschungsgemeinschaft (KN 518,1-1). Work in our own laboratory was supported by NIH Program Project 1PO1 A145897 and by a Sponsored Research Agreement between the Massachusetts General Hospital and Immerge BioTherapeutics, Inc.

References

1. United Network for Organ Sharing (UNOS). 2000 Annual Report of the US Scientific Registry of Transplant Recipients and the Organ Procurement and Transplantation Network. Department of Health and Human Services, 2001.
2. Taniguchi S, Cooper DKC. Clinical xenotransplantation — past, present and future. Ann R Coll Surg Engl 1997;79:13-9.
3. Sachs DH. The pig as a potential xenograft donor. Vet Immunol Immunopathol. 1994;43:185-91.
4. Perper RJ, Najarian JS. Experimental renal heterotransplantation: I. In widely divergent species. Transplantation 1966;4:377-88.
5. Good AH, Cooper DKC, Malcolm AJ, Ippolito RM, Koren E, Neethling FA, et al. Identification of carbohydrate structures which bind human anti-porcine antibodies: implications for discordant xenografting in man. Transplant Proc 1992;24:559-62.
6. Galili U, Shohet SB, Kobrin E, Stults CL, Macher BA. Man, apes, and Old World monkeys differ from other mammals in the expression of α-galactosyl epitopes on nucleated cells. J Biol Chem 1988;263:17755-62.
7. Oriol R, Ye Y, Koren E, Cooper DKC. Carbohydrate antigens of pig tissues reacting with human natural antibodies as potential targets for hyperacute vascular rejection in pig-to-man organ xeno-transplantation. Transplantation 1993;56:1433-42 .
8. Galili U, Mandrell RE, Hamadeh RM, et al. The interaction between the human natural anti-α-galactosyl IgG (anti-Gal) and bacteria of the human flora. Infect Immun 1998;57:1730-7.
9. Zhu A. Binding of human natural antibodies to nonalphaGal xenoantigens on porcine erythrocytes Transplantation 2000;69:2422-8.
10. Rose AG, Cooper DKC, Human PA, Reichenspurner H, Reichart B. Histopathology of hyperacute

rejection of the heart — experimental and clinical observations in allografts and xenografts. J Heart Transplant 1991;10:223–34.

11. Taniguchi S, Neethling FA, Korchagina EY, Bovin N, Ye Y, Kobayashi T, et al. In vivo immunoadsorption of anti-pig antibodies in baboons using a specific Gal(alpha)1-3Gal column. Transplantation 1996;62:1379–84.

12. Leventhal JR, Dalmasso AP, Cromwell JW, Platt JL, Manivel CJ, Bolman RM III, et al. Prolongation of cardiac xenograft survival by depletion of complement. Transplantation 1993;55:857–65.

13. Pruitt SK, Kirk AD, Bollinger RR, Marsh HC Jr, Collins BH, Levin JL, et al. The effect of soluble complement receptor type 1 on hyperacute rejection of porcine xenografts. Transplantation 1994;57:363–70.

14. Cozzi E, White DJ. The generation of transgenic pigs as potential organ donors for humans. Nat Med 1995;1:964–6.

15. Dalmasso AP, Vercellotti GM, Platt JL,Bach FH. Inhibition of complement-mediated endothelial cell cytotoxicity by decay-accelerating factor. Potential for prevention of xenograft hyperacute rejection. Transplantation 1991;52: 530–3.

16. van den Berg CW, Morgan BP. Understanding the immune protection afforded by endogenous complement regulatory molecules. Graft 2001;4: 63–65.

17. Shimizu A, Meehan SM, Kozlowski T, Sablinski T, Ierino FL, Cooper DKC, et al. Acute humoral xenograft rejection: destruction of the microvascular capillary endothelium in pig-to-nonhuman primate renal grafts. Lab Invest 2000;80:815–30.

18. Pino-Chavez G. Differentiating acute humoral from acute cellular rejection histopathologically. Graft 2001;4:60–2.

19. Bühler L, Awwad M, Basker M, Gojo S, Watts A, Treter S, et al. High-dose porcine hematopoietic cell transplantation combined with CD40 ligand blockade in baboons prevents an induced anti-pig humoral response. Transplantation 2000;69:2296–304.

20. Bühler L, Yamada K., Kitamura H, Alwayn IPJ, Basker M, Barth RN, et al. Pig kidney transplantation in baboons: anti-Gal IgM alone is associated with acute vascular rejection and disseminated intravascular coagulation. Transplantation 2001 (in press).

21. Teranishi K, Gollackner B, Bühler L, Knosalla C, Correa L, Down JD, et al. Depletion of anti-Gal antibodies in baboons by intravenous therapy with bovine serum albumin conjugated to Gal oligosaccharides. Transplantation 2001 (in press)

22. Lambrigts D, Sachs DH, Cooper DKC. Discordant organ xenotransplantation in primates: world experience and current status. Transplantation 1998;15:66:547–61.

23. Zaidi A, Schmoeckel M, Bhatti F, Waterworth P, Tolan M, Cozzi E, et al. Life-supporting pig-to-primate renal xenotransplantation using genetically modified donors. Transplantation. 1998;65:1584–90.

24. Bach FH, Ferran C, Hechenleitner P, Mark W, Koyamada N, Miyatake T, et al. Accommodation of vascularized xenografts: expression of "protective genes" by donor endothelial cells in a host Th2 cytokine environment. Nat Med 1997;3:196–204.

25. Thall AD, Maly P, Lowe JB. Oocyte Galα1,3Gal epitopes implicated in sperm adhesion to the zona pellucida glycoprotein ZP3 are not required for fertilization in the mouse. J Biol Chem 1995;270:21437–40.

26. Sandrin MS, Fodor WL, Mouhtouris E, Osman N, Cohney S, Rollins SA, et al. Enzymatic remodeling of the carbohydrate surface of a xenogenic cell substantially reduces human antibody binding and complement-mediated cytolysis. Nat Med 1995;1:1261–7.

27. Yamada K, Auchincloss H. Cell-mediated xenograft rejection. Curr Opin Organ Transplant 1999: 4; 90–4.

28. Sachs DH. Mixed chimerism as an approach to transplantation tolerance. Clin Immunol 2000;95;S63–8.

29. Kozlowski T, Shimizu A, Lambrigts D, Yamada K, Fuchimoto Y, Glaser R, et al. Porcine kidney and heart transplantation in baboons undergoing a tolerance induction regimen and antibody adsorption. Transplantation. 1999; 67;18–30.

30. Zhao Y, Swenson K, Sergio JJ, Arn JS, Sachs DH, Sykes M. Skin graft tolerance across a discordant xenogeneic barrier. Nat Med 1996;2;1211–6.

31. Yamada K, Shimizu A, Utsugi R, Ierino FL, Gargollo P, et al. Thymic transplantation in miniature swine. II. Induction of tolerance by transplantation of composite thymokidneys to thymectomized recipients. J Immunol 2000;164:3079–86.

32. Bracy JL, Sachs DH, Iacomini J. Inhibition of xenoreactive natural antibody production by retroviral gene therapy. Science. 1998;281:1845–7.

33. Cooper DKC, Lanza RP. Xeno: The Promise of Transplanting Animal Organs into Humans. New York: Oxford University Press, 2000; 1–274.

Commentary on Chapter 8

Ignazio R. Marino

The significant advances achieved in the field of organ transplantation have led to an increased demand for organs creating a wide gap between organ availability and supply. Whilst the number of transplants performed worldwide is limited by this dramatic donor shortage, alternative sources need to be explored, where a wider availability of organs would allow an expansion rather than a contraction of the indications for transplantation and at the same time a relaxation of the patient selection criteria. As discussed by Drs Knosalla and Cooper in Chapter 8, these facts clearly justify the renewed interest in xenotransplantation which has been observed in the last decade [1,2].

Before the concept of xenotransplantation advances to a clinical reality, at least three practical challenges must be overcome. The first consists of all the immunological barriers as listed in this chapter. The second issue is related to the potential risk of the introduction of novel and serious infectious organisms into the human recipient (and possibly into the human population at large) via the xenotransplant. Lastly, xenotransplantation raises issues and concerns in several different fields, most notably theological, anthropological, psychological, ethical and legal considerations. This commentary will mainly focus on the immunological issues of xenotransplantation as well as on the risk of exposing the general public to novel infectious agents, generally referred to as xenozoonoses.

In their chapter Drs. Knosalla and Cooper have explained why the pig is considered to be the most suitable animal source of organs for humans and have outlined the three main rejection mechanisms preventing the clinical application of a pig-to-human xenotransplantation procedure; namely hyperacute rejection (HAR), acute humoral xenograft rejection (AHXR) and cellular xenograft rejection (CXR). These immunological barriers are significantly more difficult to overcome in a pig-to-human xenotransplant when compared with a primate-to-human xenotransplant (e.g. baboon-to-human). On June 28, 1992 and January 10, 1993 we performed two baboon-to-human liver xenotransplantations in Pittsburgh [3]. The two patients survived respectively for 70 and 26 days. The first patient (the one who survived longer) was placed on an oral diet by the 5th post-transplant day and he spent most of his time in a regular hospital ward, briefly leaving the hospital on one occasion. This experience demonstrated that a human being may live with a baboon liver. However, while in the past non-human primates have been preferred as a source of organs for humans, the transplant community and regulatory agencies in the countries dealing with this issue are nowadays more favorably looking at the pig. This is because non-human primates potentially carry an increased risk of infection transmission and also because of a variety of other ethical and practical concerns (e.g. organ size). The truth is that in the two cases of baboon-to-human liver xenotransplantation mentioned above, it was possible to demonstrate only a single case of a baboon pathogen (a cytomegalovirus) which was apparently transferred to a patient. At any rate, this event did not result in a disease process [4] and the death of both patients was totally unrelated to any sort of xenozoonoses. In both recipients, evidence was found of an adequately functioning liver mass, sufficient to sustain life. On the other hand, even though proven feasible, the use of baboons is complicated mainly by limited availability, inadequate size of organs for adult human beings and high costs. Another non-human primate, the chimpanzee, is most likely the best donor for human transplantation of this type in biological terms, largely due to the very small genetic differences between this species and humans. In this respect, in 1963 a woman lived for 9 months without dialysis with a functioning chimpanzee kidney and died free of rejection. The endangered status of the chimpanzee, however, prevents their widespread use for clinical purposes. In the United States only 25–50 chimpanzees may be used annually in biomedical research and it is estimated that only 70 chimpanzees per year would be available worldwide as organ donors. Therefore, their use (as well as the use of other great apes such as the gorilla) would further jeopardize these species and would raise insurmountable ethical concerns without solving the organ shortage problem.

In the last ten years the use of genetic engineering has resulted in a marked improvement of the survival time of a pig organ transplanted in a non-human primate model [5,6]. Nevertheless, substantial immunological barriers still exist and strategies to prevent HAR and AHXR in a pig-to-primate need to be developed further. Although the use of genetic engineering has resulted in significant improvement in survival time for a pig organ in a non-human primate (close to 3 months), these survival times do not yet approach that of human organ allotransplantation. The ultimate goal here is obviously to obtain immunological tolerance of the graft by the recipient organism [7].

As discussed in Chapter 8, the main barrier to successful xenotransplantation of vascularized porcine organs into humans is antibody and complement-mediated HAR, mostly as a result of naturally occurring anti-Galα(1,3)Gal antibodies. This carbohydrate epitope (which is not found in humans or Old World monkeys) may be induced by gut bacteria which possess a related Galα1-3Gal structure [8]. The strategies to deal with these are considered by Drs Knosalla and Cooper and include transgenic approaches designed to reduce the antibody titer and to express either membrane-bound or soluble complement regulators; most notably CD46, CD55 and CD59. These approaches may be combined with attempts to modify the donor animals by the inactivation of their galactosyltransferase genes so as to diminish the synthesis of Galα(1,3)Gal, although this is still experimental in the pig. Such a strategy will probably also require nuclear transfer technology for the production of knockout pigs or composite transgenic technology with multiple gene transfers [9,10]. In this regard, preliminary evidence of these approaches shows that it appears to attenuate experimental hyperacute rejection. The immunology affecting non-vascularized xenotransplants, such as porcine pancreatic islets appears to be different since although antibody-mediated mechanisms are important, they are not generated through anti-Gal activity [11]. Even if these techniques are successful, additional strategies which alter the phases of vascular and chronic rejection of xenotransplanted organs will still be required and it seems unlikely at the present time that combination therapies of porcine tissue transgenic for CRP's and standard immunosuppression will enable desired levels and durations of graft survival. Here, an improved understanding of the immunological process of accommodation, (sometimes observed in ABO-mismatched allografts), where the graft endothelium becomes resistant over time to the action of specific antibodies, is needed. This process may be secondarily under the control of protective genes such as hemo-oxygenase 1 [12,13].

Successful xenotransplantation may require the induction of T cell tolerance as discussed in this chapter, with the use of deliberate mixed hemopoietic chimerism using donor and recipient bone marrow; an approach which has been used successfully in baboons to transiently suppress anti-Gal responses in marrow transplants [14]. Human-to-baboon bone marrow transplantation has already been performed at the Thomas E. Starzl Transplantation Institute laboratories, after conditioning the donor marrow with non-lethal irradiation. However, it remains to be seen if incomplete or even full chimerism will change the image of animal organs enough to make them be immunologically viewed as "allografts" by humans.

Newer approaches are of necessity complex if we are to entirely eliminate the offending epitope principally involved in xenografting. In rodents, embryonic stem cells for the production of animals which are incapable of producing the Galα1,3Gal epitope but which can still produce antibodies to it have been developed, however, at present, porcine embryonic stem cells of this type capable of germline transmission have not been able to be produced. Cloning of pigs with inactivated Gal glycosyltransferase systems by a combination of available technology (notably cloning of animals from somatic cells) and modification of candidate genes in such clones by homologous recombination may provide an alternative to stem cell approaches [15,16].

There are also a number of other concerns limiting a wide application of xenotransplantation in a clinical setting. The most important of these is the infectious disease risks posed by xenozoonoses as outlined in this chapter. The crucial question is whether in our attempts to save individual life through a xenotransplantation we are putting a larger population at risk from novel infectious disease. On one side of this debate there are those who believe that any chance of bringing new infectious organisms into the human population is far too great a risk to pay for this technology and that, as a consequence, xenotransplantation should not be performed at all [17]. On the opposite side, others are convinced that there should not be any further delay in using this technology for life-saving procedures such as transplanting an animal liver as a "bridge" solution in the treatment of a fulminant hepatitis, whilst awaiting a suitable human organ [18].

The true risk to humans of swine-related viral infection is unclear, but given views concerning the cross-species genesis of AIDS, variant Creutzfeldt-Jakob disease, chicken Hong Kong H5N1 influenza virus and the current South East Asian pandemic of Nipah virus (probably reservoired in fruit bats but transmitted to humans by swine contact and responsible for a number of recent fatal infections in Malaysia and Singapore), a general social concern seems justified [19,20]. Moreover, xenotransplantation could change the dynamics of infection by the breaching of the physical barrier towards cross-species infection (through surgical implantation), by attendant immunosuppression and by human proteins which normally modulate HAR serving as viral receptors and protecting against complement-directed anti-viral attack [21].

The sort of barrier husbandry required to render these animals virus- and microbe-free is going to be complex and expensive. Here, a number of studies have reported on the development of quality herds with high health conditions as source animals for xenotransplantation [22]. Controlled delivery by hysterotomy, the use of closed herds and careful monitoring of both animals and veterinary staff for general health status are some of the most important techniques aiming at preventing a transmission of infectious agents from animals selected as organ donors for xenotransplantation. In pigs a strict application of these rules should significantly diminish the concerns related to xenozoonoses. However, even with swine, areas of preoccupation still exist. Monitoring for ubiquitous viruses capable of virtually continuous re-infection of the herd (like the parvovirus or the circovirus) and the identification of new as yet unknown viruses in swine is a major challenge. Moreover, the delineation of innocent viruses in animals does not necessarily imply that they will remain innocent in humans.

At present, the porcine endogenous retroviruses (PERVs) are viewed as carrying the most significant risk of xenozoonoses in clinical xenotransplantation, where it has been reported that PERVs are capable of infecting human cells in vitro [23]. The importance of the PERV agent is its facility for vertical transmission, where the genome is incorporated into the genome of the host. Such a replication-competent virus has a potential for infecting totally unrelated species. These PERVs were originally detected being released from porcine renal cell cultures and are C-type γ retroviruses which share homology with murine leukemia viruses [24]. Since the types of pigs used for xenotransplantation contain at least 50+ PERVs incorporated into their genome, until these are cloned and sequenced, it will be hard to know how replication-competent they are and consequently what is their infectious potential [25]. It is so far evident that in a large cohort of patients either receiving xenografts or undergoing extra-corporeal perfusion of their blood through pig organs, that none have shown evidence of PERV infection, either by sero-conversion of PERV-antibodies (using serological assays or PCR viral genomic primers) or by the presence of PERV DNA detectable in peripheral blood monocytes. [26] This however, has been associated with the presence of porcine mitochondrial and centromeric DNA sequences in some patients often detectable for many years following extra-corporeal therapies, which suggests that these viruses have little true contagious potential. These results need, however, to be viewed with caution since PBMC's may be relatively PERV-resistant and it is possible that PERVs themselves may result in immune dysfunction [27]. The hope of breeding PERV-free animals seems, however, to be a realistic prospect for the not too distant future [28].

If, on the one hand, the obstacles discouraging the practice of xenotransplantation are well-known both to clinicians and scientists (HAR, AHXR, and xenozoonoses), there are also undeniably strong arguments in support of xenotransplantation which go beyond the mere problem of organ shortage. Xenotransplantation may offer many other clinical opportunities exceeding the simple idea of treating patients with end-stage organ diseases. In theory, a pig-to-human hepatic xenograft might be less susceptible to reinfection with hepatitis C virus or to recurrence of an autoimmune disorder, where liver xenotransplantation could be used to cure such diseases more effectively than liver allotransplantation.

It would be essentially unethical, in fact, to proceed with xenotransplantation research without putting in place strict principles which limit these new risks as much as possible. In this context, given all the clinical implications, the issue of xenotransplantation needs to be discussed in the social arena, in order to reach the widest agreement on such a delicate matter, involving philosophical, cultural, religious and scientific themes [29,30]. Such a debate will effectively parallel the recent debate which has been carried out on the legislative and parliamentary floors in many countries concerning stem cell and human embryonic cloning research. The outcomes of such legislation will not only affect the direction of approved research activity, (a restriction hitherto little experienced by researchers), but also the make-up of high quality personnel involved. The wrong decisions here will simply drive researchers to other countries or to other fields of endeavor. Individual and collective informed consent for xenotransplantation will thus require public dialogue, a process that has so far been somewhat wanting on the runaway train of legislation [31,32].

As far as our experience gathered during the Pittsburgh clinical trials mentioned herein is concerned, we feel the pressing need in the interim period to give answers to our patients. Some of the surgeons involved in the two baboon-to-human transplants, while visiting a wait-listed patient in the clinic after the June 1992 experience had been advertised, found themselves attacked by a group of demonstrators protesting against xenotransplantation. Before anyone could react, a candidate for a human-to-human liver transplant voluntarily stood up for the physicians by asking the demonstrators whether they were carrying donor cards in their wallets. None of the anti-xenotransplantation group of demonstrators turned out to be an organ donor card carrier. Although it is a poignant anecdote, we feel that we have the moral duty to try to offer our patients valid life-saving options where they exist and as human organ shortage is an unsolved problem, xenotransplantation will remain an avenue of legitimate research, experimentation and clinical practice which needs to be developed.

Acknowledgement

I acknowledge the invaluable help with the gathering of relevant articles and with the editing of the present commentary of Ms Claudia Cirillo.

References

1. Evans RW, Orians CE, Ascher NL. The potential supply of organ donors: an assessment of the proficiency of organ procurement efforts in the United States. JAMA 1992;267:239–46
2. Cooper DKC, Kemp E, Platt JL, White DJG. Xenotransplantation. The Transplantation of Organs and Tissues Between Species. Second Edition. Berlin, Heidelberg: Springer-Verlag, 1997.
3. Marino IR, Doyle HR, Nour B, Starzl TE. Baboon liver xenotransplantation in humans: clinical experience and principles learned. In: Cooper DKC, Kemp E, Platt JL, White DJG, editors. Xenotransplantation. The Transplantation of Organs and Tissues Between Species. Second Edition. Springer-Verlag: Berlin, Heidelberg, 1997; 793.
4. Michaels MG, Simmons RL. Xenotransplant-associated zoonoses: strategies for prevention. Transplantation 1994;57:1.
5. Cozzi E, White DJ. The generation of transgenic pigs as potential organ donors for humans. Nat Med 1995;1:964.
6. Dalmasso AP, Vercellotti GM, Platt JL, Bach FH. Inhibition of complement-mediated endothelial cell cytotoxicity by decay-accelerating factor. Potential for prevention of xenograft hyperacute rejection. Transplantation 1991;52:530.
7. Starzl TE, Valdivia L, Murase N, Demetris AJ, Fontes P, Rao A, et al. The biological basis of and strategies for clinical xenotransplantation. Immunol Rev 1994;141:212.
8. Galili U, Mandrell RE, Hamadeh RM, Shohet SB, Griffiss JM. Interaction between human natural anti-alpha-galactosyl immunoglobulin G and bacteria of the human flora. Infect Immun 1988;56:1730–7
9. Lambrigts D, Sachs DH, Cooper DKC. Discordant organ xenotransplantationin primates:world experience and current status. Transplantation 1998;66:547–61
10. Sandrin MS, McKenzie IFC. Recent advances in xenotransplantation. Curr Opin Immunol 1999;11:527–31
11. McKenzie IFC, Koulmanda M, Mandell TE, Sandrin MS. Pig islet xenografts are susceptible to

'anti-pig' but not Gal alpha(1,3)Gal antibody plus complement in Gal o/o mice. J Immunol 1998;161:5116-9

12. Lin Y, Soares MP, Sato K, Takigami K, Csizmadia E, Smith N, et al. Accommodated xenografts survive in the presence of anti-donor antibodies and complement that precipitate rejection of naïve xenografts. J Immunol 1999;163:2850-7

13. Soares MP, Lin Y, Anrather J, Czimadia E, Takigami K, Sato K, et al. Expression of hemo oxygenase-1 can determine cardiac xenograft survival. Nat Med 1998;4:1073-7

14. Ohdan H, Yang YG, Shimizu A, Swenson KG, Sykes M. Mixed chimerism induced without lethal conditioning prevents t cell- and anti-Gal alpha1,3Gal-mediated graft rejection. J Clin Invest 1999;104:281-90

15. Wilmut I, Schnieke AE, McWhir J, Kind AJ, Campbell KHS. Viable offspring derived from fetal and adult mammalian cells. Nature 1997;385:810-3

16. McGRath KJ, Howcroft J, Campbell KHS, Colman A, Schneike AE, Kind AJ. Production of gene-targeted sheep by nuclear transfer from cultured somatic cells. Nature 2000;405:1066-9

17. Butler D. Last chance to stop and think on risks of xenotransplants. Nature 1998;391:320-5

18. Takeuchi Y, Weiss RA. Xenotransplantation: reappraising the risk of retroviral zoonosis. Curr Opin Immunol 2000;12:504-7

19. Hahn BH, Shaw DM, De Cock KM, Sharp PM. AIDS as a zoonosis: scientific and public health implications. Science 2000;287:607-4

20. Paton NI, Leo YS, Zaki SR, Auchus AP, Lee KE, Ling AE, et al. Outbreak of Nipah-virus infection among abbatoir workers in Singapore. Lancet 1999;354:1253-6

21. Weiss RA. Transgenic pigs and virus adaptation. Nature 1988;391:327-8

22. Inverson WO, Talbot T. Definition of a production specification for xenotransplantation. Ann NY Acad Sc 1998;862:121.

23. Patience C, Takeuchi Y, Weiss RA. Infection of human cells by an endogenous retrovirus of pigs. Nat Med 1997;3:282.

24. Armstrong JA, Porterfield JS, De Madrid AT. C-type virus particles in pig kidney cell lines. J Gen Virol 1971;10:195-8

25. Rogel-Gaillard C, Bourgeaux N, Billault A, Vaiman M, Chardon P. Construction of a swine BAC library: application to the characterization and mapping of porcine type C endoviral elements. Cytogenet Cell Genet 1999;85:205-11

26. Paradis K., Langford G., Zhifeng L., Heneine W., Sandstrom P., Switzer W., et al. The Xen 111 Study Group. Search for cross-species transmission of porcine endogenous retrovirus in patients treated with living pig tissue. Science 1999;285:1236.

27. Tackle SJ, Kurth K, Denner J. Porcine endogenous retroviruses inhibit human immune cell function: risk for xenotransplantation? Virology 2000;268:87-93

28. Stoye J. P. Xenotransplantation: proviruses pose potential problems. Nature 1997;386:126.

29. Daar AS. Ethics of xenotransplantation: animal issues, consent and likely transformation of transplant ethics. World J Surg 1997;21:975-82

30. Fishman J, Sachs D, Shaikh R. editors. Xenotransplantation: scientific frontiers and public policy. Ann NY: Acad Sci, 1998;862:1-251

31. Hughes J. Xenografting: ethical issues. J Med Ethics 1998;24:18-24

32. Barker JH, Polcrack L. Respect for persons, informed consent and the assessment of infectious disease risks in xenotransplantation. Med Health Care Philos 2001;4:53-70

Commentary on Section II

Kirby I. Bland

In Chapter 5, Morrissey and colleagues fully discuss the immunologic basis of tissue typing in solid organ transplantation. This area along with the other chapters in this section combines an understanding of the clinical practice of transplantation with that of immune regulation and tolerance. As indicated by the authors, new advances in immunotherapy offer promise whereby donor-specific unresponsiveness or "tolerance" to solid organ transplantation may be realized in the near future. This elusive goal of tolerance has as its raison d'être the creation of a microenvironment or milieu in which the recipient may accept an allograft without immunosuppression, but remains immunocompetent to the ravenous infiltrations of infectious organisms and neoplastic transformation. Several animal models are in evolution whereby the limited exposure to immunosuppression within the period of engraftment provides donor-specific hyporesponsiveness (tolerance).

Despite the elegant early experiments in the 1950s and 1960s by Medawar and others in small animal models creating neonatal and fetal chimerism, only few examples exist of long-term tolerance in human organ transplantation which have permitted the cessation of immunosuppressants [1]. The Medawar model resulted in the production of acquired neonatal tolerance in which experimental, in utero exposure to splenocytes (as alloantigens) produced animals that were subsequently tolerant to skin allografts following birth [2]. This approach is now being revisited with the aid of transgenic technology.

As the authors have indicated, transplanted organs may produce in themselves a form of microchimerism whereby small aggregates of donor and recipient leucocytes become intermingled throughout the allograft and lymphatic compartments, creating an exchange of the donor and recipient antigen-presenting cells, for accommodation of the allograft [3]. Thus, microchimerism may provide value in its ability to reduce immunosuppression and thereafter to enhance long-term survival of allografts. Recent experimental models have achieved long-term allograft acceptance in Rhesus macaque primates following discontinuation of immunosuppressive agents. The encouraging work of Armstrong et al [4] and Kirk et al. [5] has invoked lymphoid depletion by co-stimulatory blockade at the time of alloantigen presentation. For nine MHC-mismatched monkeys, prolonged co-stimulatory blockade with anti-CD154 has allowed excellent renal function without evidence of acute rejection beyond one year [6]. These studies provide optimism regarding allograft transplantation in achieving tolerance without the associated toxicity of myeloablation and immune reconstitution. Although anti-donor antibodies develop in most of these primate models, (often resulting in chronic rejection), the recent significant contributions of Thomas et al [7] have shown that it is occasionally possible to induce stable primate tolerance without any maintenance immunosuppression in primate allograft transplantation. These primate tolerance-induced animals were free of clinical, histological and immuno-chemical evidence of chronic rejection in multiple primate allograft kidney recipients following induction with a unique treatment strategy. These authors have presented data to confirm donor-specific T and B-cell unresponsiveness in the face of normal IgG responses to unrelated antigenic challenge [8]. These results demonstrate the strength and specificity of tolerance by placing skin grafts from living donor and third-party donors (not frozen grafts) simultaneously, an intervention which did not breach kidney transplant tolerance in any recipient despite rejection of skin. These early data suggest that the permanent acceptance of a second kidney from the original donor without immunosuppressive drugs provides compelling evidence for "true" tolerance. One cannot ignore these relevant primate experiments as it appears that *durable* donor-specific T and B-cell tolerance holds promise to allow these investigators to proceed clinically to Phase I, II, and III human trials.

With the development of the newer immunosuppressive drugs, some have argued whether the induction of tolerance is important, however, it has a significant role in rejection-free short-term outcomes and affects the incidence of infectious and malignant complications encountered with conventional prolonged immunosuppression as discussed in Chapter 6. An improved understanding of tolerance within the context of immunosuppression is essential for the development of strategies in islet transplantation in diabetes, hepatocyte transplantation for specific metabolic disorders and in the transplantation of highly immunogenic complex structures, such as whole limbs. This area is also of great significance for the new field of xenotransplantation covered in Chapter 8 and its discussion.

Because of marked differences in rodent histocompatibility antigens and immune systems, the induction of rodent tolerance to human antigens in transgenic and knockout models will only have limited translation to the human setting of transplantation and new large animal models of solid organ transplantation are being developed all the time where MHC class I and II homology is demonstrated [9].

Strategies of the induction of mixed allogeneic chimerism particularly in large animal models like non-human primates, involves the use of complex techniques; most notably non-myeloablative whole body irradiation, pre-transplantation thymic irradiation, splenectomy and peri-transplantation donor bone marrow infusion and the use of anti-thymocyte globulins [10]. Such tolerance strategies may permit human organ transplantation where long-term immunosuppression can successfully be stopped with the creation of low grade mixed allogeneic chimerism and repopulation by small volume donor lymphocytes detectable in host peripheral blood [11]. The use of specific strategies designed to deplete T cells by anti-CD3 immunotoxin therapy is of particular advantage in cadaveric transplantation where pre-treatment is generally not feasible and anti-TNF therapies which inhibit T-cell co-stimulation or anti-CD40/CD154 ligand antibody therapy designed to inhibit macrophages which is of greater importance in the developing field of xenotransplantation.

   Clinical transplantation is dependent upon precise tissue typing to identify
determination of histocompatibility between the recipient and the donor via three
measures: (1) identification of the HLA phenotypes of both recipient and donor;
(2) determination of the degree of previous sensitization (PRA) and (3) determination of cross-compatibility. The PRA provides the tissue-typing laboratory with
an indication of the index for reactivity of the serum from the recipient towards
select HLA allele-specific protein receptors, where the greater the PRA, the greater
the likelihood of a cross-match compatibility. As discussed, no effective methods
exist to reduce preformed antibodies, whilst prevention of sensitization provides
the most efficacious methodology to maintain low PRA values. The latter can be
accomplished by reduction of blood transfusions and use of recombinant erythropoietin. Clearly, international data from North American and European transplant centers suggests a long-term salutary effect of HLA matching between the
donor and the recipient for renal transplantation. As indicated in this chapter,
HLA identical (2 haplotype-matched siblings) transplants have resulted in early
allograft function, decreased rejection probability and enhanced allograft survival,
while HLA non-identical (one haplotype matched, either sibling or parent, and
zero haplotype matched, either non-related or sibling) transplants have a reduced
survival when compared with the HLA identical variant. Outcomes of these
patients are good to excellent and these grafts function as well as those with perfectly HLA-matched cadaveric allografts.
   In clinical practice, chronic allograft dysfunction (CAD) is the principal
concern for the transplant immunologist. With the expression by vascular endothelial and smooth muscle cells of a range of mediators including epidermal
growth factor, insulin-like growth factor-1, PDGF-α, and PDGF-β, TGF-β and the
interleukins, there is a great potential for the development of new immunologic
modalities designed to prevent or limit CAD. The main hypotheses concerning
the forces driving CAD include alloantigen-dependent immunologic injury, (effectively an acute phenomenon) and donor-associated antigen-independent factors
surrounding the engraftment procedure. With regard to the first point, every HLA
mismatch results in roughly a 5 percent decline in long-term graft survival with
low rates of projected 20 year graft survival if there is complete mismatch [12,13]
Early acute rejection is the most important risk factor for the subsequent development of CAD and it is naturally hoped that as the incidence of the former episodes is reduced by new regimens of immunosuppressants that the incidence of
CAD will also decline.
   Non-immunologic risk factors for the development of CAD are also of equal
importance. Some may be preventable, (most notably prolonged cold ischaemia),
but many donor-specific factors are not controllable. This has resulted from the
use of marginal donors from older, hypertensive and diabetic sources as well as
the utilization of heart-beating donors [14]. Other factors of importance are the
relationship between renal mass and recipient body weight which practically
affects the use of pediatric kidney transplantation in adults, small female kidneys
into larger males (and possibly cross-racial transplantation), as well as age-related
glomerulosclerosis/senescence; all represented as a fundamental problem of
nephron loss [15,16].
   The immunological significance of brain death is also becoming increasingly
recognized as important in allograft preservation and delayed function. New
or additional strategies to neutralize the upregulation during cerebral cata-
strophes in peripheral organs, of cytokines, adhesion molecules and chemokines

may be needed [17]. The extent of ischaemia/reperfusion injury is equally a critical alloantigen-independent factor affecting graft function, resulting in loss of energy-dependent trans-membrane ion transport, ATP depletion and pro-inflammatory mediator and MHC up-regulation; all of which enhances graft immunogenicity. It is likely that CD4+ T-lymphocytes are the key cells involved in the acute allogeneic response and are the principal targets in immune suppression, as evidenced by monoclonal anti-CD4 antibody treatment in T-cell deficient rodent models of solid organ transplantation [18].

References

1. Burlingham WJ, Grailer AP, Fechner JH Jr, Kusaka S, Trucco M, Kocova M, et al. Microchimerism linked to cytotoxic T lymphocyte functional unresponsiveness (clonal anergy) in a tolerant renal transplant recipient. Transplantation 1995;59:1147–55.
2. Billingham R, Brent L, Medawar P. Actively acquired tolerance of foreign cells. Nature 1953, 172: 603–6.
3. Starzl TE, Demetris AJ, Murase AJ et al. Cell migration, chimerism and graft acceptance. Lancet 1992;339:1579–82.
4. Armstrong N, Buckley P, Oberley T et al. Analysis of primate renal allografts after T-cell depletion with anti-CD-CRM9. Transplantation 1998;66: 5–13.
5. Kirk AD, Harlan DM, Armstrong NN et al. CTLA4-Ig and anti-CD40 ligand prevent renal allograft rejection in primates. Proc Natl Acad Sci USA 1997;94: 8789–94.
6. Kirk AD, Burkly LC, Batty DS, Baumgartner RE, Berning JD, Buchanan K, Fechner JH Jr, Germond RL, Kampen RL, Patterson NB. Treatment with humanized monoclonal antibody against CD 154 prevents acute renal allograft rejection in nonhuman primates. Nat Med 1999;5:686–93.
7. Thomas JM, Contreras JL, Jiang XL, et al. Peritransplant tolerance induction in macaques: early events reflecting the unique synergy between immunotoxin and deoxyspergualin. Transplantation 1999;68 (11):1660–73.
8. Thomas JM, Eckhoff DE, Contreras JL et al. Durable donor-specific T and B cell tolerance in rhesus macaques induced with peritransplantation anti-CD3 immunotoxin and deoxyspergualin: Absence of chronic allograft nephropathy. Transplantation 2000;69(12):2497–2503.
9. Geluk A, Elferink DG, Slierendregt BL, Van Meijgaarden KE, de Vries RR, Ottenhoff TH, et al. Evolutionary conservation of major histocompatibility complex-DR/peptide/T cell interactions in primates. J Exp Med 1993;177:979–87.
10. Kimikawa M, Sachs DH, Colvin RB, Bartholomew A, Kawai T, Cosimi AB. Modifications of the conditioning regimen for achieving mixed chimerism and donor-specific tolerance in cynomolgus monkeys. Transplantation 1997;64:709–16.
11. Spitzer TR, Delmonico F, Tolkoff-Rubin N, McAfee S, Sackstein R, Saidman S, et al. Combined histocompatibility leukocyte antigen-matched donor bone marrow and renal transplantation for multiple myeloma with end stage renal disease: the induction of allograft tolerance through mixed lymphohematopoietic chimerism. Transplantation 1999;68:480–4.
12. Waaga AM, Rocha AM, Tilney NL. Early risk factors contributing to the evolution of long-term allograft dysfunction. Transplant Rev 1997;11:208–16.
13. Tullius SG, Tilney NL. Both alloantigen-dependent and independent factors influence chronic allograft rejection. Transplantation 1995;59:313–8.
14. Cho YW, Terasaki PI, Cecka JM. High kidney graft survival rates using non-heart-beating trauma donors. Transpl Proc 1998;30:3795–6.
15. Brenner BM, Milford EL. Nephron underdosing: a programmed cause of chronic renal allograft failure. Am J Kid Dis 1993;21:66–72.
16. Halloran P, Melk A, Barth C. Rethinking chronic allograft nephropathy: the concept of accelerated senescence. Am Soc Nephrol 1999;10:167–81.
17. Takada M, Nadeau KC, Hancock WW, Mackenzie HS, Shaw GD, Waaga AM, et al. Effects of explosive brain death on cytokine activation of peripheral organs in the rat. Transpantation 1998;65:1533–42.
18. Zwacka RM, Zhang Y, Halldorson J, Schlossberg H, Dudus L, Engelhardt JF. CD4(+) T-lymphocytes mediate ischemia/reperfusion-induced inflammatory responses in mouse liver. J Clin Invest 1997;100:279–89.

The remarkable advances of the past four decades had genesis in the significant breakthrough of the immunosuppressive properties of 6-mercaptopurine (6MP) confirmed by Schwartz and Dameshek (1959) and the additive effects of aza-thioprine (AZA) to prevent rejection of canine kidney allografts. The advances of the late 1970s with the immunological development of cyclosporine-A (CyA) by Borel and its combination with AZA and steroids allowed the remarkable achieve-ment of a 30 percent enhancement for one-year graft survival following renal transplantation above the 50 percent achieved with AZA alone. The more recent addition of tacrolimus in the 1990s to this regimen continues to challenge the role of CyA for primacy in immunosuppressive agents for prevention of graft rejec-tion. More recently, MMF, sirolimus and the new monoclonal antibodies to the IL-2 receptor are being considered for clinical trial applications. The key applica-tions of these regimens is eloquently described by Torpey, Bradley, and Fung in Chapter 6. The ability of agents like CyA and sirolimus to effect immunosuppres-sion by induction of apoptosis of immune-activated cells represents an exciting new molecular concept.

As indicated in Figure 6.1, immunosuppressive agents are classified according to the immunological position (point) at which they have molecular action in the process of T cell activation and clonal expansion. In two large prospective trials to date comparing tacrolimus with CyA, patients followed for a minimum of one year after renal transplantation were confirmed to have a reduction in biopsy-proven acute rejection from 45 percent to 25–30% when tacrolimus was added to the CyA regimen. Further, the combination has been compared in two large trials in hepatic transplantation and again was also confirmed to induce significant reduction in the frequency of acute rejections and in the number of episodes of severe or refractory rejection. The TMC study, (although not yet published), appears to confirm the benefit of tacrolimus and importantly demonstrate a survival advantage in the tacrolimus-treated patients at six months post-trans-plantation. Similar observations with tacrolimus have been noted in lung and heart transplantation.

The authors have emphasized in important randomized prospective trials that MMS represents a potent immunosuppressive agent in solid organ transplanta-tion. For renal transplantation, trials of immunosuppression with CyA and pre-dnisone with the additions of MMF or AZA, have concluded that patients in the MMF groups were significantly less likely to undergo severe or steroid-resistant rejection. Dosage of MMF above 2 grams per day is problematic, however, in that more side-effects are observed without the added benefit of reduction of rejection episodes. The Tricontinental MMF Renal Transplantation Study and the European MMF Co-operative Study, (as discussed in this chapter), also have suggested trends towards enhanced survival in the MMF- treated group. The fourth study of MMF for heart transplantation has shown only a modest reduction in the inci-dence and severity of acute rejection events but provides a reduction in patient deaths at year one (6%) when compared with an AZA-alone treated population (11%).

This area has undergone great changes in the last 10 years with current proto-cols designed to selectively inhibity different aspects of cell-mediated and cyto-kine-induced immune cascades. In general, both the calcineurin inhibitors CyA and tacrolimus ultimately block IL-2 production as a final common pathway in immune activation, with sirolimus inhibiting signal transduction in a more specific manner. Mycophenolate mofetil is used to block lymphocyte-dependent purine metabolism with the recent introduction of molecular antagonists such as anti-IL-2 receptor therapy in an attempt to limit CyA and tacrolimus-induced dose-related nephrotoxicity. The ligation of costimulatory molecules needed as second signals for T cell activation by CTLA4 Ig (a recombinant protein containing the extra-cellular domain of soluble CTLA4 fused with an IgG_1 heavy chain) results in T cell anergy and prolongs graft survival in experimental models [1]. Its effect on CAD in experimental chronic renal allograft rejection models is at present unclear [2].

The relative difficulties in measurement of the immunosuppressive effects of drugs on immunocytes in vivo has dogged preclinical drug development for use in transplantation, although recently, pharmacodynamic assays using whole blood matrices, (as opposed to purified peripheral blood lymphocyte subsets), has quantitated drug effects on immune cells over time, resulting in the in vitro peri-operative assessment of new immunospuppressants [3,4]. At present, the routine utilization of this approach is somewhat uncertain. For example, inhibition of IL-2 production in mitogen-stimulated whole blood by flow cytometric analysis during CyA and tacrolimus therapy has not shown an association with allograft outcome [5]. Assays of the rate limiting step enzyme inosine monophosphate dehydrogenase (IMPHD) involved in the metabolism of mycophenolate mofetil (MMF) have also been used in pharmacodynamic assays and it appears that its activity is inversely proportional to the main metabolite of MMF- MPA (mycophenolic acid) and that this in turn correlates with the histologic severity of allograft rejection in rodent models of heart allograft rejection [6]. The inhibition of the mammalian target of Rapamycin (mTOR) in response to sirolimus, (referred to in the chapter), acts as an assay for its ligand $p70^{s6}$-kinase which is involved in cell cycle protein production. There is, however, at present, no data to suggest that variations in $p70^{s6}$-kinase levels during sirolimus administration reflect the efficacy of sirolimus in the suppression of rejection episodes [7]. It may be that these pharmacodynamic assays will provide insight into new mechanisms of action of the standard immunosuppressive drugs as well as replace the more laborious animal allograft rejection models currently needed for the testing of new therapies.

In summary, state-of-the-art immunosuppressive agents represent powerful and promising biological agents to prevent allograft rejection and to enhance one-year graft survival which currently approaches 85 percent in many international solid-organ transplantation clinics. The selective molecular cloning and application of medicinal chemistry to develop new immunosuppressive agents holds great opportunity for transplant recipients. Unfortunately, all of the previously described agents failed to prevent the development of graft loss from chronic rejection – the major cause of allograft failure. This chapter eloquently deals with the significant and prolonged cardiovascular, oncologic and infectious complications long recognized with allograft transplantation. The more recent progress in the transplant immunology laboratory of Thomas at the University of Alabama at Birmingham (UAB) suggests that transplant tolerance represents a realistic therapeutic approach which has promise in high-order mammalian models. Prospective phase I, II, and III trials are currently being planned at UAB to test the clinical application of immune tolerance. With islet cell transplants as a primary therapy for Type I juvenile diabetes and the relevance of immunosuppression in children and its attendant complications, the authors have properly placed in perspective the clinical importance of various immunosuppressive agents and their biological implications for infectious, cardiovascular, neoplastic, and growth-impairment complications. The issues of patient compliance with immunosuppressive therapy and drug cost, although not addressed in this chapter, are subjects of profound importance for the socioeconomic consequences of long-term patient management and the resource provision for re-transplantation.

Recently, there has been a trend towards aggressive high-dose chemotherapy with either progenitor cell support or bone marrow transplantation in certain metastatic solid cancers or in their high burden disease (such as in high nodal breast cancer). The principles used in the management of these patients have been learned from the experience acquired in bone marrow transplantation for hematologic malignancies. The area of high dose chemoradiotherapy followed by bone marrow transplantation has now become the treatment of choice for patients with certain hematologic malignancies; most notably acute and chronic leukemias, lymphoma and multiple myeloma. This has permitted a higher mye-loablative chemotherapeutic dose of drugs to be administered providing rescue with genotypically matched allogeneic donor lymphocyte pools with in some cases, the production of an anti-tumour graft-versus-leukemia (GVL) result [8]. This approach has been supplemented to limit graft-versus-host disease (GVHD) by post-transplantation use of graded increments of immunogenic allogeneic donor lymphocytes (donor lymphocyte infusion; DLI) as championed by the Hadassah Hospital in Jerusalem [9]. This mixed chimerism appears to be the key to the induction of successful and durable transplantation tolerance. The use of non-myeloablative stem cell transplantation has been extended into the clinical treatment of metastatic breast carcinoma and interferon-resistant renal cell cancer with progressive pulmonary metastases [10-12]. An improved understanding of the dynamics of GVHD may permit allograft rejection in the presence of suppres-sive low dose chemotherapy in association with intermittent stem-cell inoculation. This may also allow host-versus-graft stimulation accompanied by DLI to elim-inate undesirable hematopoietic cells in hematologic malignancy or non-hemato-poietic host cells deemed to be supporting tumor resistance. These DLI donor T cells may in future work be activated non-specifically by recombinant cytokines (such as IL-2) or by in vitro exposure to specific purified tumor antigens or unpurified tumor lysates.

References

1. Judge TA, Tang A, Spain LM, Deans-Gratiot J, Sayegh MH, Turka LA. The in vivo mechanism of action of CTLA4Ig. J Immunol 1996;156:2294-9.
2. Azuma H, Chandraker A, Nadeau K, Hancock WW, Carpenter CB, Tilney NL, et al. Blockade of T-cell costimulation prevents development of experimental chronic renal allograft rejection. Proc Natl Acad Sci USA 1996;93:12439-44.
3. Dambrin C, Klupp J, Morris RE. Pharmacodynamics of immunosuppressive drugs. Curr Opin Immunol 2000;12:557-62.
4. Yatscoff RW, Aspeslet LJ. The monitoring of immunosuppressive drugs: a pharmacodynamic approach. Ther Drug Monit 1998;20:459-63.
5. van den Berg AP, Twilhaar WN, van Son WJ, van der Bij W, Klompmaker U, Slooff MJ, et al. Quantitation of immunosuppression flow cytometric measurement of intacellular cytokine synthesis. Transplant Int 1998; 11(Suppl 1):S318-21.
6. Klupp J, van Gelder T, Dambrin C, Regieli J, Boecke K, Billingham ME, et al. Mycophenolate mofetil pharmacodynamics and pharmacokinetics correlate with rejection score in a BN to LEW heterotopic heart transplant model. Transplant Proc 2001;33:2170-1
7. Gallant HL, Yatscoff RW. P70 S6 kinase assay: a pharmacodynamic monitoring strategy for rapa-mycin: assay development. Transplant Proc 1996;28:3058-61.

8. Horowitz M, Gale RP, Sondel PM, Goldman JM, Kersey J, Kolb HJ, et al. Graft-versus-leukemia reactions after bone marrow transplantation. Blood 1990;75:555–62.
9. Slavin S, Naparstek E, Ackerstein A, Kapelushnik Y, Or R. Allogeneic cell therapy for relapsed leukemia following bone marrow transplantation with donor peripheral blood lymphocytes. Exp Hematol 1995;23:1553–62.
10. Eibl B, Schwaighofer H, Nachbaur C, Marth C, Gachter A, Knapp R, et al. Evidence for a graft-vs-tumor effect in a patient treated with marrow ablative chemotherapy and allogeneic bone marrow transplantation for breast cancer. Blood 1996;88:1501–8.
11. Or R, Ackerstein A, Nagler A, Kapelushnik J, Naparstek E, Samuel S, et al. Allogeneic cell mediated immunotherapy for breast cancer after autologous stem cell transplantation: a clinical pilot study. Cytokines Cell Mol Ther 1998;4:1–6.
12. Childs R, Clave E, Plante M, Tisdale J, Barrett AJ. Successful treatment of metastatic renal-cell carcinoma with a non-myeloablative allogeneic peripheral blood progenitor cell transplant:evidence for a graft-versus-host tumor effect. J Clin Oncol 1999;17:2044–9.

In Chapter 7, Fung and Bradley define the immunologic and clinical nature of allograft rejection. As already discussed, the goal of immunosuppression must balance the development of long-term donor-specific unresponsiveness with the maintenance of an intact immunoresponsiveness to other foreign stimuli. Unfortunately, the shortage of solid organs for transplantation internationally has compelled renal transplant services to utilize organs that were formerly considered (and still continue to be) sub-optimal. Furthermore, the more liberal criteria for age inclusion and hemodynamic stability have increased the potential donor pool. As indicated in this chapter, various invasive drug support measures in donors with hemodynamic instability, (together with endocrine factors), continue to impact upon initial organ dysfunction. Additionally, non-mechanical and non-immunological parameters such as hypertension, drug interactions, cytomegalovirus (CMV) infections, ischemia-reperfusion injuries from hypotension and hyperlipidemia are known to accelerate graft loss for physiological reasons. These factors together with greater demand for utilization of organs from living donors has opened a new vista for consideration of solid organ transplantation.

Regardless of the site of the transplant center, many proven immunosuppressive protocols are available. Typically, prior to the transplant operation, high-dose corticosteroids are utilized with some clinics providing a calcineurin inhibitor as a first-line therapeutic intervention. In general, triple immunosuppressive therapy with steroids and CyA/tacrolimus or AZA/MMF is the benchmark. The latter are started typically in the postoperative transplant period; a choice between CyA versus tacrolimus is determined by the experience of the transplant nephrology group and their institutional protocols. In North America, MMF has replaced AZA in most transplant centers because of its superior protection against acute rejection and its potential long-term effects. However, for UK and European centers, the substantial cost of MMF has been prohibitive and many units only use low-dose steroids as substitution for MMF. As indicated, the application of antibodies for induction therapy remains controversial; however, ATG/OKT3 induction with CyA or tacrolimus-based triple therapy is often used in lung, heart, and intestinal transplantation. As indicated in this chapter, the comparison of U.S. trials of tacrolimus or MMF (which have also used ATG) with similar European trials, shows near-identical acute rejection rates irrespective of whether ATG is utilized. Trials with anti-CD-25 antibodies and ATG for high-risk renal transplant and cardio-thoracic patients are being planned, where recent studies do not support a contributor role for CyA and where most renal transplant units now reserve ATG only for the therapy of steroid-resistance-rejection or for induction therapy of high-risk renal patients.

A second approach is to withhold CyA/tacrolimus therapy altogether. Trials in stable patients have confirmed that gradual CyA withdrawal enhances renal function and the lipid profile, while reducing the frequency of acute rejection down to 10-20%. An alternative approach to decrease these long-term side effects is to eliminate the combination from both induction and maintenance therapies by adding only sirolimus, MMF or anti-CD25 antibodies. Unfortunately no long-term follow-up with these therapeutic approaches is currently available for transplant nephrologists and surgeons. Great promise is held in the solid-organ transplantation community for the rapid-track development of immune modulation molecules and tolerance induction which will inhibit immune responses in various stages of the organ rejection algorithm.

SECTION III

PRINCIPLES OF TUMOR IMMUNOLOGY

9. Tumor Immunobiology

Andrew P. Zbar

The Nature of the Immune Response Towards Tumors — Immunosuppression and Advanced Cancer

The idea that the immune system could restrain the progression of cancer is an old one, harking back to the work of William Coley, a surgeon at Memorial Hospital in New York in the 1890s who devised a vaccine for deliberate use in cancer patients consisting of killed erysipelas bacteria [1,2]. A few years after von Behring and Kitasato discovered antisera active in children against *Diphtheria* toxin, Hericourt and Richet reported their attempts in treating cancer patients with a range of antisera prepared in dogs and donkeys [3]. At this time, Paul Ehrlich had proposed the possibility of an anticancer vaccine or *"Zauberkugel"* (magic bullet) as he described it, where his serum-derived *"Antikorper"* (antibodies) could eliminate cancer cells [4].

It is expected that the response towards tumor cells will involve both arms of the immunologic system: namely the establishment of humoral (antibody-mediated) and cellular immunity, both directed against recognizable components of tumor-associated and tumor-specific antigens. The finding of unique tumor associated antigens (TAAs) in solid malignancies has presented a range of important targets for adoptive humoral and cellular immune therapies. Early attempts to define TAAs in murine models by immunizing mice either against spontaneous tumors or chemically (and virally) induced tumors were largely confused by general species reactivity to normal transplantation antigens. The development of syngeneic mice with identical histocompatibility antigen expression permitted cutaneous but not tumor transplantation implying the presence of tumor-specific antigenicity [5]. Most work has centred on cytotoxic T cell activity in malignant disease, since the demonstration that the ability to reject tumors could be adoptively transferred by lymphocytes and not serum.

There is considerable evidence to show that patients with advanced malignancy display impairments in cell-mediated immune systems, the extent of which correlates with clinical course and outcome [6–8]. Further evidence of such cell-mediated impairment is the recognition of prolonged homograft survival and poor delayed-type hypersensitivity (DTH) to recall antigens in patients with advanced malignancy as well as a general depression in proliferative responsiveness and IL-2 production in vitro by peripheral blood mononuclear cells when exposed to standard mitogens [7–11]. These effects have been widely demonstrated in other malignancies, most notably in patients with advanced pancreatic, breast, urological and colorectal cancer [12–19].

Division of anti-tumor immune responses into B cell and T cell reactivity directed against characterized TAAs in solid epithelial tumors assists in the understanding of general anti-tumor immunobiology as well as the mechanisms whereby tumors escape immunological recognition.

Humoral Anti-tumor Responses: Antibody Structure and the Idiotypic Network

Immunoglobulins are a diverse group of glycoproteins which bind antigenic epitopes via their variable domains located at their amino (NH_2) terminals. This process initiates a variety of distinct effector functions such as complement activation, Fc-receptor binding and placental transfer through their constant carboxyl (COOH) terminals. The basic immunoglobulin molecule structure is shown in Figure 9.1. Immunoglobulins are arranged as four polypeptide chains (two heavy and two lightchains). Light chains are approximately 220 amino acids in length with a MW of 25 kDa. The heavy chains are made up of about 450–575 amino acids and have a molecular weight of 51–72 kDa depending on their class (isotype). The combined heavy and light chains contain characteristic immunoglubulin domain motifs usually 110 amino acids in length with a specific tertiary protein structure joined by disulfide bonds and dependent upon the antibody class, there are between 4–6 domain regions. The terminal section of both the light and heavy chains show a relative degree of sequence variability and are thus referred to as the variable domains (namely V_H and V_L) containing identical antigen-binding sites on each arm. These domains demonstrate excessive amino acid variability commensurate with the diverse range of recognition antigens encountered. These latter sections are the three hypervariable or complementarity determining regions (so-called CDRs) with the remainder of the antibody chain constructed of constant regions for both chains. (C_H and C_L)

The sequences of the variable regions of each chain show that there are discrete hypervariable regions separated by relatively constant (or framework) regions. Further, these areas generally conform to several classical canonical structure types with preservation of the general secondary peptide structure [20,21]. The tertiary structure of the CDRs is complementary to that of their antigenic recognition determinant(s), referred to as their epitope(s). The actual antigen-binding site usually resides in a few specific amino acid residues projecting out from the surface of the V domain and this combined triplet of CDRs located on both the H and L chains represents the recognition antigen-binding site of the antibody molecule; referred to as the paratope. The antibody specificity is a feature of the stereochemical fit of these two molecules. This inter-relationship between epitope and paratope is shown in Table 9.1.

The epitope/paratope relationship is graphically represented in Figure 9.2 where determinants located on the antibody hypervariable regions are called idiotopes. These idiotopes can be secondarily recognized by the paratopes of second antibodies (so-called anti-idiotypic antibodies) and are able to function as either epitopes or paratopes depending on their position within a recognition-generated antibody network. Differences in constant region sequences separate

Basic antibody structure

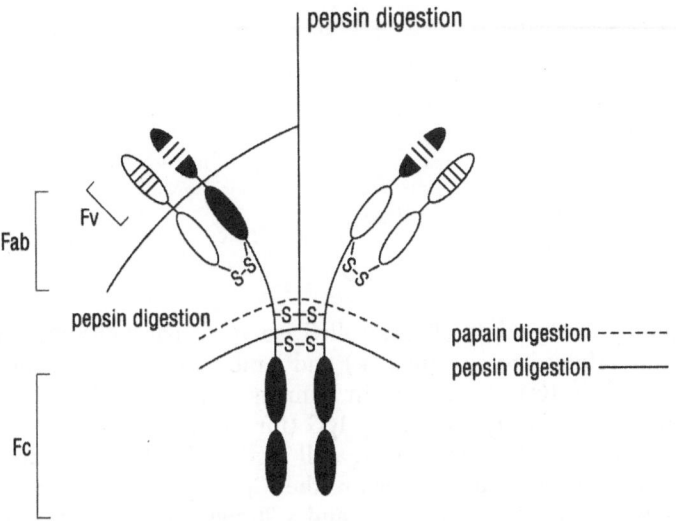

Isotypes, allotypes and idiotypes

H chain isotype	**allotype**	**idiotype**

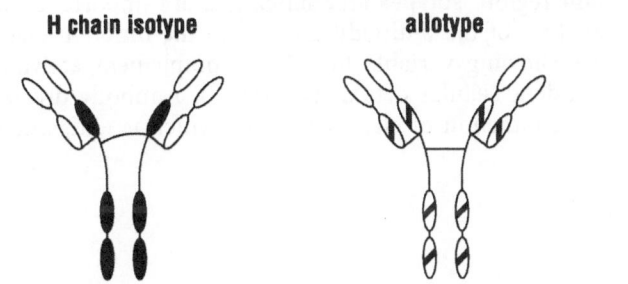 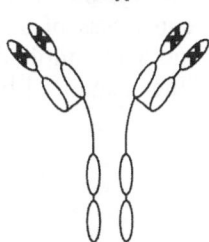

Conserved sequences in the H and/or L chain produce isotypes (classes).

Constant region allele differences produce allotypes.

Hypervariable and variable determinants constitute idiotypes.

(After Mayforth RD. Designing antibodies. Academic Press Inc San Diego 1993, with permission)

The variable regions of the H (heavy) and L (light) chains contain 3 areas of hypervariable sequence called complementarity determining regions (CDR's). The CDR constitutes the antigenic binding site (paratope). The V regions of the H and L chains constitute the Fv portion of the molecule.
The Fab region comprises the Fv's of H and L and the CH1 regions of both chains.

Papain digestion cleaves the molecule at the hinge disulfide bond producing 2 monomeric Fab's and a dimeric Fc portion.
Pepsin digestion cleaves the molecule on the carboxyl terminal side of the disulfide linkage generating an F (ab')$_2$ fragment and smaller Fc cleavage molecules. Excess pepsin digestion produces F(ab') monomers and Fv fragments.

Figure 9.1. Basic antibody structure. Reprinted from British Journal of Cancer, 77(5), Zbar AP, Lemoine NR et al., Biological therapy: approaches in colorectal cancer, 683–693, 1998, by permission of the publisher Churchill Livingstone.

Table 9.1. Interplay between antigenic determinants (epitopes) and antibody-binding or recognition determinants. (paratopes)

Term	Location	Ligand	Synonyms
Epitope	Antigen	Paratope	Antigenic determinant/Antibody binding site
Paratope	Antibody	Epitope	Hypervariable region/CDR
	HV region		Antigen binding site
Idiotope	Antibody	Anti-idiotypic	Epitope *or* Paratope
	V region	antibody paratope	

the immunoglobulins into classes called isotypes. The light chain has two principal variants referred to as kappa (κ) and lambda. (λ) In man, the κ/λ ratio is 3:2 and in mice it is 10:1 The classes in humans of immunoglobulins are determined by the heavy chain isotypes namely IgG (for γ), IgA (for α), IgM (for μ), IgD (for δ) and IgE (for ϵ). These classes are still further divided into subclasses based on amino acid sequence differences in the C_H regions with about a 30 percent sequence homology between classes and a 90 percent sequence homology between subclasses. There are marked differences between species (e.g. humans and rodents) of these varying subclasses (Figure 9.1).

These heavy chain constant region isotypes and subclasses are important since they control the effector function of the antibody class, with the different classes and subclasses of antibodies showing variable half-lives, complement activation and inducible antibody-dependent cellular cytoxicity (ADCC). Antibody diversity is further enhanced by the phenomenon of class switching, which is antigenically

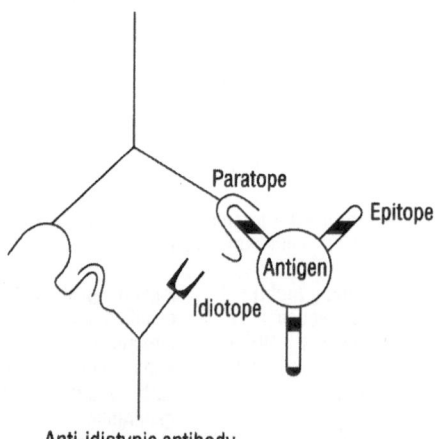

Epitopes (antigenic determinants) are recognized by primary antibody paratopes. Determinants on the V region of the primary antibody can function as "neo-epitopes" which are recognized by anti-idiotypic secondary antibodies.

Figure 9.2. Isotypes, allotypes and idiotypes. Reprinted from British Journal of Cancer, 77(5), Zbar AP, Lemoine NR et al., Biological therapy: approaches in colorectal cancer, 683–693, 1998, by permission of the publisher Churchill Livingstone.

driven, permitting B cell V_H attachment to any of the C_H regions and allowing antigenic specificity by antibody to be associated with the most suitable effector function on exposure to foreign antigens such as tumor proteins.

Historically, antibodies have been serologically defined. This view has changed with the advent of molecular genetic techniques. Antisera specific for immunoglobulins were initially discovered and screened by immunizing animals from a variety of strains and species producing the main recognition antibody determinants which have now been identified at the genetic level. The first groups were the isotypic antibodies (already mentioned) initially recognized by interspecies immunization experiments whereby recognition determinants were the constant regions of the species class. Further analyses showed serological differences in the constant regions of antibodies in the different animal strains which were referred to as allotypic determinants (or allotypes). Intraspecies immunoglobulin immunization experiments adsorbing sera with anti-allotypic and anti-isotypic antibodies showed that unique determinants recognizing components of the variable regions were present. These represented the idiotopes already referred to which can be located either on the CDR or framework regions of the variable domain. The sum of the idiotopes expressed by an antibody comprise its idiotype [22].

Immunochemistry may dictate that certain determinants on the variable regions of antigen-recognizing antibodies (so-called Ab_1 antibodies) may serve as secondary determinants for recogntion by a second tier of antibodies. These idiotopes of Ab_1 molecules function as "neo-epitopes" and are recognized by so-called anti-idiotopic (or Ab_2) antibodies as mentioned above. Because of the complexity of the variable domain, there are a range of related Ab_2 molecules and a range of recognizable idiotopes. Some of these are unique to that Ab_1 (so-called private idiotopes) and others are shared or cross reactive. (so-called public idiotopes) [23,24].

Figure 9.3 shows the subsets of postulated Ab_2 anti-idiotypic antibodies available for Ab_1 recognition. These comprise the $Ab_2\alpha$ molecules which recognize idiotopes lying outside the antigen-binding site of Ab_1 and $Ab_2\beta$ molecules which recognize idiotopes of the Ab_1 binding site. The latter represent internal images of the antigen and have been shown to possess antigen-sequence homology. Bona and Kohler [25] have also described a third Ab_2 variant (the $Ab_2\gamma$ molecule) which recognizes a portion of the Ab_1 binding site but which does not function as a true internal image. The specificity of each Ab_2 antibody is demonstrable by its ability to block Ab_1-antigen binding. The ligand binding characteristics of these inter-related molecules is shown in Table 9.2.

In 1974, Neils Jerne formulated a theory based upon the presence of a network of these anti-idiotypic antibodies which functioned as a controlling web of variable-domain molecules forming a dynamic equilibrium or idiotypic cascade [26]. He postulated that they governed the repertoire of antibody responsiveness directed against foreign antigen (such as TAA) although a separate but less-well formulated prediction of these networks was also made by Lindenmann approximately one year earlier [27]. Although Lindenmann's terminology has not become generally accepted in the same way that that of Jerne has, it is clear that Lindenmann's "homobodies" are Jerne's internal images and that his "aliotypes" are equivalent to Jerne's public idiotypes (vide supra). Similar writings are evident historically in the works of Ramseier and Rosenstein but neither had constructed an interactive network theory of antibody production as organized as that postulated by Jerne [28,29].

Table 9.2.   Ligand-binding properties of anti-idiotypic (Ab₂) antibodies

Subgroup	Ligand	Characteristics
Ab₂α	V regions ouside Ab₁ binding site	Fails to block Ab₁-antigen binding
Ab₂β	Ab₁ paratope	Blocks Ab₁-antigen binding/mimics Antigen Antigenic internal image
Ab₂γ Not an Antigenic internal image	Partial Ab₁ paratope	Partial Ab₁-antigen blockade

The Ab₂β molecules generated comprise only a small fraction of all anti-idio-typic antibodies or of the antibody pool (particularly where a xenogeneic immu-nizing Ab₁ is employed). They may be screened through their antigen-like effects; most notably by inhibiting ligand-receptor binding and eliciting an antibody response resembling the Ab₁. A further third-generation of antibody molecules may be produced amongst human repertoires in response to sufficiently immuno-genic hypervariable regions recognized on the Ab₂β antibody which resemble the TAA. They are specifically directed against the TAA and structurally resemble the Ab₁. These molecules are referred to as anti-anti-idiotypic (or auto-anti-idiotypic) antibodies and are designated as Ab₃ (Figure 9.3)[30,31].

Idiotypic cascades have been confirmed in neonatal mice immunized in experi-mental bacterial sepsis and viral disease as well as in in vivo anti-tumor immu-

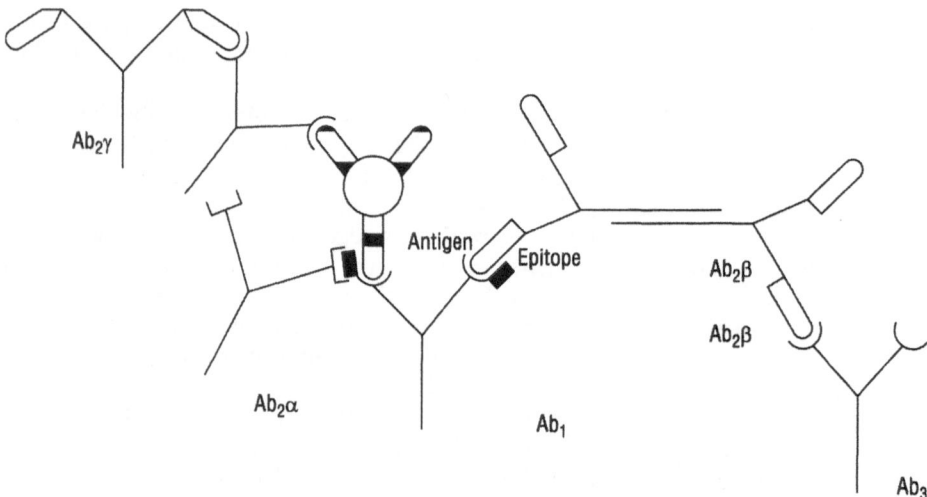

A range of anti-idiotypic antibodies are produced in response to the Ab₁ molecule. Ab₂β antibodies recognize the antigen binding site of Ab₁ and are "internal images" of the epitope.

Ab₂α antibodies recognize idiotopes which lie outside the antigen binding site of Ab₁.

Ab₂γ antibodies recognize a portion of the antigen binding site of Ab₁ but do not carry the internal image of the antigen.

An idiotype cascade results in the production of Ab₃ antibodies which resemble Ab₁ in their binding site sequence and which secondarily recognize the antigen.

Figure 9.3.   The immune network in tumor biology.

nity, although their exact clinical significance remains to be determined [32–36]. The importance of these idiotopes is that they may bear the internal images of TAAs and that administered anti-TAA antibodies (either xenogeneic or genetically constructed humanized in form) could induce primary amplified idiotypic cascades directed against weakly immunogenic tumor epitopes [37–39] These could then either induce TcR recognition determinants to lyse malignant cells through T cell/B cell interaction or be coupled to bifunctionally displayed cytotoxins or cytokines designed to destroy the tumor cell initially recognized immunologically [40,41].

The presence of these idiotypes in tumors has been demonstrated serologically since the 1950s with the production of specific inducible rabbit antisera (after removal of anti-allotypic and anti-isotypic antibodies) by immunization with mouse myeloma protein [42,43]. This type of inducible idiotypic reactivity has been shown in animals to provide a protective anti-tumor immunity to tumor load challenge in vivo when anti-idiotypic antibodies expressing the internal images of tumor-specific and tumor-associated antigens were used in vaccination [44].

The mechanisms whereby anti-idiotypic antibodies regulate antigen-driven disease might include the neutralization by Ab_2 of target Ab_1 antibodies, the direct modulation of idiotype-specific B cell antibody production, or the secondary stimulation of specific idiotype-responsive T cells and their receptors. Both human anti-idiotypic sera and primary xenogeneic anti-TAA antibody have been used in patients as passive forms of immunotherapy in advanced colorectal cancer, metastatic melanoma and haematopoietic malignancies [45].

Anti-idiotypic antibodies serve as natural agents for use in passive immunotherapy trials because of their ability to act as surrogate antigen vaccines expressing surface TAAs. In theory, they may be desirable as immunotherapeutic agents against cancer because of their specificity and the ability to serologically select them as well as their relative ease of mass production. This may be important particularly where a natural oncofoetal TAA (like CEA) may be poorly expressed on the surface of the tumor. Moreover, such therapy has the ability to induce both passive and active immunoresponsiveness with a single treatment through the induction of idiotypic cascades and without the need for custom-made therapy using autologous cells bearing idiosyncratic private idiotopes [38,46]. $Ab2\beta$ have been successfully used in animal models to trigger immunity against bacterial, viral and parasitic infections [47–50].

The importance for this therapy in solid epithelial cancer is the induction through monoclonal antibody therapy of potential immunoresponsiveness in a condition where the tumor antigen itself is relatively non-immunogenic [51]. Moreover, the induction of host-origin cascades of specific antibodies should produce a situation where cytolytic acitivity (in part through complement and ADCC means) will prove more efficient than those effector functions induced by purely xenogeneic antibodies [52].

Cell-mediated Reactivity Directed Towards Solid Epithelial Tumors

T cells recognize different epitope determinants of complex antigens such as tumor-associated proteins in a fundamentally different way to B cells. Knowledge of the intricate process of foreign antigen presentation as well as the chemistry of the T cell receptor (TcR) mechanism will assist in the development of immunological strategies which enhance antigen recognition and which may couple recognition determinants with TcR molecules in a bifunctional approach to increase tumor targeting.

The ontogeny of MHC division in the processing of foreign protein appears to relate to the immune system recognizing endogenous foreign antigen by cytotoxic lymphocyte (CTL) production (such as in viral replicants or tumor cells) and by endocytic uptake and antibody attack for non-replicating exogenous proteins. Knowledge of the intricate mechanisms involved in foreign antigen presentation will permit the development of potential genetic targets to overcome heterogeneity in relatively non-immunogenic tumors like colorectal cancer.

Intracellular and extracellular antigens are handled differently by the immune system with the development of parallel but separate mechanisms for dealing with these foreign challenges. Intracellular antigens produce processed peptides (usually 8–9 amino acids in length) which are generally presented to CD8+ (T suppressor/cytotoxic) cells by major histocompatibility class (MHC) I molecules. Extracellular antigen is processed for presentation as 15–25 amino acid length peptides to CD4+ (T helper) cells by the MHC class II molecules only found on specialized professional antigen- presenting cells such as dendritic cells, macrophages or B lymphocytes. (Figure 9.4) This phenomenon is called MHC restriction and implies that TcR recognition of MHC and antigenic peptides is related to a single receptor molecule. The activation of the TcR is a complex process which requires the presence of costimulatory signals including tyrosine kinases, interleukins and other specific costimulatory molecules. The discovery of costimulatory signals has created a model of lymphocyte activation originally developed by Bretscher and Cohn whereby processed antigen may be linked either to the MHC complex or to a costimulatory ligand in its presentation to the T cell [53]. The basic structure of the TcR is shown in Figure 9.5.

A series of these molecules have been described,most notably the B7 family [54], the ICAM group, lymphocyte function associated antigens (LFA-3),vascular cell adhesion molecules (VCAM-1) and heat stable antigens. Epithelial tumors may escape immune surveillance by failing to express B7 molecules, thus resulting in the presentation of cognate membrane antigen without costimulation. The effect of this type of presentation may result in T cell clonal anergy or deletion, antigenic desensitization or apoptosis [55,56].

An understanding of TcR-related mechanisms of foreign antigen response at the cellular level has been coupled to the consistent demonstration of T cells with specific cytotoxic function against autologous solid tumors both in vitro and in vivo [57,58]. These have been extensively demonstrated in malignant melanoma, squamous cell carcinoma, ovarian cancer, gastric cancer, renal cell cancer, glioblastoma and breast cancer [59–65]. The demonstration of tumor-specific T cells which recognize tumor-derived peptides in an MHC-restricted fashion, particularly in melanoma as well as the extraction of specific cytolytic T cells derived from lymphocytic cell infiltrates at the tumor site (so-called tumor-infiltrating lymphocytes or TILs) which have potent in vitro anti-tumor activity towards autologous tumor cells has lent further credence to the importance of a restricted group of T cells which are vital in inducing specific tumor cell killing following repeated tumor challenge [66–68]. The finding in some tumors of a clinical advantage in those cases with extensive lymphocytic infiltrate as well as the

Class I MHC antigen processing:

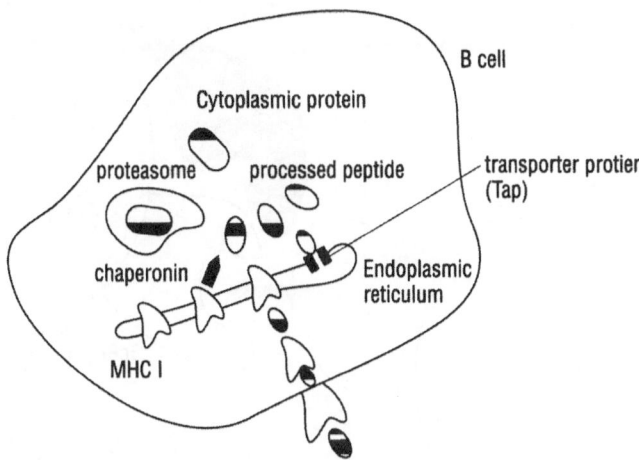

Proteasomes digest cytoplasmic foreign protein into processed peptides (8-9 amino acids in length).
These peptides adhere to the endoplasmic reticulum by polymorphic transporter proteins (Tap-1 and Tap-2). Chaperonin molecules detain empty MHC Class I molecules in the endoplasmic reticulum for association with processed antigen and transfer to the cell surface.

Class II MHC antigen processing:

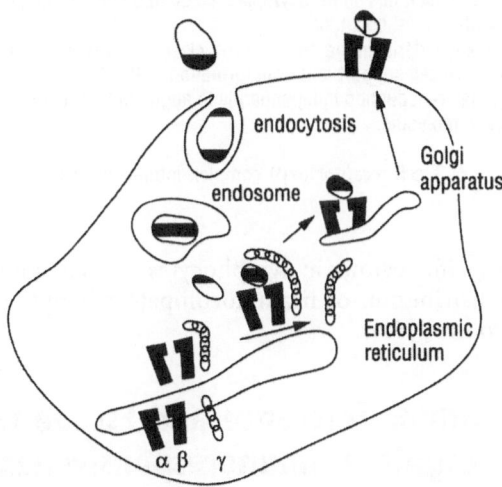

Foreign antigen is endocytosed and after processing (peptides 15-25 amino acids in length) the peptide is aggregated in the Golgi apparatus with α, β and γ components of the MHC class II molecule formed in the endoplasmic reticulum.
After complexing with foreign peptide the γ chain is degraded and the αβ heterodimer/ processed antigen is expressed on the cell surface for Th TcR recognition. The mechanism of transport of the complex from the Golgi apparatus to the cell membrane is unknown.

Figure 9.4. Mechanism of MHC molecule antigen processing. Reprinted from British Journal of Cancer, 77(5), Zbar AP, Lemoine NR et al., Biological therapy: approaches in colorectal cancer, 683—693, 1998, by permission of the publisher Churchill Livingstone.

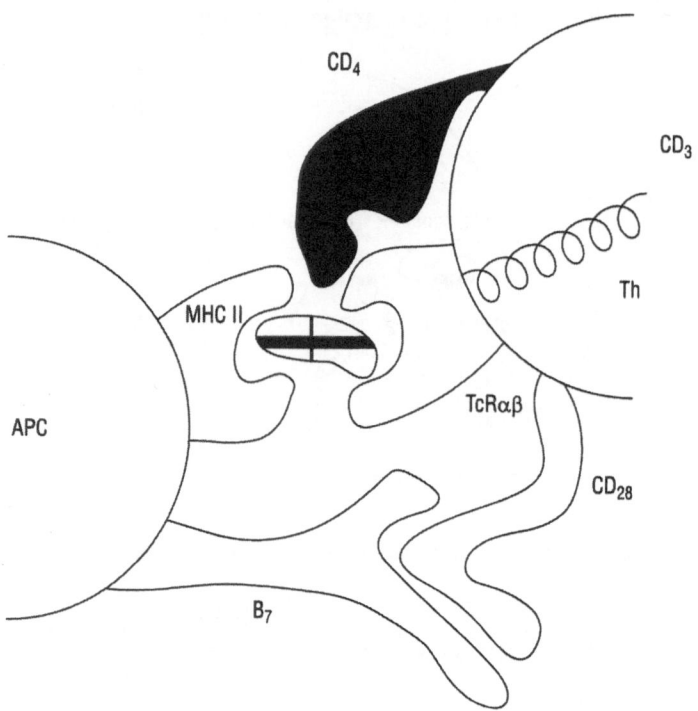

T cells have a dual specificity for MHC molecules and processed antigen. The TcR αβ is complexed with CD3 which has an intracytoplasmic component for signal transduction after occupancy with processed antigen.
The CD4 molecule secondarily interacts with MHC class II to produce local cytokines (IL-2 and IFN-γ) for Th cell support and transformation of B cells.
CD 28 initiates signal transduction independently to augment local cytokine production using B7 as a ligand molecule.

Figure 9.5.   Mechanism of T cell receptor (αβ) complex interaction with antigen presenting cell.

presence of tumor-specific cytotoxic lymphocytes in malignant ascites implies that a site-specific redistribution of immunocompetent lymphocytes may be relevant in local tumor control [69].

Mechanisms of Tumor Tolerance and Escape from Immunologic Recognition Imunoresponsiveness Towards Tumor-associated Antigen (TAA): Activation or Tolerance?

An understanding of lymphocyte ontogeny and the mechanisms involved in tolerance, may assist in improving biologic therapy directed against tumors and explain the defences some tumor cells employ to evade immunological attack. Mechanisms for thymic negative selection of T cells have been established as part of mature T cell development and as an explanation for the elimination of self-reactive repertoires [70] and knowledge of the peripheral induction of T cell tolerance as it applies to self-MHC recognition may provide clues to the immune anergy and deletion of potentially immunocompetent lymphocytes when repeatedly exposed to tumor antigen. Unlike the B cell system, the entire T cell repertoire must be formed intrathymically as there is no diversification of the TcR gene once developed [71].

Potentially dangerous antigen may elude the immune system in the periphery if presented in an immunologically priveleged site such as the CNS (or the eye), but other more complex mechanisms of peripheral T cell tolerance towards tumors must exist. Much work has been recently reported using animals transgenic for tissue-specific promoters exposed to extrathymic Class I and Class II molecules [72]. These elegant experiments have shown peripheral T cell tolerance of specific 'antigen-ignorant' clones as well as clonal deletion and there is evidence that this state of affairs is somewhat dependent upon local cytokine production [73]. Importantly, relatively high density antigen exposure (as may occur in some tumors which shed surface TAA such as colorectal cancer) has been shown in these models to induce TcR and co-receptor downregulation or apoptosis. The subsequent survival of the T cell and induction of its memory for TAA to act as a "recall" antigen also appears to depend on a complex interplay between apoptotic signals (such as Fas/Fas L, Bad and Bax) with members of the Bcl-2 family of anti-apoptotic receptors, most notably Bcl-2 and Bcl-x_L [74,75].

B cell tolerance is obviously important in the avoidance of auto-antibody development for potentially cross-reactive antigen. It is unknown whether similar mechanisms are involved in the failure by TAAs to initiate B cell presentation. Auto-antibodies to naturally occurring but over-expressed TAA may perhaps be produced but be transient, of low affinity or the wrong isotype. Experimentation with hapten-specific B cell populations has shown that tolerance may either lead to clonal deletion (so-called negative selection or clonal abortion) when exposed to high dose antigenic load or to clonal hapten-specific anergy when much smaller antigen loads are employed [55,76]. The evidence provided by animals transgenic for both a given antigen and a monoclonal B cell receptor specific for that antigen has shown that early presentation to developing B cells in the bone marrow results in maturation arrest with V region genetic editing for recognition immunoglobulins [56,77]. This may have considerable relevance for B cell repertoire development against oncofetal antigens like CEA and α-foetoprotein and will govern the antigenic dose necessary to induce optimal B cell responsiveness during monoclonal antibody therapy directed against the relevant TAA.

It is likely that high affinity antibody with a high molarity of presentable antigen favours anergy and this phenomenon may play an important part in the poor responsiveness to membrane-bound ubiquitous TAA which is merely over-represented on solid epithelial tumors. The difference with the B cell side of immunocyte development when compared to the generation of the TcR is that genes coding for the B cell receptor are subject to a very high rate of random somatic mutation, suggesting that a dual mechanism exists where antigen may be "tolerized" by a secondary B cell lineage within the developing germinal centre of lymph nodes draining the primary tumor [78].

It is also debatable how important the continuous presence of antigen is in the induction of both B and T cell memory. This may have relevance in cancers where TAA is intermittently shed from the main tumor mass and affects the need for repeated dosing against TAA with anti-tumor monoclonal antibodies [79–81].

The variability of tumors themselves also permits their escape from immune

recognition. Previously the main markers for tumor heterogeneity were morpho-
logical, biochemical and karyotypic but increasingly there is recognized to be
both molecular biological and immunohistochemical variability within tumor cell
subpopulations that may affect immunotherapeutic and chemotherapeutic
response. The multistep nature of colorectal carcinogenesis for example, proposes
many potential mechanisms for such intratumoral heterogeneity. At its simplest
level, differences in tumor differentiation and tumor DNA ploidy may be reflected
in differences in outcome where tumor aneuploidy has been shown to correlate
with overall prognosis in ovarian, renal cell, thyroid, adrenal and breast cancer
[82–85]. Potential mechanisms for immunological escape by tumor cells include
changes in the structure of crucial molecules such as MHC activation ligands,
regulators of complement activation, lytic enzyme neutralizers and adhesion
molecule receptors. In this sense the immune system contributes to the phenotypic hetereogeneity of the tumor.

In summary, the heterogeneity of MHC, costimulator and TAA expression by
the tumor as well as the timing of antigen exposure, the molar concentration,
surface expression density and solubility of antigen and the repeatedness of TAA
exposure for potentially reactive immunocytes may decide the likelihood of
immune elimination of isolated tumor deposits. The state of pre-ordained immunotolerance to TAA (as may occur towards oncofoetal antigens like CEA already
expressed in low density on normal tissues) may also be established early on in
the ontogenic lineage of immunocytes and control their cytokine-mediated recep-
tor/responder phenotype when primary tumors expressing higher density non-
mutated TAAs develop [86,87].

The recent demonstration of TILs and tumor-associated lymphocytes (TALs) in
solid tumors with impaired in vitro proliferative function and cytotoxicity has
suggested that there may be tumor-induced alteration of subcellular T cell receptor signaling [88-90]. These cells unlike normal memory T cells respond relatively
poorly to mitogens ex vivo and cannot mediate effective anti-tumor cytotoxicity
towards autochthonous tumor targets [91,92]. These changes have in part been
linked to abnormalities in the expression of the ζ chain linked to the TcR needed
for the transduction of signals delivered following T cell antigen recognition [93].
These findings have been noted in the TILs and TALs derived from colon, prostate, renal, cervical and ovarian cancers as well as melanomas and head and neck
squamous carcinomas [94–101].

The subcellular mechanims for these changes in the T cell are at present
unclear, however, there appears to be diminished intracellular calcium mobilization and altered tyrosine kinase activity following the cross linking of the TcR as
a result of tumor-induced activation of local ζ chain degradative caspases. This
appears to be linked with an aberrant stimulation of the T cell apoptotic pathway
involving the Janus family tyrosine kinases (JAKs), cytosolic latent transcription
factors (signal transducers and activators of transcription; STATs) [102–104] and
the FasL pathways [105,106].

The prospects for therapy to reverse these changes are still speculative, since
the exact derangement of normal T subcellular mechanisms is as yet poorly
understood. Potential future strategies might include the use of virally encoded T
cell gene therapy ex vivo in dysfunctional T cells for adoptive immunotherapy.
Whether these would revert to their dysfunctional state in the presence of the
tumor microenvironment is uncertain and the risks of T cell induced tumorigenesis at present are unclear.

In the more advanced stages of tumors, there appears to be a progressive induction of antigen-specific anergy among CD4 T helper cells following the injection of tumor cells expressing the cognate antigen [107] with a variation in the inherent cytokine pattern towards a Th2 profile (producing inhibitory IL-4 and IL-10) and away from the Th1 cytokine profile of IL-2 and interferon-γ production deemed to be normally necessary for tumor rejection. Our group (and others) have shown a Th2 cytokine predominance in peripheral blood mononuclear cells derived from patients with advanced colorectal cancer which is somewhat stage dependent [108,109]. Moreover, we have shown a conversion of this cytokine profile in response to standard mitogens in vitro from a Th2 to a Th1 type during to Th1 in human advanced colorectal cancer during specific murine anti-CEA therapy with a novel antibody directed at cell-based membrane bound TAA [110]. This effect is unfortunately not associated with clinical responsiveness to therapy; a result also noted by other groups in colorectal cancer using a murine syngeneic Ab$_2$ anti-idiotypic antibody [111].

Interestingly, such progressive immunodeficiency in cancer bears some resemblance to the changes noted in progressive AIDS which may be associated with a depressed DTH response, reduced CTL activity and a Th2 dominant PBMC cytokine profile [112,113]. The changes we have noted during anti-TAA specific monoclonal antibody immunotherapy mirror those changes seen in HIV-positive patients during human anti-retroviral (HAART) therapy, often predating changes in peripheral CD4/CD8 ratios [114–116].

Barriers to Monoclonal Antibody Therapy in Malignancy — a Model of Immune Evasion

Along with impairments of the host response in cancer, there are specific barriers to certain forms of immunotherapy, most notably against monoclonal antibody usage in solid malignancy. The lessons learnt from immunoprophylaxis in infectious diseases have only limited application in anti-neoplastic therapy, since in malignancy preferential reactivity with tumor cells expressing either self-antigen in high density or modified oncogenic product is often not possible. The shedding of TAA from tumors will also in theory reduce the effectiveness of antibody/tumor targeting particularly when repeated therapy is used [117].

The mechanism of tumor cell kill following monoclonal antibody therapy is controversial suggesting the induction of complement-dependent and antibody-dependent cytotoxicity or apoptosis and highlighting the importance of the treating antibody isotype in inducing a particular type of immune response [118–124]. Further, the immunological significance and biological activity of traditionally defined idiotypes as well as the structural basis of unique idiotopic complementarity for the complex multiple epitopes presented by TAAs has been brought into question [125]. Here, the specific selection of Ab$_2$ β clones may not always provide protective immunity against tumor growth in animal models as there may be differences in antigen-specificity noted between Ab$_1$ and Ab$_2$-induced Ab$_3$ antibodies. This coupled with the relative lack of sequence homology between the Ab$_2$ and its corresponding antigen imply that there may be innate problems with conventional network theory [126–130].

Debate exists concerning the enhanced specificity of human or xenogeneic monoclonal anti-idiotypic therapy in malignancy [46]. The advantages of anti-idiotypic therapy include the ability to avoid cross-species reactivity which will reduce the bioavailability of the antibody and potentially contribute to serious morbidity. In addition enhanced specificity of response is likely in situations where the tumor antigen is either difficult to purify or is only weakly immunogenic. This type of approach is less expensive than the production of idiosyncratic therapies such as inactivated autologous or allogeneic adoptive tumor cells and may in theory assist in stimulating ignorant T cell clones in situations where nominal antigen has already proven itself relatively ineffective [131].

There are many practical obstacles to successful monoclonal antibody therapy which are unique to tumors and which affect drug delivery. In infectious disease, protective immunity may on occasion be provided by a single epitope with its attendant specific antibody. In these cases it may be substantially safer to produce anti-idiotypic antibodies than to culture the infectious agent itself. This type of therapy is also useful in states where organisms produce marked genetic variation, such as in HIV infection. In tumors, however, the nature of the TAA is generally more complex and governed by a range of immunodominant epitopes with variable antigenicity.

In neoplasia, one of the problems of antibody therapy is the adequacy of appreciable monoclonal concentration in the main bulk of the tumor particularly where there is an abnormal highly permeable vasculature. Although there are substantial differences in the vasculature of autochthonous tumors and subcutaneous transplant models, this may in part explain the greater response rates to monoclonal therapy in haematopoietic malignancies as opposed to solid cancers [132–134]. Jain and colleagues have outlined the physical barriers to monoclonal antibody movement in subcutaneous animal tumor and visceral metastatic models, whereby blood flow particularly in the centre of tumor deposits is intermittent or even non-existent. Although the heterogeneity of TAA, costimulator and MHC expression by tumor cell subpopulations will affect targeting, the movement of macromolecules will also be subject to the normal convectionary and diffusionary forces dependent upon the relative interstitial and plasma concentrations and vascular surface area available within the tumor nodule. The relatively high interstitial fluid pressure found in many solid tumors consequent upon an excessively permeable vasculature in the absence of functional lymphatics works against the even distribution of such molecules and confines the treatment to the periphery of the tumor. The result is that there is a roughly inverse relationship between tumor size and monoclonal antibody uptake [132, 135–137].

Pharmacokinetic modelling has also accurately predicted restrictions in extravascular diffusion of the antibody because of perivascular binding to exposed TAA. This type of blockade will not affect immunoscintigraphic antibody targeting, (indeed it may be enhanced) however, it will disturb the therapeutic potential of immunoconjugates and immunotoxins which rely on tumor cell internalization for their effect [133,138–140].

One of the greatest difficulties with the use of murine monoclonal antibodies is the development of a human anti-murine antibody (HAMA) response to the Fc portion of the primary mouse antibody administered. The extent of this response particularly to repeated murine exposure will limit the therapeutic effect of monoclonal treatment, shorten antibody half-life,enhance clearance of antibody and potentially induce a serum sickness reaction in treated patients. The nature of the HAMA response is polyclonal with anti-isotypic and anti-idiotypic reactivity and may even affect the administration of genetically-modified human and humanized antibodies. This type of heterophilic antibody response will also interfere with assays which routinely use murine monoclonals,most notably standard serum assays of tumor markers such as CEA [141].

The finding of significant HAMA responses has resulted in the production of a range of designer antibodies such as chimaeric antibodies, V_H domain molecules, antigen-binding peptides and recombinant antibody fusion proteins [142–145]. Genetically engineered antibodies which lack Fc reactivity could be used where Fc function is not desired, such as in radioimmunolocalization to diminish background [146]. Single chain antigen binding fragments (sFv) and recombinant sFv peptides which consist of V_L and V_H domains joined by peptide linkers and expressed in large quantity by *E. coli* are being developed for imaging purposes, although problems exist both with reduced affinity compared with the parent molecule and steric hindrance of the linker peptides. Many of these newer peptides are also relatively unstable. Despite chimaerization, anti-idiotypic antibodies which recognize the murine V region are potentially still a problem [147]. Although humanization of antibodies reduces their immunogenicity, the antigen/antibody binding affinity of the parent antibody may not always be reproduced.

Summary

In summary the mechanisms employed by tumors to escape immune detection and elimination may be non-specific, antigen-related or host-related. There are also many non-specific immune aspects of dysfunction which occur in those with advanced tumors and which are not tumor-specific. These include the effects of antineoplastic therapy, radiotherapy, blood transfusion, nutritional deficieny and ageing [148–151]. Global mechanisms of suppression may occur as a result of the release of tumor immunosuppressants or growth in immunopriveleged sites. Antigen-specific mechanisms may occur as a result of loss (or heterogeneity) of TAA expression, particularly during metastasis development [152] or tolerance through ignorance, anergy or clonal deletion towards cognate "self-antigens" overexpressed or presented in mutated form on the surface of malignant cells [107,153]. This may be accompanied by MHC I downregulation, (particularly during metastasis development), probably consequent upon the progressive loss of the Class I processing machinery [148,154,155].

Somewhat depressingly for the immunotherapist devising clever new strategies to combat tumor-induced evasion of immunoelimination, there may be "naturally occurring" immunoignorant T cells and other populations of T cells capable of tumor recognition but which reach senescence without ever successfully eliminating the tumor [156–158]. This represents a difficult inherent barrier to effective therapy no matter how sophisticated the antigenic recognition or the activated T cell in vitro. It may require repeated allogeneic T cell infusion therapy of immunocompetent cells when host tumor-specific T cell repertoires become exhausted in the face of substantial tumor burden — at best a complicated and personalized therapy which may simply not be cost effective.

References

1. Coley WB. The treatment of malignant tumours by repeated inoculations of erysipelas with a report of 10 original cases. Am J Med Sci 1893;105:487
2. Coley WB. The treatment of inoperable sarcoma with the mixed toxins of erysipelas and bacillus prodigiosus. J Am Med Assoc 1898;20:389–395
3. Riethmuller G, Schneider-Gadicke E, Johnson JP. Monoclonal antibodies in cancer therapy. Curr Opin Immunol 1993; 5:732–9.
4. Ehrlich P. The collected papers of P Ehrlich. In Himmelweit F editor. Immunology and Cancer Research. Pergamon Press, 1957.
5. Old LJ, Boyse EA, Clarke DA, Carswell EA. Antigenic properties of chemically-induced tumours. Ann NY Acad Sci 1962;101:80–106.
6. Chretien PB, Crowder WL, Gertner HR et al. Correlation of preoperative lymphocyte reactivity with clinical course of cancer patients. Surg Gynecol Obstet 1973, 136:380–4.
7. Brugarolas A, Takita H. Immunological status in lung cancer patients. Chest 1973; 64:427–30.
8. Catalona WJ, Chretien PB, Trachan EE. Abnormalities of cell-mediated immunocompetence in genitourinary cancer. J Urol 1974;111:229–32.
9. Pinsky CM,El Domieri A,Caron AS et al. Delayed hypersensitivity reactions in patients with cancer. Rec Results CancerRes 1974;47:39–44
10. Kadish AS, Doyle AT, Steinhauer EH, Ghossein NA. Natural cytotoxicity and interferon production in human cancer: deficient natural killercell activity and normal interferon production in patients with advanced disease. J Immunol 1981;127:1817–22
11. Goodale RL, Springer GF, Shearen JG, Desai PR, Tegtmeyer H. Delayed-type cutaneous hypersensitivity to Thomsen-Friedenreich (T) antigen in patients wit pancreatic cancer. J Surg Res 1983; 35:293–7.
12. Funa K, Nilsson G, Jacobsson G, Alm V. Decreased natural killer cell activity and interferon production by leukocytes in patients with adenocarcinoma of the pancreas. Br J Cancer 1984;50:231–3.
13. Monson JRT, Ramsden C, Guillou PJ. Decreased interleukin-2 production in patients with gastrointestinal cancer. Br J Surg 1986;73:483–6.
14. Whittaker MG, Rees K, Clark CCG. Reduced lymphocyte transformation in breastcancer. Lancet 1971; i:892–3.
15. Guillou PJ, Brennan TG, Giles GR. Phytohaemagglutinin stimulated transformation of peripheral and lymph node lymphocytes in patients with gastrointestinal cancer. Br J Surg 1973; 60:745–9.
16. McLaughlin AP, Kessler WO, Triman K, Gittes RF. Immunological competence in patients with urologic cancer. J Urol 1974;111:233–7.
17. Fortner JG, Kim DK, Hopkins L et al. Immunologic function in patients with carcinoma of the pancreas. Surg Gynecol Obstet 1980,;150:215–8.
18. Nakayama E, Asano S, Takuwa N et al. Decreased TCGF activity in the culture medium of PHA stimulated peripheral mononuclear cells from patients with metastatic cancer. Clin Exp Immunol 1983;51:511–6.
19. Monson JRT, Guillou PJ. Immunological perspectives on pancreatic cancer and jaundice. Hepatogastroenterol 1989;36:437–41.
20. Wu TT, Kabat E. An analysis of the sequences of the variable regions of Bence-Jones proteins and myeloma light chains and their implications for antibody complementarity. J Exp Med 1970;132:211–250.
21. Chothia C, Lesk AM, Tramontano A, Levitt M, Smith-Gill S, Air G, et al. Conformations of immunoglobulin hypervariable regions. Nature (Lond) 1989;342:877–883.
22. Jefferis R. What is an idiotype? Immunol Today 1993;14:119–121.
23. Dreesman GR, Kennedy RC. Anti-idiotypic antibodies: implications of internal image-based vaccines for infectious disease. J Infect Dis 1985;151:761–765.
24. Schroeder HW, Hillson JL, Perlmutter RM. Structure and evolution of mammalian V_H families.Int Immunol 1990;2:41–50.
25. Bona CA, Kohler H. Antiidiotypic antibodies and internal images . In: JC Venter, CM Fraser and J Linstrom Editors. Monoclonal and anti-idiotypic antibodies: Probes for receptor structure and function. New York: Alan R. Liss, 1984;141–9.
26. Jerne NK. Towards a network theory of the immune system. Ann Immunol (Paris) 1974;125C: 373–389.
27. Lindenmann J. Speculations on idiotypes and homobodies. Ann Immunol (Paris) 1973;124C: 171–184.

28. Ramseier H, Lindenmann J. Aliotypic antibodies. Transplant Rev 1972;10:57-96.
29. Rosenstein RW, Musson RA, Armstrong MYK, Konigsberg WH, Richards FF. Contact regions for dinitrophenyl and menadione haptens in an immunoglobulin binding more than one antigen. Proc Natl Acad Sci (Wash) 1972;69:877-81.
30. Gaulton GN, Greene MI. Idiotypic mimicry of biologic receptors. Annu Rev Immunol 1986;4:253-80.
31. Erlanger BF. Some thoughts on the structural basis of internal imagery. Immunol Today 1989,;10:151-2.
32. Jerne NK, Roland J, Cazenave PA. Recurrent idiotopes and internal images. EMBO J 1982;1:243-7.
33. Stein KE, Soderstrom T. Neonatal administration of idiotype or antiidiotype primes for protection against Escherichia coli K13 infection in mice. J Exp Med 1984;160:1001-11.
34. Kennedy RC, Eichberg JW, Lanford RE, Dreesman GR. Anti-idiotypic antibody vaccine for type B viral hepatitis in chimpanzees. Science 1986;232:220-3.
35. Burdette S, Schwartz RS. Idiotypes and idiotypic networks. N Engl J Med 1987;317:319-224.
36. Zoller M. Alteration of idiotypic connectivity in prenatally tolerized mice. Scand J Immunol 1990;31:619-29.
37. Klinman DM,Steinberg AD. Idiotypy and autoimmunity. Arthr Rheum 1986;29:697-703.
38. Geha RS. Idiotypic interactions in the treatment of human diseases. Adv Immunol 1986;39:255-97.
39. Rossi F, Dietrich G, Kazatchkine MD. Anti-idiotypes against autoantibodies in normal immunoglobulins: evidence for network regulation of human autoimmune responses. Immunol Rev 1989;110:135-49.
40. Eichmann K, Rajewski K. Induction of T and B cell immunity by anti-idiotypic antibody. Eur J Immunol 1975;5:661-7.
41. de Gast CG, Van de Winkel JGJ, Bast BEJEG. Clinical perspectives of bispecific antibodies in cancer. Cancer Immunol Immunother 1997;45:121-3.
42. Slater RJ, Ward SM, Kunkel HG. Immunological relationships among the myeloma proteins. J Exp Med 1955;101:85-108.
43. Oudin J, Michel M. Une nouvelle forme d'allotypie des globulines du serum de lapin, apparemment liee a la fonction et la specificite des anticorps.C. R. Acad Sci 1963;257:805-8.
44. Bona CA. Idiotype network theory and its implications in anti-tumour immunity. Immun to Cancer 1989;II:215-21.
45. George AJT, Spooner RA, Epenetos AA. Applications of monoclonal antibodies in clinical oncology. Immunology Today 1994;15:559-61.
46. Durrant L. Anti-idiotypic tumor immunotherapy.Tumor Targeting 1995;1:65-6.
47. Sacks DL, Esser KM, Sher A. Immunization of mice againstAfrican trypanosomiasis using anti-idiotypic antibodies. J Exp Med 1982;115:1108-19.
48. McNamara MK, Ward RE, Kohler H. Monoclonal idiotopes vaccine against Streptococcus pneumoniae infection. Science 1984;226:1325-6.
49. Chanh TC, Dreesman GR, Kennedy RC. Monoclonal antiidiotypic antibody mimics the CD4 receptor and binds human immunodeficiencey virus. Proc Natl Acad Sci USA 1984;81:2850-4.
50. Grzych JM, Capron M, Lambert PH, Dissous C, Torres S, Capron A. An anti-idiotype vaccine against experimental Schistosomiasis. Nature (Lond)1985, 316:74-6
51. Chattopadhayay P, Starkey J, Morrow WJW, Raychaudhari S. Murine monoclonal anti-idiotype antibody breaks unresponsiveness and induces a specific antibody response to human melanoma associated proteoglycan antigen in cynomolgus monkeys. Proc Natl Acad Sci USA 1992, 89:2684-8
52. Koido T, Scheck S, Herlyn D. Induction of immunity to colon carcinoma antigen CO17-1A by monoclonal anti-idiotype (Ab2): effects of Ab2 fragmentation, carrier and adjuvant. Tumor Targeting 1995; 1:115-24.
53. Bretscher PA, Cohn M. A theory of self discrimination. Science 1970;169:1042-9.
54. Chen L, Linsley PS, Hellstrom KE. Costimulation of T cells for tumour immunity. Immunology Today 1993;14:483-6.
55. Nossal GJV, Pike BL. Clonal anergy: persistence in tolerant mice of antigen-binding B lymphocytes incapable of responsding to antigen or mitogen. Proc Natl Acad Sci USA 1980;77:1602-6.
56. Goodnow CC, Crosbie J, Adelstein S, Lavoie TB, Smith-Gill SJ, Brink RA, Pritchard-Briscoe H, Wotherspoon JS, Loblay RH, Raphael K, Trent RJ, Basten A. Altered immunoglobulin expression and functional silencing of self-reactive B lymphocytes in transgenic mice. Nature 1988;334:676-82.
57. Anichini A, Fossati G, Parmiani Clonal analysis of cytotoxic T-lymphocyte response to autologous human metastatic melanoma. Int J Cancer 1985;35:683-9.
58. Itoh K, Platsoucas CD, Balch CM. Autologous tumour specific cytotoxic T lymphocytes in the

infiltrate of human metastatic melanoma. Activation by interleukin-2 and autologous tumour cells and involvement of the T cell receptor. J Exp Med 1988;168:1419–41.

59. Ioannides CG, Platsoucas CD, Rashed S, Wharton JT, Edwards CL, Freedman RS. Tumour cytolysis by lymphocytes infiltrating ovarian malignant ascites. Cancer Res 1991; 51:4257–65.

60. Ioannides CG, Freedman RS, Platsoucas CD, Rashed S, Kim YP. Cytotoxic T cell clones isolated from ovarian tumour-infiltrating lymphocytes recognize multiple antigenic epitopes on autologous tumour cells. J Immunol 1991;146:1700–7.

61. Shimizu Y, Weidmann E, Iwatsuki S, Heberman RB, Whiteside TL. Characterization of human autumour-reactive T cell clones obtained from tumour-infiltrating lymphocytes in liver metastasis of gastric carcinoma. Cancer Res 1991; 51:6153–62.

62. Finke JH, Rayman P, Edinger M, Tubbs RR, Stanley J, Klein E, Bukowski R. Characterization of human renal cell carcinoma specific cytotoxic CD8+ T cell line. J Immunol 1992;11:1–11.

63. Miyatake S, Hanada H, Yamashita J, Yamaski T, Ueda M, Namba Y, Hanaoka M. Induction of human glioma-specific cytotoxic T lymphocyte lines by autologous tumour stimulation and interleukin-2. J Neurooncol 1986; 4:55–64.

64. Schwartzentruber DJ, Solomon D, Rosenberg SA, Topalian SL. Characterization of lymphocytes infiltrating human breast cancer: specific immune reactivity detected by measuring cytokine secretion. J Immunother 1992, 12:1–12

65. Yasumura S, Hirabayashi H, Schwartz DR, Toso JF, Johnson JT, Herberman RB, Whiteside TL. Human cytotoxic T-cell lines with restricted specificity for squamous cell carcinoma of the head and neck. Cancer Res 1993;53:1461–8.

66. Wolfel T, Klehmann E, Muller C, Schutt KH, Meyer zum Buschenfelde KH, Knuth A. Lysis of human melanoma cells by autologous cytolytic T cell clones: identification of human histocompatibility leukocyte antigen A2 as a restriction element for the three different antigens. J Exp Med 1989;170:797–810.

67. Topalian SL, Solomon D, Rosenberg SA. Tumour-specific cytolysis by lymphocytes infiltrating human melanomas. J Immunol 1989;142: 3714–25.

68. Restifo NP, Wunderlich JR. Biology of cellular immune responses. In: de Vita Jr VT, Hellman S, Rosenberg SA, editors. Biologic Therapy of Cancer. Philadelphia: JB Lippincott, 1995;3–38.

69. Brocker EB, Kolde G, Steinhausen D, Peters A, Macher E. The pattern of mononuclear infiltrate as a prognostic parameter in flat superficial spreading melanomas. J Cancer Res Clin Oncol 1984,;107:48–52.

70. Janeway CA Jr. Thymic selection: two pathways to life and two to death. Immunity 1994;1:3–6.

71. Fink PJ, Matis LA, McElligott DL, Bookman M, Hedrick SM. Correlations between T-cell specificity and the structure of the antigen receptor. Nature 1986; 321:219–26.

72. Miller JFAP, Morahan G, Allison J, Hoffman M. A transgenic approach to the study of peripheral T-cell tolerance. Immunol Rev 1991;122:103–16.

73. Miller JFAP, Morahan G. Peripheral tolerance. Annu Rev Immunol 1992;10:51–69.

74. Ju S-T, Panka DJ, Cui H, Ettinger R, El-Khatib M, Sherr DH, Stranger BZ, Marshak-Rothstein A. Fas (CD95)/FasL interactions required for programmed cell death after T-cell activation. Nature 1995;373:444–8.

75. Farrow SN, Brown R. New members of the Bcl-2 family and their protein partners. Curr Opin Genet Dev 1996;6:45–9.

76. Nossal GJV. Cellular mechanisms of immunological tolerance. Annu Rev Immunol 1983;1:33–62.

77. Hartley SB, Crosbie J, Brink R, Kantor AB, Basten A, Goodnow CC. Elimination from peripheral lymphoid tissues of self-reactive B lymphocytes recognizing membrane-bound antigen. Nature 1991, 353:765–9

Haak HR,Cornelisse CJ,Hermans J,Cobben L,Fleuren GJ. Nuclear DNA content and morphologic characteristics in the prognosis of adrenocortical carcinoma.Br J Cancer 1993;68:151–5.

78. Linton PJ, Rudie A, Klinman NR. Tolerance susceptibility of newly generating B cells. J Immunol 1991;146:4099–104.

79. Gray D, Skarvall H. B cell memory is short-lived in the absence of antigen. Nature 1988;336:70–2.

80. Gray D, Matzinger P. T cell memory is short-lived in the absence of antigen. J Exp Med 1991;174:969–74.

81. Lau LL, Jamieson BD, Somasundaram R, Ahmed R. Cytotoxic T cell memory without antigen. Nature 1994;369:648–52.

82. Rodenburg CJ, Cornelisse CJ, Heintz APM, Hermans J, Fleuren GJ. Tumour ploidy as a major prognostic factor in advanced ovarian cancer. Cancer 1987;59:317–23.

83. Hamming JF, Shelfhout LJDM,Cornelisse CJ,Van de Velde CJH,Goslings BM,Hermans J, et al. Prognostic value of nuclear DNA content in papillary and follicular thyroid cancer. World J Surg 1988; 12:503–08.

84. Hedley DW, Clark GM, Cornelisse CJ, Killander D, Kute T, Merkel D. DNA cytometry consensus conference: consensus review of the clinical utility of DNA cytometry in carcinoma of the breast. Breast Cancer Research Treatment 1993;14(5):482–5.

85. Oosterwijk E, Warnaar SO, Zwartendijk J, Van der Velde EA, Fleuren GJ, Cornelisse CJ. Relationship between DNA ploidy,antigen expression and survival in renal cell carcinoma. Int J Cancer 1988;42:703–8.

86. Pawelec G, Zeuthen J, Kiessling R. Escape from host-antitumor immunity. Crit Rev Oncog 1997;8:111

87. Pawelec G. Tumour escape from the immune response: the last hurdle for successful immunotherapy of cancer? Cancer Immunol Immunother 1999;48:343–5.

88. Whiteside TL. Signaling defects in T lymphocytes of patients with malignancy. Cancer Immunol Immunother 1999;48:346–52.

89. Buggins AG, Hirst WJ, Pagliuca A, Mufti GJ. Variable expression of CD3-zeta and associated tyrosine kinases in lymphocytes with myeloid malignancies. Br J Haematol 1998;100:784.

90. Choi SH, Chung EJ, Whang DY, Lee SS, Jang YS, Kim CW. Alteration of signal-transducing molecules in tumour-infiltratimg lymphocytes and peripheral blood T lymphocytes from human colorectal carcinoma patients. Cancer Immunol Immunother 1998;45:299.

91. Correa MR, Ochoa AC, Ghosh P, Mizoguchi H, Harvey L, Longo DL. Sequential development of structural and functional alterations in T cells from tumor-bearing mice. J Immunol 1997;158:5292.

92. Corsi MM, Maes HH, Wasserman K, Fulgenzi A, Gaja G, Ferero ME. Protection of L-oxothiazolidine-carboxylic acid of hydrogen peroxide induced CD3zeta and CD16 zeta chain down-regulation in human peripheral blood lymphocytes and lymphokine-activated killer cells. Biochem Pharmacol 1998;56:657.

93. Elsasser-Biele U, Kleist S von, Fischer R, Monting JS. Impaired cytokine production in whole blood cell cultures from patients with colorectal carcinomas as compared to benign colorectal tumors and controls. J Clin Lab Anal 1992;6:311.

94. Miescher S, Whiteside TL, Moretta L, von Fliedner V. Clonal and frequency analyses of tumor-infiltrating lymphocytes from human solid tumors. J Immunol 1987;138:4004–11.

95. Miescher S, Stoeck M, Qiao L, Barras C, Barrelet L, von Fliedner V. Proliferative and cytolytic potentials of purified human tumor infiltrating T lymphocytes. Impaired response to mitogen-driven stimulation despite T cell receptor expression. Int J Cancer 1998;42:659–66.

96. Whiteside TL, Jost LM, Herberman RB. Tumor-infiltrating lymphocytes: potential and limitations to their use for cancer therapy. Crit Rev Oncol Hematol 1992;12:25–47.

97. Whiteside TL. Tumor-infiltrating lymphocytes as anti-tumor effector cells. Biotherapy 1992;5:47–61.

98. Reichert TE, Rabinowich H, Johnson JT, Whiteside TL. Immune cells in the tumor microenvironment: mechanisms responsible for signaling and functional defects. J Immunother 1998;21:295–306.

99. Nakagomi H, Petersson M, Magnusson I, Juhlin C, Matsuda M, Mellstedt H, Taupin J-L, Vivier E, Anderson P, Kiessling R. Decreased expression of the signal-transducing ζ chains in tumor-infiltrating T cells and NK cells of patients with colorectal carcinoma. Cancer Res 1993;53:5610–2.

100. Healy CG, Simons JW, Carducci MA, DeWeese TL, Bartkowski M, Tong KP, Bolton WE. Impaired expression and function of signal-transducing zeta chains in peripheral T cells and natural killer cells in patients with prostate cancer. Cytometry 1998;32:109–19.

101. Zea AH, Brendan CD, Longo DL, Alvord WG, Strobl SL, Mizoguchi H, Creekmore SP, O'Shea JJ, Powers GC, Urba WJ, Ochoa AC. Alterations in T cell receptor and signal transduction molecules in melanoma patients. Clin Cancer Res 1995;1:1327–35.

102. Kiessling R, Wasserman K, Horiguchi S, Kono K, Sjoberg J, Pisa P, Petersson M. Tumor-induced immune dysfunction. Cancer Immunol Immunother 1999;48:353–62.

103. Leonard WJ, O'Shea JJ. Jaks and STATs: biological implications. Annu Rev Immunol 1998;16:293.

104. Pericle F, Kirken RA, Bronte V, Sconocchia G, DaSilva L, Segal DM. Immunocompromised tumor-bearing mice show a selective loss of STAT5a/b expression in T and B lymphocytes. J Immunol 1997;159:2580.

105. Rabinowich H, Reichert TE, Kashii Y, Gastman BR, Bell MC, Whiteside TL. Lymphocyte apoptosis induced by Fas ligand-expressing ovarian carcinoma cells. Implications for altered expression of T cell receptor in tumor-associated lymphocytes. J Clin Invest 1998;101:2579.

106. Suda T, Hashimoto H, Tanaka M, Ochi T, Nagata S. Membrane Fas ligand kills human peripheral blood T lymphocytes and soluble Fas ligand blocks the killing. J Exp Med 1997;186:2045.

107. Staveley-O'Carroll K, Sotomayor E, Montgomery J, Borrello I, Hwang L, Fein S, Pardoll D, Levitsky H. Induction of antigen-specific T cell anergy : an early event in the course of tumor progression. Proc Natl Acad Sci USA 1998;95:1178.

108. Pellegrini P, Berghella A-M, Del Beato T, Cicia S, Adorno D, Casciani CU. Dysregulation in Th1 and Th2 subsets of CD4+ T cells in the peripheral blood of colorectal cancer patients and involvement in cancer establishment and progression. Cancer Immunol Immunother 1996;42:1–8.

109. Zbar AP, Thomas H, Snary D et al. A phase I/II trial of vaccination with a novel murine monoclonal anti-CEA antibody in advanced colorectal cancer. Br J Surg 1999;86(Suppl 1):102–3(A).

110. Zbar AP, Snary D, Thomas H, Kmiot WA, Allen-Mersh TG. Immunoresponsiveness in metastatic colorectal cancer during anticarcinoembryonic antigen vaccination. Br J Surg 2000; 87:627(A).

111. Foon KA, John WJ, Chakraborty M, Sherratt A, Garrison J, Flett M, Bhattacharya-Chatterjee M. Clinical and immune responses in advanced colorectal cancer patients treated with anti-idiotype monoclonal antibody vaccine that mimics the carcinoembryonic antigen. Clin Cancer Res 1997;3:1267–76.

112. Barcellini W, Rizzardi GP, Borghi MO, Fain C, Lazzarini A, Meroni P-L. Th1 and Th2 cytokine production by peripheral blood mononuclear cells from HIV-infected patients. AIDS 1994;8:757–62.

113. Clerici M, Shearer G. A Th1 to Th2 switch is a critical step in the aetiology of HIV infection. Immunol Today 1993;14:107–10.

114. Clerici M, Hakim FT, Venzon DJ et al. Changes in IL-2 and IL-4 in asymptomatic HIV-seropositive individuals. J Clin Invest 1993;91:759–65.

115. Miedema F, Petit AJ, Terpstra FG et al. Immunological abnormalities in human immunodeficiency virus (HIV)-infected asymptomatic homosexual men. HIV affects the immune system before CD4+ T helper cell depletion occurs. J Clin Invest 1988;82:1908–1916.

116. Evans TG, Fitzgerald T, Gibbons DC, Keefer MC, Soucher H and the AIDS Vaccine Evaluation Group. Th1/Th2 cytokine responses following HIV-immunization in seronegative volunteers. Clin Exp Immunol 1998;111:243–50.

117. Frodin J-E, Harmenberg U, Biberfeld P, Christensson B, Lefvert A-K, Rieger A, Shetye J, Wahren B, Mellstedt H. Clinical effects of monoclonal antibodies (mAb 17-1A) in patients with metastatic colorectal cancer. Hybridoma 1988;7:309–21.

118. Herlyn D, Koprowski H. Monoclonal anticolon carcinoma antibodies in complement-dependent cytotoxicity. Int J Cancer 1981;27:769.

119. Steplewski Z, Chang TH, Herlyn M, Koprowski H. Release of monoclonal-antibody defined antigens by human colorectal carcinoma and melanoma cells. Cancer Res 1981;41:2723–7.

120. Adams DO, Hall T, Steplewski Z, Koprowski H. Tumours undergoing rejection induced by monoclonal antibodies of the IgG2a isotype containing increasing numbers of macrophages activated for distinctive form of antibody dependent cytolysis. Proc Natl Acad Sci USA 1984, 81:3506–10

121. Kipps TJ, Parham P, Punt J,Herzenberg LA. Importance of immunoglobulin isotype in human antibody-dependent cell-mediated cytoxicity directed by murine monoclonal antibodies. J Exp Med 1985;161:1–17.

122. Ortolado J, Woodhouse C, Morgan AC, Herberman RB, Cheresh DA, Reisfeld R. Analysis of effector cells in human antibody-dependent cellular cytotoxicity with murine monoclonal antibodies. J Immunol 1987; 138:3536–41.

123. Lanzavecchia A, Abrignani S, Scheidegger D, Obrist R, Dorken B,Moldenhauer G. Antibodies as antigens:the use of mouse monoclonal antibodies to focus human T cells against selected targets. J Exp Med 1988,167:345–52.

124. Trauth BC,Klas C,Peters AMJ, Matzku S,Moller P,Falk W,Debatin KM, Krummer PH. Monoclonal antibody mediated tumor regression by induction of apoptosis. Science 1989,245:301–5.

125. Kohler H, Kieber-Emmons T, Srinivasan S, Kaveri S, Morrow WJW, Muller S, et al. Revised immune network concepts. Clin Immunol Immunopathol 1989;52:104–116.

126. Bruck C, Co MS, Slaoui M,Gaulton GN, Smith T, Fields BN, Mullins JI, Greene MI. Nucleic acid sequence of an internal image-binding monoclonal anti-idiotype and its comparison of the sequence of the external antigen. Proc Natl Acad Sci USA 1986;83:6578–82.

127. Viale G, Flamini G, Grassi F, Buffa R, Natali PG, Pelagi M, et al. Idiotypic replica of an anti-human tumour-associated antigen monoclonal antibody. J Immunol 1989,143:4388–44

128. Bentley GA, Boulot G, Riottot MM, Poljak RJ. Three-dimensional structure of an idiotope-anti-idiotope complex. Nature 1990;348:254–7.

129. Raychaudhari S, Kang C-Y, Kaveri S-V, Kieber-Emmons T,Kohler H. Tumour idiotypic vaccines.VII. Analysis and correlation of structural,idiotypic and biological properties of protective and non-protective Ab2's. J Immunol 1990;145:760–7.

130. Bhattacharya-Chatterjee M, Foon KA,Kohler H. Anti-idiotype monoclonal antibodies as vaccines for human cancer. Intern Rev Immunol 1991;7:289–302.

131. Bona C,Herber-Katz E,Paul EW. Idiotype-antiidiotype regulation.I. Immunization with a levan-

binding myeloma protein leads to the appearance of auto-anti-(anti-idiotype) antibodies and to the activation of silent clones. J Exp Med 1981;153:951-67.

132. Jain RK. Haemodynamic and transport barriers to the treatment of solid tumours. Int J Radiat Biol 1990; 60:85-100(a).

133. Jain RK. Vascular and interstitial barriers to delivery of therapeutic agents in tumours. Cancer Met Rev 1990;9:253-266(b).

134. Grossbard ML,Press OW, Applebaum FR, Bernstein ID, Nadler LM. Monoclonal antibody-based therapies of leukemia and lymphoma. Blood 1992;80:863-78.

135. Hagan PL,Halpern SE, Dillman RO et al. Tumour size : effect of monoclonal antibody uptake in tumour models. J Nucl Med 1986;27:422-427.

136. Watanabe Y,Endo K, Koizumi M et al. Effect of tumour mass and antigenic nature on the biodistribution of labeled monoclonal antibodies in mice. Cancer Res 1988;49:2884-9.

137. Boucher Y, Baxter LT, Jain RK. Interstitial pressure gradients in tissue-isolated and subcutaneous tumours: implications for therapy. Cancer Res 1990;50:4478-84.

138. Fujimori K,Covell DG, Fletcher JE. A modelling analysis of monoclonal antibody percolation through tumours: a binding site barrier. J Nucl Med 1990; 31:1191-8.

139. Baxter LT,Jain RK. Transport of fluid and macromolecules in tumours.III: role of binding and metabolism. Microvasc Res 1991;51:4776-84.

140. Juweid M, Neumann R,Paik C et al. Micropharmacology of monoclonal antibodies in solid tumours: direct experimental evidence for a binding site barrier. Cancer Res 1992;52:5144-53.

141. Morton BA,O'Connor-Tressel M,Beatty BG,Shively JE,Beatty JD. Artefactual CEA elevation due to human anti-mouse antibodies. Arch Surg 1988;123:1242-6.

142. Mayforth R,Quintans J. Designer and catalytic antibodies. N Engl J Med 1990;323:173-8.

143. Winter G,Milstein C. Man-made antibodies. Nature (Lond) 1991;349:293-9

144. Fell HP,Gayle MA,Grosmaire L,Ledbetter JA. Genetic construction and characterization of a fusion protein consisting of a chimaeric F(ab') with specificity for carcinomas and human IL-2. J Immunol 1991;146:2446-2452.

145. Bird RE, Hardman KD, Jacobson JW, Johnson S, Kaufman BM, Lee SM, Lee T, et al. Single-chain antigen-binding proteins. Science 1988;242:423-6.

146. Zbar AP, Lemoine NR, Wadhwa M, Thomas H, Snary D, Kmiot WA. Biological therapy: approaches in colorectal cancer. Strategies to enhance carcinoembryonic antigen (CEA) as an immunogenic target. Br J Cancer 1998;77:683-93.

147. Bruggemann M, Winter G, Waldmann H, Neuberger MS. The immunogenicity of chimaeric antibodies. J Exp Med 1989;170:2153-7.

148. Gilboa E. How tumors escape immune destruction and what we can do about it. Cancer Immunol Immunother 1999;48:382-5.

149. Ferrone S, Marincola FM. Loss of HLA class I antigens by melanoma cells : molecular mechanisms, functional significance and clinical relevance. Immunol Today 1995;16:487.

150. Lee K-H, Panelli MC, Kim CJ et al. Functional dissociation between local and systemic immune responses during anti-melanoma peptide vaccination. J Immunol 1998;161:4183.

151. Slingluff CL. Targeting unique tumour antigens and modulating the cytokine environment may improve immunotherapy for tumors with immune escape mechanisms. Cancer Immunol Immunother 1999;48:371-3

152. Maurer MJ, Gollin SM, Martin D et al. Tumor escape from immune recognition. J Clin Invest 1996;98:1633

153. Syrigos KN, Karayiannakis AJ, Zbar A. Mucins as immunogenic targets in cancer. Anticancer Res 1999;19:5239-44

154. Gilboa E, Nair SK, Lyerly HK. Immunotherapy of cancer with dendritic-cell based vaccines. Cancer Immunol Immunother 1998;46:82

155. Seliger B, Maurer MJ, Ferrone S. TAP off — tumors on. Immunol Today 1997;18:297

156. Effros RB, Pawelec G. Replicative senescence of T lymphocytes: does the Hayflick Limit lead to immune exhaustion? Immunol Today 1997;18:450.

157. Pawelec G, Adibzadeh M, Solana R, Beckman I. The T cell in the ageing individual. Mech Ageing Dev 1997;93:35.

158. Speiser DE, Miranda R, Zakarian A et al. Self antigens expressed by solid tumors do not efficiently stimulate naïve or activated T cells: implications for immunotherapy. J Exp Med 1997;186:645.

10. Immunobiology of Cancer Metastasis*

Jerald J. Killion and Isaiah J. Fidler

Introduction

Once a diagnosis of cancer is established, the urgent question is whether it is localized or has already spread to regional lymph nodes and visceral organs. Despite improvements in early diagnosis, surgical techniques, general patient care and local and systemic adjuvant therapies, most deaths of cancer patients result from the relentless growth of metastatic disease that is resistant to conventional therapies. Surgical excision of primary neoplasms is not curative in many patients because by the time of diagnosis, metastasis may well have occurred. The major challenge for treatment of metastasis is the biological heterogeneity of cancer cells within primary lesions and especially within metastases. A wide range of genetic, biochemical, immunological and biological characteristics that differ from sub-population to subpopulation include the display of cell-surface receptors, enzymes, karyotypes, cell morphologies, growth properties, sensitivities to various therapeutic agents and the ability to invade and produce metastasis [1,2]. This heterogeneity is due to differences in etiology, origin and selection pressures. The outcome of the metastatic process depends on the interaction of metastatic cells with host homeostatic factors, which include various elements of the host immune system. The establishment and progressive growth of metastatic cells requires that they exploit, subvert and suppress, when necessary, natural host defense systems. This chapter will focus on the host-tumor interactions that result in immune modulation of tumor cell populations.

The Biology of Tumor Metastasis

Evolution of the Primary Tumor

To understand the complexity of tumor-immune system interaction, it is important to appreciate the evolution of tumor heterogeneity and its relation to meta-

* This work was supported in part by Cancer Center Support Core grant CA16672 and grant R35-CA42107 (I.J.F.) from the National Cancer Institute, National Institutes of Health.

stasis. The concept that neoplasms are heterogeneous and contain different cells with different biological properties is not new. More than a century ago, Stephen Paget [3] analyzed autopsy records of patients with breast cancer and concluded that the non-random pattern of metastasis was not due to chance. Rather, metastases resulted from the proliferation of a few tumor cells (the seed) in the favorable milieu provided by some organs (the soil) [3]. A current definition of Paget's hypothesis consists of three principles. First, as stated above, neoplasms are heterogeneous for metastatic properties. Second the process of metastasis is sequential and selective and contains stochastic features. Third, the production of clinical metastases is ultimately dependent upon and moulded by the interaction of metastatic cells with host cells and their products (reviewed in [4]).

Neoplastic transformation involves genetic alterations in the target cells, such as activation or regulation of proto-oncogenes. The subsequent alterations in cellular DNA lead to a potential myriad of processes that commit transformed cells to continued proliferation. Autonomy from normal growth control mechanisms and the diversity of cell populations within the initial primary tumor give neoplasms growth advantages in host organs. Although many neoplasms have a unicellular origin, by the time of diagnosis the lesions present a spectrum of heterogeneous properties. The initial mitogenic events of transformation associated with the transcription of oncogenes and the dysregulation of the cell cycle afforded by the loss of suppressor genes help the cell achieve growth autonomy from the host's microenvironment. For example, the eventual switching of tumors to an angiogenic phenotype, i.e., the production of a variety of chemotactic, growth and survival factors needed to induce a required vascular supply, is essential for continued expansion of the primary tumor [5,6]. These factors include the up-regulation of vascular endothelial growth factor, platelet-derived endothelial growth factor, the family of basic fibroblast growth factors, angiogenin, angiotropin, epidermal growth factor, transforming growth factor-alpha and beta, interleukins and colony-stimulating factors, as well as the expression of metalloproteinases.

Necrotic regions of the neoplasm will contain cellular products that are chemotactic for host infiltrate cells, such as leukocytes, monocytes and fixed macrophages. These "normal" infiltrate cells can produce needed growth factors and enzymes required to degrade the basement membrane and model the surrounding stroma into an architecture that allows for the migration, invasion and eventual escape of tumor cells from the confines of the primary tumor mass [7]. Eventually the primary tumor consists of multiple subpopulations of cells which manifest a multitude of functional aberrations, including metabolic, enzymatic and molecular perturbations, that result in membrane-associated changes in cell-surface structure and function [5,7].

Because these events do not occur uniformly within different regions of the primary tumor, the malignant or benign nature of the tumor cannot be determined with confidence unless multiple sections are examined. Besides, variations in the metastatic capability of different zones of dissected tumor have been described [1,8]. This zonal composition of primary tumors can influence the nature of distant metastases. It is conceivable that multi-cell aggregates from specific zones of a primary tumor may yield metastases with uniform characteristics, whereas the selective survival of single cells from other regions of the primary tumor may result in metastases with quite different properties. Hence, evolutionary forces within the primary tumor eventually select for an increasingly rich fraction of cells that are competent to survive in a new environment distant from the primary tumor. At first the migration into the lymphatics and vasculature is limited to a select population of cells, but as the size of the primary tumor becomes larger, the percentage of metastatic-competent cells becomes greater.

Sequential Events During the Pathogenesis of Metastasis

The process of cancer metastasis consists of a series of inter-related steps, each of which is rate-limiting, since a failure at any of the steps aborts the process [9]. The outcome of the process is dependent on both the intrinsic properties of the tumor cells and the responses of the host; the balance of these interactions differs from patient to patient.

The sequential steps in the formation of a metastasis are:

(a) establishment of an extensive blood supply, accomplished by the production and secretion of angiogenesis factors by tumor cells and host cells which play a key role in establishing a capillary network from the surrounding host tissue.

(b) Local invasion of the host stroma by some tumor cells occurs by several parallel mechanisms. Thin-walled venules, like lymphatic channels, offer very little resistance to penetration by tumor cells and provide the most common pathways for tumor cell entry into the circulation.

(c) Detachment and embolization of single tumor cells or aggregates occurs next, the vast majority of circulating tumor cells being readily destroyed.

(d) Once the tumor cells have survived the stresses of circulation, they must

(e) arrest in the capillary beds of distant organs by adhering either to capillary endothelial cells or to sub-endothelial basement membrane that may be exposed.

(f) Extravasation occurs next, probably by mechanisms similar to those operative during invasion, i.e., by the upregulation of degradative enzymes.

(g) Proliferation within the organ parenchyma completes the metastatic process and survival depends again upon developing a vascular network and evading host defenses intrinsic to the organ site [10].

Each of these events involves interaction between the host and tumor that continually modulate the host/immune responsiveness and shape the cancer cell phenotype needed for survival and continued growth.

The Immunology of Metastasis

Immunological Properties of Tumor Cells as Determinants of Metastasis

Rejection or Transplantation Antigens of Tumor

The classical experiments of Richmond Prehn and colleagues established the existence of tumor antigens as defined by the ability of a syngeneic host to reject transplanted, carcinogen-induced, murine tumors [11,12]. These tumor antigens were not cross-reactive with normal tissue, since immunization with normal tissue did not protect against a subsequent challenge with tumors, nor did immunization with tumor cause rejection of syngeneic tissue transplants. Of particular interest, with important implications, were the observations that individual tumors from an autochthonous host were antigenically distinct, i.e., multiple tumors from a single mouse did not necessarily give rise to transplantation immunity against individual tumors [13]. These early studies established the concepts that tumors possessed potentially unique antigens that could provoke transplantation immunity and that tumors were heterogeneous with respect to the antigenic properties of their cells. It was later shown that the immunogenic and antigenic properties of murine tumors depended upon the nature of the transforming event (e.g., carcinogens, ultraviolet light, or viruses) (reviewed in [14]).

Furthermore, spontaneous murine tumors tend to be less immunogenic than the tumors induced by carcinogens and viruses and this has been the basis for arguing that the strong antigenic features of human tumors are difficult to demonstrate. However, one cannot strictly use transplantation experiments to discern the immunogenicity of human cancers and furthermore there is overwhelming evidence that physical and chemical carcinogens underlie the etiology of most human cancers.

Expression of major histocompatibility complex (MHC) antigens are frequently altered in human and experimental tumors and in most cases, a decrease in these antigens has been reported [14,15]. Cell surface MHC molecules present peptides derived from processed proteins to the immune system. Activation of T-lymphocytes to putative tumor-specific antigens depends upon the presence of MHC antigens as well as co-stimulatory molecules that enhance immune recognition (see Chapter 9).

The loss of MHC antigens may give a selective escape advantage to tumor cells by subverting immune cell recognition and subsequent immune reactivity. This downregulation may correlate with the metastatic properties of tumor cells that arise out of viral etiology due to MHC-class restriction of immune responses against cells that display viral antigens. Gelber and colleagues [16] demonstrated that a highly metastatic and low immunogenic Lewis lung carcinoma, D122, of C57BL/6, mice expressed H-2K major MHC antigens. Transfection of H-2K region genes abrogated the metastatic properties of this cell line, suggesting that downregulation of MHC was an important prerequisite in these cells being able to form metastasis at distant sites. Mice injected with the H-2K-expressing transfectants manifested strong T-cell cytotoxicity against both parental (non-transfected) and the transfected cell line. Further insight into the role of the H-2 alleles was shown by transfection of the D122 subline with H-2D genes, which resulted in no change of the highly metastatic properties.

This phenomenon was also shown using a poorly immunogenic clone, B78H1, derived as an H-2^b-negative cell line from the murine B16 melanoma. Transfection with the H-2K^b gene decreased the ability of the cells to form lung metastasis following intravenous inoculation [17]. Again, a cytotoxic T-cell response was observed. In addition, homotypic aggregation of H-2K-transfected cells was significantly lower than that of the parental cell population, suggesting that adhesion properties of cells expressing the MHC molecules were altered.

Quantitative alterations in the display of either H-2K or the H-2D alleles may have intrinsic consequences to host responsiveness, typically mediated by T-cell recognition of tumor-specific antigens that may be present, or by recognition by natural killer (NK) cells. There is evidence that treatment of tumor cells with interferon (IFN) up-regulates the expression of MHC [18]. At the same time, this phenomenon may require a precise ratio or abundance of either the H-2K or H-2D allele, since treatment of mouse carcinoma with IFN can enhance the metastatic and tumorigenic properties of these cells, a feature that may be related to preferential display of H-2D antigens. It is believed that this may hinder recognition of tumor by NK cells that would ordinarily minimize the metastatic properties of the tumor. Evidence for this concept comes from studies such as those performed by Geldhof and colleagues [19], who transfected the mouse IFN gene into lymphoma cells. This resulted in a selective induction of H-2D antigens and concomitant enhanced metastasis. Anti-sialo-GM1 treatment of AKR mice allowed rapid metastasis of the parental and transfected cells, but the high H-2KD expressing cell line was resistant to lysis by NK cells, in contrast to the parental (or neogene transfected) cells. This result suggests that H-2KD expression may in part control NK sensitivity of tumor cells.

Alterations and reduced expression of MHC antigens in human tumors are also well documented [20,21]. This can result in decreased immune recognition and responsiveness. Other defined antigens associated with tissue-specific growth, such as differentiation antigens, or fetal antigens, (most notably alpha fetoprotein and carcinoembryonic antigen), may influence the adhesive characteristics of tumor cells and the form of homotypic emboli. These may bind to basement membranes and endothelium, which may determine a tumor's ability to metastasize [22,23].

Display of Costimulatory Molecules Required for Efficient Immune Recognition

Immune recognition and processing is carefully orchestrated by cross-linking of signal transducing, trans-membrane proteins found on T-cell populations and MHC antigens with bound antigen present on antigen-presenting cells such as dendritic cells, B-cells and macrophages. Besides the classical stabilizing molecules, such as CD8 and CD4, (which define T-cell subsets), antigen binding to the T-cell receptor (TCR) is associated with ligation of co-stimulatory molecules for efficient activation, cytokine release and subsequent maturation [24]. Several of these molecules have been characterized and are members of a family of adhesion molecules such as the integrins. For example, LFA-1 (an $\alpha3$ integrin) is found on lymphocytes and its ligand, ICAM-1, (a well-described adhesion molecule), is required for optimal T-cell stimulation. ICAM-1 may be found on antigen-presenting cells and tumor cells. Down-regulation of ICAM-1 or MHC on tumor cells may shield them from this form of complete recognition.

Poor expression of ICAM-1 is associated with metastasis via lymphatic tissues in lung cancer [25]. The best-studied system is the B-7 family of immunoglobulin-like molecules, which serve as potent co-stimulatory molecules for T-cell governed immunity. Transfection of B-7 molecules renders tumor cells highly immunogenic for immunocompetent hosts and results in induction of cytotoxic lymphocytes (CTLs), this form of antigenic alteration of tumor cells has been used as a vaccine preparation against B-7-deficient parental tumor cells in several tumor models [26,27]. An additional T-cell ligand for the B7 family is CD28, an activation molecule expressed on lymphocytes. Binding of this receptor (or its related homologue, CTLA-4) results in cytokine release and differentiation of the T-cell. CD44 is a cell surface receptor for extracellular matrix glycosaminoglycans such as hyaluronan and is abundant on lymphocytes, allowing them to adhere to endothelial cells. This molecule can serve as a focal point for lymphocyte interaction and is also expressed in variant form by tumor cells [28,29], resulting in enhanced binding within capillary and lymphatic beds and enhancing metastatic potential. Indeed, pre-operative values of soluble CD44 (variant 6) appear to be closely related to distant metastases and staging in breast cancer [30]. Overexpression of CD44 on primary malignant melanomas correlates with increased metastatic risk and reduced survival [31].

Role of Expression of Fas or Fas-Ligand in Metastasis of Tumor Cells

The Fas/Fas-ligand (Fas-L) system is involved in the induction of apoptosis and can mediate T-cell cytotoxicity (in addition to classical granzyme-mediated cell death of target cells) as well as down-regulate expansion of lymphocyte populations. Cells that express Fas are susceptible to the induction of apoptosis, e.g., Fas-expressing lymphocytes are susceptible to apoptosis in an environment rich with soluble or cell-bound Fas-L.

A number of observations indicate that tumor cell expression of Fas-L in both lymphoid and non-lymphoid malignancies can influence their ability to circumvent T-cell responses. For example, high levels of Fas-L expression correlated with aggressive disease in leukemia [32]. Whereas indolent chronic myelogeneous leukemic (CML) cells stained negative for Fas-L, from 60–100% of CML cells were positive during blast crisis phase, suggesting that rapid expansion of these cells was associated with expression of Fas-L and this expression contributed to evasion of immune responsiveness. Primary and metastatic melanomas have been extensively studied for potential correlations between metastatic potential and expression of Fas/Fas-L. It was reported that both the incidence and extent of lung metastasis of K-1735 murine melanoma was enhanced in Fas-L-deficient mice [33], supporting the concept that inactivation of Fas expression on melanoma cells could enhance their metastatic potential. However, it is not clear whether Fas expression by melanoma renders these cells sensitive to Fas-L+ cells. On the other hand, primary lesions of melanoma tend to be negative for Fas-L expression and serial studies on metastases from the same patients demonstrated an increase in Fas-L expression, but this increase was not correlated with any increase in the apoptotic index within the tumor [34]. Hence, for melanoma, it is not clear whether Fas expression confers a special sensitivity to melanoma cells or if the presence of Fas-L offers these cells protection from immune interactions mediated by the Fas/Fas-L system.

Esophageal carcinomas have been shown to express Fas-L and down-regulate Fas to escape from host immune surveillance. Shibakita et al. [35] immunohistochemically analyzed over 100 specimens of human esophageal cancer for Fas, Fas-L and CD8 expression. Strong Fas-L expression correlated with a decrease in tumor-associated CD8+ cells but not survival, whereas strong Fas expression by the tumor cells was an independent prognosticator of recurrence-free survival. A similar study revealed that Fas-L expression in greater than 25 percent of the cancer cells as determined by immunohistochemistry was associated with a higher incidence of lymph node metastasis [36]. Indeed, greater than 50 percent of the cancer cells in all cancer metastases in lymph nodes expressed Fas-L.

Interestingly, the presence of soluble Fas (sFas) in the serum of breast cancer patients correlated with a poor prognosis for both overall and disease-free survival, suggesting an immune interaction favored expansion of Fas-L-negative carcinoma or down-regulation of immune effector cells [37]. Patients with liver metastasis of breast carcinoma had the highest levels of sFas. The balance of cell-bound Fas or Fas-L, together with Fas, may regulate the dynamics of tumor cell-lymphocyte interaction and ultimately determine the ability of both neoplastic and host immune effector cell populations to expand in the presence of one another.

Selected Tumor Cell Subpopulations with Loss of Antigens

Antigen-loss variant cell populations have been demonstrated in a variety of experimental animal tumor models. This was best demonstrated by studies showing the progression of a highly immunogenic UV-induced tumor normally rejected by immunocompetent syngeneic mice to a poorly immunogenic, highly metastatic variant [38,39]. The original tumor had multiple strong trans-plantation antigens that could be defined by different T-cell clones. Passage of large numbers of this cell line into normal or immunized mice eventually resulted in the emergence of a highly malignant cell line that had lost, in a sequential fashion, many of its cytolytic T-cell specificities. Hence, progression to a highly metastatic state was paralleled by selective loss of dominant antigens that would have otherwise provoked T-cell immunity. This antigen loss can be exten-ded to the concept of antigen-modulation [40]. For example, mice immunized against the thymic leukemia antigen TL developed titers of anti-TL antibodies that were cytotoxic to TL+ leukemia cells. However, these leukemia cells often grew equally well in normal and immunized mice because of the disappearance of the TL antigen in the presence of the antibody. This type of antigen modulation constitutes a de facto loss of antigen and may help the cells evade immune reac-tivity and allow rapid metastatic spread of populations of cells with this pheno-type.

Immunological Responses of the Host as Determinants of Metastasis

Cellular Composition and Function Within the Tumor Microenvironment

One hallmark of the malignant neoplasm is the ability to invade surrounding normal stroma and host tissue. This insidious process begins by up-regulation of degradative enzymes produced by both normal host infiltrate cells and tumor cells, mainly at the periphery of the tumor cell mass [7]. This catabolism of sur-rounding cellular architecture releases stromal-bound growth factors and pro-enzymatic molecules and causes chemotactic activation of infiltrative cells, such as granulocytes, monocytes and fixed macrophages, that in turn secrete a myriad of cytokines, colony-stimulating factors, bioactive lipids and growth factors into the milieu of the tumor microenvironment (reviewed in [41]). Depending on the location, growth rate, and histological type of primary tumor, the composition of the host cell infiltrate will reflect the natural chemotactic response to differences in cellular integrity, oxygenation, local pH and products of tumor-stromal inter-actions. Inflammatory responses may then be up-regulated.

Lymphocytes, represented by the subsets of natural killer (NK) cells, or lym-phokine-activated killer cells (LAK), as well as CD4+ and CD8+ cells present within the tumor, together with macrophages, represent a first line of host defense against the proliferation of malignant cells. The quality and quantity of the immune response will be a function of how well the host recognizes, in an immunological fashion, tumor cells. In addition, lymphocytes are not merely immunocytes; they also enhance tumor growth by secreting cytokines that stimulate the proliferation of tumor cells [42]. This dual nature of the immune response (inhibition and stimulation of tumor growth) was described by Prehn, who demonstrated that the growth of tumors that induce weak anti-tumor immunity is stimulated by products of nearby lymphocytes [11,12]. Support for this hypothesis came from studies of Seung et al., who showed that a strongly antigenic UV-induced fibrosarcoma that normally regressed when implanted in syngeneic mice, could escape immune destruction by proliferating rapidly in the presence of factors released by granulocytes. This tumor escape could be prevented by pre-treatment of the mice with antigranulocyte antibody [43].

Subpopulations of cells within the tumor differ in their immunogenic properties, suggesting that different immunological responses occur within a single neoplasm. One study focused on the influence of the immune status of the host and the inherent immunogenicity of three different murine fibrosarcomas [44]. As expected, the highly immunogenic tumor formed more lung tumor nodules following intravenous injection in an immunosuppressed host than a normal (sham-suppressed) host. However, the most immunogenic tumor unexpectedly formed fewer tumor nodules in immunologically compromised hosts than that observed in normal mice. This particular observation is consistent with leukocyte-enhanced growth of the weakly immunogenic tumor [11–13].

Tumor-host Interactions in Antitumor Immunity

There is abundant evidence that primary tumors can present bona fide antigens to the immune system. Melanoma serves as a model of this phenomenon of immunogenicity of human tumor and several tumor antigens, including MAGE, MART-1/Melan A and gp100, recognized by CTL's have been isolated (reviewed in [45]). These antigens are MHC-Class I restricted [46] and the frequency of CTLs may depend on the presence of maturing cytokines, such as IFN-γ or IL-2. Similar antigens (RAGE-1, PRAME, gp75) have been described for renal cell carcinoma [47] and this initial host modeling of the tumor population may ultimately determine the nature of the metastatic phenotype. The lack of intracellular signaling caused by an absence of T-cell co-stimulation can result in immunological anergy to these self-antigens. Host infiltrate cells and tumor cells can secrete a variety of factors, such as IL-4, IL-6, IL-10, TGF-α and prostaglandins, that cause immune dysfunction within lymphocyte populations involved in antigen presentation or effector cell function [48]. Human head and neck squamous cells that secrete high levels of GM-CSF contain CD34+ natural suppressor cells, which inhibit the activity of intra-tumoral T-cells and this inhibition correlates with increased metastasis [49]. CD8$^+$ suppressor cells that inhibit LAK cell cytotoxicity have been identified in the peripheral blood of patients with advanced gastric carcinoma [50], reinforcing the notion that the balance among the lymphocyte populations and the cytokine environment together play a role in determining the ultimate metastatic burden. Even in strongly antigenic tumors, such as those induced by UV irradiation, UV radiation is immune suppressive and cytokines secreted by UV-irradiated keratinocytes (such as IL-10) can enhance antigen presentation to primarily a Th2 T-cell helper population, resulting in specific suppression of host immunity to an otherwise strongly antigenic tumor [51].

Specific T-cell Defects in Antitumor Immunity

The metastasis of a primary tumor may be enhanced by specifically impaired immune responses, such as a poor proliferative response by intra-tumoral lymphocytes or down-regulated cytolytic T lymphocyte function. In one study, tumor-infiltrating lymphocytes (TIL) had reduced CD3ξ chain levels compared to peripheral blood lymphocytes (PBL) of patients with colorectal carcinoma and this reduction correlated with increased lymph node metastasis [52]. Downstream signaling was diminished whereas the levels of p56^{lck} and p59^{fyn} protein tyrosine kinase were lower in patients than in healthy controls. Yotnda et al. [53] showed that the bone marrow of patients with acute lymphocytic leukemia contained T-cells that did not express CD40L and CD25 markers, as they would if they were from normal marrow and an increase in T-cell apoptosis was detected, suggesting an in vivo dysfunction of T-cell proliferative and cytotoxic activity. Zeta-chain defects have been described for CD4+, CD8+ and natural killer (NK) cells in a variety of patients with malignancies [54]. Low expression of this signaling pathway correlates with a significantly shorter 5-year survival for patients with advanced head and neck cancer and with decreased responsiveness of TIL cells in renal cell carcinoma. Partial loss of the lck kinase and ZAP-70 signaling molecules was detected in the PBL of melanoma patients by Maccalli et al., who concluded that soluble HLA class I molecules may contribute to this immune defect [55]. Other pathways of T-cell signaling, such as the production of IL-2 and IL-2-mediated receptor signaling, can also be altered by the presence of tumor. For example, soluble products from renal tumor explants suppressed the IL-2 and IFN-γ production of PBL and suppressed T-cell proliferation [56]. These products included gangliosides isolated from tumor cell supernatants that could also downregulate NF-κB activation and nuclear accumulation in lymphocytes. Hence, the expansion and metastasis of tumor cell populations can be altered by intrinsic and induced defects in T-cell responses. The subject of tumour-induced down-regulation of T cell receptor signaling is discussed in Chapter 12.

Natural Effector Cell Modulation of Metastasis

Natural killer and lymphocyte-activated killer cells are a group of effector cells that act non-specifically against tumor cells. The activation and expansion of these populations can be enhanced by IL-2, IL-12, and IFN-γ [57–59]. LAK cell activity can be mediated by a variety of lymphocyte subsets, including CD4+ and CD8+ cells and is generally enhanced by the presence of IL-2, whereas NK activity is not only defined by specific target cells (K562 human leukemia cells or murine YAK lymphoma cells), but by specific markers, such as the presence of a sialo-GM1 ganglioside, NK1.1 or the cell surface marker CD56 (CD57 in humans) [60].

The role of NK cells in the dissemination of murine tumors was shown by Wiltrout et al. using the Lewis lung carcinoma and B16 melanoma in syngeneic C57BL/6 mice [62]. Mice depleted of NK cells by administration of a sialo-GM1 antibody had increased lung metastasis from both cell lines following intravenous inoculation and augmentation of NK activity by maleic anhydride divinylether significantly depressed the ability of these cells to form liver and lung metastasis. Increasing the levels of Th1-type cytokines (such as

IL-2 and IL-12) simultaneously enhanced the level of NK and LAK cell activity and depressed the ability of murine carcinoma to form metastases [63]. It is well established that the ability of human tumors to grow and metastasize in severe combined immunodeficiency (SCID) and athymic (nude) mice is dependent on the site of tumor implantation and intrinsic NK activity [64,65].

Increased infiltration of NK cells in biopsy specimens from patients with gastric carcinoma correlated with fewer metastases to lymph nodes and less lymphatic invasion [66]. NK activity in patients with this type of cancer is modulated by the presence of TGF-α in their serum, suggesting that inherent non-specific immune reactivity toward tumor is dependent upon a balance of activating and down-regulating factors [67]. In colorectal adenocarcinomas matched for grade and stage, the presence of infiltrating CD57+ NK cells predicted longer disease-free survival [68] and NK cells may play a similar role in squamous cell carcinoma because PBL NK cytolytic activity was inversely associated with regional and distant metastases [69]. Lutz and Kurago [70] showed that the level of HLA class I molecules on squamous cell carcinoma cell lines correlated with cytolysis by NK-enriched PBL, suggesting that subpopulations of tumor cells may be selected for survival and ultimate metastases by this initial interaction with host immune defense.

Tumor Interactions with Host Macrophages

The tumor microenvironment is a dynamic milieu due to the local secretion of growth factors, regulatory molecules and cytokines from tumor cells, host, stromal and parenchymal cells and tumor-infiltrating cells. Macrophages are envisioned to easily traffic to local regions of inflammation and sites whose tissue architecture has been altered by progressive tumor growth. The presence of non-cytotoxic (i.e., non-activated) macrophages in neoplasms could actually enhance tumor growth [72], inasmuch as macrophages (and lymphocytes) produce many diffusible growth, angiogenic and cytotoxic factors [73]. According to the type and level of such mediators, tumor-associated macrophages (TAMs) may therefore enhance or inhibit the growth of neoplasms [11].

The population of inflammatory macrophages in growing tumors is maintained through recruitment of circulating monocytes [74] and in certain tumors, the proliferation of mononuclear phagocytes [75]. In regressing murine sarcomas, TAMs are found throughout the tumors, whereas in progressing sarcomas, they are confined to the periphery [76]. The induction time of murine tumors varies with their macrophage content; the faster growing tumors are those with fewer infiltrating macrophages. Small tumors are infiltrated by a large number of macrophages, whereas large tumors are not. On the other hand, other investigators have also concluded that the accumulation of macrophages in tumors does not necessarily correlate with the metastatic properties or immunogenicity of the tumors [74].

Macrophages can be activated by their interaction with lymphokines. Mitogen and antigen-stimulated T cells release diffusible mediators that interact with specific receptors on target cells. Lymphokines are able to render macrophages tumoricidal. These include IFN-γ, (which is able to prime macrophages for activation following the induction of a second signal such as the presence of bacteria and their products, e.g., endotoxin), IFN-α and IFN-β, which can prime macrophages in a synergistic fashion [77,78].

Activated macrophages can destroy syngeneic, allogeneic and xenogeneic tumor cells but leave normal, non-tumorigenic cells unharmed, suggesting that histocompatibility and tumor-specific antigens are not involved in this recognition [79]. In addition, differences in metastatic potential, chromosome number, resistance to chemotherapeutic agents and the antigenic properties of tumor cells, were not important factors for macrophage recognition of tumor cells (reviewed in [80]), but the cell membrane phospholipid phosphatidylserine (PS) was important for such recognition [79]. The distribution of cellular phospholipids in the bilayer membrane is extremely asymmetric; phosphatidylcholine and sphingomyelin are preferentially positioned in the outer leaflet of the lipid bilayer, whereas phosphatidylethanolamine is preferentially distributed in the inner leaflet. Normal cells contain PS only in the inner leaflet of the cell membrane. Experiments based on several lines of evidence now suggest that when PS is expressed on the outer leaflet, it serves as a recognition molecule for macrophages [80,81].

Macrophage recognition of PS correlates with their increased binding to tumor cells. The levels of PS on the outer leaflet of murine erythroleukemia cell (MELCs) and differentiated murine erythroleukemia cells (dMELCs) were measured; MELCs contained a greater density of PS on the outer leaflet than dMELCs [81]. As MELCs differentiated, they progressively lost PS from the outer leaflet of the plasma membrane and these cells were bound less by macrophages. Similar data were derived by examining the interaction of human monocytes with three human tumorigenic cell lines [82].

Collectively, these results indicate that activated macrophages recognize and destroy neoplastic cells without injuring non-tumorigenic cells [80]. The mechanism for this recognition is non-immunologic and requires cell-to-cell contact. Because activated macrophages can destroy phenotypically diverse tumor cells, (including cells resistant to killing by other host defense mechanisms), the appearance of tumoricidal macrophages in the environment of primary and metastatic tumors is one of the first events that impact the growing population of tumor cells.

Lymphoid-mediated Angiogenesis

Angiogenesis is essential to homeostasis and its regulation by lymphoid cells, such as T-lymphocytes, macrophages and mast cells is well documented [83,84]. A local inflammatory reaction characterized by T-lymphocytes and macrophages is often associated with invasive cutaneous melanoma and an intense inflammatory reaction is often associated with increased risk of metastasis, suggesting that angiogenesis induced by inflammation may contribute to tumor progression and metastasis.

Immunological events involved in physiological angiogenesis occur subsequent to wound healing [85]. Systemic chemotherapy has been shown to retard wound healing, possibly by decreased immune response; whether this is mediated by inhibition of angiogenesis is not clear. We have investigated the role of tumor vascularization and its effect on tumor growth in immunosuppressed mice. The growth of weakly immunogenic B16 melanoma was retarded in myelosuppressed mice compared with control mice [86]. Further evidence implicating myelosuppression in the retardation of tumor growth and vascularity was obtained from adriamycin-pre-treated animals injected with normal spleen cells one day before implantation of colon cancer cells into the wall of the colon. Tumor growth in these mice was comparable to control mice [87].

Macrophages produce factors that act directly to influence angiogenesis-linked endothelial cell functions. In vitro studies have shown that macrophages produce more than 20 molecules that induce endothelial cell proliferation, migration and differentiation [88]. Macrophages can also modulate angiogenesis by modifying the extracellular matrix through the direct production of matrix components or through the production of proteases. In addition, macrophages can release thrombospondin-1 [89] and angiostatin [90] which in turn suppress angiogenesis.

Recently, we examined the mechanism for generation of angiostatin, an angiogenesis inhibitor isolated from plasma of mice bearing Lewis lung carcinoma (3LL) [91]. We found that the generation of angiostatin by subcutaneous tumors required the presence of macrophages and directly correlated with their metalloelastase activity [90]. The addition of plasminogen to 3LL cells cultured in vitro did not result in generation of angiostatin, whereas the addition of plasminogen to co-cultures of macrophages and 3LL cells did. Elastase activity in macrophages was up-regulated by the cytokine GM-CSF. GM-CSF secreted by 3LL cells significantly enhanced the production of elastase by macrophages and hence the generation of angiostatin from plasminogen. These data suggest that elastase released from tumor-infiltrating macrophages is responsible for the angiostatin production in this tumor model and the angiogenesis-inhibiting role of macrophages.

Conclusions

The progressive growth of a primary tumor sets into motion regulatory events that govern tissue architecture and control of local cell proliferation. Primary neoplasms contain metastatic subpopulations of tumor cells. This heterogeneity extends to immunological properties of the tumor cells to include the alteration of major histocompatiblity antigens, loss of co-stimulatory molecules, secretion of immmunosuppressive cytokines and rapid generation of variant populations that can circumvent normal host defenses.

In turn, the host response to aberrant cell populations consists of natural surveillance mechanisms by lymphocytes that seek cells with low amounts of MHC antigen and an abundance of infiltrate cells that may produce inflammatory cytokines and consequently a non-specific control of tumor populations. Ultimately, they give rise to cytotoxic lymphocytic responses against bona fide tumor antigens. However, this response can be subverted at the level of the tumor microenvironment, which may actually supply the tumor with needed growth factors and products for angiogenesis.

The ability of unique populations of tumor cells to establish metastasis depends on the balance of homeostatic mechanisms that control the growth and spread of cells with altered growth properties, the abnormal membrane display of cellular antigens and the ability of rapidly growing tumor cells to establish autonomy from host responsiveness. The challenge of immunotherapy is to overcome these obstacles.

References

1. Fidler IJ, Poste, G. The cellular heterogeneity of malignant neoplasms: implications for adjuvant chemotherapy. Semin Oncol 1985;12:207–22.
2. Fidler IJ, Balch CM. The biology of cancer metastasis and implications for therapy. Current Prob Surg 1987;24:131–233.
3. Paget S. The distribution of secondary growths in cancer of the breast. Lancet 1889;1:571–3
4. Fidler IJ. Critical factors in the biology of human cancer metastasis: GHA Clowes Memorial Award lecture. Cancer Res 1990;50:6130–8.
5. Folkman J. How is blood vessel growth regulated in normal and neoplastic tissue? GHA Clowes Memorial Award lecture. Cancer Res 1986;46:467–73.
6. Fidler IJ, Ellis LM. The implications of angiogenesis for the biology and therapy of cancer metastasis. Cell 1994;79:185–8.
7. Liotta LA, Stetler-Stevenson WG. Tumor invasion and metastasis: an imbalance of positive and negative regulation. Cancer Res 1991;51:5054s–9s.
8. Fidler IJ, Hart IR. Biological and experimental consequences of the zonal composition of solid tumors. Cancer Res 1981;41:3266–7.
9. Poste G, Fidler IJ. The pathogenesis of cancer metastasis. Nature 1979;283:139–46.
10. Folkman J, Klagsbrun M. Angiogenic factors. Science 1987;235:44–447.
11. Prehn RT. The immune reaction as a stimulator of tumor growth. Science 1972;176:170–
12. Prehn RT. Stimulatory effects of immune reactions upon the growth of untransplanted tumors. Cancer Res 1994;54:908–14.
13. Prehn RT. An immunostimulation theory of tumor development. Transplant Rev 1971;7:26–54.
14. Schreiber H. Tumor Immunology. In: Paul W editor. Fundamental Immunology, 2nd edn. New York: Raven Press, 1989; 923–55.
15. Tanaka K, Yoshioka T, Bieberich C et al. Role of the major histocompatibility complex class I antigens in tumor growth and metastasis. Ann Rev Immunol 1988;6:359–80.
16. Gelber C, Plaksin D, Vadai E et al. Abolishment of metastasis formation by murine tumor cells transfected with "foreign" H-2K genes. Cancer Res 1989;49:2366–73.
17. De Giovanni C, Palmeri G, Nicoletti G et al. Immunological and non-immunological influence of H-2K^b gene transfection on the metastatic ability of B16 melanoma cells. Int J Cancer 1991;48:270–6.
18. Ramani P, Balkwill FR. Enhanced metastasis of a mouse carcinoma after in vitro treatment with murine interferon-gamma. Int J Cancer 1987;40:830–4.
19. Geldhof AB, VandenDriessche T, Opdenakker G et al. Introduction of the interferon gamma gene into mouse T lymphoma cells with low MHC class I expression results in selective induction of H-2Dk and concomitant enhanced metastasis. Cancer Immunol Immunother 1996;42:329–38.
20. Bernards R. Suppression of MHC expression in cancer cells. Trends Genet 1987;3:298–301.
21. Nicolson GL. Metastatic tumor cell interactions with endothelium, basement membrane, and tissue. Curr Opin Cell Biol 1989;1:1009–19.
22. Gasic GJ. Role of plasma, platelets and endothelial cells in tumor metastasis. Cancer Metastasis Rev 1984;3:99–127.
23. Weiss L. Cell adhesion molecules: a critical examination of their role in metastasis. Invasion Metastasis 1994–1995;14:192–7.
24. Schreiber H. Tumor immunology. In: Paul W editor. Fundamental Immunology. New York: Raven Press, 1991; 1143–78.
25. Passlick B, Pantel K, Dubuschok B et al. Expression of MHC molecules and ICAM-1 on non-small cell lung carcinomas: association with early lymphatic spread of tumor cells. Eur J Cancer 1996;32:141–5.
26. Geldhof AB, Raes G, Bakkus M et al. Expression of B7-1 by highly metastatic mouse T lymphoma induces optimal natural killer cell-mediated cytotoxicity. Cancer Res 1995;55:2730–3.
27. Ostrand-Rosenberg S, Baskar S, Patterson N et al. Expression of MHC class II and B7-1 and B7-2 costimulatory molecules accompanies tumor rejection and reduces the metastatic potential of tumor cells. Tissue Antigens 1996;47:414–21.
28. Lesley J, Hyman R, English N et al. CD44 in inflammation and metastasis. Glycoconj J 1997;14:611–22.
29. Ilangumaran S, Borisch B, Hoessli DC. Signal transduction via CD44: role of plasma membrane microdomains. Leuk Lymphoma 1999;35:455–69.
30. Sheen-Chen SM, Chen WJ, Eng HL et al. Evaluation of the prognostic value of serum soluble CD44 in patients with breast cancer. Cancer Invest 1999;17:581–5.

31. Dietrich A, Tanczos E, Vanscheidt W et al. High CD44 surface expression on primary tumours of malignant melanoma correlates with increased metastatic risk and reduced survival. Eur J Cancer 1997;33:926–30.

32. Lickliter JD, Kratzke RA, Nguyen PL et al. Fas ligand is highly expressed in acute leukemia and during the transformation of chronic myeloid leukemia to blast crisis. Exp Hematol 1999;27:1519–27.

33. Owen-Schaub LB, van Golen KL, Hill LL et al. Fas and Fas ligand interactions suppress melanoma lung metastasis. J Exp Med 1998;188:1717–23.

34. Terheyden P, Siedel C, Merkel A et al. Predominant expression of Fas (CD95) ligand in metastatic melanoma revealed by longitudinal analysis. J Invest Dermatol 1999;112:899–902.

35. Shibakita M, Tachibana M, Dhar DK et al. Prognostic significance of Fas and Fas ligand expressions in human esophageal cancer. Clin Cancer Res 1999;5:2464–9.

36. Younes M, Schwartz MR, Ertan A et al. Fas ligand expression in esophageal carcinomas and their lymph node metastases. Cancer 2000;88:524–8.

37. Ueno T, Toi M, Tominaga T. Circulating soluble Fas concentration in breast cancer patients. Clin Cancer Res 1999;5:3529–33.

38. Urban JL, Kripke ML, Schreiber H. Step-wise immunological selection of antigenic variants during tumor growth. J Immunol 1986;137:3036–41.

39. Wettstein PJ, Bailey DW. Immunodominance of the immune response to "multiple" histocompatibility antigens. Immunogent 1982;16:47–58.

40. Boyse EA, Old LJ, Luell S. Antigenic properties of experimental leukemia. II. Immunological studies in vivo with C57Bl/6 radiation-induced leukemias. J Natl Cancer Inst 1963;31:987–95.

41 Orr FW, Wang HH, et al. Interactions between cancer cells and the endothelium in metastasis. J Pathol 2000;190:310–29.

42. Fidler IJ. Lymphocytes are not only immunocytes. Biomed 1980;32:103.

43. Seung LP, Seung SK, Schreiber H. Antigenic cancer cells that escape immune destruction are stimulated by host cells. Cancer Res 1995;55:5094–500.

44. Fidler IJ, Gersten DM, Kripke ML. Influence of immune status on the metastasis of three murine fibrosarcomas of different immunogenicities. Cancer Res 1979;39:3816–21.

45. Castelli C, Rivoltini L, Andreola G et al. T-cell recognition of melanoma-associated antigens. J Cell Physiol 2000;182:323–31.

46. Osanto S. Vaccine trials for the clinician: prospects for tumor antigens. Oncologist 1997;2:284–99.

47. Neumann E, Englesberg A, Decker J et al. Heterogeneous expression of the tumor-associated antigens RAGE-1, PRAME, and glycoprotein 75 in human renal cell carcinoma: candidates for T-cell-based immunotherapies? Cancer Res 1998;58:4090–5.

48. Elgert KD, Alleva DG, Mullins DW. Tumor-induced immune dysfunction: the macrophage connection. J Leukoc Biol 1998;64:275–90.

49. Young MR, Wright, MA, Lozano Y et al. Increased recurrence and metastasis in patients whose primary head and neck squamous cell carcinomas secreted granulocyte-macrophage colony-stimulating factor and contained CD34+ natural suppressor cells. Int J Cancer 1997;74:69–74.

50. Koyama S, Fukao K. Phenotypic analysis of nylon-wool-adherent suppressor cells that inhibit the effector process of tumour cell lysis by lymphokine-activated killer cells in patients with advanced gastric carcinoma. J Cancer Res Clin Oncol 1994;120:240–7.

51. Ullrich SE. Does exposure to UV radiation induce a shift to a Th-2-like immune reaction? Photochem Photobiol 1996;64:254–8.

52. Choi SH, Chung EJ, Whang DY et al. Alteration of signal-transducing molecules in tumor-infiltrating lymphocytes and peripheral blood T lymphocytes from human colorectal carcinoma patients. Cancer Immunol Immunother 1998;45:299–305.

53. Yotnda P, Mintz P, Grigoriadou K et al. Analysis of T-cell defects in the specific immune response against acute lymphoblastic leukemia cells. Exp Hemotol 1999;27:1375–83.

54. Whiteside TL. Signaling defects in T lymphocytes of patients with malignancy. Cancer Immunol Immunother 1999;48:346–52.

55. Maccalli C, Pisarra P, Vegetti C et al. Differential loss of T cell signaling molecules in metastatic melanoma patients' T lymphocyte subsets expressing distinct TCR variable regions. J Immunol 1999;163:6912–23.

56. Rayman P, Uzzo RG, Kolenko V et al. Tumor-induced dysfunction in interleukin-2 production and interleukin-2 receptor signaling: a mechanism of immune escape. Cancer J Sci Am 2000;6:S81–7.

57. Ortaldo JR, Mason A, Overton R. Lymphokine-activated killer cells. Analysis of progenitors and effectors. J Exp Med 1986;164:1193–1205.

58. Ortaldo JR. Human cytotoxic effector cells: definition and analysis of activity. Allergol Immunonopathol 1991;19:145–156.

59. Inverardi L, Witson JC, Fuad SA et al. CD3 negative "small agranular lymphocytes" are natural killer cells. J Immunol 1991;146:4048–52.
60. Mason LH, Mathieson BJ, Ortaldo JR. Natural killer (NK) cell subsets in the mouse. NK-1.1+/LGL-1+ cells restricted to lysing NK targets, whereas NK-1.1+/LGL-1- cells generate lymphokine-activated killer cells. J Immunol 1990;145:751–9.
61. Ortaldo JR, Winkler-Pickett R, Mason AT et al. The Ly-49 family: regulation of cytotoxicity and cytokine production in murine CD3$^+$ cells. J Immunol 1998;160:1158–65.
62. Wiltrout RH, Herberman RB, Zhang SR et al. Role of organ-associated NK cells in decreased formation of experimental metastases in lung and liver. J Immunol 1985;134:4267–75.
63. Takeda K, Seki S, Ogasawara K et al. Liver NK1.1+ CD4+ alpha beta T cells activated by IL-12 as a major effector in inhibition of experimental tumor metastasis. J Immunol 1996;56:3366–73.
64. Hanna N. Expression of metastatic potential of tumor cells in young nude mice is correlated with low levels of natural killer cell-mediated cytotoxicity. Int J Cancer 1980;26:675–80.
65. Yano S, Nishioka Y, Izumi K et al. Novel metastasis model of human lung cancer in SCID mice depleted of NK cells. Int J Cancer 1996;67:211–7.
66. Ishigami S, Natsugoe S, Tokuda K et al. Prognostic value of intratumoral natural killer cells in gastric carcinoma. Cancer 2000;88:577–83.
67. Yoon SJ, Heo DS, Kang SH et al. Natural killer cell activity depression in peripheral blood and ascites from gastric cancer patients with high TGF-beta 1 expression. Anticancer Res 1998;18:1591–6.
68. Coca S, Perez-Piqueras J, Martinez D et al. The prognostic significance of intratumor natural killer cells in patients with colorectal carcinoma. Cancer 1997;79:2320–8.
69. Schantz SP, Ordonez NG. Quantitation of natural killer cell function and risk of metastatic poorly differentiated head and neck cancer. Nat Immunol Cell Growth Reg 1991;10:278–88.
70. Lutz CT, Kurago ZB. Human leukocyte antigen class I expression on squamous cell carcinoma cells regulates natural killer cell activity. Cancer Res 1999;59:5793–9.
71. Mantovani A, Bottazzi B, Colatta F et al. The origin and function of tumor-associated macrophages. Immunol Today 1992;13:265–70.
72. Nathan CF Secretory products of macrophages. J Clin Invest 1987;79:319–26.
73. Evans R. Macrophages and neoplasms: new insights and their implications in tumor immunobiology. Cancer Metastasis Rev 1982;1:227–43.
74. Mantovani A . Tumor-associated macrophages. Curr Opin Immunol 1992; 2:689–94.
75. Russell SW, Gillespie GY. Nature, function, and destruction of inflammatory cells in regressing and progressing Moloney sarcomas. J Reticuloendothelial Soc 1997;22:159–68.
76. Saiki I, Dunegan MA, Fann AV et al. Regulatory effects on macrophages of human recombinant interferon-α. J Interfer Res 1986;6:603–11.
77. Pace JL. Synergistic interactions between IFN-α and IFN-β in priming murine macrophages for tumor cell killing. J Leukoc Biol 1986;44:514–20.
78. Fidler IJ, Schroit AJ. Recognition and destruction of neoplastic cells by activated macrophages: discrimination of altered self. Biochim Biophys Acta 1988;948:151–73.
79. Fidler IJ. Targeting of immunomodulators to mononuclear phagocytes for therapy of cancer. Adv Drug Del Rev 1988;1:69–106.
80. Ratner S, Schroit AJ, Vinson SB et al. Analogous recognition of phospholipids by insect phagocytes and mammalian macrophages. Proc Soc Exp Biol Med 1986;182:272–6.
81. Pak CC, Fidler IJ. Activated macrophages distinguish undifferentiated-tumorigenic from differentiated-nontumorigenic murine erythroleukemia cells. Differentiation 1989;41:49–55.
82. Utsugi T, Schroit AJ, Connor J et al. Elevated expression of phosphatidylserine in the outer membrane leaflet of human tumor cells and recognition by activated human blood monocytes. Cancer Res 51:3062–6.
83. Polverini PJ, Leibovich JS. Induction of neovascularization in vivo and endothelial proliferation in vitro by tumor-associated macrophages. Lab Invest 1984;51:635–42.
84. Leek RD, Harris AL, Lewis CE. Cytokine networks in solid human tumors: regulation of angiogenesis. J Leukoc Biol 1994;56:423–35.
85. Sunderkötter C, Steinbrink K, Goebeler M et al. Macrophages and angiogenesis. J Leukoc Biol 1994;55:410–22.
86. Gutman M, Singh RK, Yoon S et al. Leukocyte-induced angiogenesis and subcutaneous growth of B16 melanoma. Cancer Biother 1994;9:163–70.
87. Yoneda J, Killion JJ, Bucana CD et al. Angiogenesis and growth of murine colon carcinoma are dependent on infiltrating leukocytes. Cancer Biother Radiopharm 1999;14:221–30.
88. Polverini PJ. How the extracellular matrix and macrophages contribute to angiogenesis-dependent diseases. Eur J Cancer 1996;32A:2430–7.

89. Lingen MW, Polverini PJ, Bouck N. Inhibition of squamous cell carcinoma angiogenesis by direct interaction of retinoic acid with endothelial cells. Lab Invest 1996;74:476–83.
90. Dong Z, Kumar R, Yang X, Fidler IJ. Macrophage-derived metalloelastase is responsible for the generation of angiostatin in Lewis lung carcinoma. Cell 1997;88:801–10.
91. O'Reilly MS, Holmgren L, Shing Y et al. Angiostatin: a novel angiogenesis inhibitor that mediates the suppression of metastases by a Lewis lung carcinoma. Cell 1994;79:315–28.

11. The Radioimmunoscintigraphy and Radioimmunotherapy of Human Cancer: Current Concepts and Future Developments

Thomas M. Behr and Martin Béhé

Introduction

More than half a century ago, radioactive iodine was introduced as one of the first radiopharmaceuticals in the history of medicine. It was used (and still is), to stage and treat patients with differentiated thyroid cancer. Presently, besides surgery, radioiodine therapy has become the standard mode of therapy for differentiated thyroid cancer and has led to a dramatic improvement in the five- and ten-year survival rates in this disease (Figure 11.1) [1]. The underlying principle in thyroid cancer is that the gland retains the iodine-accumulating features of benign thyroid tissue, (due to the maintained expression of the sodium iodine symporter molecule in the cell membrane). Unfortunately, no other human cancer type has shown relevant sodium iodine symporter expression which could be used for radioiodine diagnosis or therapy. Therefore, over the past decades, much effort has been spent on developing and exploiting other mechanisms designed to assist in the accumulation of intra-tumoral radionuclides for diagnostic and therapeutic purposes.

In this context, the introduction of radiolabeled antibodies as specific tools to systemically target malignant tumors for clinical diagnosis and therapy dates back almost 25 years [2]. In these early beginnings, rather enthusiastic hopes were associated with such a molecular recognition approach. Over time, however, some doubts arose that monoclonal antibodies may really fulfill the hopes of the predicted "magic bullet" (*zauberkugel*) of Paul Ehrlich [3]. Although many of the problems associated with their clinical use have been solved [4] and in some cancers, most notably hematologic neoplasms, they have become the third standard mode of (systemic) treatment alongside chemotherapy and external beam radiation therapy, their large molecular weight and size impairs bioavailability. The rapid pharmacokinetics which would be desirable for obtaining both high and homogenous uptake in the target (tumor) with simultaneous rapid clearance from non-target ("background") tissues are sometimes difficult to achieve. A comparably slow targeting of the tumor and slow clearance from the blood and normal tissues results in only

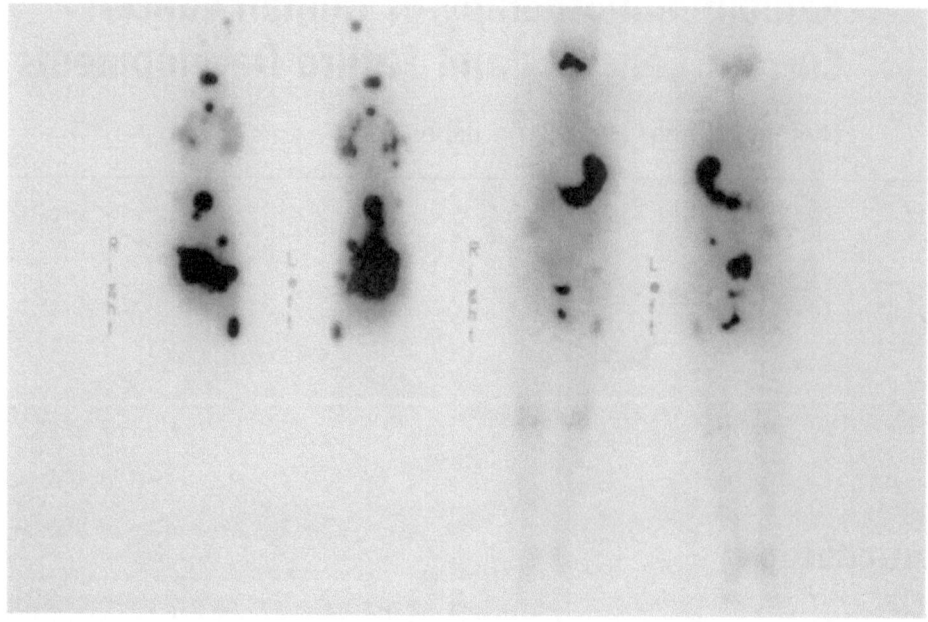

Figure 11.1. Staging and therapy of differentiated thyroid cancer by sodium (radio-)^{131}iodide as proto-type for all nuclear medical approaches for tumor imaging and therapy: the left whole-body scans show widespread metastatic disease (to lymph nodes, the lungs, liver and bone) on the occasion of the first therapy cycle. The scans on the right show a good partial remission after several therapy cycles.

moderate radio-localization indices in diagnostic application and effectively low tumor/non-tumor radiation dose ratios when used therapeutically [4].

An early approach to overcome these problems was to create smaller molecular recognition units with similar sensitivity and specificity [5]. Accordingly, antibody fragments (Fab′, F(ab′)$_2$, scFv etc.) have been derived and developed, often providing advantages over the complete IgG molecule, with recent evidence showing that the smaller the molecular weight of the antibody fragment, the higher the radio-localization indices and the better the therapeutic windows achieved [4,5]. Nevertheless, these antibody-derived fragments still have molecular weights of several thousand Daltons. Furthermore, the immunogenicity of these xenogeneic proteins (mostly of murine origin), frequently results in specific anti-rodent immune responses (e.g., human anti-mouse antibodies (HAMA) formation), which has been a big problem preventing antibody re-administration. The chimerization or even humanization by means of genetic engineering and improvements in radiochemistry have led, in the meantime, to improvements in the diagnostic and therapeutic results of these engineered antibodies.

The recent development of radiolabeled regulatory peptides has also opened up new horizons in diagnostic and therapeutic nuclear oncology [6]. Regulatory peptides are small, readily diffusable and potent natural substances with a wide spectrum of receptor-mediated actions in humans. High affinity receptors for these peptides are (over-) expressed in many neoplastic tissues and these receptors may therefore represent promising new molecular targets for cancer diagnosis and therapy. Finally, therapy itself using radiopharmaceuticals rather than the diagnostic approach alone has gained increasing momentum in the nuclear medicine and oncological community [4]. The purpose of this review is to give a short overview of these recent developments.

Diagnostic Application of Monoclonal Antibodies and Peptides in Human Solid and Hematologic Tumors

Monoclonal Antibodies Directed Against Tumor-associated Antigens for the Diagnosis and Staging of Solid Tumors

Various tumor-associated and tumor-specific antigens have served as target molecules for radioimmunodetection, including carcinoembryonic antigen (CEA), TAG72-4, prostate-specific antigen (PSA). Historically, CEA was one of the first target molecules identified (Figure 11.2) [2].

In a recent study, we assessed the clinical relevance of immunoscintigraphy with ^{99m}Tc-labeled anti-CEA antigen-binding antibody fragments in the follow-up of patients with colorectal carcinoma [5]. We especially aimed at investigating the role of immunoscintigraphy in the assessment of surgical resectability with a combination of conventional imaging methods, such as ultrasound, computed tomography and magnetic resonance imaging which are used in the routine follow-up of patients with colorectal carcinoma. This study was undertaken to evaluate immunoscintigraphy with ^{99m}Tc-labeled anti-CEA antigen-binding Fab' fragment alone or combined with conventional imaging methods. Twenty-two patients, operated on for colorectal carcinoma and suspected of having a recurrence, underwent scintigraphy with the ^{99m}Tc-labelled anti-CEA-Fab' and whole-body single-photon emission computed tomography (SPECT). All results were compared with those using computed tomography and in 19 of the patients, with histological findings at re-resection or biopsy. The potential influence of the scintigraphic results on surgical management was analyzed retrospectively with respect to the pre-operative estimate of tumor resectability. In this study, the lesion-based sensitivity of immunoscintigraphy was 94 percent and the diagnostic accuracy was 92 percent, both being unrelated to the CEA-serum level (i.e., the detectability of lesions requires CEA expression by the tumor cells, but does not depend on serum CEA levels). When CT and immunoscintigraphy were concordant regarding resectability, this estimate was correct in all instances. But in cases of discordance, the results of immunoscintigraphy were verified operatively in 88 percent of cases. In no patient was there measurable immune reaction with the formation of HAMA against the Fab' fragments, in contrast to other complete murine antibodies. These results indicate that immunoscintigraphy together with SPECT can achieve reliable and sensitive localization of recurrent tumor lesions. The combination of immunoscitigraphy with conventional imaging techniques may also theoretically improve the non-invasive estimation of surgical resectability.

Although a clear diagnostic benefit could be demonstrated in this and a number of other studies, by far the higher diagnostic sensitivity as well as the better target-to-non-target ratios of ^{18}FDG positron emission tomography [7] has led to the almost complete replacement of diagnostic immunoscintigraphy with, (where available), PET scanning (vide infra).

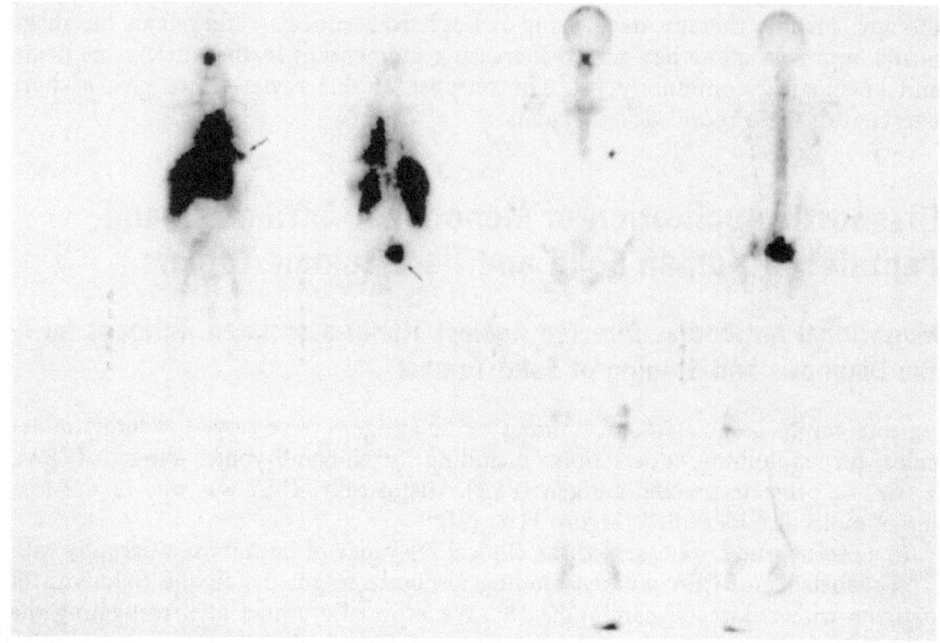

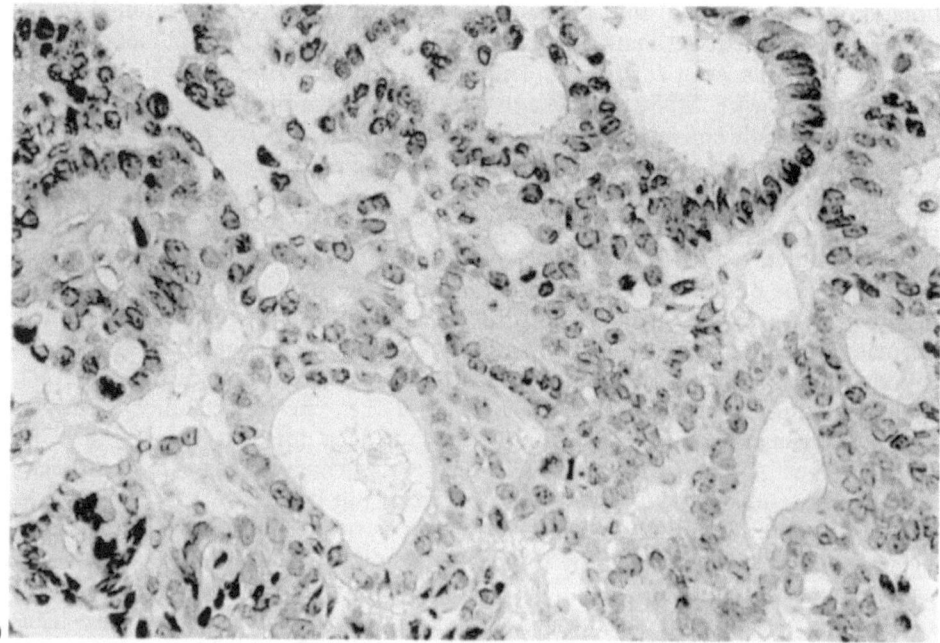

Figure 11.2. Anti-CEA immunoscintigraphy of metastatic colorectal cancer: (a)the whole-body scan at 24 h after the administration of ^{99m}Tc-labeled BW431/26 (murine anti-CEA IgG$_1$) shows intense uptake in a local recurrence as well as a distant bone metastasis in a rib (left panel, arrows), confirmed by a subsequently performed bone scan (right panel). (b) Biopsy and histology confirms both lesions as a rectal adenocarcinoma metastatic to the bone.

Monoclonal Antibodies Directed Against Tumor-associated Antigens for Diagnosing and Staging Hematological Neoplasms

In contrast to its emerging role in the therapy of hematologic neoplasms, radio-immunoscintigraphy has only played a marginal role in their detection and staging. This may partly be due to the fact that these malignancies do not express tumor-specific surface antigens, but only those present on normal blood-borne and progenitor cells. This would necessitate large amounts of protein to overcome the antigenic sink caused by these normal cells within the bone marrow, spleen and circulating blood. Since CD22 is quantitatively less expressed than other (e.g., CD20) surface antigens of B cells, it is the only target that has been successfully used for diagnostic purposes to date [8,9].

In a recent study, the value of ^{67}Ga citrate scanning as a transferrin receptor agent was compared with a ^{99m}Tc-labeled anti-CD22 Fab' fragment (LL2) in patients with low- and high-grade B-cell non-Hodgkin's lymphoma (NHL) (Figure 11.3) [9]. Thirteen patients with histologically confirmed NHL were examined prospectively with both radiopharmaceuticals within one week. The results of immunoscintigraphy were compared with those of ^{67}Ga citrate scanning and the clinical and radiological workup (computed tomography, ultrasound, and magnetic resonance imaging) of the patients. The overall sensitivity of ^{67}Ga citrate and ^{99m}Tc-labeled LL2 fragment was 80 percent respectively in a total of 43 lesions. Low-grade lymphoma patients had a higher sensitivity for LL2 imaging (82% versus 71%), whereas in high-grade lymphoma patients, ^{67}Ga citrate scanning was more sensitive than the LL2 Fab' (100% versus 75%).

Again, however, by far the higher diagnostic sensitivity as well as the better target-to-non-target ratios of ^{18}FDG positron emission tomography has led to the almost complete replacement of diagnostic immunoscintigraphy using ^{67}Ga citrate with PET and more recently with ^{18}FDG-PET (Figure 11.4) [10,11]. FDG acts as a glucose analog and, thus allows for imaging of the greatly enhanced glucose metabolism within malignant tumor cells, which mostly rely on anaerobic glycolysis instead of aerobic glucose oxidation as already recognized by the biochemist and Nobel laureate Warburg more than 70 years ago [12].

Bone Marrow Scintigraphy for the Staging of Malignant Conditions

In several studies, immunoscintigraphy of hematopoietic bone marrow was compared with conventional bone scanning in patients with malignant disease [13]. Since so-called bone metastases uniformly start their existence as bone marrow lesions only affecting the bone structure later during their development, it may be assumed that the detection of focal bone marrow lesions may be more sensitive than bone scintigraphy for the staging of bone-seeking neoplastic diseases.

In one of the early studies, out of 141 patients, 40 had breast cancer (Figure 11.5), 25 prostatic carcinoma, 14 kidney or bladder cancer, 13 bronchial carcinoma, 39 malignant lymphoma and 10 multiple myeloma [13]. A total of 18,800 skeletal regions were evaluated. Marrow scans showed more metastatic lesions than bone scanning in all patient subgroups [13]. Computed tomography was concordant with bone marrow scintigraphy in 83.3 percent of 323 skeletal sites. Bone marrow scans in 30 control patients with fever of unknown origin were abnormal only in 3 patients and in only 7 out of 2,135 skeletal regions examined.

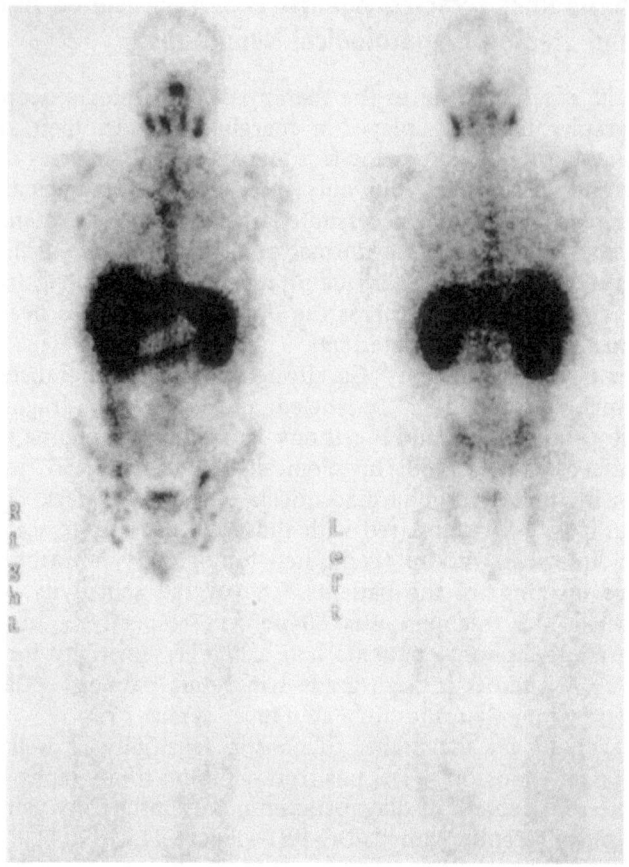

Figure 11.3. Immunoscintigraphy of non-Hodgkin's lymphoma with ^{99m}Tc-labeled Fab' fragments of the anti-CD22 antibody LL2: the whole-body scan in a patient with malignant macroglobulinemia (Waldenström's disease) shows, at 24 h p.i., uptake in multiple involved lymph node regions (parailiac, periaortic, mediastinal, axillary, submindibular and in both tonsils) as well as uptake in the involved and expanded bone marrow.

In patients with malignant lymphoma, bone marrow histology or aspiration cytology was concordantly positive in 14 and concordantly negative in 17 patients. Thus, immunoscintigraphy of hematopoietic bone marrow provides a reliable, sensitive and safe approach for non-invasive detection of metastatic spread to the skeleton.

Prognostic Information Obtained by Monoclonal Antibody Scanning

Despite some advantages of ^{18}FDG-PET, immunoscintigraphy may still add some prognostic information not obtainable from other diagnostic procedures, as we have shown, e.g., in the case of medullary thyroid cancer (MTC) [14,15]. We recently compared the sensitivity and diagnostic accuracy of immunoscintigraphy with anti-CEA antibodies and receptor-targeted imaging by using somatostatin

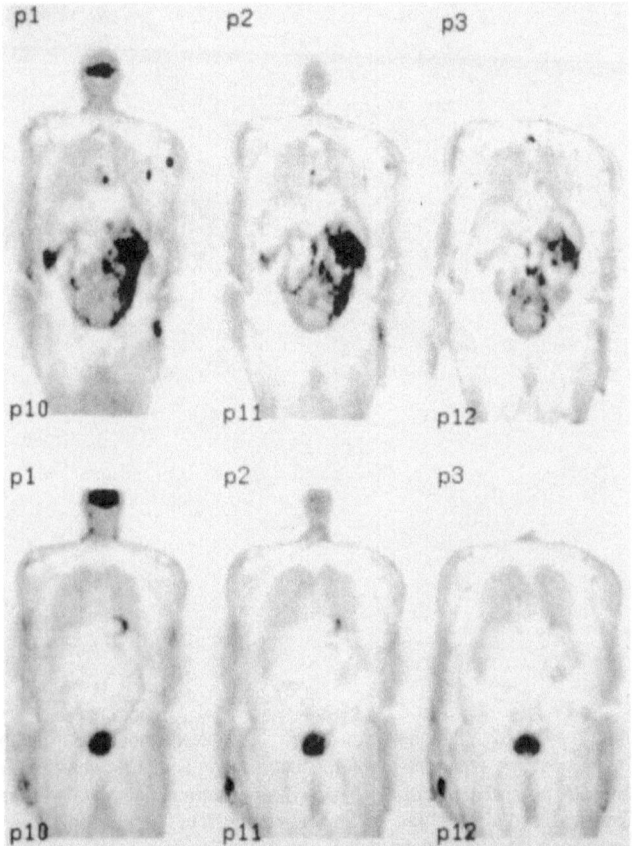

Figure 11.4. ^{18}F-FDG-PET in a patient with non-Hodgkin's lymphoma with mediastinal and axillary lymph node as well as abdominal wall involvement before (upper panel) and after high-dose chemotherapy (lower panel), the latter indicating a complete remission. Normal uptake, due to high physiological glucose metabolism is essentially confined to the brain, myocardium and the urinary bladder (the latter functioning as an excretory organ for the radiopharmaceutical).

analogs for the detection of recurrent or metastatic MTC [14,15]. Additionally, we tried to assess whether there may be correlations between the scintigraphic behavior in both imaging modalities and the patients' prognosis. A total of 26 patients with MTC were examined (Figure 11.6). Ten suffered from known disease, 14 from occult metastatic MTC and two patients were free of disease at the time of presentation (as indicated by normal serum calcitonin levels after pentagastrin stimulation).

In patients with known disease, the overall lesion-based sensitivity was 86 percent for anti-CEA immunoscintigraphy. In contrast, octreotide was unable to target any tumor in patients with rapidly-progressing disease, as well as to detect distant metastases (resulting in an overall sensitivity of only 47%). However, in in all patients with occult MTC, anti-CEA antibodies as well as the somatostatin analog ^{111}In-DTPA-octreotide were able to localize at least one

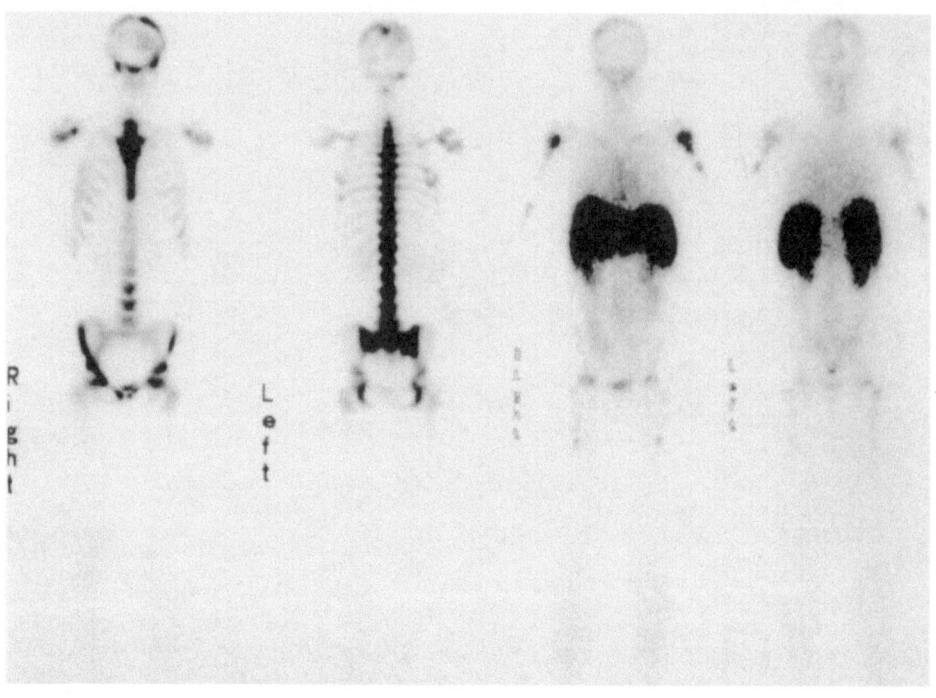

Figure 11.5. Bone marrow scintigraphy with the ^{99m}Tc-labeled monoclonal antibody BW250/183 (murine anti-NCA95 IgG$_1$) shows replacement of the bone marrow in the whole central regions (right panel) of a woman with advanced metastatic breast cancer, corresponding to a "super scan" in bone scintigraphy (left panel). Blood-forming red marrow is confined to the humerus and femurs, whereas there is almost no such hematopoietic activity left in the ribs, spine or pelvis.

lesion (patient-based sensitivity virtually 100%) (Figure 11.6). In patients with post-surgically persisiting hyper-calcitoninemia, cervical lymph node metastases were identified as the most frequent site of disease, whereas in patients with occult and slowly progressing disease several years after primary surgery, immunoscintigraphy and octreotide showed bilateral involvement of mediastinal lymph nodes (the so-called "chimney sign") (Figure 11.7) [14–16]. Tumor/non-tumor ratios were usually higher with octreotide in these latter cases. With anti-CEA antibodies, the highest tumor/non-tumor ratios were observed in clinically aggressive, rapidly progressing disease. We have concluded from this data that for the detection of occult MTC, anti-CEA immunoscintigraphy and octreotide seems to have a sensitivity which is superior to conventional diagnostic modalities, especially when used in combination. However, better detection rates are achieved with anti-CEA antibodies (probably corresponding to a higher tissue CEA expression), in more aggressive forms of MTC, whereas somatostatin receptor expression with normal CEA plasma levels and weaker antibody targeting is associated with a more benign clinical course. These data are in good accordance with the study of Busnardo et al. [17], who showed that rising CEA and at the same time constant or decreasing calcitonin serum levels were associated with a poor prognosis. These data also confirm that of Mendelsohn et al. [18] who analyzed the

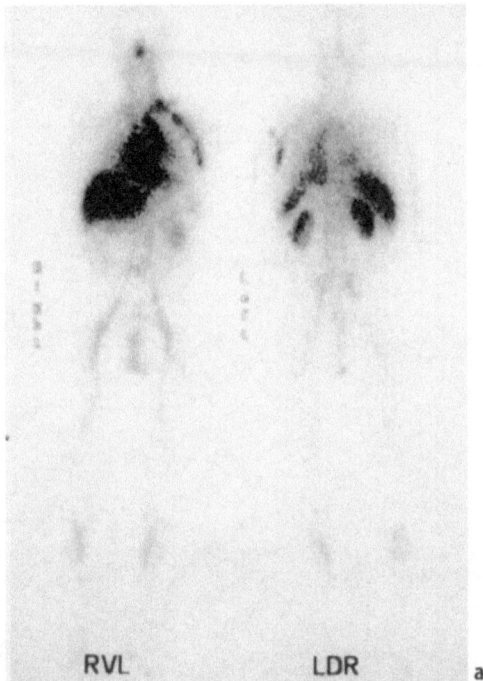

RVL   LDR   a

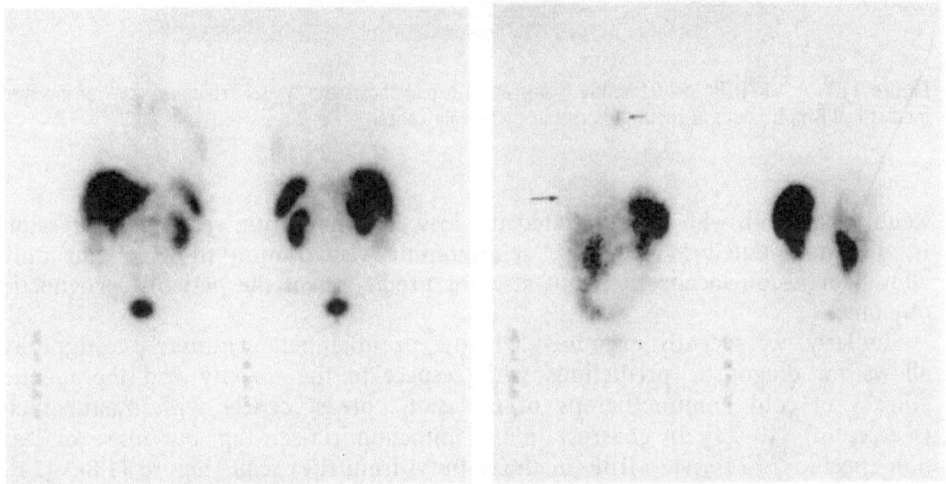

b   c

Figure 11.6. Whole-body scans of a patient with medullary thyroid cancer metastatic to cervical, axillary, mediastinal lymph nodes, the liver and the bone marrow: (a) Immunoscintigraphy with ^{99m}Tc-labeled BW431/26 (murine anti-CEA IgG$_1$). (b) as compared with somatostatin receptor scintigraphy with ^{111}In-DTPA-pentetreotide (scans at 24 h p.i. each).

relationship between tissue CEA and calcitonin expression and immunohistochemical tumor aggression, where there was a clear increase of CEA and decrease of calcitonin expression with progressive de-differentiation. Finally, our scintigraphic in vivo findings confirm the in vitro receptor autoradiographic data of

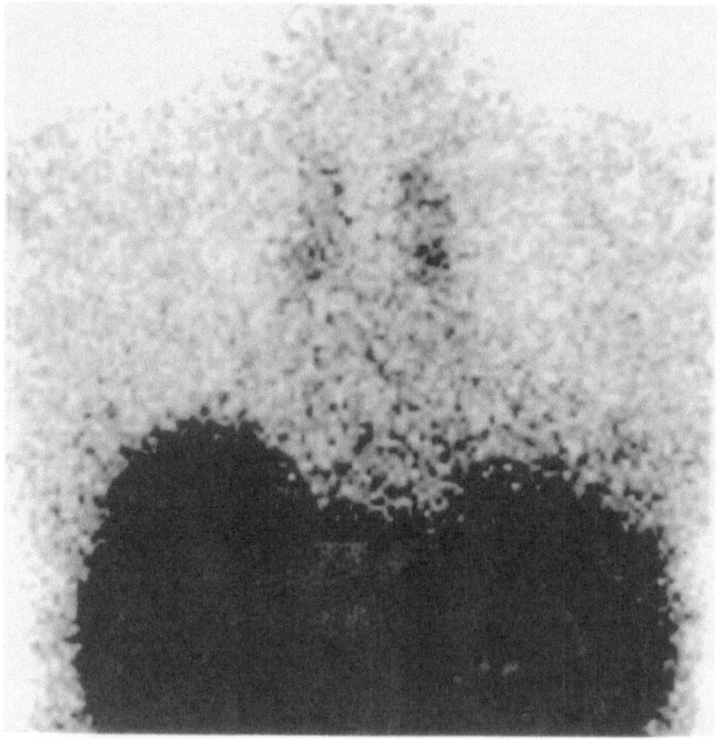

Figure 11.7. ^{111}In-DTPA-pentetreotide (scans at 24 h p.i.) shows the typical "chimney sign" of involved mediastinal lymph nodes in metastatic medullary thyroid cancer.

Reubi et al. [19], who demonstrated the loss of somatostatin receptor expression in de-differentiated MTC. Thus, scintigraphic visualization of MTC not only allows for lesion localization, but also for prediction of the patient's prognostic outcome.

Similarly, we recently examined whether pre-therapeutic immunoscintigraphy allows for diagnostic predictions with respect to the toxicity and therapeutic efficacy of cold immunotherapy of metastatic breast cancer with trastuzumab (Herceptin) [20–23]. In contrast to the mitochondria-seeking, but more or less non-specific ^{99m}Tc-sesta-MIBI (methoxy-butyl-isonitrile) scan (Figure 11.8a) [24], trastuzumab (Herceptin, Genentech, San Francisco, CA) is a monoclonal antibody (human IgG$_1$), directed against the c-erbB-2 proto-oncogene product [20–22]. It has been approved for immunotherapy of HER2/neu receptor-expressing breast cancer and is discussed in Chapter 17. Objective response rates of between 17–53% have been observed [20–22]. Slamon et al. [21] have demonstrated that the addition of trastuzumab to anthracycline/cyclophosphamide or paclitaxel chemotherapy regimens in women with metastatic breast cancer over-expressing the HER2/neu receptor is associated with significantly higher response rates, longer times to disease progression, longer durations of response and longer survival rates than is achieved with the respective chemotherapeutic regimen alone [21]. A pathophysiologically poorly understood cardiotoxicity is the major, potentially

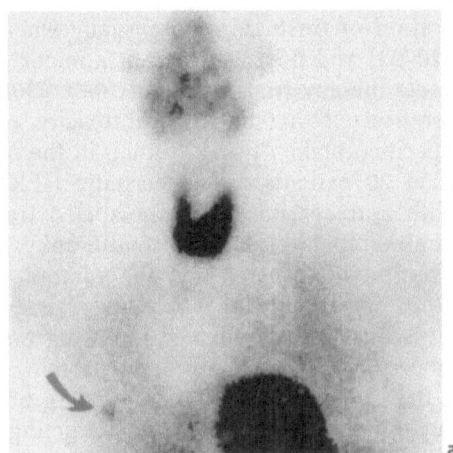

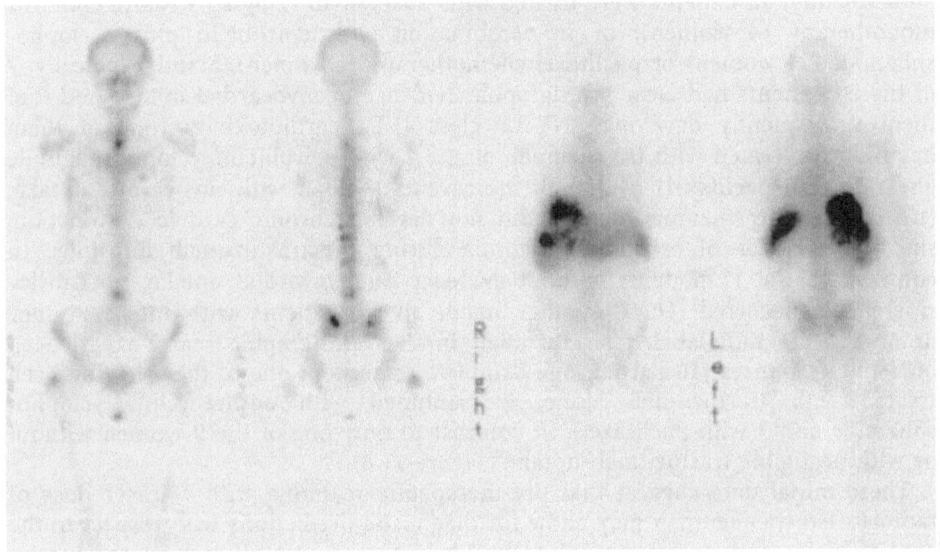

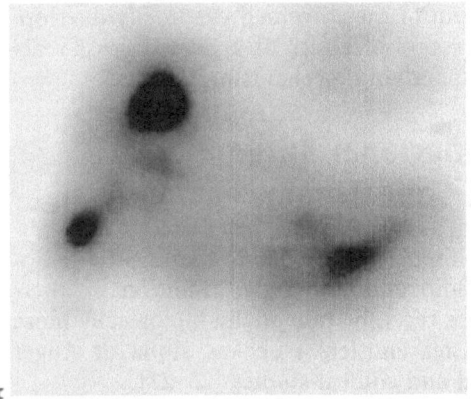

Figure 11.8. Non-specific versus antigen-specific targeting of breast cancer (a) Uptake of ^{99m}Tc-sestamibi in a primary tumor in the right breast. MIBI is a mitochondria-seeking agent that is taken up in especially mito-chondria-rich tissues, such as breast cancer. (b)Targeting of multiple HER2/neu over-expressing liver and bone (marrow) lesions with ^{111}In-trastuzumab (right panel; cf. left: bone scan in the same patient). Also note the myocardial uptake in this particular patient (c).

dose-limiting complication of trastuzumab especially when used in combination with anthracyclines [20–23] and this may present a major challenge to the design of adjuvant breast cancer therapy trials using this monoclonal antibody.

Since we have hypothesized that both cardiotoxicity and anti-tumor efficacy may be related to a specific uptake of trastuzumab in the myocardium and tumor respectively, we studied 20 patients with metastatic HER2/neu receptor-expressing breast cancer with a tracer dose of radiolabeled trastuzumab in order to determine whether pre-therapeutic external scintigraphy may allow for cardiotoxicity prediction. Immunohistochemically, the tumors of all patients stained 2+–3+ for the HER2/neu receptor [23]. Whole-body and single-photon emission computed tomography scans were performed following the injection of 5–7 mCi ^{111}In-DTPA-trastuzumab (5mg of total antibody protein). This tracer dose was co-administered with the initial loading dose of 4mg/kg body weight, since dose-finding studies had suggested that optimal tumor targeting was seen at this level, whereas lower amounts led to a rapid hepatic clearance of the immunoconjugate. Subsequently, all patients were treated with trastuzmab (2mg/kg weekly) either as monotherapy (4 women), or in combination with epirubicin plus cyclophosphamide (11 women) or paclitaxel chemotherapy (5 women). Scintigraphically, 7 of the 20 patients had clear scintigraphic evidence of myocardial uptake and 6 of them subsequently developed NYHA class II-IV cardiotoxicity (one of them having been treated with trastuzumab alone, 4 with epirubicin/cyclophosphamide and one with paclitaxel). Although the seventh woman with myocardial uptake, (treated with trastuzumab alone), did not develop chronic cardiac dysfunction, she had episodes of cardiac arrhythmia during the trastuzumab infusions. In contrast, in the 13 patients without evidence of myocardial uptake, no cardiac side-effects occurred. On the other hand, all 11 patients with intense tumor uptake of the radiolabeled trastuzumab in the scintigraphic scans experienced objective responses (10 partial, one complete remission; one of them having been treated with trastuzumab alone, 7 combined with anthracycline/cyclophosphamide and 3 with paclitaxel), in contrast to only one of the 9 women without or with negligible trastuzumab uptake (Figure 11.8).

These initial data suggest that pre-therapeutic scanning with a tracer dose of radiolabeled trastuzumab may allow for diagnostic predictions with respect to the cardiotoxicity and potentially, also the likely therapeutic efficacy of the monoclonal antibody in metastatic breast cancer. The latter is more easily explained, since it obviously reflects specific HER2 targeting in tumor sites, which is dependent upon more physiological factors in vivo than just antigen expression. The targeting of trastuzumab to the myocardium of those women eventually developing cardiac side-effects, suggests the expression of HER2 or a related cross-reactive antigen in the patients' heart as one underlying mechanism.

Therapeutic Application of Monoclonal Antibodies in Hematological Neoplasms and Solid Tumors

Table 11.1 gives an overview of the most important potentially therapeutic radionuclides used for radioimmuno- and/or radiopeptide-therapy. Traditionally, therapeutic isotopes are beta emitters, but more recently, potentially biologically more potent, so-called high linear energy transfer emitters (such as alpha or Auger electron emitters) have entered pre-clinical and clinical studies [25–27].

Table 11.1. Important potentially therapeutic radionuclides used for radioimmunotherapy (RIT)

Radionuclide	t½ (h)	Mode of decay	Decay energy	(MeV_max)	Mean path length in tissue (mm)
frequently used radionuclides:					
Iodine-131	193.0	β⁻	β⁻	0.610	0.4
			γ	0.364	
Yttrium-90	64.1	β⁻	β⁻	2.28	2.5
less frequently used radionuclides:					
Copper-67	61.9	β⁻	β⁻	0.577	0.4
			γ	0.185	
Lutetium-177	161.0	β⁻	β⁻	0.497	0.3
			γ	0.210	
Rhenium-186	90.6	β⁻	β⁻	1.074	1.1
			γ	0.137	
Rhenium-188	17.0	β⁻	β⁻	2.120	2.4
			γ	0.155	
Iodine-125	60.1 d	EC	Auger e⁻	0.025	in the nm-μm range
			γ	0.035	
Bismuth-213 / Polonium-213	45 min	β⁻/α	α	8.380	≤ 0.1
			γ	0.440	

Radioimmunotherapy of Non-Hodgkin's Lymphoma and Other Hematological Neoplasms

Due to the exquisite radiosensitivity of hematological neoplasms where there is a higher accretion of radiolabeled macromolecules (e.g., monoclonal antibodies) than usually seen in solid tumors, non-Hodgkin's lymphoma (NHL) has become one of the most successful targets for a radioimmunotherapeutic approach. Table 11.2 shows a selection of the most important clinical studies, the target antigens, radionuclides and monoclonal antibodies used in this tumor with the reported response rates. Although impressive results have been obtained with conventional régimes respecting the bone marrow as the dose-limiting organ, even more spectacular long-term remissions (?"cures") have been obtained using myeloablative high-dose approaches modeled according to high-dose myeloablative chemotherapeutic regimens (Figure 11.9, Table 11.2).

The results of radioimmunotherapy in NHL are so encouraging [28–44] that this modality has become a standard mode of treatment for these disorders and the first radiolabeled anti-CD20 antibodies will very soon be approved as drugs for treating NHL by the regulatory agencies of Europe and the United States.

Radioimmunotherapy of Solid Tumors

Whereas in non-Hodgkin's lymphoma, radioimmunotherapy (RIT) is becoming a standard modality of treatment, in solid tumors it is still in its experimental stages [4]. A traditional target cancer for this approach has been colorectal cancer. Table 11.3 provides an overview of some recent RIT studies in this tumor type. The five-year survival of colorectal cancer patients with surgically unresectable metastases

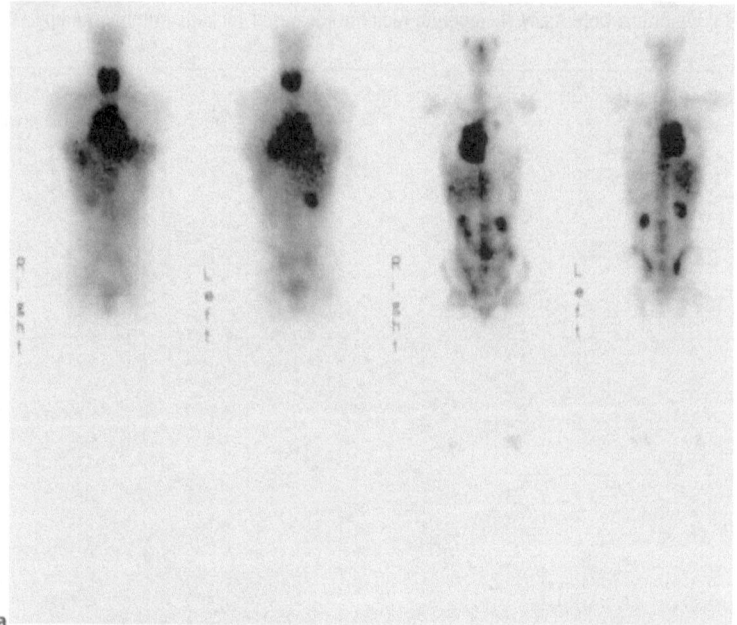

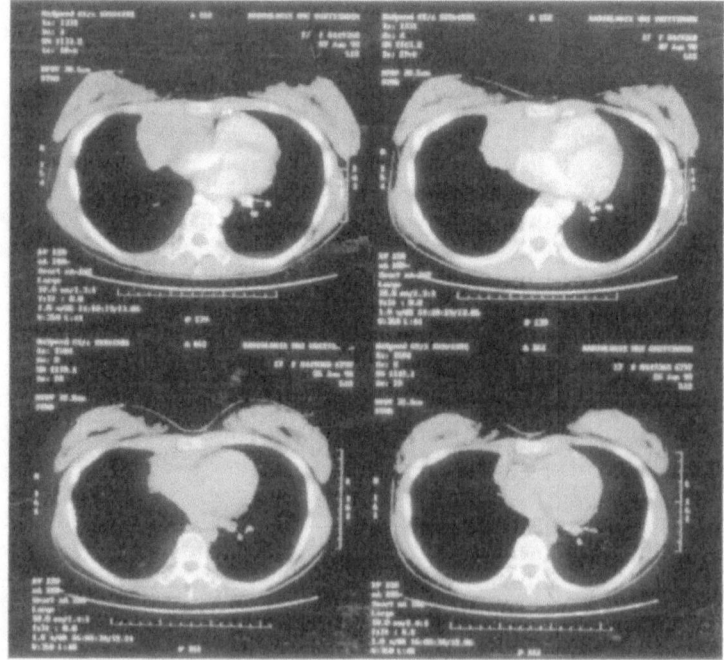

Figure 11.9. Radioimmunotherapy (RIT) of non-Hodgkin's lymphoma in a patient with high-grade NHL: (a) Targeting of ^{131}I-C2B8 (anti-CD20, left panel) as compared with ^{67}Ga citrate scanning (right panel), showing good uptake in the involved mediastinal lymph nodes, pararenal nodes and the involved bone marrow. (b) Therapeutic response in the mediastinal mass already noted at three weeks after high-dose, myeloablative ^{131}I-C2B8 therapy.

Table 11.2. Clinical radioimmunotherapy (RIT) studies in malignant B-cell non-Hodgkin's lymphoma

Radionuclide (cumul. mCi)	target antigen	antibody	(cumul). mg	number of cycles	number of eval. patients	response rate (CR+PR)	ref.
Non-myeloablative ("low-dose"):							
[131]I (26–1044)	HLA-DR	Lym-1	(8–676)	1–16	57	54% (11CR,20PR)	[28,29]
[131]I (50–267)	HLA-DR	Lym-1	(30–67)	1–2	13	31% (4PR)	[30]
[131]I (6–343)	CD22	LL2	(0.2–157)	1–7	12	33% (2CR,2PR)	[31]
[131]I (15–59)	CD22	LL2	(54–139)	1	10	20% (1CR,1PR)	[32]
[131]I (25–161)	CD37	MB-1	(40)	1	10	30% (1CR,2PR)	[33]
[131]I (38–161)	CD20	B1	(15–1565)	1–2	47	72% (16CR,18PR)	[34]
[131]I (90–200)	CD21	OKB7	(25)	3–4	18	6% (1PR)	[35]
[67]Cu (131–388)	HLA-DR	Lym-1	(135–288)	1–4	3	66% (1CR,1PR)	[28]
[90]Y (10–54)	anti-idiotypic		(1000–4050)	1–4	9	33% (2CR,1PR)	[36]
[90]Y (14–22)	CD20	B1	(2–110)	1	4	50% (1CR,1PR)	[37]
[90]Y (20–53)	CD20	2B8	(55–294)	1–2	14	79% (5CR,6PR)	[37]
Myeloablative ("high-dose"):							
[131]I (280–785)	CD20	B1	(58–1168)	1	29	93% (23CR,4PR)	[39]
[131]I (608)	CD20	1F5	(274)	1	1	100% (1PR)	[38,40]
[131]I (234–628)	CD37	MB-1	(275–970)	1	6	100% (6CR)	[38,40]
[131]I (232)	anti-idiotypic		(1000)	1	1	100% (1CR)	[37]
[131]I (145–323)	CD22	LL2	(97–111)	1	7	29% (2PR)	[32]
[131]I (225–495)	CD20/22	IDEC-2B8/LL2	(25–220)	1	10	90% (7CR,2PR)	[42,43]
[90]Y (20)	CD20	B1		1	3	33% (1PR)	[37]
[131]I (261–495)	CD20	C2B8	(2.5–10 mg/kg)	1	7	100% (6CR,1PR)	[70]
(pilot phase II in mantle cell NHL)							

is close to zero, despite the development of several new chemotherapeutic agents. Therefore, novel therapeutic strategies are warranted. Whereas RIT has shown disappointing results in "bulky disease" in solid tumors, pre-clinical results in small volume disease appear promising [45,46]. Our group has worked extensively on the radioimmunotherapeutic treatment of colorectal cancer over the past few years. The aim of one of our recent studies was to evaluate, in a phase-I/II trial, the therapeutic efficacy and dose-limiting toxicity of RIT in colorectal cancer patients with small volume disease. Forty colorectal cancer patients with low burden disease (all lesions ≤2.5 cm) were entered into a mCi/m^2-based dose escalation study with the ^{131}I-labeled murine anti-CEA MAb, F023C5, which belongs to the IgG$_1$ subtype [45]. The patients were given single injections, starting at 50 mCi/m^2 and escalating in 10 mCi/m^2 increments with the maximum tolerated dose (MTD) being defined as the dose level at which ≤ 1/6 patients develop a grade-4 myelotoxicity.

Thirty-one of the 40 patients had lesions known from radiological investigations (CT and/or MRI), with 9 patients having occult disease, (as suggested by elevated and/or rising tumor markers; CEA, CA19-9 without radiological correlates). At mean red marrow doses of 0.45 cGy/mCi, myelotoxicity was dose-limiting and a fairly good correlation between the red marrow doses and resulting toxicities was found. At 110 mCi/m^2 (i.e., the MTD), patients regularly developed

Table 11.3. Some recent radioimmunotherapy (RIT) studies in colorectal cancer

Antigen	antibody	nuclide	activity	nr. of patients	clinical results	ref.
TAG-72	CC49 IgG *phase-I*	[131]I	$15 \rightarrow 75$ mCi/m^2	24	no objective responses	[71]
	CC49 IgG *phase-II*	[131]I	75 mCi/m^2	15	no objective responses	[72]
A33	A33 IgG	[131]I	$15 \rightarrow 90$ mCi/m^2	23	3/23 "minor/mixed response"	[73]
	A33 IgG	[125]I	$50 \rightarrow 350$ mCi/m^2	21	4/21 "minor/mixed response"	[74]
17–1A	ch17–1A IgG	[125]I	$20 \rightarrow 250$ mCi	28	no objective responses	[75]
CEA	NP-4 IgG	[131]I	$44 \rightarrow 268$ mCi	57	1/35 PR, 11/35 "minor/mixed"	[76]
	NP-4 F(ab')$_2$	[131]I	$70 \rightarrow 296$ mCi	13	6/13 "minor/mixed response"	[77]
	cT84.66 IgG	[90]Y	5 mCi/m^2	3	no objective responses	[78]
	F6 F(ab')$_2$	[131]I	87–300 mCi	10	1/9 PR, 2/9 "minor/mixed"	[79]
	F023C5 IgG	[131]I	$50 \rightarrow 130$ mCi/m^2	40	1/31 CR, 7/31 PR, 12/31 "minor/mixed"	[45]
	hMN–14 IgG *phase-I*	[131]I	$40 \rightarrow 60$ mCi/m^2	12	2/11 PR, 5/11 "minor/mixed"	[46]
	hMN-14 IgG *phase-II*	[131]I	60 mCi/m^2	30	3/19 PR, 8/19 "minor/mixed" 7/9 adjuvant relapse-free	[47]

grade-3 toxicity and at 120 mCi/m^2 2/6 patients had a grade-4 leucopenia or thrombocytopenia. Tumor doses increased exponentially with decreasing tumor sizes (up to 185 cGy/mCi in a 0.5 cm lung lesion). In the 31 patients with radiologically documented lesions, one had a complete, 7 had partial remissions (corresponding to an objective response rate of 26 percent) and 12 patients (i.e., 39 percent) experienced stabilization of their previously rapidly progressing disease; lasting up to and beyond 18 months. The majority of patients showed a significant (i.e., >50%) decrease of tumor marker levels in their blood. Thus, myelotoxicity is the only dose-limiting toxicity of the ^{131}I-labeled monoclonal anti-CEA antibody F023C5. The MTD has been reached at 110 mCi/m^2, which became the dose level of the phase-II arm. Although many patients were treated below this dose level, the observed anti-tumor effects are encouraging. Re-treatment, however, does not seem to be an option since almost all patients developed HAMA as a consequence of the first therapy injection.

It was anticipated that the humanization of antibodies would avoid HAMA formation and could lead to improved therapeutic results. As a result, 12 colorectal cancer patients with small volume disease metastatic to the liver (all lesions ≤2.5 cm) were entered into a mCi/m^2-based phase-I dose escalation study with ^{131}I-labeled humanized version of the high-affinity anti-CEA antibody MN-14, hMN-14 [46]. The patients were given single injections, starting at 50 mCi/m^2 and escalating in 10-mCi/m^2 increments as before. The MTD (as previously defined) was reached at 60 mCi/m^2 of hMN-14 (at 70 mCi/m^2, 2/3 grade-4 myelotoxicities). In 11 assessable patients, 2 had partial remissions (corresponding to an objective response rate of 18%) and 5 (45%) had minor/mixed responses or experienced stabilization of previously rapidly progressing disease.

Based on these encouraging results, the aim of the subsequent phase-II trial was to evaluate the therapeutic efficacy of this ^{131}I-labeled humanized anti-CEA antibody in colorectal cancer patients with small volume disease or in an adjuvant setting [47]. Here, 30 colorectal cancer patients with small volume metastatic disease (n=21, all lesions ≤3.0 cm, all being chemo-refractory to 5-fluorouracil/folinic acid) or in adjuvant setting (n=9), were entered at 4–6 weeks after surgical resection of liver metastases with curative intention. The patients were given a single injection of ^{131}I-hMN-14 IgG at the 60 mCi/m^2 dose level. Follow-up was obtained at three-monthly intervals for up to 36 months. At a mean blood-based red marrow dose of 3.0 ± 1.3 cGy/mCi, myelotoxicity was the only toxicity observed, but only one of 28 assessable patients developed transient grade-4 thrombocytopenia. In 19 assessable out of the 21 patients with radiologically documented lesions, 3 experienced partial remissions and 8 showed minor responses (Figure 11.10) of up to 15 months; corresponding to an objective response rate of 16 percent and an overall response rate of 58 percent with a

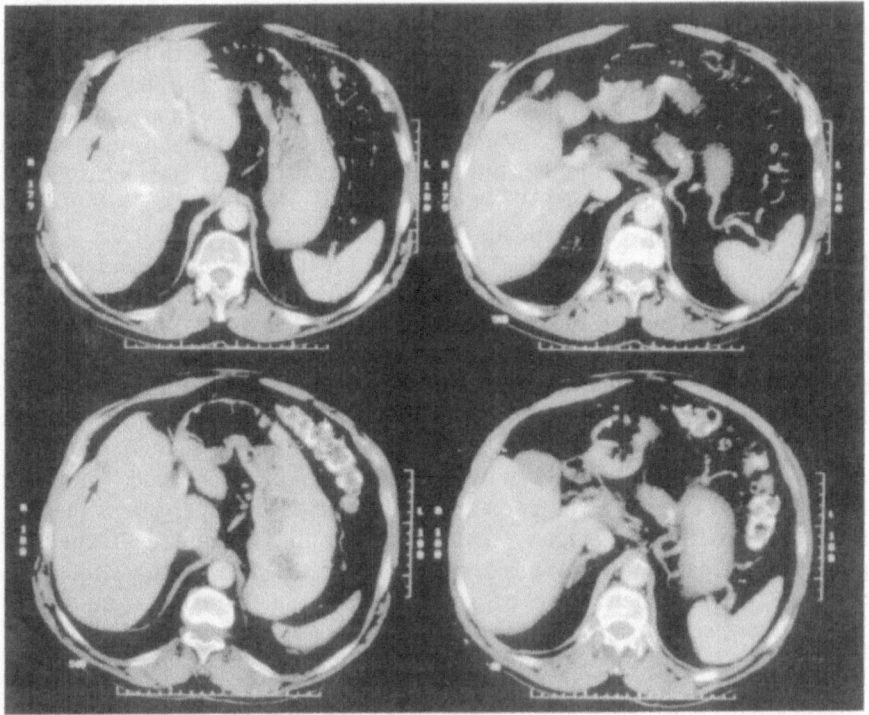

Figure 11.10. Therapeutic partial response (PR) of a small-volume liver metastasis of colorectal cancer to radioimmunotherapy with a humanized ^{131}I-labeled anti-CEA IgG (clone hMN-14).

mean duration of response of 9 months. Seven out of 9 patients in the adjuvant setting have remained free of disease for up to 36 months, with one patient relapsing at 6 months and another at 30 months. This is compared with the relapse rate in a non-randomized historical control group from our institution receiving chemotherapy which was 67 percent over the same time period. Five patients with radiologically documented lesions, having experienced at least disease stabilization as a consequence of radioimmunotherapy, were re-treated at the same 60 mCi/m^2 dose level between 8–16 months after the first therapy. No evidence of increased toxicity was observed with no hematological toxicity > grade 3. Two of 4 assessable of these re-treated patients experienced partial remissions with one achieving disease stabilization as a consequence of the second radioantibody therapy injection.

These data suggest that RIT is a safe and effective form of therapy in small volume disease and potentially in an adjuvant setting for colorectal cancer. Toxicity is restricted to mild and transient leukopenia and thrombocytopenia. Moreover, in relapse, re-treatment appears to be a feasible option with at least a likely probability of response. A prospective randomized comparison with standard chemotherapy is obviously now indicated following these initial results with similarly encouraging therapeutic effects being also noted in initial RIT trials in MTC and ovarian cancer (Figure 11.11) [48,49,50] (see Chapter 16).

Recent Pre-clinical and Experimental Findings in Radioimmunotherapy

Recent experimental data suggests that RIT with high linear energy transfer (LET) radiation may have therapeutic advantages over low-LET (e.g., β⁻-) emissions and that fragments may be more effective in controlling tumor growth than IgG [25,51–53]. The aim of our recent experimental work was to assess the toxicity and anti-tumor efficacy of RIT with the α-emitter ^{213}Bi/^{213}Po as compared with the β-emitter ^{90}Y, linked to a monovalent Fab′ fragment in a colon cancer xenograft model in nude mice [25]. Biodistribution studies of ^{213}Bi- or ^{88}Y-labeled BzDTPA-conjugated Fab′ fragments of the monoclonal antibody CO17-1A were performed in nude mice bearing subcutaneous human colon cancer xenografts. ^{213}Bi was obtained from an "in-house" ^{225}Ac/^{213}Bi generator. It decays by β⁻- and 440 keV-γ-emission with a t$_{1/2}$ of 45.6 min to the ultra-short lived α-emitter, ^{213}Po (t$_{1/2}$ 4.2 s).

For therapy, the mice were injected either with ^{213}Bi- or ^{90}Y-labeled CO17-1A Fab′, whereas control groups were left untreated. The MTD of each agent was then determined. The mice were treated with or without inhibition of the renal accumulation of antibody fragments, with D-lysine, bone marrow transplantation, or a combination of both. Myelotoxicity and second-organ toxicities, as well as tumor growth, were monitored at weekly intervals. In accordance with kidney uptake values of as high as 80 percent of the injected dose per gram, the kidney was the first dose-limiting organ with the use of both ^{90}Y- and ^{213}Bi-labeled Fab′ fragments. Application of D-lysine decreased the renal dose by more than 3-fold. Accordingly, myelotoxicity then became dose-limiting with both conjugates. By using D-lysine protection, the MTD of ^{90}Y-Fab′ was 250 Ci and the MTD of ^{213}Bi-Fab′ was 700 Ci, corresponding to blood doses of 5–8 Gy (as representatives of the red marrow doses). Additional bone marrow transplantation allowed for an increase of the MTD of ^{90}Y-Fab′ to 400 Ci and for ^{213}Bi-Fab′ to 1100 Ci, respectively and at these dose levels, no biochemical or histological evidence of renal damage was observed (kidney doses <35 Gy). At equitoxic dosing, ^{213}Bi-labeled

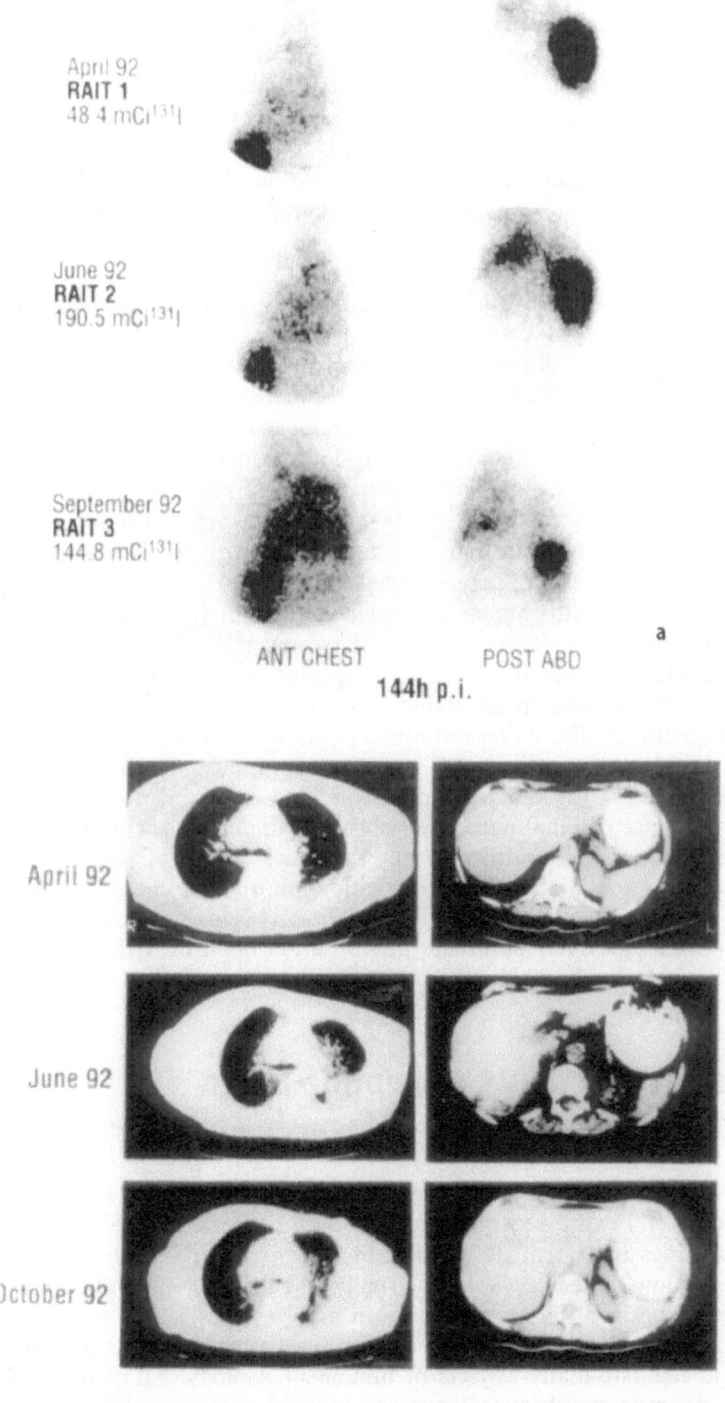

Figure 11.11. Therapeutic response of a large liver metastasis of medullary thyroid cancer to several cycles of anti-CEA radioimmunotherapy with ^{131}I-MN-14 anti-CEA F(ab')$_2$ fragments (in contrast, note the concomitant progression of a malignant pleural effusion).

Fab' fragments were significantly more effective than ^{90}Y-labeled conjugates (p < 0.01). These data show that RIT in an experimental model with α-emitters may be therapeutically more effective than the conventional β-emitters traditionally used. Surprisingly, maximum tolerated blood doses were at 5–8 Gy, with very similar results using the high-LET α-emitters as those obtained with low-LET β-emitters. Due to its short physical $t_{1/2}$ ^{213}Bi appears as especially suitable for use in conjunction with fast-clearing fragments [25,53].

Elevated renal uptake and extended retention of radiolabeled antibody fragments and peptides is a problem in the therapeutic application of such agents. Over the past years, another focus of our research has been to develop suitable methods designed to reduce renal accretion. In these studies, it has been shown that the kidney uptake of antibody fragments in animals can be reduced by the systemic application of cationic amino acids and their derivatives in a dose-dependent manner by almost one order of magnitude, whereas the uptake in all other organs, as well as in the tumor, remains essentially unaffected [53]. A similar reduction in renal retention is achieved for all intracellularly-retained radionuclides (e.g., radiometals) or radio-iodinated immunoconjugates, as well as for smaller peptides. Lysine is usually the preferred agent and its D- and L-isomers are equally effective whether given intra-peritoneally or orally. Amino sugars are also effective, but their N-acetyl derivatives, (lacking a positive charge), are not efficacious. Basic polypeptides also appear to be effective, with their potency increasing with increasing molecular weight (i.e., the amount of positive charges per molecule). Urine analysis of treated individuals shows the excretion of unmetabolized, intact fragments or peptides, in contrast to mostly low molecular weight metabolites in untreated controls.

In therapeutic studies using radiometal-conjugated Fab fragments, the kidney is the first dose-limiting organ [53]. Application of cationic amino acids enables a substantial increase in their maximum tolerated dose and no biochemical or histological evidence of renal damage is observed under these conditions. As was the case in animals, in pilot clinical trials, the renal uptake of patients injected with Fab' fragments concomitantly given with amino-acids could be decreased significantly, whereas the uptake of all other organs remained unaffected. Such strategies can thus effectively eliminate the radiation nephrotoxicity of these antibody fragments.

Recent Developments of Peptide-based Radiopharmaceuticals for Diagnosis and Therapy

Table 11.4 gives an overview of some typical receptors for regulatory peptides which are (over-) expressed on various human cancers. Physiologically, these regulatory peptides that form the natural ligands for their receptors are very potent molecules of low molecular weight (usually less than 30–40 amino acids long) [6]. They are synthesized mainly in the brain and gastrointestinal tract, but also play a role in the peripheral nervous and immune systems and are produced and secreted to regulate many aspects of human physiology. All of them bind to and act through trans-membrane G protein-coupled receptors. In contrast to larger molecules, such as monoclonal antibodies or other proteins, they have the advantage of easily penetrating into all tissues, with the only exception of the brain.

Table 11.4. Typical receptors for regulatory peptides which are (over-)expressed by human tumors

Peptide Receptor	Tumor Types
Somatostatin receptor	neuroendocrine tumors (carcinoids etc.) small cell lung cancer medullary thyroid cancer various tumors of the nervous system lymphoma (NHL, Hodgkin's disease)
VIP receptor	various adenocarcinomas (stomach, colon, pancreas, lung etc.) small cell lung cancer neuroendocrine tumors lymphoma
CCK-B receptors	medullary thyroid cancer small cell lung cancer stromal ovarian cancer astrocytoma (potentially gastrointestinal adenocarcinomas [stomach, colon, pancreatic cancers])
CCK-A receptors	gastroenteropancreatic tumors meningiomas, neuroblastomas
Substance-P receptors	medullary thyroid cancer small cell lung cancer breast tumors peri- and intratumoral vessels
Bombesin/GRP receptors	small cell lung cancer colonic cancer glioblastoma
Neurotensin receptors	pancreatic cancer prostate cancer small cell lung cancer
GnRH receptors	breast cancer prostate cancer
Glp-1 receptors	insulinoma, small cell lung, medullary thyroid cancer

Due to their relative hydrophilia, the blood-brain barrier is non-permeable to these peptides in either direction, therefore, the central nervous system and the periphery (e.g., the gastrointestinal tract) form two independent regulatory systems which can use the same messenger molecules without any danger of a confusing interaction (the neuro-gastric axis).

On the background of their action as flexible messenger molecules, their rapid degradation and fast inactivation, is of utmost importance for clinical use. Due to ubiquitously occurring peptidases, most of them are extremely short-acting and for their use as (radio-) pharmaceuticals, these short half-lives act as obstacles, since many do not even reach their intended targets. Most peptide research has thus been heavily involved in the development of metabolically stable peptides for clinical use.

Further pre-requisites for a peptide for human in vivo scintigraphy or even therapeutic application include a high affinity (usually in the nano- or sub-nano-molar range) to a receptor target as well as a high target specificity. The specificity problem is even more pronounced when developing metabolically stabilized, synthetic peptides. Frequently, several polymorphisms of the various receptors exist, (which is often genetically determined), whereas the respective natural ligands bind with similar or even equal affinity to all subtypes. Here, chemically modified synthetic analogs often display strong selectivity for only one or, at best, a few of these clinically relevant receptor subtypes.

Somatostatin Receptor Scintigraphy

As is the case with other regulatory peptides, somatostatin forms a whole family of structurally related peptides [54]. The two most important physiological members are 14 (SS-14) and 28 (SS-28) amino acids long [55,56] (Figure 11.12). These peptides naturally occur in a number of organs, including the central nervous system, the hypothalamo-pituitary axis, the gastrointestinal tract, (including the pancreas) and throughout the immune system. The members of the somatostatin family exert inhibitory effects on a wide spectrum of physiological functions, including hormone secretion or mitosis, although the anti-proliferative effects are mainly seen in cell culture and clinical results have mostly been disappointing [56]. Furthermore, numerous tumors in animals and humans express somatostatin receptors with 5 human somatostatin receptor subtypes being characterized so far [56,57]. All are typical G-protein coupled with 7 trans-membrane domains, functionally inhibiting adenylate cyclase. All naturally occurring members of the somatostatin family have very short half-lives in serum, but bind to all 5 receptor subtypes with equal or similar affinity. The molecular modifications during the development of octreotide as a metabolically stable somatostatin analog (Figure 11.12) were conserved the high affinity to the sst2 and sst5 receptor subtypes, but have lost binding specificity for both subtype 1 and 4, (their affinity to sst3 receptors being moderate, at best) [56]. Besides the central nervous system, relevant amounts of peripheral somatostatin receptors are expressed on lymphocytes and activated leukocytes, causing a prominent uptake of somatostatin analogs in the normal spleen (cf. Fig. 11.12b). Some somatostatin receptor expression is encountered in the liver and the kidneys as well. However, the physiological uptake of ^{111}In-DTPA-D-Phe^1-octreotide in these organs is probably mainly due to some loss of indium by hepatic chelation and non-specfic peptide uptake by renal tubular cells (cf. Fig. 11.12b).

Extensive clinical studies involving several thousands of patients have shown that the major clinical application of somatostatin receptor scintigraphy is in the detecetion and the staging of gastroenteropancreatic neuroendocrine tumors (carcinoids) [56,58–60]. This tumor entity is rather rare, with an annual incidence of approximately 0.7 cases per 100,000. However, although the term "carcinoid" suggests a homogeneous pathological entity, they are quite heterogeneous in terms of histological differentiation, hormone production, biological and clinical behaviour. A more embryologically oriented classification system

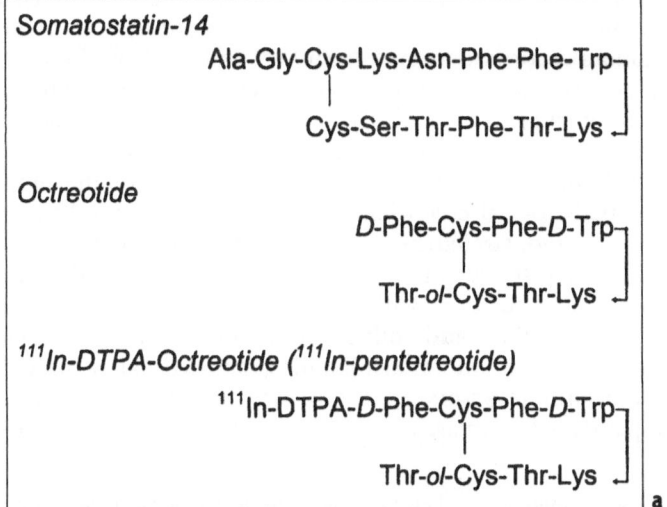

Somatostatin-14

Ala-Gly-Cys-Lys-Asn-Phe-Phe-Trp ┐
               |
Cys-Ser-Thr-Phe-Thr-Lys ┘

Octreotide

D-Phe-Cys-Phe-*D*-Trp ┐
          |
Thr-*ol*-Cys-Thr-Lys ┘

^{111}In-DTPA-Octreotide (^{111}In-pentetreotide)

^{111}In-DTPA-*D*-Phe-Cys-Phe-*D*-Trp ┐
                    |
Thr-*ol*-Cys-Thr-Lys ┘

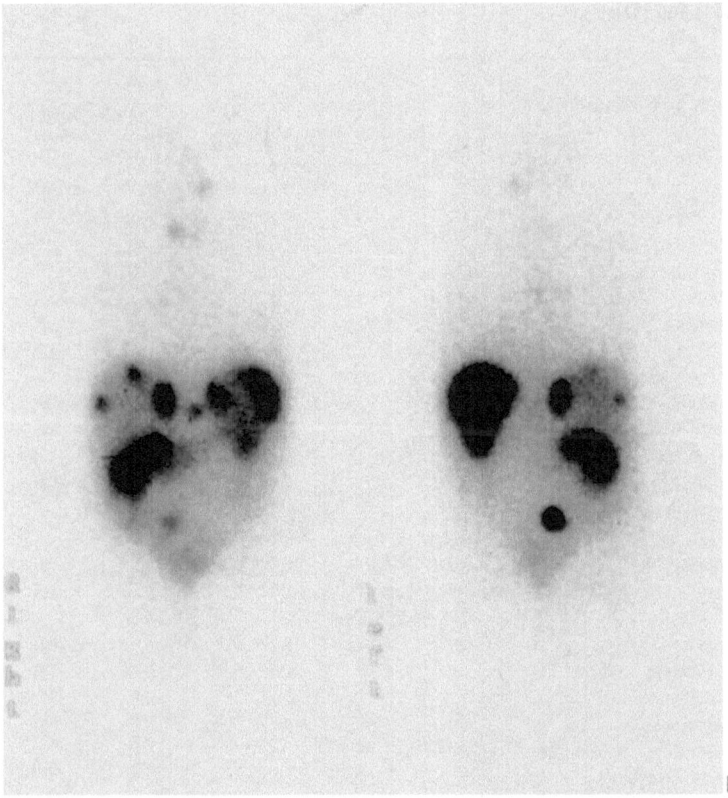

Figure 11.12. Somatostatin receptor scintigraphy: (a) Structure of natural somatostatin-14, as compared with its metabolically stabilized analog octreotide, and its radiolabeled analog, ^{111}In-pentetreotide. (b) ^{111}In-pentetreotide scan in a patient with a gastroentero-pancreatic neuroendocrine tumor metastatic to the liver.

distinguishes foregut (respiratory tract, thymus) from midgut (jejunum, ileum, right colon) and hindgut (left colon, rectum) tumors, but divides pancreatic endocrine tumors according to their hormonal activity (gastrinomas, insulinomas, VIPomas, glucagonomas, somatostatinomas etc.). Somatostatin receptor scintigraphy has been shown to visualize the vast majority of these tumor types, including primary tumors and metastases. Table 11.5 provides an overview of the sensitivity of ^{111}In-DTPA-D-Phe^1-octreotide scintigraphy in these tumors and various other pathological conditions as compared with the "true" somatostatin receptor status, demonstrated by in vitro autoradiography. In accordance with their high in vitro somatostatin receptor expression, outstanding diagnostic accuracies have been achieved with somatostatin receptor scintigraphy in pituitary tumors, carcinoids and other gastroenteropancreatic neuronendocrine tumors (with the exception of insulinomas, approximately only half of which express somatostatin receptors, in accordance with the 50 percent scintigraphic sensitivity), paraganglionomas, phaeochromocytoma and neuroblastoma (as well

Table 11.5. Sensitivity of ^{111}In-DTPA-D-Phe^1-octreotide scintigraphy in vivo as compared with the in vitro receptor status (both data are from different patient cohorts; modified from [54] and [57])

Tumor type or pathological condition	In vivo scintigraphy No.	(Sensitivity)	In vitro receptor status No.	(Sensitivity)
Pituitary tumors:				
GH producing	7/10	70%	45/46	98%
TSH producing	2/ 2	100%	n/d	
Non-functioning	12/16	75%	n/d	
Carcinoids	74/78	95%	55/62	88%
Gastrinoma	13/14	93%	6/ 6	100%
Insulinoma	13/28	46%	18/27	67%
Exocrine pancreatic tumors	0/24	0%	0/12	0%
Unclassified APUDoma	15/20	75%	4/ 4	100%
Paraganglioma	42/42	100%	4/ 4	100%
Pheochromocytoma	13/15	87%	38/52	73%
Neuroblastoma	8/ 9	89%	15/23	65%
Differentiated thyroid cancer:				
Follicular	5/ 6	83%	n/d	
Papillary	2/ 3	67%	n/d	
Medullary thyroid cancer	24/35	69%	10/26	38%
Small cell lung cancer	38/38	100%	4/ 7	57%
Non-small cell lung cancer	42/42	100%	0/17	0%
Breast cancer	47/69	68%	33/72	46%
Meningioma	14/14	100%	54/55	98%
Astrocytoma	4/ 6	67%	14/17	82%
Non-Hodgkin's lymphoma	93/112	83%	26/30	87%
Hodgkin's disease	39/40	98%	2/ 2	100%
Sarcoidosis	29/29	100%	3/ 3	100%
Wegener's granulomatosis	4/ 4	100%		
Tuberculosis	9/ 9	100%	2/ 2	100%
Sjögren's syndrome	4/ 5	80%	n/d	
Rheumathoid arthritis	14/14	100%	6/ 7	86%

as other tumors of neural origin such as meningioma) and certain granulomatous diseases. Despite widespread somatostatin receptor expression, clinical results in lymphoma (Hodgkin's and non-Hodgkin's disease) are mostly disappointing, with only rather weak tumor-to-background ratios.

Approximately half of small cell lung (SCLC) and medullary thyroid cancers (MTC) express somatostatin receptors, but although no receptor expression is found in non-small cell lung cancers, many of these latter tumors can be visualized by octreotide scintigraphy. This has been partially attributed to somatostatin receptor expression in intra- and peri-tumoral vessels and by intra-tumoral leukocytes [61]. Interestingly, in both, medullary thyroid and small cell lung cancers, somatostatin receptor expression is frequently inversely related to the tumor's degree of differentiation, where the sensitivity in detecting the primary tumor is outstandingly high (>90%), but where more than half of the metastases have lost somatostatin receptor expression [62]. Thus, scintigraphic visualization of MTC or SCLC not only allows for primary lesion localization, but also possibly for the prediction of the patient's prognostic outcome. Due to its higher metabolic stability for therapeutic radionuclides, a DOTA derivative of Tyr^3-octreotide, called DOTATOC, has recently been developed for therapeutic application, although clinical trials are awaited [63,64].

Other Regulatory Peptides, e.g., Gastrin Analogs

The outstanding sensitivity of pentagastrin stimulation in detecting metastatic MTC, suggests widespread expression of the corresponding receptor type on human MTC. This receptor is also present in most cases of SCLC and in a variety of other solid tumors [65,66]. The aim of our recent work has been to systematically screen and optimize suitable radioligands for targeting cholecystokinin (CCK-B) and related receptors in vivo in a pre-clinical model. A variety of CCK/gastrin-related peptides, all having in common the C-terminal receptor binding sequence Trp-Met-Asp-PheNH$_2$, have been studied [67–69]. They were radioiodinated by the Iodogen or Bolton-Hunter procedures. The peptides tested were members of the gastrin or CCK families, (or possessed characteristics of both), which differ only by the intramolecular position of a tyrosyl moiety (occurring in native or sulfated form). Their stability and affinity were tested and their biodistribution and therapeutic efficacy were studied in nude mice, bearing subcutaneous human MTC xenografts. DTPA-derivatives of suitable peptides were synthesized and evaluated, labeled with ^{111}In. All members of the CCK or gastrin family were stable in serum (with a $t_{1/2}$ of several hours at 37° C) and the stability of those peptides was highest when they bore N-terminal pGlu residues (e.g., big gastrin, gastrin-I, caerulein etc.) or D-amino acids. In accordance with their comparably low affinity, non-sulfated members of the CCK family showed fairly low uptake in the tumor and other CCK-B receptor-expressing tissues (e.g., the stomach). Sulfated CCK derivatives performed significantly better, but additionally displayed a high uptake in normal, CCK-A receptor-expressing tissues (such as the liver, gallbladder, pancreas and bowel). The best tumor uptake and tumor-to-non-tumor ratios were obtained with members of the gastrin family, due to their selectivity and affinity for the CCK-B receptor subtype. Pilot therapy experiments in human MTC-bearing animals have shown significant anti-tumor efficacy when compared with untreated controls.

¹¹¹In-labeled DTPA derivatives showed excellent targeting of CCK-B receptor-expressing tissues in animals and also in a normal human volunteer [67–69]. Twenty patients with metastatic MTC, (9 with occult disease), have been recently studied by our group with CCK-B receptor scintigraphy. All had undergone ultrasonography, whole-body CT and MRI, as well as bone scanning and somatostatin receptor scintigraphy. CCK-B receptor scintigraphy was performed with 3–5 mCi (111–185 MBq) of an ¹¹¹In-labeled DTPA-derivative of minigastrin (13 amino acids long; affinity in the nM range). Whole-body scans were performed at 10 min, 1, 4, and 24 h, SPECT at 4 and 24 h p.i. The normal organ uptake of the radiopeptide was confined to the stomach and (to a much lesser extent, the gallbladder) as a result of CCK-B receptor binding as well as to the kidneys. No physiological uptake was observed in any other organ, such as the liver or spleen. Strong uptake in the gastric mucosa represents the only extra-cerebral tissue with high physiological CCK-B receptor expression. The major excretion pathway is renal, but its renal retention was significantly lower than that observed with ¹¹¹In-DTPA-octreotide. All tumor manifestations known from conventional imaging were clearly visualized as early as 1 h p.i., with increasing tumor-to-background ratios over time; where at least one lesion was detected in all patients with occult disease (patient-based sensitivity virtually 100%) (Figure 11.13). Among these

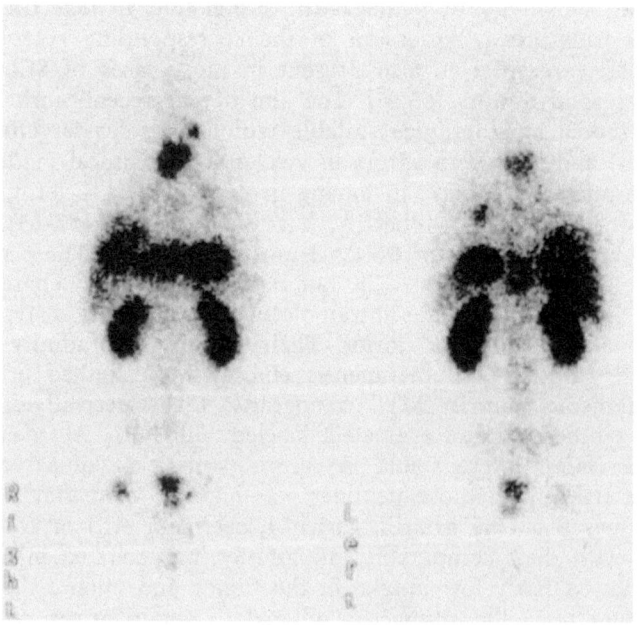

Figure 11.13. Cholecystokinin-B / gastrin receptor scintigraphy in a patient with advanced metastatic medullary thyroid cancer: physiological uptake in the stomach and kidneys, pathological uptake in a local recurrence, lymph node, pulmonary, hepatic and bone / bone marrow metastases (scan at 24 h p.i.).

cases were local recurrences, lymph node, pulmonary, hepatic, splenic and bone metastases. Therefore, CCK-B receptor ligands appear to be a promising new class of receptor binding peptides for the staging of known and occult metastatic MTC. DOTA derivatives of this receptor have similarly been developed for therapeutic application in patients with advanced disease (e.g., labeled with ^{90}Y) and further clinical studies, (diagnostic as well as therapeutic), are ongoing.

These radiolabeled regulatory peptides have opened up new horizons in nuclear oncology for diagnosis and therapy. Due to their low molecular weight and good tissue penetration properties, their high affinity for their receptor, as well as the fact that after receptor binding, they are internalized into the tumor cells and they are promising candidates not only for staging, but also for internal radionuclide therapy of various cancer types. Only a minority of the huge number of potentially useful regulatory peptides and peptide families has been more or less thoroughly investigated so far and future work will probably reveal a multitude of potentially clinically useful peptide-based radioligands. In contrast to monoclonal antibodies, (which can be raised theroretically against any surface structure of any given tumor cell), regulatory peptides need a specific receptor on the target cell surface, most importantly, for internalization.

Conclusions

Whereas the clinical role and importance of diagnostic immunoscintigraphy is decreasing in many tumors, (due in part to the outstanding sensitivity of FDG-PET), it may play a role with respect to prognostic predictions in some cancer types (e.g., MTC or breast cancer). Radioimmunotherapy (RIT) has crossed the threshold to become a standard mode of therapy in hematologic malignancies, but initial results in solid tumors also appear promising. A variety of peptide-based radioligands is currently also under development for use in specialized tumors. These radiolabeled regulatory peptides have created new opportunities for the nuclear oncologist in specialized cancer diagnosis and therapy.

Acknowledgements

The authors' pre-clinical as well as clinical studies have been supported over the years by various grants from the Deutsche Forschungsgemeinschaft (German Research Foundation), the Deutsche Krebshilfe (German Cancer Research Fund), the Directorate General of the European Union, and the National Cancer Institute (National Institutes of Health) of the United States of America.

The authors would like to take the opportunity to express their gratitude to all their previous and present collaborators and coworkers, graduate students and last but not least, technologists. Without their diligence, experimental skills, ideas, creativity and support, our group would not have been able to achieve many of our recent observations and discoveries.

This chapter is dedicated to my (TMB) mother, Dr. Gertrud Behr, in an attempt to acknowledge her constant support, encouragement, and compassion, as well as to Dr. Bernd von Garmissen for his reliable friendship, intellectual and emotional support and for his encouragement, which sometimes also includes the encouragement to take and pursue unorthodox paths in research and life.

References

1. Biersack HJ, Grünwald F. Thyroid Cancer. Berlin/Heidelberg/New York:Springer Verlag, 2001.
2. Goldenberg DM, DeLand F, Kim E, Bennett S, Primus FJ, van Nagell JR Jr, et al. Use of radiolabeled antibodies to carcinoembryonic antigen for the detection and localization of diverse cancers by external photoscanning. N Engl J Med 1978;298:1384–6.
3. Mach JP, Carrel S, Forni M, Ritschard J, Donath A, Alberto P. Tumor localization of radiolabeled antibodies against carcinoembryonic antigen in patients with carcinoma: a critical evaluation. N Engl J Med 1980;303:5–10.
4. Behr TM, Goldenberg DM, Becker WS. Radioimmunotherapy of solid tumors: a review "Of Mice and Men". Hybridoma 1997;16:101–7.
5. Behr TM, Goldenberg DM, Scheele JR, Wolf FG, Becker W. Klinische Relevanz der Immunszintigraphie mit ^{99m}Tc-markierten Anti-CEA-Fab'-Fragmenten in der Nachsorge des kolorektalen Karzinoms: Chirurgische Resektabilitäts-Beurteilung aus der Kombination mit konventioneller Bildgebung. Dtsch Med Wschr 1996;122:463–70.
6. Behr TM, Behe W, Becker W. Diagnostic applications of radiolabeled peptides in nuclear endocrinology. Q J Nucl Med 1999;43:268–80.
7. Bombardieri E, Aliberti G, de Graaf C, Pauwels E, Crippa F. Positron emission tomography (PET) and other nuclear medicine modalities in staging gastrointestinal cancer. Semin Surg Oncol 2001;20:134–46.
8. Goldenberg DM, Horowitz JA, Sharkey RM, Hall TC, Murthy S, Goldenberg H, et al. Targeting, dosimetry, and radioimmunotherapy of B-cell lymphomas with iodine-131-labeled LL2 monoclonal antibody. J Clin Oncol 1991;9:548–64.
9. Becker WS, Behr TM, Cumme F, Rossler W, Wendler J, Kern PM, et al. ^{67}Ga citrate versus ^{99m}Tc-labeled LL2-Fab' (anti-CD22) fragments in the staging of B-cell non-Hodgkin's lymphoma. Cancer Res 1995;55:5771–3.
10. Front D, Israel O. The role of Ga-67 scintigraphy in evaluating the results of therapy of lymphoma patients. Semin Nucl Med 1995;25:60–71.
11. Buchmann I, Reinhardt M, Elsner K, Bunjes D, Altehoefer C, Finke J, Moser E, Glatting G, Kotzerke J, Guhlmann CA, Schirrmeister H, Reske SN. 2-(fluorine-18)fluoro-2-deoxy-D-glucose positron emission tomography in the detection and staging of malignant lymphoma. A bicenter trial. Cancer 2001;91:889–99.
12. Warburg O. The metabolism of tumors. London: Constable, 1930.
13. Reske S, Kartsens J, Sohn M, Glockner W, Buell U. Bone marrow immunoscintigraphy compared with conventional bone scintigraphy for the detection of bone metastases. Acta Oncol 1993;32:753–761.
14. Behr TM, Gratz S, Markus PM, Dunn RM, Hüfner M, Schauer A, Fischer M, Munz DL, Becker H, Becker W. Anti-carcinoembryonic antigen antibodies versus somatostatin analogs in the detection of metastatic medullary thyroid carcinoma: Are carcinoembryonic antigen and somatostatin receptor expression prognostic factors? Cancer 1997;80:2436–57.
15. Behr TM, Becker W. Metabolic and receptor imaging of metastatic medullary thyroid cancer: does anti-CEA and somatostatin-receptor scintigraphy allow for prognostic predictions? Eur J Nucl Med 1999;26:70–1.
16. Behr TM, Gratz S, Markus PM, Dunn RM, Hüfner M, Becker H, Becker W. Enhanced bilateral somatostatin receptor expression in mediastinal lymph nodes ("chimney sign") in occult metastatic medullary thyroid cancer: a typical site of tumor manifestation? Eur J Nucl Med 1997;24:184–91.
17. Busnardo B, Girelli ME, Simioni N, Nacamulli D, Bosetto E. Nonparallel patterns of calcitonin and carcinoembryonic antigen levels in the follow-up of medullary thyroid carcinoma. Cancer 1984;53:278–85.
18. Mendelsohn G, Wells Jr SA, Baylin SB. Relationship of tissue carcinoembryonic antigen and calcitonin to tumor virulence in medullary thyroid carcinoma. Cancer 1984;54:657–62.
19. Reubi JC, Chayvialle JA, Franc B, Cohen R, Calmettes C, Modigliani E. Somatostatin receptors and somatostatin content in medullary thyroid carcinomas. Lab Invest 1991;64:567–73.
20. Pegram MD, Lipton A, Hayes DF, Weber BL, Baselga JM, Tripathy D, et al. Phase II study of receptor-enhanced chemosensitivity using recombinant humanized anti-p185 HER2/neu monoclonal antibody plus cisplatin in patients with HER2/neu-overexpressing metastatic breast cancer refractory to chemotherapy treatment. J Clin Oncol 1998;16:2659–71.
21. Slamon DJ, Leyland-Jones B, Shak S, et al. Use of chemotherapy plus a monoclonal antibody against HER2 for metastatic breast cancer that overexpresses HER2. N Engl J Med 2001;344:783–92.
22. Eisenhauer EA. From the molecule to the clinic — inhibiting HER2 to treat breast cancer (Editorial). N Engl J Med 2001:344;841–2.

23. Behr TM, Béhé M, Wörmann B. Does external scintigraphy allow for predictions with respect to the toxicity and therapeutic efficacy of trastuzumab therapy of HER2/neu expressing breast cancer? N Engl J Med 2001;344 in press.

24. Khalkhali I, Villanueva-Meyer J, Edell SL, Connolly JL, Schnitt SJ, Baum JK, et al. Diagnostic accuracy of ^{99m}Tc-sestamibi breast imaging: multicenter trial results. J Nucl Med 2000;41:1973–9.

25. Behr TM, Béhé M, Stabin MG, Wehrmann E, Apostolidis C, Molinet R, et al. High-linear energy transfer (LET) alpha versus low-LET beta emitters in radioimmunotherapy of solid tumors: therapeutic efficacy and dose-limiting toxicity of ^{213}Bi- versus ^{90}Y-labeled CO17-1A Fab' fragments in a human colonic cancer model. Cancer Res 1999;59:2635–43.

26. Behr TM, Sgouros G, Stabin MG, Béhé M, Angerstein C, Blumenthal RD, et al. Studies on the red marrow dosimetry in radioimmunotherapy: an experimental investigation of factors influencing the radiation-induced myelotoxicity in therapy with beta-, Auger/conversion electron-, or alpha-emitters. Clin Cancer Res 1999;5:3031–43.

27. Jurcic JG, McDevitt MR, Sgouros G, Ballangrud Å, Finn RD, Geerlings MW, et al Targeted alpha-particle therapy for myeloid leukemias: A phase I trial of bismuth-213-HuM195 (anti-CD33). Blood 1997;90(Suppl.):504a.

28. DeNardo GL, DeNardo SJ. Treatment of B-lymphocyte malignancise with ^{131}I-Lym-1 and ^{67}Cu-2IT-BAT-Lym-1 and opportunities for improvement. In: Goldenberg DM (Hrsg.). Cancer Therapy with Radiolabeled Antibodies. Boca Raton: CRC Press, 1995; S217–27.

29. Lewis JP, DeNardo GL, DeNardo SJ. Radioimmunotherapy of lymphoma: a UC Davis experience. Hybridoma 1995;14:115–20.

30. Meredith RF, Khazaeli MB, Plott G. Comaprison of diagnostic and therapeutic doses of ^{131}I-Lym-1 in patients with non-Hodgkin's lymphoma. Antib Immunoconj Radiopharm 1993;6:1–11.

31. Goldenberg DM, Horowitz JA, Sharkey RM, Hall TC, Murthy S, Goldenberg H, et al Targeting, dosimetry and radioimmunotherapy of B-cell lymphomas with iodine-131-labeled LL2 monoclonal antibody. J Clin Oncol 1991;9:548–64.

32. Juweid M, Sharkey RM, Markowitz A, Behr T, Swayne LC, Hansen HJ, et al. Treatment of Non-Hodgkin's lymphoma with radiolabeled murine, chimeric, or humanized LL2, an anti-CD22 monoclonal antibody. Cancer Res 1995;55:5899–907.

33. Kaminski MS, Fig LM, Zasadny KR, Koral KF, DelRosario RB, Francis IR, et al. Imaging, dosimetry, and radioimmunotherapy with iodine 131-labeled anti-CD37 antibody in B-cell lymphoma. J Clin Oncol 1992;10:1696–711.

34. Kaminski MS, Zasadny KR, Francis IR, Fenner MC, Ross CW, Milik AW, et al.. Iodine-131-anti-B1 radioimmunotherapy for B-cell lymphoma. J Clin Oncol 1996;14:1974–81.

35. Czuczman MS, Straus DJ, Divgi CR, Graham M, Garin-Chesa P, Finn R, et al. Phase I dose-escalation trial of iodine 131-labeled monoclonal antibody OKB7 in patients with non-Hodgkin's lymphoma. J Clin Oncol 1993;11:2021–9.

36. White CA, Halpern SE, Parker BA, Miller RA, Hupf HB, Shawler DL, et al. Radioimmunotherapy of relapsed B-cell lymphoma with yttrium-90 anti-idiotype monoclonal antibodies. Blood 1996;87:3640–3649.

37. Davis TA, Knox SJ. Radioimmunoconjugate therapy of non-Hodgkin's lymphoma. In: Grossbard ML (Hrsg.). Monoclonal Antibody-Based Therapy of Cancer. New York: Marcel Dekker Inc., 1998; S113–36.

38. Press OW, Eary JF, Appelbaum FR, Martin PJ, Badger CC, Nelp WB, et al. Radiolabeled-antibody therapy of B-cell lymphoma with autologous bone marrow support. N Engl J Med 1993;329:1219–24.

39. Press OW, Eary JF, Appelbaum FR, Martin PJ, Nelp WB, Glenn S, et al. Phase II trial of ^{131}I-B1 (anti-CD20) antibody therapy with autologous stem cell transplantation for relapsed B cell lymphoma. Lancet 1995;346:336–40.

40. Press OW, Eary JF, Appelbaum FR, Bernstein ID. Treatment of relapsed B cell lymphoma with high-dose radioimmunotherapy and bone marrow transplantation. In: Goldenberg DM (Hrsg.). Cancer Therapy with Radiolabeled Antibodies. CRC Press, Boca Raton 1995; S. 229–237.

41. Badger CC, Eary JF, Brown S. Therapy of lymphoma with I-131-labeled anti-idiotype antibodies (anti-id). Proc AACR 1987;28:388.

42. Behr TM, Holler E, Gratz S, Wörmann B, Sharkey RM, Dunn RM, Hiddemann W, et al. CD22 is a suitable target molecule for detection and high-dose, myeloablative radioimmunotherapy with the monclonal antibody LL2 in acute lymphatic leukemia and Waldenström's macroglobulinemia. Tumor Targeting 1998;3:32–40.

43. Behr TM, Wörmann B, Gramatzki M, Riggert J, Gratz S, Béhé M, Griesinger F, Sharkey RM, Kolb HJ, Hiddemann W, Goldenberg DM, Becker W. Radioimmunotherapy with humanized anti-CD22 or chimeric anti-CD20 antibodies in a broad spectrum of B-cell associated malignancies: low-

versus high-dose, myeloablative regimens in acute lymphatic leukemia, high- and low-grade non-Hodgkin's lymphoma, and macroglobulinemia. Clin Cancer Res 5 (1999), 3304–3314.

44. Davis TA, Knox SJ. Radioimmunoconjugate therapy of non-Hodgkin's lymphoma. In: Grossbard ML (Hrsg.). Monoclonal Antibody-Based Therapy of Cancer. Marcel Dekker Inc., New York 1998, S. 113–136.

45. Behr TM, Memtsoudis S, Vougioukas V, Liersch T, Gratz S, Schmidt F, et al. Radioimmunotherapy of colorectal cancer in small volume disease and in an adjuvant setting: preclinical evaluation in comparison to equitoxic chemotherapy and initial results of an ongoing phase-I/II clinical trial. Anticancer Res 1999;19:2427–32.

46. Behr TM, Salib AL, Liersch T, Behe M, Angerstein C, Blumenthal RD, Fayyazi A, Sharkey RM, Ringe B, Becker H, Wörmann B, Hiddemann W, Goldenberg DM, Becker W. Radioimmunotherapy of small volume disease of colorectal cancer metastatic to the liver: preclinical evaluation in comparison to standard chemotherapy and initial results of a phase I clinical study. Clin Cancer Res 1999;5:3232–42.

47. Behr TM, Liersch T, Greiner-Bechert L, Griesinger F, Béhé M, Markus PM, et al. Radioimmunotherapy of small volume disease of metastatic colorectal cancer: results of a phase-II trial with the ^{131}I-labeled humanized anti-CEA antibody, hMN-14. Cancer, in press.

48. Juweid M, Sharkey RM, Behr T, Swayne LC, Rubin AD, Hanley D, et al. Targeting and initial radioimmunotherapy of medullary thyroid carcinoma with ^{131}I-labeled monoclonal antibodies to carcinoembryonic antigen. Cancer Res 1995;55:5946–51.

49. Juweid M, Sharkey RM, Behr T, Swayne LC, Herskovic T, Pereira M, et al. Radioimmunotherapy of medullary thyroid cancer with iodine-131-labeled anti-CEA antibodies. J Nucl Med 1996;37:905–11.

50. Hird V, Maraveyas A, Snook D, Dhokia B, Soutter WP, Meares C, et al. Adjuvant therapy of ovarian cancer with radioactive monoclonal antibody. Br J Cancer 1993;68:403–6.

51. Behr TM, Memtsoudis S, Sharkey RM, Blumenthal RD, Dunn RM, Gratz S, et al. Experimental studies on the role of antibody fragments in cancer radio-immunotherapy: Influence of radiation dose and dose rate on toxicity and anti-tumor efficacy. Int J Cancer 1998;77:787–95.

52. Behr TM, Sgouros G, Vougiokas V, Memtsoudis S, Gratz S, Schmidberger H, et al. Therapeutic efficacy and dose-limiting toxicity of Auger-electron vs. beta emitters in radioimmunotherapy with internalizing antibodies: evaluation of [125]I- vs. ^{131}I-labeled CO17-1A in a human colorectal cancer model Int J Cancer 1998;76:738–48.

53. Behr TM, Goldenberg DM, Becker W. Reducing the renal uptake of radiolabeled antibody fragments and peptides for diagnosis and therapy: present status, future prospects and limitations. Eur J Nucl Med 1998;25:201–12.

54. Reubi JC. Regulatory peptide receptors as molecular targets for cancer diagnosis and therapy. Q J Nucl Med 1997;41:63–70.

55. Reubi JC. Neuropeptide receptors in health and disease: The molecular basis for in vivo imaging. J Nucl Med 1995;36:1825–35.

56. Behr TM, Gotthardt M, Barth A, Béhé M. Imaging tumors with peptide-based radioligands. Q J Nucl Med 2001;45 (in press).

57. Reubi JC, Landolt AM. High density of somatostatin receptors in pituitary tumors from acromegalic patients. J Clin Endocrinol Metab 1984;59;1148–51.

58. Reubi JC. Neuropeptide receptors in health and disease: The molecular basis for in vivo imaging. J Nucl Med 1995;36:1825–35.

59. Krenning EP, Kwekkeboom DJ, Pauwels S, Kvols LK, Reubi JC. Somatostatin receptor scintigraphy. In: Freeman LM (ed.). Nuclear Medicine Annual 1995. New York: Raven Press, 1995; 1–50.

60. Krenning EP, Kwekkeboom DJ, Bakker WH, Breeman WA, Kooij PP, Oei HY, et al. Somatostatin receptor scintigraphy with [111In-DTPA-D-Phe1]- and [123I-Tyr3]-octreotide: the Rotterdam experience with more than 1000 patients. Eur J Nucl Med 1993;20:716–731.

61. Denzler B, Reubi JC. Expression of somatostatin receptors in peritumoral veins of human tumors. Cancer 1999;85:188–98.

62. Bohuslavizki KH, Brenner W, Gunther M, Eberhardt JU, Jahn N, Tinnemeyer S, et al. Somatostatin receptor scintigraphy in the staging of small cell lung cancer. Nucl Med Commun 1996;17:191–6.

63. Otte A, Jermann E, Béhé M, Goetze M, Bucher HC, Roser HW, et al. DOTATOC: a powerful new tool for receptor-mediated radionuclide therapy. Eur J Nucl Med 1997;24:792–5.

64. Paganelli G, Zoboli S, Cremonesi M, Bodei L, Ferrari M, Grana C, et al. Receptor-mediated radiotherapy with ^{90}Y-DOTA-D-Phe3-Tyr3-octreotide. Eur J Nucl Med 2001;28:426–34.

65. Reubi JC, Waser B. Unexpected high incidence of cholecystokinin / gastrin receptors in human medullary thyroid carcinomas. Int J Cancer 67 (1996), 644–647.

66. Reubi JC, Schaer JC, Waser B. Cholecystokinin(CCK)-A and CCK-B / gastrin receptors in human tumors. Cancer Res 1997;57:1377–86.
67. Behr TM, Jenner N, Radetzky S, Behe M, Gratz S, Yucekent S, et al. Targeting of cholecystokinin-B/gastrin receptors in vivo: preclinical and initial clinical evaluation of the diagnostic and therapeutic potential of radiolabelled gastrin. Eur J Nucl Med 1998;25 :424–30.
68. Behr TM, Jenner N, Béhé M, Angerstein C, Gratz S, Raue F, et al. Radiolabeled peptides for targeting of cholecystokinin-B/gastrin receptor expressing tumors: from preclinical development to initial clinical results. J Nucl Med 1999;40:1029–44.
69. Behr TM, Béhé M, Angerstein C, Gratz S, Mach R, Hagemann L, et al. Cholecystokinin-B/gastrin receptor binding peptides: preclinical development and evaluation of their diagnostic and therapeutic potential. Clin Cancer Res 1999;5:2124–38.
70. Behr TM, Griesinger F, Riggert J, Gratz S, Béhé M, Kaufmann CC, et al. High-dose myeloablative radioimmunotherapy of mantle cell non-Hodgkin's lymphoma with the ^{131}I-labeled chimeric anti-CD20 antibody C2B8 and autologous stem cell support: results of a pilot study. Cancer, in press.
71. Divgi CR, Scott AM, Dantis L, Capitelli P, Siler K, Hilton S, et al. Phase I radioimmuno-therapy trial with iodine-131-CC49 in metastatic colon carcinoma. J Nucl Med 1995;36:586–92.
72. Murray JL, Macey DJ, Kasi LP, Rieger P, Cunningham J, Bhadkamkar V, et al. Phase II radioimmunotherapy trial with ^{131}I-CC49 in colorectal cancer. Cancer 1994;73:1057–66.
73. Welt S, Divgi CR, Kemeny N, Finn RD, Scott AM, Graham M, et al. Phase I/II study of iodine 131-labeled monoclonal antibody A33 in patients with advanced colon cancer. J Clin Oncol 1994;12:1561–71.
74. Welt S, Scott AM, Divgi CR, Kemeny NE, Finn RD, Daghighian F, et al. Phase I/II study of iodine 125-labeled monoclonal antibody A33 in patients with advanced colon cancer. J Clin Oncol 1996;141787–97.
75. Meredith RF, Khazaeli MB, Plott WE, Spencer SA, Wheeler RH, Brady LW, et al. Initial clinical evaluation of iodine-125-labeled chimeric 17-1A for metastatic colon cancer. J Nucl Med 1995;36:2229–33.
76. Behr TM, Sharkey RM, Juweid ME, Dunn RM, Vagg RC, Ying Z, et al. Phase I/II clinical radioimmunotherapy with an ^{131}I-labeled anti-CEA murine IgG monoclonal antibody. J Nucl Med 1997;38:858–70.
77. Juweid ME, Sharkey RM, Behr TM, Swayne LC, Dunn R, Siegel J, et al. Radioimmunotherapy of patients with small-volume tumors using iodine-131-labeled anti-CEA monoclonal antibody NP-4 F(ab')$_2$. J Nucl Med 1996;37:1504–10.
78. Wong JY, Williams LE, Yamauchi DM, Odom-Maryon T, Esteban JM, Neumaier M, et al. Initial experience evaluating [90]yttrium-radiolabeled anti-carcinoembryonic antigen chimeric T84.66 in a phase I radioimmunotherapy trial. Cancer Res 1995;55:5929–34.
79. Ychou M, Pelegrin A, Faurous P, Robert B, Saccavini JC, Guerreau D, et al. Phase-I/II radioimmunotherapy study with Iodine-131-labeled anti-CEA monoclonal antibody F6 F(ab')$_2$ in patients with non-resectable liver metastases from colorectal cancer. Int J Cancer 1998;75:615–9.

12. Cell-mediated Dysregulation in Malignancy and Its Therapeutic Immunopotentiation

Theresa L. Whiteside

Introduction

Cell-mediated immunity is thought to be largely responsible for detection and elimination of intracellular pathogens, which are inaccessible to humoral factors. Both natural and adaptive immunity play an important role in maintaining vigilance against viruses, fungi and other invading pathogens. In addition, cells of the immune system are responsible for regulation of the immune responses, including humoral responses, and maintaining homeostasis. This regulatory role of immune cells is central to our well-being, as excessive or suppressed immune responses are associated with the development of disease. Autoimmunity is a manifestation of excessive response against self antigens, a transplant rejection is a result of an aggressive immune response to foreign antigens; infections become chronic because of insufficient or ineffective immune mechanisms and development of cancer is associated with the partly disabled immune system.

Many years ago, a concept of immune surveillance was developed by Sir McFarlane Burnet, which attributed to immune cells the role of a guardian protecting the host against cancer development [1]. Thus cancer developed because the immune system malfunctioned. This concept has been sustained by observations that in immunodeficient animals or individuals, a high frequency of lymphoproliferative diseases were encountered [2] or that patients treated with immunosuppressive drugs developed malignancies with greater frequencies than those encountered in the control populations [3]. While the immunosurveillance theory has focused attention on a relationship between the immune system and cancer, it has not found support in the light of new knowledge. Today, cancer progression is viewed as a series of genetic and molecular alterations, leading to the emergence of cells, which initially are not perceived as a "danger signal" by the immune system [4] and later become resistant to immune intervention. Immune selection results in the elimination of altered tissue cells which are recognized by the immune system and in proliferation of those cells that escape recognition. Thus, from the earliest stages of tumorigenesis, tumor cells develop means of escape from recognition by immune cells. Seen in this context, the successful tumor avoids immune surveillance by overcoming natural defenses and inducing T-cell tolerance. The mechanisms used by the tumor to disarm the immune system have been under intense investigation in recent years. The understanding of molecular mechanisms underlying tumor-induced immunosuppression is crucial for immunotherapy of cancer. Up to now, immunotherapy has had little impact on the treatment of human cancer, primarily because complete responses have been relatively infrequent and the reasons for failure of immunotherapy in most patients and its success in only a few remain unclear.

In view of a considerable progress made recently in our understanding of molecular mechanisms governing the development of immune responses, it is now possible to set down several basic principles of tumor immunology as follows:

1. Tumors develop in the presence of the normal immune system in the host and immune cells are rendered ineffective, eliminated or used as a source of growth factors by the developing tumor.
2. Tumors express antigens, which are recognized by T cells but in most cases these are self epitopes, which are poorly immunogenic.
3. Tumors can be eradicated by manipulations of the immune system, leading to recognition and elimination of the tumor by immune effector cells.

Components of the Anti-tumor Immune Response

Immune responses to the tumor have been extensively investigated in vivo in tumor-bearing animals as well as in patients with cancer [5,6]. The general consensus of these studies appears to be that tumors express at least three types of antigens recognized by the immunocompetent host:

(a) MHC-restricted tumor-associated peptides shared by histologically-distinct tumors and silent in normal tissues, with the exception of germ cells in the testes and ovaries, such as MAGE 1 or 3, BAGE, GAGE and many others [7].
(b) differentiation-specific antigens exemplified by melanoma- and melanocyte-associated tyrosinase, MART1/Melan A or gp 100 [8].
(c) unique antigens generated by point mutations in ubiquitously expressed genes, which regulate key cellular functions, such as MUC-1, CDK4, FLICE or β-catenin [9–11].

These TAAs are clearly recognized by the host immune cells, as the presence of both antibodies and specific cell-mediated responses has been documented in tumor-bearing humans as well as animals [9,10]. This means that tumor antigens can engage an immune response, i.e., are "antigenic." However, the immune response generated appears to be ineffective in eliminating the tumor, either because the necessary components of this response are missing or because the tumor manages to avoid it. Therefore, TAA are operationally non-immunogenic or, at best, weakly immunogenic. This is not surprising, as most TAA overexpressed or inappropriately expressed by human tumors are unmutated differentiation or "self" antigens, which do not function as tumor-rejection antigens. Many of these antigens, notably TAA in melanoma, have been identified and characterized using T cells as specific probes and are referred to as "T-cell-defined" antigens [10]. The role of these antigens in immunotherapy remains controversial.

In addition to TAA-specific responses, tumors induce non-MHC-restricted, inflammatory responses in the host, especially at the time when tissue necrosis develops, leading to the accumulation of granulocytes and macrophages at the site of tumor or metastatic growth. As in most chronic diseases, both non-specific and specific components of the host response play a role in the control of tumor growth and metastasis, with some components, e.g., natural killer (NK) cells, PMN and macrophages thought to participate in the early phase of the response, prior to the appearance of tumor-specific T or B cells. The latter are essential for the development of immunologic memory. Both tumor-specific CTL and helper (CD4+) T cells as well as antibodies (Abs) are essential for antitumor effector functions [9,12]. NK cells could also be engaged in elimination of those tumor cells which fail to express individual MHC molecules and thus are not recognized by tumor-specific T cells [13].

For an effective immune response against the tumor to develop, a number of cellular interactions must take place at the right place and at the right time. Thus, expression of TAA by the tumor is not sufficient to drive the response. Such TAA have to be "biologically screened" and presented to immune cells by antigen-presenting cells (APC). Dendritic cells (DC) are responsible for processing and presentation of TAA to lymphocytes [14]. In most cases, these events occur in lymph nodes, whose anatomical structure facilitates antigen-presenting functions of DC in the T cell-rich paracortical regions and maturation of antibody-producing plasma cells in the medulla [15]. When TAA-sensitized T cells leave the lymph node environment, they make their way via the lymphatics to the site(s) of the tumor and presumably arrive there as primed but not necessarily fully differentiated effector cells. It is also likely, but so far not proven, that the DC which localize at the tumor site (referred to as tumor-associated DC or TADC) represent TAA to accumulating primed lymphocytes, inducing their activation, proliferation and maturation into anti-tumor effector cells. In addition, these TADC mediate sensitization with TAA of any naïve T cells that might be present at the tumor site. Thus, interactions between the tumor-infiltrating T lymphocytes (TIL) and tumor-resident DC (TADC) are essential for driving the local immune response and for generation of anti-tumor effector cells. Survival of both T cells and DC is enhanced by reciprocal signaling between these two cell types. A number of molecules expressed on the surface of hematopoietic and tumor cells and referred to as co-stimulatory receptor-ligand pairs participate in mediating these interactions [16]. Stimulatory signals delivered to immune cells via these molecules are essential for an effective immune response to develop.

A schematic representation of cellular interactions involving tumor and hematopoietic cells at the tumor site can be found in Figure 12.1. In order for these interactions to result in an anti-tumor immune response, the cells have to cooperate and the signals regulating the response have to be delivered at the right time. The interactions are orchestrated and carefully regulated at the cellular and molecular levels and dysfunction of any one component of the network will result in an inappropriate, absent or defective immune response. Also, because these interactions are complex, a possibility exists for multiple defects in more than one cellular component of the network. It is also important to emphasize that local immune responses, similar to those depicted in Figure 12.1, are a component of the simultaneously ongoing systemic response to the tumor and the composition, number as well as the state of activation/differentiation of the cellular infiltrate at the local site will tend to vary, depending on the systemic immune response to

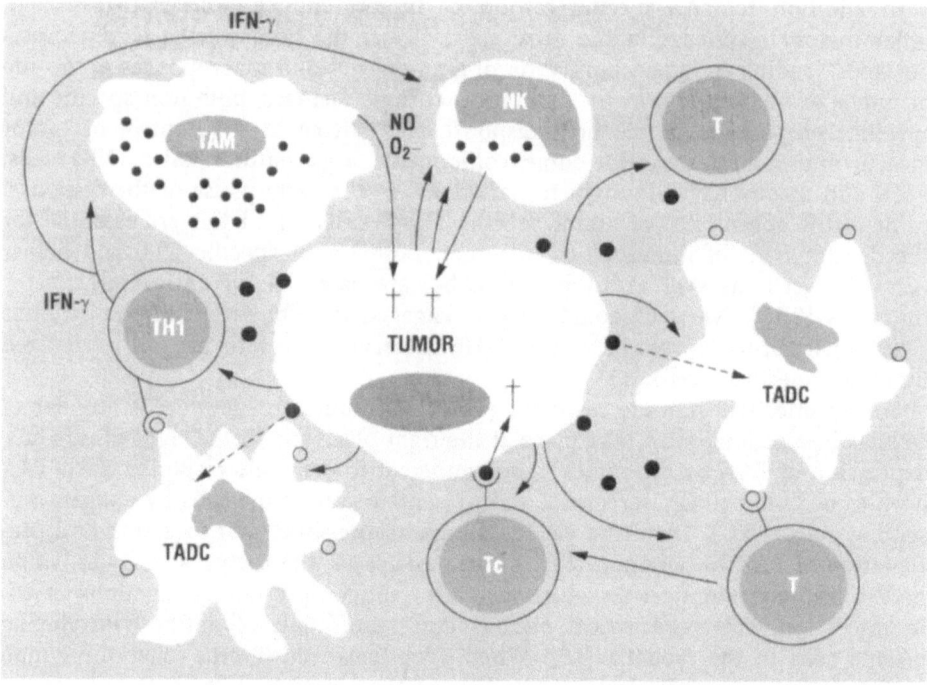

Figure 12.1. A schema of cellular interactions between the tumor and hematopoietic cells in the tumor microenvironment. Abbrreviations: TAM=tumor associated macrophages; TADC=tumor associated dendritic cells; Tc=cytolytic T cells; Th1=Thelper cell; NK=natural killer cell; + lysis of tumor cells; → antigen uptake; ● tumor antigen; ○ processed antigen.

TAA. At the same time, immunotherapy experience indicates that locoregional delivery of immunostimulatory agents often results in systemic activation of immune responses [17]. Thus, the locoregional and systemic immune responses to the tumor are intimately linked.

Tumor-induced Suppression of Immune Cells

Early experiments, dating back more than 30 years, provided evidence that tumors can alter functions of immune cells. In these experiments, supernatants of various tumor cells were found to suppress proliferation and/or cytotoxicity of normal human PBMC in vitro (reviewed in [18]). These observations from several independent laboratories demonstrated that immunosuppressive factors were produced by human tumors but not by normal tissue cells. In some cases, these soluble factors were subsequently partially purified from supernatants of tumor cells [19]. Over the years, the number of tumor-associated factors with immuno-suppressive activity grew to include those listed in Table 12.1. The list is not complete, as other factors described in the literature but not completely characterized are not included. Table 12.1 contains several categories of inhibitory factors (cytokines, retroviral-like peptides, over-produced normal metabolites,

Table 12.1. Molecularly-defined tumor-derived immunoinhibitory factors[a]

1. The TNF family ligands	Induce leukocyte apoptosis via the TNF family receptors
FasL	Fas
TRAIL	TRAIL-Rs
TNF	TNFR1
2. Small molecules	
Prostaglandin E_2 (PGE$_2$)	Inhibits leukocyte functions through increased cAMP [82, 83]
Histamine	Inhibits leukocyte functions through increased cAMP [83]
Epinephrine	Inhibits leukocyte functions through increased cAMP [83]
INOS	Promotes or inhibits Fas-mediated apoptosis by regulation of NO levels [83]
H_2O_2	Has pro-oxidant activity, increases cAMP levels, causes apoptosis in NK cells, inhibits tumor-specific CTL [83]
3. Cytokines/Growth factors	
TGF-β	Inhibits perforin and granzyme mRNA expression; inhibits lymphocyte proliferation [84, 85]
IL-10	Inhibits production of IL-1β, IFN-γ IL-12 and TNFα [86, 87]
GM-CSF	Promotes expansion of immunosuppressive tumor-associated macrophages [88]
VEGF	Inhibits maturation of DC [42]
4. Viral-related products	
p15E	Inhibits production of IFN-γ, IL-2, TNFα, IL12, upregulates
(CKS-17 synthetic peptide)	IL-10 synthesis [21, 89]
EBI-3	Inhibits IL-12 production [90]
	(homologue of IL-12 p40)
5. Tumor-associated gangliosides	Inhibit IL-2 dependent lymphocyte proliferation or induce apoptotic signals [91]

[a] A partial list of immunosuppressive factors selected to demonstrate their diversity and a wide spectrum of effects on immune cells. Reproduced with modifications from Whiteside and Rabinowich [92].

iNOS) and this suggests that numerous possibilities for inhibition of immune cells exist in cancer patients. Indeed, tumor-induced inhibition might be mediated by several distinct mechanisms. Some of the inhibitory factors may be associated with the surface of tumor cells, while others are released into the tissue and peripheral circulation. In a few cases, tumor-derived inhibitory factors have been purified and are available as synthetic proteins/peptides, e.g., the retroviral-related p15E-derived peptides [20,21]. Not all of the immunosuppressive factors listed in Table 1 are made by all human tumors. More likely, tumors vary in their ability to express and produce the inhibitory molecules and tumors which are strongly immunosuppressive are able to produce several different factors. It is reasonable to conclude that the microenvironment of the developing, and especially of the advanced, tumor is not supportive of immune effector cells and may, in fact, induce their dysfunction or even death. Furthermore, in view of the evidence that at least some of the tumor-derived factors are present in the peripheral circulation [22,23], it is highly likely that not only local but also systemic interference with immune/inflammatory responses occurs in patients with malignancies.

Functions of Immune Cells in the Tumor Microenvironment

If tumors are responsible for inducing immunosuppression in cancer patients, then immune effector cells most intimately associated with the tumor will likely be most strongly affected. Those not in contact with the tumor may only be minimally or not at all immunosuppressed. This, in fact, appears to be the case, as indicated by studies of human tumor-infiltrating lymphocytes (TIL). These cells have been studied extensively in various human tumors (reviewed in [24]) and much is known about their phenotypic and functional characteristics. When freshly isolated from surgical specimens, TIL appear to be mainly CD3+ T cells, which are activated, as judged by expression of various activation markers on the cell surface and which contain variable proportions of CD8+ and CD4+ T cells. They are almost exclusively CD45RO+ memory T cells (reviewed in [24,25]). However, in spite of their activation phenotype, TIL freshly isolated from surgical tumor biopsies have been found to be functionally impaired [26–30]. In comparison to autologous peripheral blood lymphocytes or those isolated from tissues distant from the tumor, TIL have been consistently poorly-responsive or unresponsive to the usual T-cell activating stimuli, when tested in various functional in vitro assays at the population or single-cell level (see Table 12.2). Table 12.2 summarizes evidence accumulated to date for functional deficiencies observed in fresh TIL isolated from a wide variety of human tumors. Proliferation in response to mitogens, antigens or cytokines and anti-tumor cytotoxicity were found to be depressed in TIL [24] anti-tumor and CD8+ T cells separated from human solid tumors by flow cytometry had more extensive functional defects than CD4+ T cells [26]. The cytokine profile of fresh TIL is also different from that of normal T cells: levels of mRNA for IL-2 and IFN-γ as well as expression of the respective proteins were significantly decreased or absent in these cells [31,32]. More recently, defects in Ca^{++} mobilization and reduced expression of signaling molecules, especially the ζ and ε chains associated with TcR on TIL have been documented in several laboratories, including our own [33–38]. Others have demonstrated abnormalities in NF-κB binding activity in TIL and peripheral T cells obtained from patients with cancer [39]. In aggregate, these data indicate that the apparently activated T-cells derived from tumor sites or tumor-involved human lymph nodes are functionally compromised and do not behave like normal activated T cells.

Table 12.2. Effects of the tumor microenvironment on functions of lymphocytes

1. Activates proteolytic enzymes in infiltrating leukocytes [38].
2. Induces NF-κB degradation in tumor-associated lymphocytes [39].
3. Induces signaling defects in lymphocytes at the tumor site and in the blood [36,93,94].
4. Inhibits Ca^{++} flux in tumor-associated lymphocytes [45].
5. Alters cytokine expression: induces depression of TH1 responses [20].
6. Inhibits lymphocyte proliferation and other functions by inducing the pro-oxidant state [83,95].
7. Inhibits leukocyte migration [96].
8. Induces apoptosis in tumor-associated leukocytes through the Fas/FasL-mediated pathway [45].
9. Favors expansion of immunosuppressive macrophages [97].

Functional impairments are also present in other effector cells which accumulate at the tumor site. While TIL have been studied extensively, much less information is available about DC in the tumor microenvironment. Nevertheless, several recent reports indicate that these TADC are also functionally defective, especially in their antigen-presenting functions [40–42]. Tumor-associated macrophages (TAM) have also been found to contain various functional defects relative to their counterparts obtained from non-tumor inflammatory sites [43, 44]. Mononuclear cells obtained from sites of inflammation and studied in parallel with TAMs do not exhibit these defects [43].

Co-incubation of Lymphocytes with Tumor Cells

If the tumor is the culprit in inducing signaling and functional defects in lymphocytes entering its microenvironment, then a series of simple in vitro experiments would be expected to provide indications about the events taking place in situ. Freshly-isolated or cultured tumor cells can be incubated with normal allogeneic or autologous lymphocytes for various periods of time to determine whether defects in lymphocyte signaling or other lymphocyte functions can be detected following co-incubation. We observed reduced expression of the ζ chain in T cells by Western blots and by flow cytometry after 24h of such co-culture [38]. Evidence has been obtained from these type of in vitro studies that activated lymphocytes are especially susceptible to tumor-induced inhibition, that the inhibition is non-MHC restricted and that pre-incubation of T lymphocytes with a peptide aldehyde, LLnL (which inhibits both lysosomal and proteasomal peptidase activity), prevents degradation of signaling molecules in these lymphocytes (H. Rabinowich, unpublished data). These data indicate that tumor cells can induce activation of intracellular peptidases in T lymphocytes, which are then responsible for degradation of signal-transducing proteins, including the ζ chain. We have shown, using RT-PCR, that mRNA for the ζ chain is detectable at nearly normal levels in those TIL which have reduced CD3-ζ chain expression. This finding supports the conclusion that the tumor may directly induce post-translational modifications of signal-transducing proteins in tumor-associated lymphocytes [38,45]. The possibility had to be considered that activation of intracellular proteases, which was responsible for the loss or reduction in the ζ chain expression, may be a part of the apoptotic cascade initiated in T cells by the contact with tumor cells. Indeed, in the same type of co-incubation experiments we also observed that DNA fragmentation was detectable in a significant proportion of lymphocytes incubated in the presence of tumor cells (38,45). Thus, not only signaling defects but apoptosis could be induced in lymphocytes co-incubated with tumor cells. Furthermore, the ζ chain itself has been identified as a substrate for caspases, the family of enzymes responsible for executing apoptosis or cell death (46). A computer-assisted analysis of the amino acid sequence of ζ protein revealed the presence of sites sensitive to cleavage by caspases. Subsequent experiments revealed that the ζ chain is a substrate for caspases 3 and 7, which cleave it into smaller fragments (46). Therefore, activation of caspases in lymphocytes interacting with the tumor (and perhaps also other death inducing molecules) can lead to low or absent expression of the TCR-associated ζ chain.

Biologic Significance of the ζ Chain Down-regulation

Much attention has been devoted lately to the ζ chain down-regulation in activated T lymphocytes [47]. As shown in Figure 12.2, ζ is the signaling protein of
the TcR complex. As such, it plays a major role in TcR-mediated activation of T
cells. It has been determined that there are six phosphorylation sites or ITAMS
(immune receptors tyrosine-based activation motifs) on each of the two ζ chains
in the TcR (see Figure 12.2). The effective TcR signal induces ordered successive
phosphorylation of all six ITAMS. Interactions of correctly assembled TcR on the
cell surface with the APC presenting a cognate MHC-peptide complex triggers the
receptors. The process of T-cell triggering is self-limited, and down-regulation of
triggered TcR involves a loss of ζ protein. The mechanisms responsible for this
loss are not clear, although internalization and lysosomal degradation of TcR,
including the ζ chain, have been observed in experiments involving human T-cell
clones specific for tetanus toxoid peptides [48]. The T cells then proceed to
replace the internalized receptors on the cell surface and to interact again with the
immunogenic peptide. As indicated above, lysosomal degradation may not be the
only mechanism of cellular degradation of ζ. Nevertheless, it is important to note

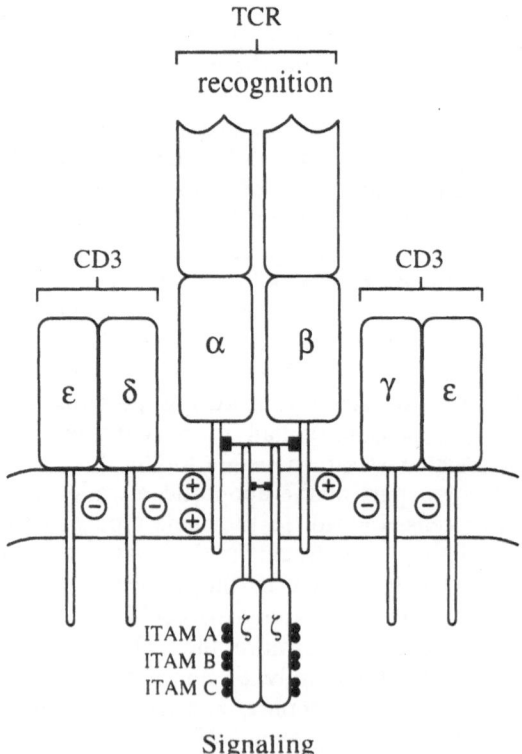

Figure 12.2. Schematic representation of T cell receptor expressed on the surface of T lymphocytes.
Note that the ζ chain homodimer is a signaling component of the complex. A single ζ chain contains
three ITAMS, each incorporating 2 phosphotyrosines. Upon full T-cell activation, all six tyrosines become
phosphorylated.

that chronic antigenic stimulation via TcR may lead to prolonged or even permanent down-regulation of ζ expression and to partial or complete T-cell anergy.

The question remains whether T-cell dysfunction associated with absent ζ or low expression of ζ is biologically significant for the tumor-bearing host. It has been observed that only mice with methylcholantrene-induced transplantable tumors which grow slowly, have compromised immune responses, including low ζ expression in T and NK cells [49]. In contrast, animals with rapidly growing tumors had reasonably normal immune responses and showed no or little ζ chain down-regulation in lymphocytes [49]. These observations are interpreted to indicate that a slow, chronic nature of host-tumor interactions, similar to that in patients with cancer, is associated with immunosuppression. As cancer is a chronic disease, immunosuppression observed in patients with advanced malignancy could be a by-product of chronic antigenic stimulation, incorporating aspects of activation-induced cell death (AICD), tumor-induced cell death (TICD) as well as immunologic "exhaustion." While ζ down-regulation is seen in only a proportion of patients with cancer, its presence appears to be a poor prognostic factor. For example, ζ chain expression was measured in TIL present in biopsies of oral carcinoma obtained from 138 patients for whom a follow-up of >5 yrs. was available [50]. Absent or low expression of ζ in TIL was detected in 32 percent of tumors and was significantly associated with a high tumor stage (T3 or T4) as well as with nodal involvement [50]. In oral carcinoma patients with advanced disease, normal expression of ζ in TIL was predictive of a significantly better 5-year survival independent of other established prognostic parameters [50]. Thus, expression of ζ in TIL was identified as an independent prognostic factor in oral carcinoma. ζ may also be a marker of response to biologic therapy, based on the finding that among 19 patients with ovarian carcinoma receiving intraperitoneal interleukin-2 (IL-2) therapy, 9 clinical responders to therapy had normal ζ expression in circulating T cells prior to therapy, while in 10 non-responders to IL-2, ζ expression was significantly decreased (I. Kuss, T.L. Whiteside, unpublished). This observation reinforces our initial impressions that in patients with cancer, ζ may be a marker of immune competence in individuals most likely to respond favorably to biotherapy and it emphasizes a need for further studies of this intriguing possibility. It is apparent from these and other studies that biologic consequences of decreased or absent ζ expression in immune cells could be profound, due to the key role this protein plays in T-cell receptor (TcR) signaling.

Evidence for Lymphocyte Apoptosis in Cancer Patients

Recent in vitro experiments have demonstrated that co-incubation with autologous tumor cells leads to DNA fragmentation in a proportion of activated T lymphocytes, presumably by the mechanism similar or identical to activation-induced cell death (AICD). Alternatively, it is possible that tumor is directly responsible for inducing apoptosis in TIL (TICD). The biologic significance of this finding was confirmed when TUNEL assays (which detect DNA fragmentation) were performed in human tumor biopsies and tumor-involved lymph nodes [45]. Contrary to expectations firmly based on years of in vitro experiments with activated effector cells which killed susceptible tumor cell targets, it was not tumor cells but TIL and DC that were positive in TUNEL assays [45]. Control normal tissues or tumor-uninvolved tissues obtained from patients with cancer contained no or only few apoptotic lymphocytes [45]. This unexpected finding was subsequently confirmed, using tumor tissues from a variety of patients with cancer [38, 51–53] and it was possible to document, by performing TUNEL assays in conjunction with immunostaining for CD3 or for CD80, that DNA fragmentation occurred in T cells or DC, respectively [38]. Evidence has been recently provided that T lymphocytes in the peripheral blood of patients with malignancies show significantly enhanced spontaneous apoptosis when incubated ex vivo. A short incubation in culture media reveals the presence of DNA breaks in a significantly larger proportion of these cells as compared with normal peripheral blood lymphocytes [54,55]. More sensitive assays (Annexin V binding or caspase-3 activity) which detect early apoptotic cells, also show that the number of such pre-apoptotic cells is higher in patients with cancer than in normal donors [54]. The observation that up to 80 percent of T cells in the peripheral circulation of patients with melanoma express Fas versus fewer than 30 percent in most normal controls [54] suggests that the majority of activated T cells may be destined to die by means of activation-induced cell death (AICD).

One unanswered question about immune cells in patients with cancer concerns the preferential sensitivity of tumor-specific CTL to apoptosis [56]. The availability of labeled tetramers specific for HLA-restricted peptides allows for evaluation by flow cytometry of the presence of tumor peptide-specific T cells in the circulation of patients with cancer [57,58]. Preliminary studies, using HLA-A0201 tetramers specific for tyrosinase and peripheral blood T lymphocytes of a patient with melanoma, indicated that peptide-specific T cells were dysfunctional, while EBV-specific T cells functioned normally [57]. This observation suggests that CD8+ T cells specific for tumor-associated peptides may be preferentially targeted for dysfunction or even death. With advances in the tetramer technology, future studies will be able to elucidate the fate of tumor-specific CTL and CD4+ T cells in patients with cancer.

Mechanisms Responsible for Effector Cell Apoptosis in the Tumor Microenvironment

The findings of multiple functional defects and evidence for apoptosis in immune effector cells isolated from the tumor site or peripheral circulation of patients with advanced malignancies have generated a great deal of controversy as to the mechanisms responsible for these phenomena. The possibility that they represent artifacts induced by PMN- or monocyte-derived proteases activated during tissue or blood processing has been considered [59] and is thought to be unlikely in view of in situ results, which document the presence of dysfunctional or apoptotic effector cells in tumor-involved tissues. At the same time, it is apparent that T lymphocyte or TAM populations isolated from tumors, lymph nodes or body fluids of patients with cancer are not all irreversibly damaged, as recovery of proliferative and cytolytic functions occurs in response to cytokines ex vivo in a subset of these cells upon their removal from the tumor site. Some investigators have been successfully utilizing TIL obtained from patients with melanoma or ovarian carcinoma as a source of T cells specific for TAA (reviewed in [25]). Nevertheless, earlier limiting-dilution studies with human TIL have indicated that only a small subset of T cells retains or recovers the ability to proliferate in response to IL-2 in culture [28, 60–62]. Thus, it appears that in any TIL population, a spectrum of tumor-induced functional abnormalities might exist. Some effector cells or their precursors in the population are not defective and are either protected from or not sensitive to apoptosis. These effector cells can be rescued and expanded following removal from the tumor site or upon exposure to exogenous cytokines. In addition, these effector cells may be selectively increased in number at the tumor site.

Recent studies of apoptosis in immune cells suggest that death of activated T cells or AICD is an essential part of an immune response, necessary for regulation of a potentially destructive expansion of powerful effector cells. In this mode, T cells achieving a high level of activation and expressing the TNF-family receptor-ligand pairs become sensitive to Fas-mediated death [22,63]. There is evidence that crosslinking of Fas with agonistic Abs, kills only activated T cells and that activated T cells express increased levels of Fas [64]. Thus in lymphocytes, sensitivity to Fas-mediated death is a regulated phenomenon, in which both IL-2 and antigenic stimulation play a crucial role. Thus, in AICD, IL-2 is a potentiating cytokine, which at appropriate concentrations and in the presence of relevant antigen enhances the Fas/FasL pathway in activated T cells. AICD is induced by repeated or chronic antigenic stimulation and neither co-stimulatory molecules nor the Bcl-2 family members can rescue T cells from AICD. Furthermore, TH1 cells appear to be more sensitive to AICD than TH2 cells.

With respect to T cells in the tumor microenvironment, it is clear that they are exposed to excess of TAA and chronic or repeated antigenic stimulation. As indicated above, they are primed and activated and they prominently express Fas on their cell surface [38,45]. Thus, these lymphocytes might be particularly sensitive to AICD via, e.g., the Fas/FasL pathway. However, expression of IL-2 in the tumor has been repeatedly shown to be very low or absent both at the message and protein level [31,32]. TIL in situ do not appear to produce IL-2 and newer evidence indicates that IL-2R transcription is reduced and IL-2 mRNA translation is defective in TIL obtained from human breast carcinomas [65]. If IL-2 is required for the assembly or functionality of the Fas death complex in lymphocytes [66,67], then it becomes questionable to what extent AICD is responsible for the demise of T cells in the tumor. A somewhat different but related mechanism may be envisioned, in which the tumor not only induces lymphocyte dysfunction, including the reduced ability to produce IL-2 and IFN-γ [32], but also capitalizes on expression of the TNF family receptors on TIL. A variety of freshly-harvested or cultured human tumor cells were examined for expression of FasL and have consistently documented expression of surface and/or cytosolic FasL [38,68]. In a recently-completed study, we have demonstrated that human SCCHN not only contain mRNA and intracytoplasmic FasL but express FasL on the cell surface [68,69]. The FasL expressed on the tumor cell surface is biologically active, as it participates in inducing death of activated T cells co-incubated with an excess of the tumor cells [68,69]. Apoptosis of these T cells was blocked in the presence of an antagonistic anti-Fas Ab (ZB4) and anti-FasL Ab (4H9) as well as FasFc [38], and it was also completely inhibited by pre-incubation of lymphocytes with caspase inhibitors Z-VAD-FMK or Z-DEVD-FMK. Addition of a metalloproteinase inhibitor (BB-94) to these co-cultures significantly increased the level of lymphocyte apoptosis, suggesting that surface expression of FasL and its activity are in part regulated by metalloproteinases [68,69]. Soluble FasL, presumably cleaved from the tumor cell surface by metalloproteinases, is present in tumor cell super-natants and sera of some patients with cancer [23,50]. It is thus likely that TIL which directly interact with tumor cells are killed via the Fas-death complex. The fact that tumor cells nearly always vastly exceed the number of TIL or TADC in vivo explains, in part, how the local environment might facilitate tumor-induced apoptosis of immune effector cells rather than AICD in these infiltrating cells.

However, this interpretation is not universally accepted. The presence of FasL on some human tumors, including melanoma, is controversial, and its role in apoptosis of effector cells in the tumor microenvironment is intensely debated at the present time [70,71]. Also, it is important to remember that TRAIL and other TNF family ligands are also expressed on human tumors and are likely to partici-pate in the events occurring during interactions of the tumor with immune effec-tor cells [72].

Immunotherapy and Protection of Effector Cells from Tumor-induced Dysfunction

In view of the evidence for immune dysfunction in the tumor microenvironment, one of the objectives of immunotherapy is to identify and evaluate therapeutically promising strategies for protection of immune cells from death. Although therapy with cytokines such as IL-2, IFNs or IL-12 has been used by many investigators to treat malignancies in recent years (reviewed in 73), it has never been specifically directed toward preventing death of immune effector cells. On the contrary, the rationale behind cytokine therapies has been the up-regulation of antitumor func-tions of immune effector cells, especially T cells specific for TAA. In retrospect, it seems that attempts to up-regulate functions of cells that are dying are not likely to succeed. A new strategy for cytokine delivery and perhaps new cytokines are necessary to rescue the dying cells or, better, to protect them from death-inducing signals. For example, providing DC or DC transduced with cytokine genes might be effective in preventing apoptosis in effector cells.

Immunotherapy of cancer with cytokines, ex vivo activated immune cells, vac-cines and more recently, peptide or genetically-modified vaccines, has been under study for almost 30 years. Partial or complete responses, which have lasted for several years in some patients, have been documented in a proportion of patients with advanced disease (10–30%, depending on the type of cancer as well as the center in which therapy is given). In addition, in a substantial but variable pro-portion of patients, stabilization of the disease and up-regulation of non-specific as well as specific immune responses have been observed (reviewed in [74]). These results indicate that immune therapies with biologic agents might result in the amelioration of the disease progression. Unfortunately, however, many patients have not shown any demonstrable benefits from immunotherapy [74]. Thus, the question remains as to why only some and not most cancer patients respond to immunotherapies and why tumor-specific immune responses have been so difficult to demonstrate in various in vitro monitoring assays.

Recent progress in tumor immunology has led to novel insights about func-tions and interactions of the immune cells (T, B, NK, MF and DC) and molecules expressed on these cells, which determine the development and efficacy of anti-tumor immune responses. In addition, a better understanding of molecular signals and mechanisms involved in the generation of productive immune responses in general, has focused attention on those molecular events that occur or do not occur in the tumor microenvironment. The realization that immune cells undergo apoptosis in tumors has led to a search for the mechanism(s) responsible for this death and was instrumental in singling out the TNF family of receptors and ligands as one class of factors mediating tumor-induced apoptosis [75, 76]. This realization was prefaced by the recognition of the Fas/FasL pathway and its role in maintaining immune privilege at sites such as the anterior chamber of the eye, the brain, the testis or the thyroid gland [77–79]. The notion that tumors might also be able to protect themselves from immune effector cells by inducing their death was both appealing and supported by the extensive evidence that these effector cells are dysfunctional in the tumor microenvironment [80] (Table 12.2). It also provided a reasonable explanation for a limited success of adoptive immunotherapy with activated effector cells in patients with cancer [81]. However, it has now become necessary to confirm that the newly-identified mechanisms leading to apoptosis of immune cells apply to tumor-effector cell interactions. If immune effector cells die in the tumor and if the rate of their demise exceeds that of survival, then it might be surmised that tumor-induced apoptosis of immune cells might be an important prognostic parameter. This hypothesis has to be tested. The potential ability of immunotherapies to protect effector cells from apoptosis might be related to the clinical response and this hypothesis can be formally examined. The question of how to best protect immune cells from premature tumor-induced apoptosis becomes the essential, but so far inadequately explored, goal of cancer immunotherapy.

There is a certain degree of urgency associated with implementation of new strategies for immunotherapy of cancer in view of extensive vaccination efforts on-going worldwide in patients with melanoma, renal cell, prostate, colon, ovarian and breast carcinomas as well as other malignancies. These clinical trials (largely initiated in patients with advanced metastatic disease) are not likely to yield optimal results if only a proportion of the vaccine-induced, tumor-specific effector cells survive in vivo. Moreover, if a proportion of specific T cells or DC are preferentially killed and if the level of apoptosis exceeds that of effector cell influx into the tumor or their generation within the secondary lymphoid sites, anti-tumor vaccines may be ineffective. To avoid likely disappointments, it might be necessary to combine vaccinations with therapies providing protection of T-cells from tumor-induced apoptosis. Preliminary evidence from pre-clinical animal models as well clinical trials, indicate that DC as well cytokines can protect immune effector cells from apoptosis in the tumor microenvironment.

References

1. Burnet FM. Immunological surveillance in neoplasia. Transplantation Rev 1971;7:3–25.
2. Hanto D, Frizzera G, Gajil-Peczalski, K, and Simmons R. Epstein-Barr virus, ummunodefficiency, and B cell lymphoproliferation. Transplantation 1985;39:461–72.
3. Starzl T E, Nalesnik MA, Porter KA, Ho M, et al. Liver stability of lymphomas and lymphoproliferative lesions developing under cyclosporine-steroid therapy. Lancet 1985;1:583–7.
4. Fuchs EJ, Matzinger P. Is cancer dangerous to the immune system? Semin Immunol. 1996;8:271–80.
5. Monach PA, Meredith SC, Siegel CT, Schreiber H. A unique tumor antigen produced by a single amino acid substitution. Immunity 1995;2:45–9.

6. Boon T, Coulie PG, Van der Eynde B. Tumor antigens recognized by T cells. Immunol Today 1997;6:267–8.

7. Van der Eynde B, Van der Bruggen P. T-cell defined tumor antigens. Current Opinion in Immunol 1997;9:684–93.

8. Cox A, Skipper J, Chen Y, Henderson RA, et al. Identification of a peptide recognized by five melanoma-specific human cytotoxic T cell lines Science 1994;264:716–9.

9. Henderson RA, Finn OJ. Human tumor antigens are ready to fly. Adv Immunol 1996;62:217–56.

10. Boon T, Old LJ. Cancer tumor antigens. Current Opinion in Immunol. 1997;9:681–3.

11. Mandruzzatto S, Brasseur F, Andry G, Boon T, Van der Bruggen P. A CASP-8 mutation recognized by cytolytic T lymphocytes on a human head and neck carcinoma. J Exp Med 1997;186:785–93.

12. Sahin U, Turecio P, Pfzeundschuch M. Serological identification of human tumor antigens. Current Opinion in Immunol 1997;9:709–16.

13. Whiteside TL, Herberman RB. Role of natural killer cells in immune surveillance of cancer. Current Opinion in Immunol 1995;7:704–10.

14. Celluzzi CM, Mayordomo JI, Storkus WJ, Lotze MT, Falo LD. Peptide-pulsed dendritic cells induce antigen specific CTL-mediated protective tumor immunity. J Exp Med 1996; 183:283–7.

15. Gretz JE, Anderson AO, Shaw S. Cords, channels, corridors and conduits: critical architectural elements facilitating cell interactions in the lymph node cortex. Immunol Rev 1997;156:11–24.

16. Allison JP, Hurwitz AA, Leach DR. Manipulation of costimulatory signals to enhance anti-tumor T cell responses. Current Opinion in Immunol 1995;7:682–6.

17. Whiteside TL, Letessier E, Hirabayashi H, Vitolo D, Bryant J, Barnes L, et al. Evidence for local and systemic activation of immune cells by peritumoral injections of interleukin 2 in patients with advanced squamous cell carcinoma of the head and neck. Cancer Res 1993;53:5654–62.

18. Whiteside TL, Rabinowich H. The role of Fas/FasL in immunosuppression induced by human tumors. Cancer Immunol. Immunother 1998;46:175–84.

19. Ebert EC, Roberts AI, O'Connell SM, Robertson FM, Nagase H. Characterization of an immunosuppressive factor derived from colon cancer cell. J Immunol 1987;138:2161–8.

20. Haraguchi S, Good RA, James-Yarish M, Cianciolo GJ, Day NK. Differential modulation of Th1- and Th2-related cytokine mRNA expression by a synthetic peptide homologous to a conserved domain within retroviral envelope protein. Immunology 1995;92:3611–5.

21. Cianciolo GJ, Copeland TD, Oroszlan S, Snyderman R. Inhibition of lymphocyte proliferation by a synthetic peptide homologous to retroviral envelope proteins. Science 1985;230:453–5.

22. Nagata S, Goldstein P. The Fas death factor. Science 1995;267:1449–56.

23. Tanaka M, Itai T, Adachi M, Nagata S. Downregulation of FasL by shedding. Nature Med 1998;4:31–6.

24. Whiteside TL. Tumor-Infiltrating Lymphocytes in Human Malignancies, Austin, TX: R.G. Landes Co., 1993.

25. Whiteside TL, Parmiani G. Tumor-infiltrating lymphocytes: their phenotype, function and clinical use. Cancer Immunol Immunother 1994;39:15–21.

26. Miescher S, Stoeck M, Qiao L, Barras C, Barrelet L, von Fliedner V. Preferential clonogenic deficit of CD8+ T lymphocytes infiltrating human solid tumors. Cancer Res 1988;48:6992–8.

27. Miescher S, Stoeck M, Qiao L, Barras C, Barrelet L, vonFliedner V. Proliferation and cytolytic potentials of purified human tumor-infiltrating T lymphocytes. Impaired response to mitogen-driven stimulation despite T-cell receptor expression. Int J Cancer 1988;42:659–66.

28. Miescher S, Whiteside TL, Moretta L, von Fliedner V. Clonal and frequency analysis of tumor-infiltrating T lymphocytes from human solid tumors. J Immunol 1987;138:4004–11.

29. Miescher S, Whiteside TL, Carrell S, von Fliedner V. Functional properties of tumor infiltrating and blood lymphocytes in patients with solid tumors: Effects of tumor cells and their supernatants on proliferative responses of lymphocytes. J Immunol 1986;136:1899–1907.

30. Whiteside TL. Tumor-infiltrating lymphocytes as antitumor effector cells. Biotherapy 1992;5:47–61.

31. Vitolo D, Zerbe T, Kanbour A, Dahl C, Herberman RB, Whiteside TL. Expression of mRNA for cytokines in tumor-infiltrating mononuclear cells in ovarian adenocarcinoma and invasive breast cancer. Int J Cancer 1992;51:573–80.

32. Rabinowich H, Suminami Y, Reichert TE, Crowley-Nowick P, Bell M, Edwards R et al. Expression of cytokine genes or proteins and signaling molecules in lymphocytes associated with human ovarian carcinoma. Int J Cancer 1996;68:276–84.

33. Finke JH, Zea AH, Stanley J, Longo DL, Mizoguchi H, Tubbs RR, et al. Loss of T-cell receptor ζ chain and p56[lck] in T-cell infiltrating human renal cell carcinoma. Cancer Res 1993;53:5613–6.

34. Matsuda M, Petersson M, Lenkei R, Raupin J-L, Magnusson I, Mellstedt H, et al. Alterations in

the signal-transducing molecules of T cells and NK cells in colorectal tumor-infiltrating gut mucosal and peripheral lymphocytes: correlation with the stage of the disease. Int J Cancer 1995;61:765–72.

35. Mizoguchi H, O'Shea JJ, Longo DL, Loeffler CM, McVicar DW, Ochoa A. Alterations in signal transduction molecules in T lymphocytes from tumor bearing mice. Science 1992;258:1795–8.

36. Nakagomi H, Petersson M, Magnusson I, Juhlin C, Matsuda M, Mellstedt H, et al. Decreased expression of the signal-transducing ζ chains in tumor-infiltrating T-cell and NK cells of patients with colorectal carcinoma. Cancer Res 1993;53:5610–2.

37. Lai P, Rabinowich H, Crowley-Nowick PA, Bell MC, Mantovani G, Whiteside TL. Alterations in expression and function of signal transduction proteins in tumor associated NK and T lymphocytes from patients with ovarian carcinoma. Clin Cancer Res 1996;2:161–73.

38. Rabinowich H, Reichert TE, Kashii Y, Bell MC, Whiteside TL. Lymphocyte apoptosis induced by Fas ligand-expressing ovarian carcinoma cells: implications for altered expression of TcR in tumor-associated lymphocytes. J Clin Invest 1998;101:2579–88.

39. Li X, Liu J, Park J-K, Hamilton TA, Rayman P, Klein E, et al. T cells from renal cell carcinoma patients exhibit an abnormal pattern of NFκB specific DNA binding activity. Cancer Res 1994;54:5424–9.

40. Lopez DM, Watson GA. Aberrant antigen presentation by macrophages from tumor-bearing mice is involved in the down-regulation of their T cell responses. J Immunol 1995;3124–34.

41. Gabrilovich DI, Corak J, Ciernik IF, Kavanaugh D, Carbone DP. Decreased antigen presentation by dendritic cells in patients with breast cancer. Clin Cancer Res 1997;3:483–90.

42. Gabrilovich, DI, Chen HL, Girgis KR, Cunningham T, Meny GM, Nadaf S, et al. Production of vascular endothelial growth factor by human tumors inhibits the functional maturation of dendritic cells. Nature Medicine 1996;2:1096–103.

43. Mantovani A, Bottazzi B, Colotta F, Sozzani S, Ruco L. The origin and function of tumor-associated macrophages. Immunol. Today 1992;13:265–70.

44. Mantovani A. Tumor-associated macrophages in neoplastic progression: a paradigm for the *in vivo* function of chemokines. Lab Investigation 1994;71:5–16.

45. Reichert TE, Rabinowich H, Johnson JT, Whiteside TL. Human immune cells in the tumor microenvironment: mechanisms responsible for signaling and functional defects. J Immunother 1998;21:295–306.

46. Gastman BR, Johnson DE, Whiteside TL, Rabinowich H. Caspase-mediated degradation of TCR-ζ chain. Cancer Res 1999;59:1422–7.

47. Whiteside TL. Signaling defects in T lymphocytes of patients with malignancy. Symposium-in-writing. Cancer Immunol Immunother 1999; 48:346–52.

48. Valitutti S, Müller S, Salio M, Lanzavecchia A. Degradation of T cell receptor (TCR)-CD3-ζ complexes after antigenic stimulation. J Exp Med 1997;185:1859–64.

49. Horiguchi S, Petersson M, Nakazawa T, Kanda M, Zea AH, Ochoa AC et al.. Primary chemically induced tumors induce profound immunosuppression concomitiant with apoptosis and alterations in signal transductio in T cells and NK cells. Cancer Res 1999;59:2950–6.

50. Reichert, TE, Day, R., Wagner, E., Whiteside, TL Absent or low expression of the ζ chain in T cells at the tumor site correlates with poor survival in patients with oral carcinoma. Cancer Res 1998;58:5344–7.

51. Hahne M, Rimoldi D, Schroter M, Romero P, Schreier LE, French P, et al. Melanoma cell expression of Fas (Apo-1/CD95) ligand: Implications for tumor immune escape. Science 1996;274:1363–6.

52. Keane MM, Ettenberg SA, Lowrey GA, Russell EK, Lipkowitz S. Fas expression and function in normal and malignant breast cell lines. Cancer Res 1996;56:4791–8.

53. Niehans GA, Brunner T, Frizelle SP, Liston JC, Salerno CT, Kanpp DJ, et al. Human lung carcinomas express Fas ligand. Cancer Res 1997;57:1007–12.

54. Saito T, Dworacki G, Gooding, W, Lotze M, Whiteside TL. Spontaneous apoptosis of CD8+ T lymphocytes in the peripheral blood of patients with advanced melanoma. Clin Cancer Res 2000 (In Press).

55. Saito T, Kuss I, Dworacki G, Gooding W, Johnson JT, Whiteside TL. Spontaneous *ex vivo* apoptosis of peripheral blood mononuclear cells in patients with head and neck cancer. Clin Cancer Res 1999;5:1263–73.

56. Walker PR, Saas P, Dietrich PY. Role of Fas Ligand (CDS95L) in immune escape: the tumor cell strikes back. J Immunol 1997;158:4521–4.

57. Lee PP, Yee C, Savage PA, Fong L, Brockstedt D, Weber JS, et al. Characterization of circulating T cells specific for tumor-associated antigens in melanoma patients. Nature Med 1999;5:677–85.

58. Pittet MJ, Valmori D, Dunbar PR, Speiser DE, Liénard D, Lejeune F, et al.. High frequencies of

naïve melan-A/MART-1-specific CD8+ T cells in a large proportion of human histocompatibility leukocyte antigen (HLA)-A2 individual. J Exp Med 1999;190:705–15.

59. Aoe T, Okamoto Y, Saito T. Activated macrophages include structural abnormalities of the T-cell receptor-CD3 complex. J Exp Med 1995;181:1881–6.

60. Mukherji B, MacAlister TJ. Clonal analysis of cytotoxic T-cell response against human melanoma. J Exp Med;158:240–5.

61. Shimizu Y, Iwatsuki S, Herberman RB, Whiteside TL. Clonal analysis of tumor-infiltrating lymphocytes from human primary and metastatic liver tumors. Int J Cancer 46:878–883.

62. Whiteside TL, Miescher S, Hurlimann J, von Fliedner V. Separation, phenotyping and limiting-dilution analysis of T-lymphocytes infiltrating human solid tumors. Int J Cancer 1986;37:803–11.

63. Tanaka M, Suda T, Takahashi T, Nagata S. Expression of the functional soluble form of human Fas ligand in activated lymphocytes. EMBO J 1995;14:1129–35.

64. Suda T, et al. Expression of the Fas Ligand in cells of T-cell lineage. J Immunol 1995;154:3806–3813.

65. Lopez CB, Rao TD, Feiner H, Shapiro R, Marks JR, and Frey AB. Repression of interleukin-2 mRNA translation in primary human breast carcinoma tumor-infiltrating lymphocytes. Cell Immunol 1998;190:141–55.

66. Lenardo M. Interleukin-2 programs mouse alpha/beta T lymphocytes for apoptosis. Nature 1991;353:858–61.

67. Esser MT, Dinglasan RD, Krishnamurthy B, Gullo CA, Graham MB, Braciale VL. Interleukin 2 (IL-2) induces Fas ligand/Fas (CD95L/CD95) cytotoxicity in CD8+ and CD4+ T lymphocyte clones. J Immunol 1997;158:5612–8.

68. Gastman BR, Atarashi Y, Reichert TE, Saito T, Balkir L, Rabinowich H, et al. Fas Ligand is expressed on human squamous cell carcinomas of the head and neck and it promotes apoptotis of T lymphocytes. Cancer Res 1999;59:5356–64.

69. Gastman BR, Johnson DE, Whiteside TL, Rabinowich H. Activation of caspase-3 and cleavage of Bcl-2 in tumor-induced apoptosis of T lymphocytes. 1998 (Submitted).

70. Chappel DB, Zaks TZ, Rosenberg SA, Restifo NP. Human melanoma cells do not express Fas (Apo-1/CD95) Ligand. Cancer Res 1999;59:59–62.

71. Chappel DB, Restifo NP. T cell-tumor cell: a fatal interaction? Cancer Immunol Immunother 1998;279:6–10.

72. Zhang XD, Franco A, Myers K, Gray C, Nguen T, Hersey P. Relaxation of TNF-related apoptosis-inducing ligand (TRAIL) receptor and FLICE-inhibitory protein expressio to TRAIL-induced apoptosis of melanoma. Cancer Res 1999;59:2747–53.

73. Lotze MT. Cytokines and the Treatment of Cancer. In: Weir, Herzenberg, Herzenberg, Blackwell, editors. The Handbook of Experimental Immunology, 5th Edition. Cambridge, MA: Blackwell Sciences, Inc., 1996; Chapter 199: pp 199.1–199.25.

74. Lotze MT, Rubin JT, Whiteside TL, Herberman RB. Cytokine and cellular-mediated immunotherapy of cancer. In: Rich RR, Fleisher TA, Schearer WT, Strobert W. editors. Clinical Immunology. Principles and Practice, Vol. 2. St. Louis: Morby, 1996; 1919–30.

75. O'Connell J, Bennett MW, O'Sullivan GC, Collins JK, Shanahan F. The fas counterattack: a molecular mechanism of tumor immune privilege. Mol Medicine 1997;3:294–300.

76. O'Connell J, O'Sullivan GC, Collins JK, Shanahan F. The Fas counterattack: fas-mediated T cell killing by colon cancer cells expressing Fas ligand. J Exp Med 1996;184:1075–82.

77. Griffith TS, Ferguson TA. The role of FasL-induced apoptosis in immune privilege. Immunol Today 1997;18:240–244.

78. Griffith TS, Brunner SM, Fletcher SM, Green DR, Ferguson TA. Fas ligand-induced apoptosis as mechanism of immune privilege. Science 1995;270:1189–92.

79. Giordano C, Stassi G, DeMaria R, et al. Potential involvement of Fas and its ligand in the pathogenesis of Hashimoto's thyroiditis. Science 1997;275:960–3.

80. Sulitzeanu D. Immunosuppressive factors in human cancer. Adv Cancer Res 1993;60:247–71.

81. Whiteside TL. Cellular adoptive therapy of cancer: expectations and reality. In Chouaib S. editor, Biotherapy of Cancers: from Immunotherapy to Gene Therapy. Paris: Editions INSERM, 1998; 239–55.

13. Colorectal Tumor Immunity

Lindy G. Durrant, Ian Spendlove and Judith M. Ramage

Introduction

There have been many successes for immunotherapy, including BCG for treatment of bladder cancer, recombinant cytokine/tumor infiltrating lymphocyte (TIL) therapy and the use of monoclonal antibodies such as Herceptin, that target growth factor receptors and induce apoptosis. However, more recent studies have led to a better understanding of the molecular basis for immune recognition of cancer. Many tumor antigens have been identified and numerous vaccination approaches have been tested in the clinic leading to new insights into the complexity of tumor immunity. Although vaccination results in stimulation of T cell responses, this appears to be rarely associated with tumor regression. This relative lack of response may be due to only partial activation of T cells which proliferate but do not acquire full effector function as well as to the tumor environment which is hostile to the incoming T cell infiltrate. The challenge for the future will be to fully activate anti-tumor immunity whilst combating the profoundly tolerogenic tumor environment.

Tumor Antigens

Screening of cDNA expression libraries with either T cell clones or high titer serum IgG from cancer patients has allowed the identification of a large number of tumor antigens [1–3]. According to their expression pattern, function or genetic origin, these antigens can be classified into 5 categories; Cancer Testis (CT) antigens (e.g. MAGE, NY-ESO-1), differentiation antigens (MelanA/MART-1, tyrosinase, gp100), mutated antigens (K-ras, p53, Caspase 8, CDF-4), over-expressed "self" antigens (CEA 17-1A, CD55, p53, EGFr) and viral antigens (HPV, EBV). As viruses have not been implicated in the etiology of colorectal cancer, they have no role to play as colorectal cancer targets. CT antigens are ideal targets as the genes encoding them are silent in normal cells except for germ line cells, which do not express HLA molecules. However, although cancer testis antigens may be useful in melanoma therapy, their expression on colorectal tumors is much more heterogeneous, making them poor targets. Similarly, mutated gene products are poor targets as they are only suitable in a minority of patients with the appropriate mutation that can be expressed on a permissive HLA haplotype. Tissue differentiation antigens that escape immune tolerance may be appropriate colorectal cancer targets as are over-expressed self-antigens. In the latter case it is of interest that most of the epitopes recognized by patients T cells are only of moderate affinity. This is probably because T cells which recognize high affinity self-epitopes have been deleted in the thymus or tolerized in the periphery as already discussed elsewhere in this book. Over-expression of these antigens by tumors allows the moderate affinity epitopes to reach the activation threshold for T cell activation and thus normally silent T cells become activated. Moderate affinity CD8 epitopes are also poor immunogens, as they do not compete effectively with higher affinity epitopes for occupation of Class I major histocompatibility (MHC) antigens. An elegant solution to this problem is to mutate anchor residues in order to give higher affinity MHC binding without alteration of T cell receptor recognition [4].

Vaccination Approaches

T cell epitopes can be presented as peptides, proteins and DNA or integrated into attenuated viruses (Table 13.1). All of these approaches have been tried in clinical trials with varying degrees of success. Peptides have consistently stimulated cytotoxic lymphocyte (CTL) responses against a variety of antigens and in combination with IL-2 give more objective clinical remissions when compared with IL-2 treatment alone. Many of the remissions associated with peptide vaccination are partial and transient. This may be related to the rapid proteolytic digestion of peptides that fail to sustain an immune response. Approaches to stabilize peptides by adding lipid tails or to present them complexed with heat shock proteins may be more effective [5]. A further reason for poor clinical responses may be due to the observation that although immunization increases the frequency of antigen specific cells, (as measured by tetramer staining), very few of these CD8 cells develop into full effector cells capable of lytic function and expressing perforin. This has highlighted the need to also stimulate antigen-specific CD4 responses to help maintain immune reactivity against the tumor. Indeed in studies where peptides from several target antigens were used, patients frequently made a response to only a single peptide and this was commonly associated with the ability of the peptide to also stimulate an inflammatory CD4 response [6]. Partial remissions were often associated with re-growth of tumors lacking the target antigen. This is a particular problem if the target antigen is not essential for tumor survival and suggests that targeting antigens involved in tumor progression, (such as p53), may be a more attractive anti-tumor strategy. Targeting several antigens would also help alleviate this problem but this requires careful epitope selection to avoid immunodominance [7].

Recombinant proteins have been effective at stimulating antibody responses but are poor T cell immunogens. An alternative approach may be to immunize patients with antigen/antibody complexes, since a recent study has shown that these target the high affinity Fc receptor (CD64) located on dendritic cells, allowing efficient processing and presentation of T cell epitopes on both Class I and II MHC molecules [8]. Furthermore, Fc endocytosis also activates dendritic cells to present co-stimulatory molecules. Thus Fc targeting of activated dendritic cells results in a 1,000 fold increase in efficiency of antigen processing and presentation [9].

Table 13.1. Different Vaccine Approaches

Vaccines	Advantage	Disadvantage	Future
Peptides	Good CTL responses in vivo	Short half-life in vivo as they are rapidly degraded	Add lipid tails. Complex to heat-shock proteins.
		Poor clinical responses as CD8 cells not fully activated	Link to peptides that stimulate anti-tumor CD4 responses
		Target single epitopes that can lead to antigen loss variants	Multi-epitopic peptide vaccines
Recombinant Proteins	Several B and T Cell epitopes	Proteins are only taken up by APCs by pinocytosis, a very inefficient process that rarely results in Class I presentation	Target proteins to CD64 receptors either as antigen-antibody complexes or as anti-idiotypic antibodies. CD64 receptor internalization allows Class I and II MHC presentation and induces costimulation.
Viral vectors	Good Class I presentation	Neutralizing antibodies quickly remove the virus from the circulation	Non-mammalian viruses may circumvent this problem but may present competing epitopes.
Naked DNA	Good Class I and II presentation	May integrate into genome	Sub-unit DNA vaccines.

Many groups have tried to improve the immunogenicity of proteins by encoding the antigens within viruses or bacteria. These approaches have been disappointing in the clinic as many patients have pre-existing neutralizing antibodies that quickly remove the virus from the circulation. The use of non-mammalian viruses may circumvent this problem, however, these complex viruses have many immunodominant epitopes that compete with the tumor epitopes.

As the duration of immunization determines the magnitude of the immune response, DNA immunization is an attractive approach. DNA vaccination most closely mimics viral infection as following injection, antigen presenting cells can be directly transfected giving efficient priming of CTL responses. Although antigen-presenting cells transfected by the DNA plasmid may not survive for long periods of time, the plasmid is also taken up by mycocytes (im) or keratinocytes (id) that continue to secrete protein for long periods of time. The protein can be secondarily taken up by antigen presenting cells to stimulate both helper and antibody responses and to boost the CTL response. DNA vaccination against both HIV and malaria has been successfully used in combination with Modified Vaccinia Anchoria (MVA) vaccination to stimulate CTL responses [10]. Similar approaches are currently being tested in cancer with 8 linked tumor specific CTL epitopes encoded within a plasmid and an MVA construct. T cell clones to each CTL epitope recognize target cells transfected with the MVA construct. Furthermore, vaccination with DNA and then the MVA construct stimulates CTL responses in HLA-A2 transgenic mice to all 8 epitopes. This approach demonstrates that with careful selection of T cell epitopes it is possible to avoid immunodominance and stimulate T cell response against a range of antigens thus avoiding selection of antigen loss tumor variants. Considerable success has also been found with B cell idiotype scFv DNA vaccination, showing complete tumor regression in mouse models. These vaccines encode a tetanus toxoid helper epitope to aid in the stimulation of antibody responses and clinical trials are currently underway. It will be of interest to see if similar encouraging results can be generated against solid tumors or indeed if it will be necessary to modify this approach to also stimulate antigen specific CD4 and CD8 cells.

Colorectal Tumor Microenvironment

The colorectal tumor microenvironment is hostile to infiltrating immune cells taking part in immunosurveillance since the normal colon protects itself from the damaging effects of Th1 cellular immune responses in part by releasing immune inhibitory factors such as TGFβ and prostaglandins.

Immunosurveillance

Until recently it has remained controversial as to whether the immune system could actually recognize in situ tumors, since early studies in nude mice failed to demonstrate enhanced susceptibility to tumor growth. Both cellular and antibody responses recognizing tumor antigens could be demonstrated in a range of patients and many tumors showed classical signs of immune avoidance, such as loss of MHC and antigen processing function. Studies in γIFN receptor knockout, STAT-1 knockout mice or RAG2$^{-/-}$ deficient mice, (that lack all T, NKT and B lymphocytes), showed that they all had an enhanced susceptibility to both carcinogen-induced and spontaneous tumors. Furthermore, the tumors which developed in the absence of lymphocytes were more immunogenic than those arising in immunocompetent mice. Thus immunosurveillance can prevent tumor growth, however, if tumors persist despite anti-tumor immunity, they acquire other mechanisms to resist immune attack.

Colorectal Tumor Growth (Figure 13.1)

In the development of a colorectal cancer, small tumors growing as a nest of cells are unlikely to stimulate much of an immune response, as they present no danger to the host. However, when the tumor reaches a certain size, cells undergo necrosis, which may activate dendritic cells to migrate to lymph nodes and present tumor antigens to T cells. Effector T cells may then return and attack the growing tumor (immunosurveillance). Tumor cells may actively escape this attack by losing antigen or down-regulating antigen presentation on MHC molecules. Furthermore, solid tumors frequently arise in tissues that protect themselves from the damaging consequences of Th1 immune responses by releasing factors such as TGFβ and PGE-2. As the tumor continues to develop, hypoxia within necrotic

1) Small tumor — No danger

— No immune response

2) Growing tumor "necrosis"

— As the tumor grows central cells become necrotic and release intracellular components that activate dendritic cells to migrate to lymph nodes and stimulate immunosurveillance. This either results in tumor death or the tumor fights back by losing MHC, antigen or releasing suppressive factors such as TGFβ and PGF.

3) Angiogenesis

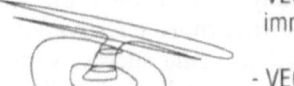

— Tumor produces VEGF to promote angiogenesis

— VEGF inhibits dendritic cell activation and immunosurveillance is switched off

— VEGF also stimulates production of complement regulatory proteins resulting in tumor resistant to antibody responses

4) Metastasis

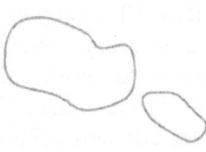

— Advanced tumors become increasingly resistant to immune attack

SOLUTION: Stimulate strong inflammatory Th1 responses in early tumors

Figure 13.1. Colorectal tumor growth.

TUMOUR GROWTH AND ANGIOGENESIS METASTASIS

areas may stimulate the production of vascular endothelial growth factor (VEGF) to induce new blood vessel formation. VEGF can also inhibit the activation of dendritic cells [11] and presentation of tumor antigen in the absence of co-stimulation, effectively induces peripheral tolerance and which may stimulate other regulatory T cells. VEGF also stimulates the expression of the complement regulatory proteins CD55 and CD46 in cells within the tumor microenvironment. The binding of C3b to CD46 on macrophages also stimulates IL-10 production and the switch from cytolytic Th1 to relatively immunosuppressive Th2 responses. Furthermore, our recent studies have suggested that extracellular CD55 not only deactivates complement but also inhibits T cell proliferation and cytokine secretion, resulting in an intra-tumoral anti-inflammatory environment.

The final stage of tumor development, once a good blood supply has been established, is to bring in B cells to the tumor site which can bind shed antigen and stimulate humoral immunity. This model is consistent with the observation from SEREX studies that high titer serum IgG responses to tumor antigens are most frequently found in the late stage bulky solid epithelial malignancies. However, these antibodies do not control tumor growth as the tumor cells are protected from complement lysis by expression of complement regulatory proteins and from antibody-dependent cellular cytotoxicity (ADCC) by the anti-inflammatory environment that fails to allow extravasation of NK cells and macrophages.

Thus tumors which survive the initial immune response become increasingly resistant to further attacks. One approach may be to reverse the anti-inflammatory environment at the tumor site thus allowing more effective extravasation of immune effector cells. In this context Coley had some success with direct intra-tumor injection of a bacterial cocktail known as "Coley's toxin". Unfortunately, due to several deaths from septicemia, this practice was stopped. More recently live-attenuated *Salmonella typhimurium* have been injected into patients. This bacterium localizes and grows in anoxic regions, such as the center of tumors. It remains to be seen if this approach will stimulate appropriate Th1 inflammatory responses at the tumor site. An alternative approach is to vaccinate patients to produce tumor specific Th1 cells which can provide help for the induction and maintenance of CD8 cells and play a broader role in mediating the activation of dendritic cells, macrophages and eosinophils [12–15]. Initial results obtained in mice appear to support this concept [16,17]. Furthermore, several recent reports have suggested that CD4 cells can mediate direct killing of class II-expressing tumor cells [18].

Thus the optimum cancer vaccine should stimulate CD4 responses that home to the site of the tumor and that initiate an inflammatory cascade which aids recruitment of competent effector cells into the tumor to reverse the Th2 environment imposed by the tissue in which the tumor arose. These CD4 cells also help in the production of CD8 cells that are the most efficient cellular killers. The vaccine should stimulate both CD4 and CD8 responses against a range of target antigens to avoid selection of antigen loss variants. Similarly, targeting antigens that are essential for tumor survival will help prevent the development of these antigen loss variants. Targeting tumor suppressor genes is an attractive approach here where it may be possible to target proteins over-expressed by the tumor cells which protect them from inflammatory responses by complement regulatory proteins. This approach may have the dual effect of killing tumor cells and reversing the hostile tumor environment. An alternative way of over-coming the tumor environment may be to target tumor endothelial cells as antigen heterogeneity, MHC loss and resistance to apoptosis that are associated with transformed epithelial cells are unlikely to be a problem with endothelial cells. Furthermore even limited damage to the tumor vasculature results in large-scale destruction of tumor cells and a highly inflammatory environment. These and other approaches for colorectal tumor immunotherapy will be discussed in more detail in the next section.

New Approaches in Anti-tumor Therapy for Colorectal Cancer

Whole Cell Vaccines

There has been some reported success immunizing patients with their own tumor cells admixed with a "danger" signal. In a non-randomized study, Dukes' stage B and C colorectal cancer patients were immunized with irradiated autologous tumor cells mixed with Newcastle disease virus, 3 times, at 2-week intervals beginning 6–8 weeks after surgery. The survival for all patients ($n = 48$) at 2 years was 98 percent, compared with 74 percent for matched historical controls ($n = 661$). The corresponding figures for Dukes' stage C were 95 percent and 62 percent respectively [19]. Using a similar protocol, Hagmuller et al. reported a 3-year survival of 88 percent ($n = 50$) for stage B colorectal carcinoma and 87 percent ($n = 41$) for stage C, compared with survival of 56 percent for historical controls at the same clinic [20]. Great caution must be exerted in drawing conclusions from these non-randomized studies which report survival benefits. Encouraging results have been obtained from one randomized study although the numbers are very small. Dukes' stage B2-C3 colon cancer patients were immunized 3 times with irradiated autologous tumor cells admixed with BCG. With a median follow-up of 93 months, there was a significant improvement in survival ($p = 0.03$) and disease-free survival ($p = 0.04$) for immunized patients ($n = 24$) in a prospective randomized study [21].

One problem with this approach is the limitation on the number of immunizations that can be given due to the number of autologous tumor cells that are obtained when the tumor is resected. This can be overcome by the use of allogeneic tumor cell lines that are presented to T cells via the patient's own antigen presenting cells (APCs). The other problem with whole cell vaccines is that they present a large number of potential peptides from a wide range of antigens. The peptides with the highest affinities for MHC will therefore predominate. Moreover, T cells recognizing high affinity self epitopes may have been deleted in the thymus.

Carcinoembryonic Antigen Vaccines

Carcinoembryonic antigen (CEA) is one of the best characterized tumor marker antigens and it is extensively expressed in humans in the majority of colorectal, gastric and pancreatic carcinomas. The first evidence that T cells from cancer patients could recognize and respond to CEA was demonstrated by in vitro immunization with anti-idiotypic antibody which mimics CEA [22]. An antibody recognizing an antigen might also bind specifically to the combining site of a second antibody. This second, or anti-idiotypic, antibody can therefore be a mimic of the original epitope and can be used to induce immune responses that recognize either anti-idiotypic antibody or antigen. (See Chapter 9)

A Phase I clinical trial with another anti-idiotypic antibody, 3H1, (which mimics CEA), in advanced colorectal cancer, has demonstrated anti-CEA antibody responses in 9/12 patients, with four patients showing T cell proliferative responses to CEA. Toxicity was limited to local reaction with mild fever and chills [23]. In a new study treating patients with minimal residual disease, 9/12 patients showed T cell responses to both the anti-idiotypic antibody and CEA. This vaccine failed, however, to elicit CTL responses, necessitating the development of recombinant CEA for use as an immunogen. Two clinical studies have been carried out using recombinant CEA. Two of five breast cancer patients showed CEA-specific proliferative responses and one also had a CEA-specific delayed-type hypersensitivity (DTH) response [24]. In the second study, the addition of the cytokine granulocyte-macrophage colony-stimulating factor (GM-CSF) that recruits more dendritic cells from the bone marrow, enhanced the proliferative responses to CEA from 2/6 patients to 6/6 patients. No toxicity was observed [25] but no CTL responses were observed either.

There are several T cell epitopes that have been identified within CEA, so this is not the problem with this approach, but lack of CTLs must be due to inefficient antigen processing for class I presentation. To overcome this problem the CEA gene has been inserted into the vaccinia genome (rV-CEA). A phase I study of this construct in patients with metastatic carcinoma showed, for the first time, that it was possible to induce cytolytic T cell responses to CEA which killed tumor cells [26]. Unfortunately, the immune response to the vaccinia inhibited replication of the administered recombinant virus at subsequent immunizations and therefore it was not possible to boost the primary immune response to CEA with the vaccinia construct. Animal studies have suggested that priming with rV-CEA and then boosting with either recombinant CEA or specific CEA peptides is a very efficient immunization protocol and clinical trials are currently being planned. It is possible to identify the relevant peptide stimulating the CTLs and show that it was only expressed in CEA and not non-cross reactive antigen, a CEA-related protein, thus giving the desired tumor specificity. It is also possible to increase the efficiency of T cell stimulation by changing one of the amino acids within the peptide. This change does not affect binding of the peptide to MHC so it is assumed that it allows better recognition by the T cells which can still recognize and kill tumor cells expressing the unmodified epitope [27]. More recently a clinical trial has shown that priming with rV-CEA and then boosting 3–8 times with avipox-CEA in the presence of GM-CSF and low dose IL-2 results in 6/6 advanced cancer patients showing increasing frequencies of CEA-specific CD8 cells. New trials in patients with minimal residual disease are planned [28].

A novel approach to vaccination that has been very successful in infectious diseases is polynucleotide immunization. DNA or RNA can be immunized by intramuscular injection whereby the myocytes take up the DNA and express the gene product [29]. The released protein is taken up by APCs which migrate to the draining lymph nodes and present antigen to the T cells. An alternative route of immunization is by intradermal injection whereby it is presumed Langerhans cells (skin dendritic cells) take up the DNA. This will lead to a continuous intracellular production of protein antigens that may be presented in association with class I MHC molecules, thus eliciting adequate CTL responses. DNA may also be combined with genes for cytokines, such as IL-2, IL-6 or IL-7, or GM-CSF, in order to enhance the immune response generated [30].

Work has shown that mice may be immunized with a plasmid encoding the full length of complementary DNA for CEA [31]. Evidence of humoral and cellular responses against the glycoprotein were seen in all of the five mice immunized and three generated CEA-specific memory T cells. In addition, a further two had IL-2/IL-4 release in response to CEA. Clearly, evidence exists supporting this approach as a potential vaccine strategy. Approval has been granted for a phase I trial of polynucleotide CEA vaccination in colorectal cancer.

Vaccines Based upon Oncogenes or Tumor Suppressor Genes

Mutant oncogenes can offer the possibility of tumor-specific vaccines, but their use will be limited to patients with the appropriate MHC phenotype who express the relevant mutation. Mutations in codon 12 of K-ras are frequently found in pancreatic adenocarcinomas [32]. Mutant p21 ras is therefore a tumor-specific antigen that can be recognized by human T cells [33]. Synthetic ras peptides have been used in conjunction with APCs as a vaccine for pancreatic cancer with encouraging results. This approach could also be applied to colorectal carcinomas which show mutations in codon 12 of K-ras. As an alternative to peptide vaccination it is possible to clone the peptide epitope as a minigene and use this DNA as the immunogen. Minigenes coding for a single epitope derived from mutant p53 have been shown in a mouse model to elicit specific CTL [34].

An exciting new approach to target the adenomatous polyposis coli (APC) gene has been described. Mutations in this gene are one of the earliest changes in colon cancer and result in expression of a truncated APC protein. This is due to either a point mutation that produces a premature stop codon or to small deletions or insertions which produce frameshift mutations. The latter is very interesting for vaccine design as it usually causes a new reading frame which produces a stop codon within about 50 codons and results in a completely novel protein with which it may be possible to induce an immune response [35]. Mice immunized with these fragments have strong specific T cell immunity.

Heat Shock Protein Vaccines — Interesting but Impractical?

Heat shock proteins (HSPs) have been considered as potential vaccines as they are produced in cells in response to stress and are therefore one of the candidate proteins which may constitute the "danger" signal required to activate dendritic cells. Peptides bind to HSPs during the normal physiological degradation of proteins [36]. They therefore contain a wide variety of peptides (6–35 mers) non-covalently bound to, or "chaperoned" by, the HSP. One consequence of this phenomenon is that HSP preparations contain the entire repertoire of peptides generated in a cell. The repertoire consists of self-peptides and antigenic peptides, thus HSPs derived from tumor are complexed with peptides derived from tumor antigens. Vaccination of animals with tumor-derived HSP-peptide complexes results in protective immunity. The main problem with this approach is that a customized, patient-specific vaccine is required. More recently groups have loaded HSPs with specific peptides raising the possibility of designing a vaccine for a group of patients. In the context of the latter approach it has also been shown that HSPs bind to CD91 on dendritic cells, resulting in co-stimulation and also allowing presentation of its peptide load on class I MHC molecules [37]. The HSP appears to bind to the CD91 receptor on activated dendritic cells and allow access of peptides to class I and class II MHC presentation pathways.

Monoclonal Antibody Vaccines

Monoclonal Antibodies Mimicking 17-1A

CO17-1A is a 37–49 kDa antigen present on over 90 percent of colorectal cancers. In a landmark paper by Riethmuller and colleagues, passive immunotherapy with the murine IgG_{2A} monoclonal antibody 17-1A was shown to prolong survival in patients with minimal residual colorectal cancer [38]. The success of this approach is probably related to treatment of patients with low tumor burden. These results are currently being tested in two large multi-center trials in Europe and the United States using the antibody Panorex. This therapy may be effective as the monoclonal antibody binds directly to the tumor cell and stimulates antibody-dependent cellular cytotoxicity. It may also stimulate an immune cascade of anti-idiotypic antibodies. Recent work has shown that an anti-idiotypic response (Ab2) and an auto-anti-idiotypic titer (Ab3) to 17-1A correlates with tumor response [39]. Twenty-four patients with metastatic colorectal cancer were treated with Mab 17-1A. After completion of therapy, five of the patients developed peripheral blood T cells specifically recognizing human anti-Mab 17-1A idiotypic antibodies. These same five patients were the only ones in the study who had any objective tumor regression following Mab therapy. The association between the presence of anti-idiotypic reactive T cells and clinical response was statistically significant.

Rather than treat patients with an antibody to stimulate an anti-idiotypic response, 30 patients with advanced colorectal cancer have been immunized with a goat polyclonal anti-idiotypic antibody to CO17-1A in a study by Herlyn et al. [40]. Humoral responses were seen and all showed evidence of Ab3 production. This antibody showed identical binding of tumor cells as that observed with Ab1, confirming its specificity. Six patients showed partial clinical remission and a further seven arrest of metastases following treatment. Of these 13 patients nine also received chemotherapy, making conclusions about the efficacy of Ab2 therapy somewhat contentious. A follow-up trial by the same group used a different goat polyclonal antibody in 12 patients who had undergone resection of their primary tumor [41]. Six of these patients developed antibodies against the anti-idiotypic antibody and two had antigen-specific T cells. In addition, seven of the original 12 showed tumor remissions which lasted between 1.1 and 4.1 years post-immunization.

More recently, animal studies with the mouse homologue of 17-1A have shown that it is only possible to cause tumor regression if animals are immunized with whole antigen expressed within adenovirus and not with antigen alone or anti-idiotypic antibodies. This correlates with the induction of CTLs. The viral construct allows intracellular production of the antigen that is efficiently processed and presented by class I MHC [42].

Monoclonal Antibodies Mimicking CD55

A human monoclonal anti-idiotypic antibody, 105AD7 has been cloned by our group from a cancer patient receiving diagnostic radioimmunoscintigraphy who had prolonged survival with liver metastases. 105AD7 recognizes the combining site of 791T/36 mouse monoclonal antibody and thus mimics the 791Tgp72 antigen expressed on many colorectal cancers [43]. It was shown that in animals, 105AD7 at low doses stimulates DTH responses to tumor cells expressing 791Tgp72 antigen [44]. At higher doses in the presence of Freund's adjuvant it could also induce antibodies that recognize 791Tgp72 antigen. We have conducted a Phase I clinical study in advanced colorectal cancer patients, which showed that the anti-idiotype was non-toxic, and stimulated T cell responses that recognized tumor cells expressing 791Tgp72 antigen [45]. A non-randomized analysis with historical controls suggested that patients receiving 105AD7 appeared to survive longer than contemporary unimmunized patients, but this has not been confirmed in a recent double blind randomized trial. In contrast, a neoadjuvant trial, in which patients were immunized at tumor diagnosis prior to operation and boosted post-operatively, showed good evidence of infiltration of helper T cells and NK cells within immunized as compared to control tumors [46, 47]. Furthermore, this was associated with a 3-fold increase in tumor cell apoptosis [48].

In this system it was important to identify the target antigen. 791Tgp72 antigen was therefore affinity-purified from an over-expressing tumor cell line and N-terminal amino acid sequencing revealed identity with CD55. 791Tgp72 was subsequently cloned, sequenced and expressed and it was shown to have an identical sequence to the complement regulatory protein CD55 [49]. It binds the C3 convertases of both the classical and alternative complement pathways thereby inhibiting deposition of C3b and assembly of the MAC complex. (See Chapter 1) It was an unexpected target for the 105AD7 cancer vaccine as it is a molecule expressed by a wide variety of normal cells to protect them from bystander killing by complement. However, radiolabeling imaging with the 791T/36 monoclonal antibody had shown good localization within tumor tissue. Expression of CD55 was therefore studied on tumor cells and was found to be over-expressed by 2-100 fold [50]. Furthermore, colorectal cancer patients whose tumors had high levels of CD55 had a poor prognosis. These results suggest that CD55 over-expression confers protection on the growing tumor and is therefore a very interesting target for a cancer vaccine. The paradox would be that if the vaccine is effective, tumor cells over-expressing CD55 will be killed and remaining tumor cells with low or no CD55 expression should be sensitized to complement mediated lysis.

Although there was some evidence of CD8 responses in patients immunized with 105AD7 these were weak. Patients showed post-immunization increases in their CD8RA/RO ratios (a measure of T cell memory phenotype) and in a rectal cancer study, enhanced killing of autologous tumor cells that was unrelated to NK killing was shown in 3/4 patients immunized with 105AD7. However in a larger trial studying 105AD7-induced tumor infiltration, although significant increases in CD4 and NK cells were observed in 105AD7-treated patients when compared with controls, no significant CD8 infiltration into the tumors was observed. These results suggested that although 105AD7 may contain CTL epitopes, the antibody was predominantly stimulating a CD4 response. Numerous studies have shown that DNA vaccination results in good CTL responses and therefore 105AD7 was reconfigured as a DNA vaccine. The variable regions of the heavy and light chains were joined by a 16 or 5 amino acid linker to form either scFv or dimeric DNA constructs. Similarly the CDRH3 region of 105AD7 was spliced to its leader region to form a minigene construct. In contrast to the anti-idiotypic protein, all three DNA constructs induced CTL responses, however, the dimeric construct was the most effective.

For patients with the appropriate HLA types 105AD7 still remains an attractive vaccine. Although CTLs are important immune effector cells, antigen specific CD4 responses are essential for initiating and amplifying inflammatory responses within tumors, allowing extravasation of both NK and CD8 cells. It was therefore important to ensure that the powerful inflammatory responses stimulated by the 105AD7 protein were not lost in the DNA vaccines. Both the dimeric and scFv constructs stimulated CD4 cells secreting γIFN and mouse IgG2a antibodies, suggesting that the DNA vaccines were stimulating Th1 responses in addition to CTL reactivity. These results would suggest that 105AD7 DNA vaccine should be even more effective in the clinic than the current protein vaccine.

Monoclonal Antibodies Binding to Growth Factor Receptors — EGF and VEGF

Following on the success of Herceptin, a monoclonal antibody that binds to the Her-2/neu receptor, several monoclonal antibodies have been developed that block the interaction of a growth factor with its receptor. The EGF receptor is a particularly attractive target as it is over-expressed by a wide range of tumors including 60–80% of colorectal cancers. Binding of EGF to this receptor not only stimulates cell growth but also stimulates angiogenesis and cell survival [51]. Thus antibodies that block binding of EGF inhibit tumor growth and angiogenesis and can also result in apoptosis. Their great clinical utility has been when used in combination with chemotherapy, where 20 percent of colorectal cancer patients who have failed irinotecan therapy, (a topoisomerase inhibitor), have been shown to respond to the combination of irinotecan and an anti-EGF receptor antibody (unpublished results). Similar encouraging results have been shown with a monoclonal antibody that binds to the KDR receptor which acts as the ligand for the important angiogenic growth factor VEGF. Clinical trials in colorectal cancer patients have shown good synergy with the anti-KDR antibody when combined with conventional chemotherapy [52].

Endothelial Vaccines

The possibility of targeting antigens over-expressed on tumor vasculature has been recently explored in our laboratory. The aim was to target moderate affinity epitopes that may have escaped T cell deletion or tolerance and then to mutate them to higher affinity immunogens. If this proved possible, endothelial-directed vaccines would offer a number of potential advantages over epithelial-directed vaccines. Even limited damage to the tumor vasculature results in large-scale destruction of tumor cells and strong inflammatory responses and the target cells become accessible to the immune system. Barriers posed by the tumor microenvironment (already alluded to) such as antigen heterogeneity,

MHC loss and resistance to apoptosis that are associated with transformed epithelial cells are unlikely to be a problem with normal endothelial cells.

CD55, KDR and the endothelial cell-specific tyrosine kinase receptor, Tie-2 have been screened by our group using computer-aided motif predictions for possible HLA-DR epitopes (unpublished observations). Peptides have therefore been identified that should stimulate helper T cells. To avoid cross-reactivity peptides were selected from these regions of the molecule that were unique to each antigen. Peptides were also selected from regions of the molecules that were homologous between humans and mice to allow therapeutic evaluation of the vaccines in mouse models. The Tie-2 peptides were predicted to stimulate T cells in donors expressing HLA-DR 1,3,4,7 and HLA-Dr 1,3,7 phenotypes respectively. Using a range of unimmunized donors, the predictions were confirmed with lymphocytes from all permissive donors showing proliferation. Furthermore, a 20 amino acid peptide stimulated γIFN but not IL-4, indicating that it was stimulating Th1 responses. A recombinant protein of the first Tie2-Ig domain stimulated proliferation responses in all donors. Using limited dilution, T cell clones have been generated that are specific for the Tie2-Ig domain. Therefore there is a repertoire of T cells in healthy individuals able to recognize endothelial antigens.

Using these computer-aided motif predictions for HLA-A2, peptides unique to Tie-2, KDR and CD55 have been identified. As these receptors are self-antigens, peptides that bound with moderate affinity were selected, as it was predicted that peptides binding with high affinity would be deleted in the thymus or anergised in the periphery by normal endothelial cells. To allow for therapeutic evaluation of vaccines in mouse models, peptides were selected from regions of Tie-2 and KDR that were homologous between mouse and humans. These peptides were initially screened in vitro for their ability to stimulate primary CTL responses. Although the culture conditions were very efficient at stimulating CTL responses to a high affinity influenza peptide, no CTL responses to the endothelial peptides were generated. This may have been due to lack of a T cell repertoire, poor priming of CTL responses with moderate affinity epitopes or to a very low precursor frequency of näive T cells that were not efficiently expanded in vitro. To answer these questions a colony of HLA-A2 transgenic mice were established. The human HLA-A2 transgenic mice are an excellent model for testing the efficacy of these vaccines as the mouse T cells have been educated on an HLA-A2 background and because human and mouse Tie-2 and KDR have a high degree of homology. Immunization of these transgenic mice with the moderate affinity peptides still failed to stimulate CTL responses. To increase the predicted binding affinity of these peptides for MHC, the amino acids 1 or 9 were changed to preferred HLA-A2 anchor residues. Using the TAP-deficient cell line T2, increases in MHC stabilization with mutated peptides compared to native peptides were demonstrated. Immunization of HLA-A2 transgenic mice with the mutant peptides resulted in the generation of CTL responses that recognized both modified and wild type peptides. CTL epitopes from Tie-2, KDR and CD55 have all been successfully identified proving that there is a T cell repertoire in transgenic mice that recognizes normal endothelial antigens and suggesting that a similar repertoire could exist in humans. The toxicity and efficacy of endothelial vaccines of this type are now being screened in an animal model prior to entering clinical trials in patients.

References

1. Boon T, Vanderbruggen P. Human tumor antigens recognized by T-lymphocytes. Journal Of Experimental Medicine1996;183:725–9.
2. Rosenberg SAA New era for cancer immunotherapy based on the genes that encode cancer antigens. Immunity 1999;10:281–7.
3. Sahin U, Tureci, O, Pfreundschuh, M. Serological identification of human tumor antigens, Curr. Opin. Immunol.1997,9: 709–716.
4. Rosenberg SA, Yang JC, Schwartzentruber DJ, Hwu P, Marincola FC, Topalian S, et al. Immunologic and therapeutic evaluation of a synthetic peptide vaccine for the treatment of patients with metastatic melanoma. Nature Medicine1998;4: 321–7.
5. Moroi Y, Mayhew M, Trcka J, Hoe MH, Takechi Y, Hartl FU, et al. Induction of cellular immunity by immunization with novel hybrid peptides complexed to heat shock protein 70. Proc Natl Acad Sci 2000;97:3485–90.
6. Jager E, Ringhoffer M, Dienes HP, Arand M, Karbach J, Jager D, et al. Granulocyte-macrophage-colony-stimulating factor enhances immune-responses to melanoma-associated peptides in-vivo. International Journal Of Cancer 1996;67:54–62.
7. Belz GT, Stevenson PG, Doherty PC. Contemporary analysis of MHC-related immunodominance hierarchies in the CD8+ T cell response to influenza A viruses. J Immunol 2000;165:2404–9.
8. Regnault A, Lankar D, Lacabanne V, Rodriquez A, Thery C, Rescigno M, et al. Fcγ receptor-mediated induction of dendritic cell maturation and major histocompatibity complex class I restricted antigen presentation after immune complex internalization. J Exp Med 1999;189: 371–80.
9. Sallusto F, Lenig D, Mackay CR, Lanzavecchia A. Flexible programs of chemokine receptor expression on human polarized T helper 1 and 2 lymphocytes. J Exp Med 1998;187:875–83.
10. Hanke T, McMichael AJ. Design and construction of an experimental HIV-1 vaccine for a year-2000 clinical trial in Kenya. Nature Medicine 2000;6:951–60.
11. Gabrilovich DI, Chen HL, Girgis KR, Cunningham HT, Meny GM, Nadaf S, et al. Production of vascular endothelial growth factor by human tumors inhibits the functional maturation of dendritic cells, Nature Medicine 1996;2:1096–103.
12. Ossendorp F, Mengede E, Camps M, Filius R, Melief CJM. Specific T helper cell requirement for optimal induction of cytotoxic T lymphocytes against major histocompatibility complex class II negative tumors. J Exp Med 1998;87:693–702.
13. Ridge JP, Di Rosa F, Matzinger P. A conditioned dendritic cell can be a temporal bridge between a CD4 T-helper and a T killer cell, Nature 1998;393:474.
14. Hung K, Hayashi R, Lafond-Walker A, Lowenstein C, Pardoll D, Levitsky H. The central role of CD4+ T cells in the antitumor immune response, J Exp Med 1998;188:2357–68.
15. Greenberg PD, Kern DE, Cheever MA. Therapy of disseminated murine leukemia with cyclophosphamide and immune Lyt-1+, 2- T cells. Tumor eradication does not require participation of cytotoxic T cells. J Exp Med 1985;161:1122–34.
16. Pardoll DM. Cancer vaccines. Nature Medicine 1998;4:525–31.
17. Toes REM, Ossendorp F, Offringa R, Melief CJM. CD4 T Cells and their role in antitumor immune responses, J Exp Med 1999;189:753–6.
18. Manici S, Sturniolo T, Imro MA, Hammer J, Sinigaglia F, Noppen C et al. Melanoma cells present a MAGE-3 epitope to CD4+ cytotoxic T cells in association with histocompatibility leukocyte antigen DR11. J Exp Med 1999;189:871–6.
19. Ockert D, Schirrmacher V, Beck N, Stoelben E, Ahlert T, Flechtenmacher J, Hagmuller E, Buchcik R, Nagel M, Saeger HD. Newcastle disease virus-infected intact autologous tumor cell vaccine for adjuvant active specific immunotherapy of resected colorectal carcinoma. 1: Clin Cancer Res 1996;Jan;2(1):21–8.
20. Hagmuller E, Beck N, Ockert D, Schirrmacher V. Adjuvant therapy of liver metastases: active specific immunotherapy. 1: Zentralbl Chir 1995;120(10):780–5.
21. Shirrmacher V, Ahler T, Bastert G. Workshop: active specific immunotherapy with tumour cell vaccines J Cancer Res Clin Oncol 1995;121:487–9.
22. Durrant LG, Denton GWL, Jacobs E, Mee M, Moss R, Austin EB, et al. An idiotypic replica of carcinoembryonic antigen inducing cellular and humoral responses directed against human colorectal tumors. International Journal Of Cancer 1992;50:811–6.
23. Foon KA, Chakraborty M, John WJ, Sharratt A, Kohler H, Bhattaoharya-Chatterjee, M. Immune response to the carcinoembryonic antigen in patients treated with an anti-idiotype antibody vaccine. J Clin Invest 1995;96:334–42.

24. Conry RM, Seleh MN, Schlom J, LoBuglio AF. Human immune response to carcinoembryonic antigen tumor vaccines, J Immunother 1995;18:137.
25. Fagerberg J, Samanci A, Yi O, Strigard K, Frodin J, Wahren B, et al. Recombinant carcinoembryonic antigen and granulocyte-macrophage colony-stimulating factor for active immunization of colorectal carcinoma patients. J Immunother 1995;18:132.
26. Tsang KY, Zaremba S, Nieroda CA, Zhu MZ, Hamilton JM, Schlom J. Generation of human cytotoxic T-cells specific for human carcinoembryonic antigen epitopes from patients immunized with recombinant vaccinia-cea vaccine. J Natl Cancer Inst 1995;87:982-90.
27. Zaremba S, Barzaga E, Zhu M, Soares N, Tsang K-Y, Sclom J. Identification of an enhancer agonist cytotoxic T lymphocyte peptide from human carcinoembryonic antigen. Cancer Res 1997;57: 4570-7.
28. Marshall JL, Hoyer RJ, Toomey MA, Faraguna K, Chang P, Richmond E, et al. Phase I study in advanced cancer patients of a diversified prime-and-boost vaccination protocol using recombinant vaccinia virus and recombinant nonreplicating avipox virus to elicit anti-carcinoembryonic antigen immune responses. J Clin Oncology 2000;18:3964-73.
29. Whalen RG, Davis HL. Short analytical review. DNA-mediated immunization and the energetic immune response to hepatitis B surface antigen. Clin Immuno. Immunopathol 1995;75:1-12.
30. Irvine KR, Rao JB, Rosenberg SA, Restifo NP. Cytokine enhancement of dna immunization leads to effective treatment of established pulmonary metastases, Journal of immunology 1996;156:238-45.
31. Conry RM, Lobuglio AF, Kantor J, Schlom J, Loechel F, Moore SE, et al. Immune-response to a carcinoembryonic antigen polynucleotide vaccine. Cancer Res 1994;54:1164-8.
32. Gjertsen MK, Bakka A, Breivik J, Solheim BG, Soreide O, Thorsby E, et al. Vaccination with mutant ras peptides and induction of T-cell responsiveness in pancreatic carinoma patients carrying the corresponding RAS mutation, Lancet 1995;346:1399-400.
33. Jung S, Schluesener HJ. Human T lymphocytes recognize a peptide of single point-mutated, oncogenic ras proteins. J Exp Med 1991;173:273-6.
34. Ciernik IF, Yanuck M, Berzofsky JA, Carbone DP. Expression of a mutant P53 epitope fused with the adenovirus E3 leader sequence in tumor-cells overcomes Gamma-Ifn dependence of lysis by p53-specific Ctl. Journal of Cellular Biochemistry 1995;163-163.
35. Townsend A, Ohlen C, Rogers M, Edwards J, Mukherjee S, Bastin J. Source of unique tumour antigens. Nature 1994;371:662.
36. Blachere N.E, Udono H, Janetzki S, Li Z, Heike M, Srivastava PK. Heat-shock protein vaccines against cancer. J of Immunother 1993;14:352-6.
37. Binder RJ, Harris ML, Menoret A, Srivastava PK. Saturation, competition and specificity in interaction of heat shock proteins (hsp) gp96, hsp90, and hsp70 with CD11b+ cells. J Immunol 2000;165:2582-7.
38. Riethmuller G, Scheidergadicke E, Schlimok G, Schmiegel W, Raab R, Hoffken K, et al. Randomized trial of monclonal-antibody for adjuvant therapy of resected Dukes-C colorectal carcinoma. Lancet 1994;343:1177-83.
39. Fagerberg J, Hjelm AL, Ragnhammar P, Frodin JE, Wigzell H, Mellstedt H. Tumor-regression in monoclonal antibody-treated patients correlates with the presence of anti-idiotype-reactive T-lymphocytes, Cancer Research 1995;55:1824-7.
40. Herlyn D, Wettendorff M, Schmoll E, Iliopoulos D, Schedel I, Dreikhausen U, et al. Anti-idiotype immunization of cancer-patients — modulation of the immune-response, Proceedings of the National Academy of Sciences of the United States of America 1987;84:8055-9.
41. Somasundaram R, Zaloudik J, Jacob L, Benden A, Sperlagh M, Hart E, et al. Induction of antigen specific T and B cell immunity in colon carcinoma patients by anti-idiotypic antibody. J Immunol 1995;155:3253-61.
42. Li WP, Berencsi K, Basak K, Somansundaram R, Ricciardi RP, Gonczol E, et al. Human colorectal cancer (CRC) antigen Co17/GA733 encoded by adenovirus inhibits growth of established CRC cells in mice. J of Immunol 1998;159:763-9.
43. Austin EB, Robins RA, Durrant LG, Price MR, Baldwin RW. Human monoclonal anti-idiotypic antibody to the tumour associated antibody 791T/36, Immunol 1989;67:525-30.
44. Austin EB, Robins RA, Durrant LG, Baldwin RW. A human monoclonal antiidiotypic antibody with potential for induction of antitumor immunity. British Journal Of Cancer 1990;62:533.
45. Denton GWL, Durrant LG, Hardcastle JD, Austin EB, Sewell HF, Robins RA. Clinical outcome of colorectal-cancer patients treated with human monoclonal antiidiotypic antibody. Int J Cancer 1994;57:10-4.
46. Maxwell-Armstrong CA, Durrant LG, Scholefield JH. Immunotherapy for colorectal cancer. American Journal of Surgery 1999;177:344-8.
47. Durrant LG, Spendlove I, Buckley DJ, Robins RA. 105AD7 cancer vaccine stimulates anti-tumour

helper and cytotoxic T cell responses in HLA-A1,3,24 and HLA-DR 1,3,7 colorectal cancer patients. Int J Cancer 2000;85:87–92.

48. Schwann A, Robins RA, Maxwell-Armstrong CA, Scholefield JH, Durrant LG. Vaccine-induced Apoptosis: A Novel Clinical Trial End Point?. Can Res 2000;60:3132–6.

49. Spendlove I, Li L, Potter V, Christiansen D, Loveland B, Durrant LG. A therapeutic human anti-idiotypic antibody (105AD7) mimics CD55 (decay accelerating factor) in three distinct regions. Eur J Immunol 2000 (submitted).

50. Li L, Spendlove I, Morgan J, Durrant L.G. CD55 is over-expressed in the tumour environment. British J Can 2001;84:80–6.

51. Shaheen RM, Ahmad SA, Liu W, Reinmuth N, Jung YD, Tseng WW, Drazan KE, Bucana CD, Hicklin DJ, Ellis LM. Inhibited growth of colon cancer carcinomatosis by antibodies to vascular endothelial and epidermal growth factor receptors. 1: Br J Cancer 2001 Aug 17;85(4):584–9.

52. Witte L, Hicklin DJ, Zhu Z, Pytowski B, Kotanides H, Rockwell P, Bohlen P. Monoclonal antibodies targeting the VEGF receptor-2 (Flk1/KDR) as an anti-angiogenic therapeutic strategy. 1: Cancer Metastasis Rev 1998 Jun;17(2):155–61.

14. The Immunotherapy of Renal Cell Carcinoma

Paul Nathan and Martin Gore

Introduction

Renal cell carcinoma (RCC) is one of the most immunogenic of solid epithelial tumors. Spontaneous regression of metastatic disease is well documented and a variety of biological therapies result in objective responses, with a small proportion of patients obtaining long-term complete remissions.

Spontaneous Regression

Spontaneous regressions of renal cell cancer were initially described in 1928 by Bumpus [1] with the literature being first reviewed in 1966 [2]. Estimation of the overall incidence of spontaneous regression is difficult given reporting bias and the frequent absence of histological confirmation, [3] however, the largest series estimate that rates are less than 1 percent [4,5]. Most reports describe the resolution of pulmonary metastases, although disease regression in bone [6], brain [7,8], liver [9] and lymph nodes [10] has also been reported. The majority of these reports describe regression following nephrectomy. It should be stressed that given the low incidence of spontaneous regression, this phenomenon is not in itself an indication for nephrectomy when metastatic disease is present. Two studies have investigated immunological parameters pre- and post-nephrectomy, both finding that patients had lower proportions of T helper cells than normal and that these tended to normalize post-nephrectomy [11,12].

Most authors have assumed that the mechanism of spontaneous regression is immunologically mediated and although this would seem to be the most likely mechanism, it is not proven. Definitive data is difficult to produce because of the low frequency of spontaneous regression and problems of correlating clinical findings with in vitro assays. One report, however, showed that in vitro measurement of lymphokine activated killer (LAK) cell activity and mixed lymphocyte culture (MLC) cytotoxicity in a patient showed no significant increase in activity [13] but this appears to be an isolated observation.

The activity of immunomodulators in the treatment of renal cell carcinoma is

295

supporting evidence for the importance of the immune system in this tumor type and trials of immunotherapy in this disease are described in this chapter.

The Role of Surgery in Immunotherapy of RCC

Radical nephrectomy remains the definitive treatment for primary RCC and still has an important place in the management of metastatic disease. Even though the incidence of spontaneous remission in nephrectomised patients in one series was 0.6 percent [14] which is twice that in a non-nephrectomised series [15], the overall number of events is very small and the difference is likely to be explained by reporting bias. The data suggests that even if nephrectomy induced spontaneous regression, 199 patients with metastatic disease would need to be nephrectomised to result in a single responder [16].

The indications for nephrectomy in the metastatic patients would include [17]:

1. Large primary tumor which is causing symptoms in the presence of small volume metastatic disease in an otherwise fit patient.
2. Large primary tumor which is likely to be symptomatic before metastatic disease causes significant clinical problems in an otherwise fit patient.
3. Immunotherapy clinical trial protocol requiring prior nephrectomy.

There is some evidence that the chance of effective stimulation of anti-tumor responses is inversely proportional to tumor bulk. There is, however, scanty evidence for an up-regulation of anti-tumor immunity post-nephrectomy. Some defects in natural killer (NK) cell and LAK cell activity have been shown to be partly reversed in one study, but the clinical significance of this observation is unclear [18].

Prognostic Indicators

A number of studies have identified the following features as important prognostic factors in metastatic RCC [19–22].

i)   >24 month disease-free interval between initial nephrectomy and the appearance of metastatic disease.
ii)   Single site metastatic disease.
iii) ECOG performance status = 0.

There was a strong suggestion from case-controlled studies that there was a survival benefit for patients with good prognostic features [19,20]. A more recent analysis of prognostic factors in 670 patients with advanced renal cell cancer identified the following variables as being associated with poor survival [23].

i)   Low Karnofsky performance status (<80 percent)
ii)   High lactate dehydrogenase (LDH: $>1.5x$ upper limit of normal)
iii) Low haemoglobin (below lower limit of normal)
iv)   High corrected serum Ca^{2+}
v)   Absence of nephrectomy

The criteria below have been used to categorise patients into the following prognostic groups.

i)   Favourable risk (no risk factors) — 25 percent of patients.
ii) Intermediate risk (1–2 factors) — 53 percent of patients.
iii) Poor risk (>3 factors) — 22 percent of patients.

Group A had a median survival of 20 months, group B a median survival of 10 months and group C a median survival of 4 months. Care should therefore be exercised in selecting those patients who are most likely to benefit from biological and bio-chemotherapy. Patients with bad prognostic features, particularly those with a poor performance status, should perhaps not be exposed to the side effects of biotherapy. The principal cytokine therapies employed in advanced RCC include the interferons and interleukins.

Interferons

Interferons are a heterogeneous group of glycoproteins classified into α, β and γ types. All interferons appear to have a combination of anti-viral and immuno-regulatory activity and interferons α and β also have anti-proliferative effects affecting normal and malignant cells. Interferon γ stimulates macrophages and up-regulates MHC class II expression on antigen-presenting cells as well as modulating T and B cell responses. The precise mechanisms of action that are responsible for clinical anti-tumor activity have not been fully defined [24].

Interferon-α (IFN-α) was first shown to have activity against RCC in 1983 [25,26]. Quesada and colleagues reported 19 patients who received 3×10^6 U interferon-α/day intramuscularly and 5 patients obtained a partial response [26]. IFN-α appears to have the most activity of all interferons in RCC [27] and although the mode of action is at present poorly understood, it is probably a combination of stimulation of cell-mediated cytotoxicity, direct anti-proliferative anti-tumor activity and an anti-angiogenesis effect.

A number of phase II studies reporting the activity of IFN-α in RCC have shown objective responses in the order of 10–20% with median response durations of 6–10 months and complete responses in only 1 percent of patients [27–30]. A multi-center, randomized MRC trial has recently demonstrated that this activity of IFN-α translates into a statistically significant survival advantage. Three hundred and fifty patients were randomized to receive IFN-α subcutaneously at 10 MIU/m^2 for 12 weeks or oral medroxyprogesterone acetate (MPA) at 300mg daily for 12 weeks. In an intention to treat analysis, 111 patients had died in the IFN-α group versus 125 deaths in the MPA arm. This represented a statistically significant survival advantage of 12 percent (95 percent CI 3–22%) at 1 year for patients treated with IFN-α and a 2.5 month improvement in median survival [31].

Objective responses to IFN-α are frequently delayed and can take up to 11 months to occur [32]. However, most patients who are going to respond have done so by about 3 months and it would be unlikely for a patient who initially progressed on treatment to respond at a later date. There is little evidence available on the optimum duration of treatment and most centres continue for as long as the response is maintained, toxicity permitting. The mechanisms of subsequent

Table 14.1. Randomized trials of immunotherapy vs. non-immunotherapeutic regimens in renal cell carcinoma

Reference	patient no's	Treatments	Survival advantage or overall response rate (OR)	Significant?
MRC [31]	350	IFN-α vs MPA	12% IFN-α arm survival advantage	yes 95% CI 3–22%
Atzpodien [64]	78	IL-2/5-FU/IFN-α vs tamoxifen	39% biochemotherapy OR vs 0% tamox.	yes 95% CI 24–55% vs. 0–9%.
Steineck [29]	60	IFN-α vs MPA	7% vs 3%	no, survival benefit unevaluable due to cross over
Kriegmar [30]	76	IFN-α + vinblastine vs MPA	22% IFN-α arm vs 0%	yes

treatment failure are also poorly understood. There may be generation of anti-interferon antibodies which have been demonstrated and although their production may theoretically be related to the development of relapse their precise clinical importance is unclear [33]. A number of studies have assessed the dose-response curve of IFN-α in RCC where chronic dosing appears to have more activity than intermittent dosing. In a grouped analysis of 17 studies assessing dosage, doses <5 MIU/day resulted in a response rate of 11 percent whereas doses of 5–10 or >10 MIU/day resulted in response rates of 20 and 15 percent respectively [34]. There is no evidence to support regimes with higher doses than 10MIU/m^2. A recent meta-analysis of 8 randomised studies totalling 525 patients has shown that IFN-α-containing regimes have a higher overall response rate (24 percent: range 10–46%) when compared with those regimes not utilizing IFN-α (17 percent: range 5–30%) [35].

The toxicity of interferon-α is also dose and route of administration-dependent. Interferon-α is generally well tolerated and may be self-administered sub-cutaneously on an out-patient basis. There is increased activity with alternative routes of administration but there is a higher incidence of side effects when IFN-α is given intravenously. In one study 97 patients were randomized to receive IFN-α subcutaneously (2×10^6 IU/m^2 3 x weekly) or intra-venously (30×10^6 IU/m^2 for 5 days every 3 weeks, ref [35]). Grade 3 toxicity occurred much more frequently in those patients receiving intra-venous IFN-α. Subcutaneous regimes are widely used and at doses of 5–10 MIU influenza-like symptoms are the main side effect, although these usually last less than 3 weeks. Administration at night appears to alleviate the side-effects of IFN-α, although occasionally gastro-intestinal symptoms including anorexia, vomiting and changes in taste become dose-limiting. Rarely myelosuppression, hepatic and CNS side-effects are seen, although these mainly occur when high-dose parenteral regimes are used.

There has recently been a great deal of interest in the activity of interferon-α conjugated with a polyethylene glycol (PEG) molecule [36]. This conjugation increases the plasma half-life of the agent, enhances the biological activity of the interferon and allows for once weekly administration but a disadvantage of

Table 14.2. Randomised immunotherapy trials in renal cell carcinoma comparing immunotherapeutic regimens

Reference	Patient no's	Treatments	Survival advantage or overall response rate (RR)	Significant?
Muss et al [35]	97	IFN-α sc or iv	10% RR sc vs 7% iv	no
De Mulder et al [38]	102	IFN-α vs IFN-α + IFN-γ	13% RR IFN-α alone vs. 4% RR combination	no
Yang et al [43]	125	IL-2 iv high vs low dose	20% RR high dose vs 15% RR low dose	no
Yang et al [49]		IL-2 high dose iv vs intermediate dose iv vs low dose sc	16% RR high dose vs 4% RR int. vs 11% RR low dose	no
McCabe et al [52]	69	IL-2 high dose vs IL-2 + LAK	8% IL-2 alone RR vs 13% combination	no
Atkins et al [58]	99	high dose IL-2 +/- IFN-α	11% RR combination vs 17% IL-2 alone	no
Negrier et al [60]	425	IFN-α vs IL-2 vs IFN-α + IL-2	18.6% RR combination, 7.5% IFN & 6.5% IL-2	yes
Pyrhönen et al [73]	79	IFNα/vinblastine vs vinblastine	16.5% RR combination vs 2.5% vin. alone	yes p=0.0025
Motzer et al [74]	284	IFN-α/cis-retinoic acid vs IFN-α	11% RR combination vs 6% IFN alone	no

PEG-IFN-α may be longer duration side-effects. A number of clinical trials are currently underway evaluating this new agent. Interferon α has also been used in combination with interferon γ and with tumor necrosis factor (TNF). Despite promising early in vitro and in vivo patient data, neither combination has demonstrated an advantage in terms of efficacy [38,39].

Interleukin 2

IL-2 is a highly biologically active cytokine that is the principal stimulator of T cell growth and which has profound effects on T cell, B cell and macrophage activity. In the early 1980s, IL-2 was shown be a potent in vitro stimulator of the generation of cytotoxic T lymphocytes (CTL) and non-T cell receptor-restricted LAK cells, both of which lyse in vitro tumor targets. IL-2 alone was also shown to have in vivo anti-tumor activity in a large number of murine experiments as was the adoptive transfer of in vitro-generated LAK cells and CTL into mice bearing a variety of tumor burdens.

IL-2 was assessed in patients with RCC given the perceived immunogenicity of this tumor and promising early results were obtained by Rosenberg and colleagues at the NCI. An overall response rate of 22 percent was reported with bolus doses of IL-2 and long-term remissions (>3 years) were obtained in some patients [40]. However, most subsequent studies have reported overall response rates of only 10–15%. Rosenberg utilized high doses (600,000–720,000 IU/kg every 8 hrs on days 1–5 and 15–19) and toxicities were severe. The principal problems encountered included capillary leak syndrome and associated hypotension which resulted in many patients requiring aggressive inotropic support during treatment. There were also renal, hepatic, cardio-respiratory and haematological toxicities but experience proved that these were all manageable given appropriate patient selection and support during treatment [41,42]. Serious and potentially life-threatening IL-2-related toxicities appear short-lived and generally reverse within hours to days of stopping treatment. In a randomised comparison of high versus low dose IL-2, 125 patients received IL-2 by intra-venous bolus at doses of either 710,000 IU/kg or 72,000 IU/kg [43]. Patients in the high dose arm had a significantly increased incidence of grade 3 and 4 thrombocytopenia, malaise and hypotension with 52 percent of courses requiring inotropic support as opposed to 3 percent in the low dose arm. Patients in the low dose group had a 7 percent complete (CR) and an 8 percent partial (PR) response rate whist those in the high dose group had a 3 percent CR and a 17 percent PR, although these differences did not reach statistical significance. The 12 month survival figures for the two groups were also comparable at 74 percent in the low dose and 78 percent in the high dose arms.

In an effort to further reduce IL-2 associated toxicities, a number of sub-cutaneous regimes have been assessed using low dose subcutaneous IL-2 (15–20 million IU daily for 5 days) on an out-patient basis [44–46]. Low dose regimes are certainly much better tolerated. However, it is still unclear which regime produces the most durable clinical responses. A direct comparison of high dose intra-venous, intermediate dose intra-venous and low dose sub-cutaneous IL-2 produced response rates of 16 percent, 4 percent and 11 percent respectively [47]. Dose intensity may be a further variable that correlates with response. In one phase II study in 20 patients, a dose intensity below 1440 MIU/m2/year correlated with failure to achieve a complete response (p < 0.01) [48]. Recently, inhaled IL-2 has been shown to have efficacy with reduced toxicity in selected patients with pulmonary metastases. This is a local treatment and appears to not be effective at more distant sites [49].

Alternative high dose protocols using continuous infusions of IL-2 have also been examined. Overall response rates are similar and toxicities are less severe [50,51]. Some of these reports are not, however, strictly comparable, since in some of the early studies, IL-2 was administered as part of an adoptive strategy with the transfer of in vitro generated LAK cells. Peripheral blood lymphocytes from patients were expanded in vitro using high doses of IL-2 before being infused back into the patient with additional systemic doses of IL-2. Response rates initially appeared higher when compared to high dose single agent IL-2 treatment (33 percent vs. 24 percent) [40], although later studies have failed to show a difference between these two treatments [52,53].

The adoptive transfer of in vitro expanded tumor-infiltrating lymphocytes (TILs) has also been investigated but there is no evidence that this strategy is associated with an improvement in efficacy [54]. Currently there is no convincing evidence to justify the use of adoptive transfer either of LAK or TILs, most studies showing similar activity to high dose IL-2 alone with a high expense and technical expertise required for the generation of the former therapies.

Some patients clearly benefit from IL-2 based therapy with durable complete responses being achieved. The durability of response may be increased by high dose intra-venous IL-2. Of the 17 patients achieving a complete response (7 percent) in a large study of 255 patients [55], the median duration had not been reached by the time of update publication (range 7–107 months). It should, however, also be remembered that the majority of patients treated with IL-2 do not respond. Attention has therefore focused on combinations of cytokines with or without the addition of chemotherapeutic agents.

Combination IL-2 and IFN-α Therapy

The activity of both IFN-α and IL-2 in RCC led to the investigation of the efficacy of using these agents in combination. In vitro and in vivo animal data had shown a synergistic relationship between the two cytokines [56]. Initial phase II studies were performed using sub-cutaneous IFN-α in combination with intra-venous bolus, intra-venous continuous infusion and sub-cutaneous IL-2 regimes. Although the first phase I study using a high-dose IL-2/IFN-α combination in 35 patients demonstrated a 31 percent response rate [57], later studies showed no evidence for additional activity of IFN-α with high dose IL-2 with or without LAK cell therapy [58,59]. There was, however, significantly increased toxicity using this combination and therefore studies were conducted utilizing IFN-α in combination with lower doses of IL-2.

Recently combination IL-2–IFN-α treatment has been assessed in a randomized trial by Negrier and colleagues [60]. 425 patients were randomized to receive IFN-α (18mU sub-cutaneously 3 weekly for 10 weeks) or IL-2 (18mU/m2 intra-venously in 5 day cycles as 2 induction and 4 maintenance cycles) or both IL-2 and IFN-α (at a lower dose of 6mU). Response rates after 10 weeks on an intention-to-treat analysis were 6.5 percent IL-2, 7.5 percent IFN and 18.6 percent in the combined group. There was, however, no difference in overall survival between the two groups.

Attempts to define host responses induced by these treatments have proved difficult although there is some evidence of an increase in NK cell activity [61]. In addition, the generation of thyroid auto-antibodies has been correlated with increased survival. In a study of 329 unselected patients, 60 (18 percent) were found to have anti-thyroglobulin and anti-microsomal thyroid auto-antibodies and the presence of auto-antibody correlated with prolonged survival ($p < 0.0001$) [62]. It has been suggested that the development of auto-antibodies is a measure of a breaking of tolerance to tumor and self antigens.

Biochemotherapy

Renal cell carcinoma is very resistant to conventional chemotherapy. However, there has been much recent interest in combining cytotoxic agents with biological therapies which have proven to be active in vitro against this tumor.

Atzpodien and colleagues first demonstrated increased response rates combining IL-2 and IFN-α with 5-Fluorouracil (5-FU), a well tolerated pyrimidine analogue that interferes with thymidylate synthesis [63]. Treatment was given on an outpatient basis with 8 weeks of IFN-α (6–9 mU/m2 1-3 times weekly sub-cutaneously), IL-2 (5-20 mU/m2 3 times weekly sub-cutaneously for 4 weeks) and 5-FU (750mg/m2 intra-venously weekly for 4 weeks). Of the first 35 patients reported, a response rate of 49 percent was demonstrated [63]. Subsequent phase III studies reported slightly lower response rates although a number showed an apparent advantage over IFN/IL-2 dual therapy. In a randomised study the same group compared the activity of the IL-2/IFN/bolus 5-FU against tamoxifen in 78 patients [64]. There was a 39 percent response rate in the biochemotherapy group vs. 0 percent in the tamoxifen group, with an impressive statistically significant improvement in survival. Median overall survival was not reached in the bio-chemotherapy group after 42 months vs. a median overall survival of 14 months in the tamoxifen treated group.

Our group has investigated the use of continuous ambulatory intra-venous 5-FU incombination with IFN-α and IL-2 [65,66]. 55 patients received IL-2 (10MIU/ m^2 sub-cutaneously twice daily on days 3,4,5 during week 1 and 4, 5MIU/m^2 days 1,3,5 week 2 and 3), IFN-α (6MIU/m^2 on day one for week 1 and 4; days 1,3,5 on week 2 and 3; 9MIU/m^2 on weeks 5-8) and protracted venous infusion (PVI) 5-FU (200mg/m^2/day on weeks 5-9). Objective responders or those with stable disease received a further 9-week cycle. A response rate of 38 percent was seen in evalu-able patients with a 29 percent response rate on an intention to treat basis [66]. Interestingly the majority of these patients were in a poor or moderate prognostic group with 47 patients having disease at more than one site and 26 patients having an ECOG performance status of 1.

Good responses to 5-FU containing biochemotherapy have been reported by other groups [67,68] although not all reports have been able to demonstrate any significant advantage with the addition of 5-FU to an IFN-α/IL-2 combination [69,70]. It is likely that this is a reflection of differences between protocols in the scheduling of the cytokines and in patient selection.

Additional chemotherapeutic agents used for RCC include vinblastine which is now being added to the IFN-α/IL-2 combination given the apparent advantage that biochemotherapy has over biotherapy alone; the early data looks promising [71,72]. Pyrhönen and colleagues have recently shown in a randomized trial that the combination of vinblastine and IFN-α is superior to vinblastine alone. There was a statistically significant increase in survival and overall response rate in patients receiving IFN-α and chemotherapy [73]. The 79 patients receiving bio-chemotherapy had a median survival of 67.6 weeks compared with 37.8 weeks for the 81 patients receiving vinblastine alone (p=0.0049).

Cis-retinoic acid has also been reported to have activity in combination with IFN-α in small-scale phase II trials and has recently been assessed in a rando-mized phase III study of 284 patients with advanced RCC [74]. There was no dif-ference in time to progression, survival or response rates between patients treated with IFN-α alone or IFN-α + cis-retinoic acid. There is an ongoing randomized study that is investigating the incorporation of cis-retinoic acid into the IL-2/IFN-α/5-FU regimes.

Other Immunotherapeutic Approaches

An alternative approach to aid the interaction between killer cell and target is to use bi-specific antibodies that have binding sites specific for both effector and target cells. In an in vitro study, bi-specific antibodies were constructed that have binding sites for the EGF receptor (over-expressed on a number of RCC cell lines) and antibody Fc receptors [75]. The bi-specific antibodies showed enhanced cytotoxicity when compared with conventional anti-EGF receptor antibodies in the presence of effector cells.

The recognition that dendritic cell-mediated antigen presentation is the most effective way of inducing cellular immune responses has led to interest in a variety of new immunotherapy approaches. Granulocyte-macrophage colony stimulating factor (GM-CSF) is a cytokine that stimulates the number and activity of dendritic cells and several groups are evaluating whether there is any benefit of adding this agent to existing therapies. Naughton and colleagues [76] used GM-CSF (1.25 mcg/kg sub-cutaneously days 1-5, week 1, 2.5 mcg/kg sub-cutaneously days 1-5 weeks 2 and 3) in combination with IL-2 (15MIU sub-cutaneously days 3-5 week 1, days 2-5 weeks 2 and 3) and assessed the levels of circulating dendritic cells. The regimen was well tolerated with no grade 3 or 4 toxicities being reported. An alternative approach is to "pulse" dendritic cells in vitro with candidate tumor antigens before adoptively transferring these primed cells back into the patient. In a recent study 12 patients received dendritic cell vaccines prepared by harvesting peripheral blood mononuclear cells after stimulation with GM-CSF. Dendritic cells were then pulsed with antigens from cell lysates of cultured autologous tumor cells along with the immunogenic adjuvant keyhole-limpet haemocyanin (KLH). Dendritic cells were administered by 3 intra-venous infusions at monthly intervals. Generation of anti-tumor cell and KLH immunity was demonstrated in vitro and the infusions were well tolerated [77]. The clinical effects of this customized therapy are awaited.

Attempts to identify tumor antigens that are recognised by CTL are an important component of these approaches and may result in more specific tumor vaccines being developed. For example, a number of tumor specific CTL have been shown to recognise members of the heat shock protein (hsp) family [78] and trials are underway with hsp-based vaccines [79]. These proteins are thought to act as "chaperones" for tightly bound immunogenic peptides aiding their passage through subcellular compartments where a single chaperone preparation may contain a number of differing immunogenic peptides. In a preliminary report, 29/33 evaluable patients completed weekly intra-dermal vaccinations on 4 occasions; one patient achieved a CR and 3 PRs were obtained with 18 patients showing stable disease. No significant toxicities were reported [78]. Small-scale trials of a variety of autologous tumor vaccines have been performed without any demonstrable benefit [80,81]. A prospective randomised study of a vaccine consisting of autologous tumor cells in combination with bacillus Calmette-Guerin (BCG) in 120 patients demonstrated the generation of vaccine-specific immunity as defined by cutaneous delayed-type hypersensitivity reactions (DTH) but without any advantage in disease-free or overall survival at a follow-up of 5 years [80].

Gene therapy is also being used to administer cytokines that have proven to be active in RCC. Administration of the IL-2 gene in a lipid particle delivery system (liposome) has shown encouraging early results, [82] where 17 patients, (of whom 14 were evaluable), were treated with plasmid DNA encoding the IL-2 gene. Two treated patients had partial responses lasting > 16 months. The use of adenoviral vectors has also being studied in vitro and tumor-infiltrating lymphocyte (TIL) cultures have been infected with adenoviral constructs containing the IL-2 gene. Genetically-modified TILs producing IL-2 showed enhanced anti-tumor activity against autologous renal cell tumor cultures in vitro in this preliminary study [83].

Conclusion

Renal cell carcinoma is one of the most immunogenic of human solid tumors. Standard therapy in fit patients consists of single agent IL-2 or IFN-α. Response rates, progression-free interval and overall survival are similar with both modalities although there is the suggestion that there are more durable complete remissions with IL-2-based regimes. Current efforts are focused on optimising biotherapy treatment protocols and exploring ways of increasing the efficiency of biochemotherapy, particularly those regimens containing 5-FU. In addition, the data suggesting high response rates with biochemotherapy provide a good rationale for the development of immunologically-based maintenance strategies.

However, it should be remembered that even with the promising early results of biochemotherapy, the majority of patients with metastatic disease do not respond to treatment and the majority of responders eventually relapse and die. There is therefore the need to identify those patients who will benefit from treatment, to find methods to reduce treatment toxicities and to develop more active therapies. The identification of CTL-specific tumor vaccines and the potential of cytokine gene therapy is an important area of on-going and future research.

References

1. Bumpus HC. The apparent disappearance of pulmonary metastasis in a case of hypernephroma following nephrectomy. J Urol 1928;2:185–91.
2. Everson TC. Cole WH. Spontaneous regression of cancer. Philadelphia:W.B. Saunders, 1966.
3. Kavoussi LR, Levine SR, Kadmon D, et al. Regression of metastatic renal cell carcinoma: A case report and literature review. J Urol 1986;135:1005–7.
4. Bloom HGJ. Regression of renal cancer. Cancer 1973;32:1066–71.
5. Snow RM, Schellhammer PF. Spontaneous regression of renal cell carcinoma. Urology 1982;20:177–81.
6. Kerble K, Pauer W. Spontaneous regression of osseous metastasis in renal cell carcinoma. Aust N Z J Surg 1993;63(11):901–3.
7. Omland H, Fossa SD. Spontaneous regression of cerebral and pulmonary metastases in renal cell carcinoma. Scand J Urol Nephrol. 1989;23(2):159–60.
8. Guthbjartsson T, Gislason, T. Spontaneous regression of brain metastases secondary to renal cell carcinoma. Scand J Urol Nephrol 1995;29(2):215–7.
9. Ritchie AW, Layfield LJ, deKernion JB. Spontaneous regression of liver metastasis from renal cell carcinoma. J Urol 1988;40(3):596–7.
10. de la Figuera M, Biosca M, Garcia-Bragado F. et al. Spontaneous regression of bilateral hilar lymphadenopathy in renal cell carcinoma. Eur J Resp Dis 1985;67(2):133–5.
11. Ritchie AW, James K, Micklem HS, Chisholm GD. Lymphocyte subsets in renal cell carcinomas — a sequential study using monoclonal antibodies. Br J Urol 1984;56(2):140–8.
12. Dadian G, Riches PG, Henderson DC, et al. Immunological parameters in peripheral blood of patients with renal cell carcinoma before and after nephrectomy. Br J Urol 1994;74(1):15–22.
13. Abskar YA, Chou TH, Redman BG. Spontaneous remission of renal cell carcinoma: a case report and immunological correlates. J Urol 1994;152:156–7.
14. Possinger K, Wagner H, Beck R, et al. Renal cell carcinoma. Contrib Oncol 1988;30:195–207.
15. Snow R.M, Schellhammer P.F. Spontaneous regression of renal cell carcinoma. Urology 1982;20:177–81.
16. Gore ME. Advances in management of renal cell carcinoma. Recent advances in urology/andrology 6:81–102.
17. Chowdhury S, Gore ME. The management of metastatic renal cell carcinoma. Urological Cancer Abstracts 1999;4:2–5.
18. Dadian G, Riches P, et al. Immunological parameters in peripheral blood of patients with renal cell carcinoma before and after nephrectomy. Br J Urol 1994;74:15–22.

19. Fossa S, Jones M, Johnson P, et al. Interferon-alpha and survival in renal cell carcinoma. Br J Urol 1995;76:286–90.33.
20. Jones M, Philip T, Palmer P, et al. The impact of interleukin-2 on survival in renal cancer: a multivariate analysis. Cancer Biother 1993;8:275–88.
21. Elson PJ, Witte RS, Trump DL. Prognostic factors for survival in patients with recurrent or metastatic renal cell carcinoma. Cancer Res 1988;48:7310–3.
22. Palmer PA, Vinke J, Philip T. et al. Prognostic factors for survival in patients with advanced renal cell carcinoma treated with recombinant interleukin-2. Ann Oncol 1992;3:475–80.
23. Mazumdar M, Bacik J, Motzer RJ. Survival-based prognostic stratification of 670 patients with advanced renal cell carcinoma treated on successive clinical trials at memorial sloan-kettering cancer centre. ASCO 1999;18:A1263.
24. Kalvakolanu DV, Borden EC. An overview of the interferon system: signal transduction and mechanisms of action. Cancer Invest 1996;14:25.
25. deKernion JB, Sarna G, Figlin R. The treatment of renal cell carcinoma with human leukocyte alpha-interferon. J Urol 1983;130:1063.
26. Quesada JR, Swanson DA, Trindade A. Renal cell carcinoma: antitumor effects of leukocyte interferon. Cancer Res 1983;43:940.
27. Horoszewicz JS, Murphy GP. An assessment of the current use of human interferons in therapy of urological cancers. J Urol 1989;142:1173–80.
28. Minasian LM, Motzer RJ, Gluck L, Mazumder M, Vlamis V, Krown SE. Interferon alfa-2a in advanced renal cell carcinoma: treatment results and survival in 159 patients with long-term follow-up. J Clin Oncol 1993;11:1368–75.
29. Steineck G, Strander H, Carbin BE, et al. Recombinant leucocyte interferon alpha-2A and medroxyprogesterone in advanced renal cell carcinoma. Acta Oncol 1990;29:155–62.
30. Kriegmar M, Oberneder R, Hofsetter A. Interferon alpha and vinblastine versus medroxyprogesterone acetate in the treatment of metastatic renal cell carcinoma. Urology 1995;45:758–62.
31. Medical Research Council Renal Trial Collaborators. Interferon-alpha and survival in metastatic renal cell carcinoma: early results of a randomized controlled trial. Lancet 1999;353(9146):14.
32. Muss HB. Interferon therapy for renal cell carcinoma. Semin Oncol 1987;14:36–42.
33. Quesada JR, Rios A, Swanson D. Antitumor activity of recombinant-derived interferon alpha in metastatic renal cell carcinoma. J Clin Oncol. 1985;3:1522.
34. Muss HB. The role of biological response modifiers in metastatic renal cell carcinoma. Semin Oncol 1988;15(suppl 5):30–4.
35. Hernberg M, Pyrhönen S, Muhonen T. Regimens with or without Interferon-α as treatment for metastatic melanoma and renal cell carcinoma: an overview of randomized trials. J Immunotherapy 1999;22(2):145–54.
36. Muss HB, Constanzi JJ, Leavitt R, et al. Recombinant alfa interferon in renal cell carcinoma: a randomised trial of two routes of administration. J Clin Oncol 1987;5:1083.
37. Bukowski R, Ernstoff M, Gore M, et al. Phase I study of polyethylene glycol (PEG) Interferon Alpha-2B (PEG INTRON) in patients with solid tumors. ASCO 1999;18:A1719.
38. De Mulder PH, et al. EORTC (30885) randomised phase III study with recombinant interferon alpha and recombinant interferon alpha and gamma in patients with advanced renal cell carcinoma. Br J Cancer 1995;71(2):371–5.
39. Niijima T, et al. Combination therapy with natural type human tumor necrosis factor (MHR-24) and human lymphoblastoid interferon-alpha (MOR-22) against renal cell carcinoma — a multiclinic cooperative early phase II study. Hinyokika Kiyo — Acta Urologica Japonica 1982;38(10):1201–7.
40. Rosenberg SA, Lotze, MT, Yang JC, et al. Experience with the use of high dose interleukin-2 in the treatment of 652 cancer patients. Ann Surg 1989,210:474–85.
41. Margolin KA, Raynor MJ, Hawkins MB, et al. Interleukin 2 and lymphokine-activated killer cell therapy of solid tumors: analysis of toxicity and management guidelines. J Clin Oncol 1989;7:486.
42. Siegel JP, Puri RK. Interleukin-2 toxicity. J Clin Oncol 1991;9:694.
43. Yang JC, Topalian SL, Parkinson DR. et al. Randomised comparison of high-dose and low-dose intravenous interleukin-2 for the therapy of metastatic renal cell carcinoma: an interim report. J Clin Oncol 1994;12:1572.
44. Sleijfer D, Janssen R, Willemse P, et al. Subcutaneous (s.c.) interleukin-2 (il-2) (Cetus) in patients (pts) with metastatic renal cell cancer (RCC). Proc Am Soc Clin Oncol 1991;10:517.
45. Lopez, Hanninen E, Kirchner H, Atzpodien J. Interleukin-2 based home therapy of metastatic renal cell carcinoma: risks and benefits in 215 consecutive single institution patients. J Urol 1996;155:19.
46. Tagliaferri P, Barile C, Caraglia M, et al. Daily low-dose subcutaneous recombinant interleukin-2

by alternate weekly administration: antitumor activity and immunomodulatory effects. Am J Clin Oncol 1998;21(1):48–53.

47. Yang JC, Rosenberg SA. An ongoing prospective randomised comparison of interleukin-2 regimens for the treatment of metastatic renal cell cancer. Cancer J Sci Am 1997;3(suppl 1):S79–84.

48. Oleksowicz L, Dutcher JP. A phase II trial of dose-intensive interleukin-2 in metastatic renal cell carcinoma. J Cancer Res Clin Oncol 1999;125(2):101–8.

49. Huland E, Heinzer H, Huland H. Treatment of pulmonary metastatic renal-cell carcinoma in 116 patients using inhaled interleukin-2 (IL-2). Anticancer Researsc 1999;19(4A):2679–83.

50. Gold PJ, Thompson JA, Markowitz DR, et al. Metastatic renal cell carcinoma: long-term survival after therapy with high-dose continuous-infusion interleukin-2. Cancer J Sci Am 1997;3(suppl 1):S85–91.

51. Gore ME, Galligioni E, Keen CW, et al. The treatment of metastatic renal cell carcinoma by continuous intravenous infusion of recombinant interleukin-2. Eur J Cancer 1994;30A(3):329–33.

52. McCabe MS, Stablein D, Hawkins MH. The modified group C experience — phase III randomised trials of IL-2 vs IL-2/LAK in advanced renal cell carcinoma and advanced melanoma. Proc Am Soc Clin Oncol 1991;10:714.

53. Rosenberg SA, Lotze MT, Yang JC, et al. Prospective randomised trial of high-dose interleukin-2 alone or in conjunction with lymphokine activated killer cells for the treatment of patients with advanced cancer. J Natl Cancer Inst 1993;85:622.

54. Hanson J, Petit R, Walker M, et al. Tumor infiltrating lymphocyte therapy (TIL) for metastatic renal cancer (RC) using interleukin-2 (IL-2). Proc Am Soc Clin Oncol 1992;11:682.

55. Fisher RI, Rosenberg SA, Sznol M, et al. High-dose aldesleukin in renal cell carcinoma: long-term survival update. Cancer J Sci Am 1997;3(suppl 1):S70–2.

56. Mule JJ, Rosenberg SA. Combination cytokine therapy: experimental and clinical trials. In: DeVita VT, Hellman S, Rosenberg SA editors. Biologic Therapy of Cancer, Philadelphia: JB Lippincott, 1991; 197.

57. Rosenberg SA, Lotze MT, Yang JC, et al. Combination therapy with interleukin-2 and alpha-interferon for the treatment of patients with advanced cancer. J Clin Oncol 1989;7:1863

58. Atkins MB, Sparano J, Fisher RI. Randomized phase II trial of high-dose interleukin-2 either alone or in combination with interferon alfa-2b in advanced renal cell carcinoma. J Clin Oncol 1993;11:661.

59. Aronson FR, Sznol M, Atkins MB, et al. A phase II trial of interleukin-2, interferon-alpha and lymphokine-activated killer cells for advanced renal cell carcinoma. Proc Am Soc Clin Oncol 1990;9:183.

60. Negrier S, Escudier B, et al. Recombinant human interleukin-2, recombinant interferon-alpha or both in metastatic renal cell carcinoma. N Engl J Med 1998;338:1272–8.

61. Molto L, Carballido J, Manzano L, et al. Immunological changes in peripheral blood mononuclear cells of patients with metastatic renal cell carcinoma after low doses of subcutaneous immunotherapy with IFN-alpha-2b and IL-2. J Immunotherapy 1999;22(3):260–7.

62. Franzke A, Peest D, Probst-Kepper M, et al. Autoimmunity resulting from cytokine treatment predicts long-term survival in patients with metastatic renal cell cancer. J Clin Oncol 1999;17(2):529–33.

63. Atzpodien J, Kirchner H, Hanninen EL. Interleukin-2 in combination with interferon-alpha and 5-fluorouracil for metastatic renal cell cancer. Eur J Cancer 1993;29A(suppl 5):S6–8.

64. Atzpodien J, Kirchner H, et al. Results of a randomised clinical trial comparing sc interleukin-2, sc interferon-alpha and bolus iv 5-fluorouracil against oral tamoxifen in progressive metastatic renal cell carcinoma. Proc ASCO 1997;16:A1164.

65. Vaughan M, Johnston S, et al. A phase 2 study of subcutaneous IL-2, alpha interferon (IFN) and prolonged venous infusional (P.V.I.) 5-FU in patients with metastatic renal cell carcinoma. Br J Cancer 1997;76(suppl 1):50.

66. Allen M, Vaughan M, Johnston S, et al. Protracted venous infusion 5-Fluorouracil (PVI 5-FU) in combination with subcutaneous (sc) interleukin-2 (IL-2) and alpha interferon (IFN) in patients with metastatic renal cell cancer: A phase II study. Proc ASCO 1999;18:A1274.

67. Samland D, Steinbach F, Reiher F, et al. Results of immunochemotherapy with interleukin-2, interferon-alpha2 and 5-fluorouracil in the treatment of metastatic renal cell cancer. Eur Urology 1999;35(3):204–9.

68. Elias L, Binder M, Mangalik A, et al. Pilot trial of infusional 5-fluorouracil, interleukin-2 and subcutaneous interferon-alpha for advanced renal cell carcinoma. Am J Clin Onc 1999;22(2):156–61.

69. Ravaud A, Audhy B, et al. Subcutaneous interleukin-2, interferon alfa-2a and continuous infusion of fluorouracil in metastatic renal cell carcinoma: a multicenter phase II trial. J Clin Oncol. 1998;16(8):2728–732.

70. Escudier B, Theodore C, et al. 5-Fluorouracile does not add any benefit to cytokine treatment in metastatic renal cell carcinoma. Proc ASCO 1999;18:A1303.
71. Naglieri E, Gebbia V, Durini E, et al. Standard interleukin-2 (IL-2) and interferon-alpha immunotherapy versus an IL-2 and 4-epirubicin immuno-chemotherapeutic association in metastatic renal cell carcinoma. Anticancer Research 1998;18(3B):2021–6.
72. Pectasides D, Varthalitis J, Kostopoulou M, et al. An outpatient phase II study of subcutaneous interleukin-2 and interferon-alpha-2b in combination with intravenous vinblastine in metastatic renal cell cancer. Oncology 1998;55(1):10–5.
73. Pyrhönen S, Salminen E, Ruutu M, et al. Prospective randomized trial of interferon alfa-2a plus vinblastine versus vinblastine alone in patients with advanced renal cell cancer. J Clin Onc 1999;17(9):2859–67.
74. Motzer RJ, Murphy BA, et al. Randomized phase III trial of interferon alfa-2a (IFN) versus IFN plus 13-cis-retinoic acid (CRA) in patients (pts) with advanced renal cell carcinoma (RCC). Proc ASCO 1999;18:A1271.
75. Elsasser D, Stadick H, Stark S, et al. Preclinical studies combining bispecific antibodies with cytokine-stimulated effector cells for immunotherapy of renal cell carcinoma. Anticancer Research 1999;19(2C):1525–8.
76. Naughton MJ, Haug J, DiPersio J, et al. A phase II study of dendritic cell mobilization with GM-CSF in conjunction with IL-2 as immunotherapy for renal cell carcinoma (RCC), an initial report. Proc ASCO 1999;18:A1344.
77. Holtl L, Rieser C, Papesh C, et al. Cellular and humoral immune responses in patients with metastatic renal cell carcinoma after vaccination with antigen pulsed dendritic cells. J Urol 1999;161(3):777–82.
78. Gaudin C, Kremer F, Angevin E, et al. A hsp70-2 mutation recognized by CTL on a human renal cell carcinoma. J Immunol 1999;162(3):1730–8.
79. Amato RJ, Murray L, Wood L, et al. Active specific immunotherapy in patients with renal cell carcinoma (RCC) using autologous tumor derived heat shock protein — peptide complex 96 (HSPP-96) vaccine. Proc ASCO 1999;18:A1278.
80. Galligioni E, Quaia M, Merlo A, et al. Adjuvant immunotherapy treatment of renal carcinoma patients with autologous tumor cells and bacillus Calmette-Guerin: five-year results of a prospective randomised study. Cancer 1999;77(12):2560–6.
81. Repmann R, Wagner S, Richter A. Adjuvant therapy of renal cell carcinoma with active-specific immunotherapy (ASI) using autologous tumor vaccine. Anticancer Research 1997;17(4B):2879–82.
82. Figlin R, Galanis E, Thompson J, et al. Direct gene transfer of a plasmid encoding the IL-2 gene (Leuvectin) as treatment for patients with metastatic renal cell carcinoma (RCC). Proc ASCO 1999;18:A1662.
83. Mulders P, Tso CL, Pang S, et al. Adenovirus-mediated interleukin-2 production by tumors induces growth of cytotoxic tumor-infiltrating lymphocytes (TILs) against human renal sell carcinoma. J Immunotherapy 1998;21(3):170–80.

15. The Immunotherapy of Bladder Cancer

Konstantinos N. Syrigos and Anastasios J. Karayiannakis

Introduction

Bladder Cancer is the fifth most common cancer in the Western World, with a projected estimate of 55,000 new cases in 2001 in the United States. It accounts for about 6.3 percent of all new cases of cancer amongst men, with the lifetime risk of being diagnosed with bladder cancer around 3.5 percent. In the United Kingdom, bladder cancer is the second most common urological malignancy, with an estimated 13,000 new cases and 5,500 deaths from this disease occurring each year [1].

Seventy percent of bladder tumors are superficial at initial presentation and are managed by endoscopic resection (TURBT). Unfortunately, 70 percent of superficial tumors recur and 25 percent of them progress to advanced grade and detrusor muscle invasion. The unpredictability of the progression pattern has led to the extensive use of intravesical therapies, following therapeutic resection of superficial bladder cancer. Indeed, although the incidence of bladder cancer in the USA increased by 26 percent from 1956 to 1990, the mortality has declined by 8 percent following the introduction of bacille Calmette-Guerin (BCG) immunotherapy and of cisplatinum-based chemotherapy regimens [2].

Superficial bladder cancer represents an almost ideal model for the application of cancer immunotherapy, since it allows the direct contact between the biological agent, (administered intravesically) and the malignant urothelium. Furthermore, as systemic absorption is minimal, theoretically high doses of the agent could by used with little systemic side-effects. Intravesical administration of BCG in patients with superficial bladder cancer (SBC) is the first and probably the most successful example of cancer immunotherapy. In fact, it was as early as 1929 when Pearl reported that patients with tuberculosis had significantly fewer bladder tumors than controls. But it was not until 1976 that Morales used intravesical instillations of BCG in the definitive treatment of SBC [3]. Since that report, several studies have confirmed the decrease in the recurrence and progression rate of SBC with the application of BCG. Other agents such as keyhole limpet hemocyanin (KLH), bropirimine and interferons have also shown promise as effective immunotherapeutic agents.

This chapter reviews these various intravesical immunotherapeutic agents in the treatment of bladder cancer along with the immunological concepts involved in therapy.

BCG

BCG is a non-specific immune stimulant. When applied intravesically, live myco-bacteria attach to the urothelial lining, facilitated by the fibronectin of the extra-cellular matrix. BCG is also internalized into bladder tumor cells, following specific activation of integrins. Thus, bacterial cell surface glycoproteins are attached to urothelial cell membranes, displaying antigenic epitopes which mediate the immune response. In fact, it has been demonstrated that BCG administration increases the expression of HLA-DR antigens on the surface of tumor cells.

The anti-neoplastic effect of BCG is the result of a combination of enhanced activity of various arms of the immune system. It induces non-specific inflammation of the urothelium, activating macrophages, T lymphocytes, B lymphocytes and natural killer (NK) cells. Intravesical BCG results in stimulation of local cyto-kine production, (most notably, IL-1, IL-2, IL-6, INF-γ and TNF-α), which can be measured in the urine for many hours following bladder instillation. BCG also induces a type II cytokine immune response mediated by IL-1, IL-4 and IL-10, which activate the cytotoxic cells (predominantly macrophages and T-helper cells) and subsequently develop an efficient anti-tumor response, where the lamina propria becomes infiltrated with immunologically active CD4 and CD8 cells. The in vitro motility of neoplastic cells is also decreased, following the interaction of BCG with the extra-cellular matrix fibronectin.

In conclusion, BCG-mediated inflammation is a localized phenomenon, which does not involve specific immunity, although changes in the peripheral blood are also seen, including heightened immunoproliferative response to BCG antigen in vitro and production of BCG-specific antibodies [2,4].

Immune stimulation requires multiple treatments and usually peaks following the sixth instillation in patients who have not had other prior therapies. In patients with a history of previous BCG intravesical treatment, in subsequent BCG courses, immune stimulation generally peaks by the third instillation. With continued treatment or increased doses, close to the maximum tolerated dose of BCG, the immune response is ultimately suppressed, because of the evolution of complex immune regulatory mechanisms. When induced, BCG immune stimulation persists for many months.

Carcinoma in situ

BCG immunotherapy is the only approved intravesical treatment of carcinoma in situ (CIS). Complete response rates following BCG intravesical treatment are as high as 72 percent, compared with only 50 percent for chemotherapy [5]. More than 60 percent of patients with complete response to BCG remain disease-free for up to 5 years, compared with only 20 percent of patients treated with chemotherapy [6]. Studies are in progress to investigate whether periodical administration of BCG would further improve these results [7].

Papillary Transitional Cell Carcinoma

A T1 lesion is defined as a tumor invading the lamina propria. Such tumors have the potential to recur and progress despite adequate resection and about two-thirds of the patients presenting with T1 disease will develop tumor recurrences within the first 5 years of their follow-up. Up to 30 percent of them will progress to muscle invasion at 1 year [8,9] and this aggressive biological behavior has an impact on overall survival [10]. The original tumor reflects the recurrence potential, since T1 tumors have a 7-fold progression rate, compared with Ta tumors. The original tumor also reflects the status of the remaining urothelium where patients with T1 lesions successfully excised are at increased risk of producing recurrent tumors with a more aggressive phenotype [11]. These observations provide the rationale for adjuvant therapies in order to decrease the recurrence and progression rate of T1 tumors. In fact, BCG is the most effective intravesical agent in increasing disease-free interval and prolonging survival. All six randomized trials performed comparing BCG immunotherapy after complete excision, with surgery alone have demonstrated a 38 percent reduction in recurrence rates (29 percent vs. 67 percent respectively). When compared with intravesical chemotherapy, (generally thiotepa, doxorubicin or Mitomycin C-MMC), BCG has demonstrated its superiority both in terms of the recurrence rates of tumor (20 percent vs. 33 percent respectively) and the disease-free interval (36 vs. 20 months respectively).

Nevertheless, although BCG seems to decrease recurrence and progression in patients with T1 tumors, half of the patients treated with BCG will ultimately progress if followed up for more than six years. Moreover, it is clear that not all patients benefit from BCG and a better understanding of the biology of T1 tumors will allow the assessment of patients who will require a more aggressive approach.

BCG Treatment Schedules

The optimal dosage and treatment schedule of BCG has not yet been defined. The current recommended low dose of 75 mg of BCG is effective, at least for patients with low malignant potential; providing acceptable toxicity. With regard to the management after initial treatment with BCG, two different approaches have been investigated. The first is an additional induction course after an initial complete response. A second course of BCG is also indicated in a select group of patients who develop positive cytology or a positive biopsy specimen within 6 months following the initial treatment. An alternative approach is maintenance therapy using three weekly instillations at 3, 6, 12, 18, 24, 30, and 36 months, aiming to achieve better local tumor control [11].

BCG Toxicity

BCG therapy is well tolerated by the majority of patients (>95 percent). Many of the adverse reactions caused by BCG therapy are related to the desired immunological response that is so important in its efficacy. Most patients experience mild dysuria, haematuria, fever and urinary frequency, which typically begin after the third instillation, as a consequence of the inflammatory response of the urothelium. This mild "cystitis" can usually be managed with acetaminophen and diphenhydramine. If the symptoms persist, patients may be given 300 mg isoniazid orally daily. Systemic absorption of BCG may occur, especially if patients develop gross haematuria and it is advisable to postpone further BCG administrations until the hematuria has resolved. The current recommendation is to wait at least 1 week after TURBT or biopsy before re-commencing BCG treatment [12].

Major adverse reactions are relatively uncommon. BCG sepsis, following traumatic catheterization with bleeding is the most important and often it is difficult to distinguish it from patients with simple BCG fever. Therefore, it is recommended that patients with fever lasting more than 48 hours must be admitted and placed on oral isoniazid 300 mg and rifampicin 600 mg per day. Once the fever has resolved, most patients can return to BCG intravesical therapy at a reduced dose, after receiving isoniazid for 1 day prior to treatment. If BCG sepsis is documented, antibiotics are given for 3–6 months, depending on the severity and duration of symptoms [12,13]. Other serious complications include granulomatous prostatitis, urethral obstruction, arthralgia, rash, pneumonitis and rarely hepatitis [13].

BCG Immunotherapy — Concluding Remarks

BCG is the most effective therapy for CIS of the bladder, while a significant number of patients with T1 lesions achieve a decreased recurrence and progression rate when treated with BCG. There is no definitive recommendation regarding the optimum dose and the administration schedule of BCG. Randomized trials are in progress to answer whether a second course of BCG after initial response and a maintenance therapy are beneficial for patients with high-risk superficial tumors [2,11].

Keyhole Limpet Hemocyanin

Keyhole Limpet Hemocyanin (KLH) is a nonspecific immune stimulator, with lack of any evident toxicity. It is a highly antigenic respiratory pigment isolated from the keyhole limpet mollusk *(Megathura creaulata)*. KLH initiates a cellular as well as a humoral immune response where it is recognized by macrophages. KLH induces a delayed-type hypersensitivity reaction and an increased local secretion of IL-1α in the urine. In an animal model, KLH therapy has demonstrated a reduction in tumor growth and prolongation of survival [14,15]. Intravesical administration of 2, 10 or 50 mg of KLH resulted in a 45 percent complete response (25 of 51 patients) and 21 percent partial responses (12 of 51 patients in one study by Lamm et al [16]. Response to KLH appears better in patients with CIS and in a further study by the same authors 6 weeks of intravesical treatment induced complete responses in 58 percent of patients [2]. When compared with intravesical chemotherapy (Mitomycin C), KLH resulted in less tumor recurrences of superficial TCC [17].

Bropirimine

Bropirimine (2-amino-5-bromo-6-phenyl-4-3H-pyrimidone) is an oral immunomodulator, which stimulates the production of endogenous cytokines such as INF-α2b, IL-2 and TNF. It also elicits cellular immune responses, with B-cell proliferation and activation of macrophages, lymphokine-activated killer cells (LAK) and NK cells [18]. It has shown its efficacy in the therapy of CIS and in patients treated for residual disease. The best responders are those who have not received prior intravesical therapy, with complete response rates approaching 70 percent in this group. The duration of responses ranges from 3 to 30 months, with a mean duration of 6 months [19,20]. The above data support the role and efficacy of bropirimine in the treatment of bladder cancer and provide the background for additional clinical trials.

Interferons

Interferons are biologic response modifiers, produced primarily by leukocytes, with anti-tumor and anti-proliferative properties. They induce antigen/antibody interactions, mediated by class I MHC antigens. Furthermore, INF-γ increases the expression of class I and class II MHC molecules by the tumor, facilitating differentiation of tumor-specific B and T lymphocytes and activating NK cells directed against the tumor.

Intravesical interferon therapy is very well tolerated, even when given in high concentrations. This has prompted several investigators to examine whether interferons could be used to prevent tumor recurrence and progression following TURBT. The results have been rather disappointing with intravesical interferon α-2b administration in patients with grade II TCC after TUR, resulting in between 21-37% recurrence rates over a 2 year follow-up. Up to 25 percent of these recurrences have significant muscle invasion with a mean interval until treatment failure of only 9.4 months on average [21,22]. Furthermore, in a randomized prospective clinical trial by Portillo et al. of 45 patients treated with IFN α-2b compared with 45 controls, the relapse rate for the interferon group was higher than the control group (53.8 percent vs. 51.2 percent respectively) after 43 months of follow-up [23]. A recent contrary dose-escalation study performed by Giannakopoulos et al. has demonstrated a significant advantage of adjunct intravesical interferon α-2b when compared with TURBT alone, suggesting that dose intensity may be important [24].

In an alternative therapeutic strategy, various studies have examined the ability of interferon to eliminate existing tumors or CIS. In one of the early studies, Oliver and co-workers failed to achieve any response in the CIS patients, whilst 75 percent of the patients with superficial disease responded (38 percent with complete response) [25]. In a further study by DiStasi et al., recombinant interferon α-2a was administered intralesionally in 15 patients with superficial papillary transitional cell carcinoma, with 5 patients (6.7 percent) having a complete response and 6 (40 percent) showing a partial response at a mean follow-up of 19.3 months [26].

Few clinical trials have investigated the therapeutic or prophylactic use of interferon-β. or interferon-γ. No complete responses have been observed and only minimal partial responses of short duration have been reported [27-29].

In conclusion several studies have been performed in patients with TCC, with the intravesical application of various interferons, before or after transurethral resection. Unfortunately, as there is an inconsistency in the type of interferon, the dosing and scheduling, it is difficult to judge their effectiveness. Studies are currently performed to investigate the potential role of interferons in combined application with intravesical chemotherapy or BCG.

Conclusions

The intravesical application of BCG in bladder cancer patients presenting with superficial disease is probably the most successful clinical example of anti-neoplastic immunotherapy available. BCG immunotherapy is the only approved intravesical treatment for carcinoma in situ, achieving complete response rates of about 70 percent. BCG is also the most effective intravesical agent in increasing disease-free interval and prolonging survival in patients with T1 bladder tumors, but it is also associated with significant toxicity and a tumor relapse rate of between 20–40 percent. Other agents, such as Keyhole Limpet Hemocyanin and Bropirimine are currently under clinical evaluation, whilst the interferons, (particularly recombinant interferon α-2b), have demonstrated encouraging efficacy against recurrent superficial transitional cell carcinoma and CIS. Investigation is currently in progress to identify the group of patients most likely to benefit from intravesical immunotherapy, while alternative therapeutic strategies with the combination of more than one agent are now also being considered for the clinical setting of bladder tumor sub-groups.

References

1. Silverman DT, Rothman N, Devesa SS. Epidemiology of bladder cancer. In: Syrigos KN, Skinner DG, editors. Bladder cancer: biology, diagnosis and management. London: Oxford University Press, 1999; 11–55.
2. Hall D, Battin J, Nseyo UO, Lamm DL. Immunotherapy of bladder cancer. In: Syrigos KN, Skinner DG, editors. Bladder cancer: biology, diagnosis and management. London: Oxford University Press, 1999; 345–58.
3. Morales A, Eidenger D, Bruce AW. Intracavitary bacillus Calmette-Guerin in the treatment of superficial tumors. J Urol 1976;116:127.
4. Patard JJ, Saint F, Velotti F, et al. Immune response following intravesical bacillus Calmette-Guerin instillations in superficial bladder cancer: A review. Urol Res 1998;26:155.
5. Herr HW. Carcinoma in situ of the bladder. Semin Urol 1983;1:15.
6. Lamm DL. Carcinoma in situ. Urol Clin North Am 1992;19:573.
7. Lamm DL, Crawford ED, Blumenstein B. SWOG 8795: A randomized comparison of BCG and mitomycin C prophylaxis in stage Ta and T1 transitional cell carcinoma of the bladder. J Urol 1993;149:275.
8. Heney NM, Ahmed S, Flanagan MJ, et al, for the National Bladder Cancer Collaborative Group A (NBCCGA). Superficial bladder cancer: Progression and recurrence. J Urol 1983;130:1083.
9. Pagano F, Garbeglio A, Milani C, et al. Prognosis of bladder cancer. I. Risk factors in superficial transitional cell carcinoma. Eur Urol 1987;13:145.
10. Jakse G, Loidl W, Seeber G, et al. Stage T1, grade 3 transitional cell carcinoma of the bladder: An unfavorable tumor? J Urol 1987;137:39.
11. Dalbagni G, Herr HW. Current use and questions concerning intravesical bladder cancer group for superficial bladder cancer.
12. Koukol SC, DeHaven JL, Riggs DR, Lamm DL. Drug therapy of BCG sepsis. Urol Res 1995;22:373.
13. Kritstjansson M, Green P, Manning HL. Molecular confirmation of BCG as the cause of pulmonary infection following urinary tract instillation. Clin Infect Dis 1993;17:228.
14. Lamm DL, De Haven JI, Riggs DR, et al. Immunotherapy of murine bladder cancer with keyhole-limpet hemocyanin (KLH). J Urol 1993;149:648 .
15. Lamm DL, Haven JL, Riggs DR. KLH immunotherapy of murine bladder cancer. Urol Res 1993;21:7.
16. Lamm DL, Morales A, Grossman HB. KLH immunotherapy of papillary and in situ transitional cell carcinoma of the bladder. A multicenter phase I-II clinical trial. J Urol 1996;155:1405A.
17. Jurinicic CD, Englemann U, Gasch J, et al. Immunotherapy in bladder cancer with keyhole-limpet hemocyanin: A randomized study. J Urol 1988;139:723.
18. Lotzova E, Savary CA, Stringfellow DA. Pyrimidones: new molecules with cancer therapeutic potential and interferon-inducing capacity are strong inducers of murine natural killer cells. J Immunol 1983;130:965.
19. Sarosdy MF, Lowe BA, Schellhammer PF. Bropirimine immunotherapy of bladder CIS. Phase II results of an oral interferon inducer. Proc Annu Meeting ASCO 1994;13:719A.
20. Sarosdy MF, Lowe BA, Schellhammer PF. Oral bropirimine immunotherapy of carcinoma in situ of the bladder: results of a phase II trial. Urology 1996;48:21.

21. Kostakopoulos A, Deliveliotis C, Mavromanolakis E, et al. Intravesical interferon alpha-2b administration in the treatment of superficial bladder tumors. Eur Urol 1990;18:201A.
22. Bartoletti R, Massimini G, Criscuolo D, et al. Interferon alpha 2a in superficial bladder cancer prophylaxis: Toleration and long-term follow-up. A phase I-II study. Anticancer Res 1991;11:2167A.
23. Portillo J, Martin B, Hernandez R, et al. Results at 43 months' follow up of a double-blind, randomized, prospective clinical trial using intravesical interferon alpha-2b in the prophylaxis of stage pT1 transitional cell carcinoma of the bladder. Urology 1997;49:187.
24. Giannakopoulos S, Gekas A, Alivizatos G, et al. Efficacy of escalating doses of intravesical interferon alpha-2b in reducing recurrence rate and progression in superficial transitional cell carcinoma. Br J Urol 1998;82:829.
25. Oliver RTD, Waxman JH, Kwok H, et al. Alpha lymphoblastoid interferon for noninvasive bladder cancer. Br J Cancer 1986;53:432.
26. DiStasi SM, Vergilli G, Vespasiani G, et al. Intralesional alpha interferon therapy in papillary superficial transitional cell carcinoma of the bladder: A pilot study. Br J Urol 1993;71:422.
27. Geboers ADH, van Bergen TNLM, Oosterlinck W. Gamma-interferon in the therapeutic and prophylactic management of superficial bladder cancer. J Urol 1987;137:276.
28. Migliari R, el Demiri M, Muscas G, et al. Intravesical installation of beta-interferon in the treatment of bladder cancer. Br J Urol 1992;70:169.
29. Niijima T. Intravesical treatment of bladder cancer with recombinant human interferon-beta: Intravesical GKT-beta chemotherapy research group. Cancer Immunol Immunother 1989;30:81.

16. Immunotherapy of Ovarian Cancer

Steve Nicholson

Introduction

There is no established role for immunotherapy in the management of epithelial ovarian cancer. The amount of research in this area is extensive, however, with some reports predating the introduction of efficacious platinum-based chemotherapy. The goals remain an improvement in response rates and (more realistically) the maintenance of responses by immunological means. An overview of both conventional ovarian cancer management and the immune environment of the peritoneum is provided before detailing clinical trial results and considering future developments.

Conventional Treatment of Carcinoma of the Ovary

Surgery

Surgery provides both histological confirmation of epithelial ovarian cancer, accurate staging and the first element of treatment. Surgery should, where possible, involve bilateral salpingo-oophorectomy and total abdominal hysterectomy, together with infra-colic omentectomy. The objective is cytoreductive; i.e. to remove as much tumour as possible, with a clear survival advantage (where optimal surgical cytoreduction has been achieved), regardless of histologic tumor type [1].

The vogue for "second-look" surgery was largely abandoned in the 1980s, when no survival advantage was found to accrue to patients who had residual disease resected after chemotherapy [2]. There has, however, been a resurgence of interest in "interval debulking" for patients in whom optimal primary surgery was not initially possible, where recent studies have shown that such patients who are rendered operable by preliminary cycles of chemotherapy may have a survival advantage if definitive surgery is performed before continuing with the remaining chemotherapeutic cycles [3].

Radiotherapy

Radiotherapy for ovarian carcinoma has been superseded by the emergence of cisplatin. The toxicity of whole abdominal external beam radiotherapy compared with that of chemotherapy led to experimentation with the intraperitoneal use of radiocolloids; the rationale for which is considered below (section 1.2.4). Comparisons with chemotherapy still, however, showed fewer side effects for the latter [4]. Selected patients undoubtedly benefited from irradiation in the pre-chemotherapy era [5], however the addition of radiotherapy to chemotherapy has not been shown overall to be beneficial, even where it is used as consolidation therapy for patients who achieve complete remission [6].

Chemotherapy

Stage Ia and Ib tumours are usually treated by surgery alone, but of the remainder almost all patients should be offered chemotherapy in either the adjuvant or the palliative setting. Platinum-based drugs (cisplatin and carboplatin) have supplanted alkylating agents (melphalan, chlorambucil, treosulfan) as the mainstay of chemotherapy for ovarian cancer. This is based upon both improved response rates and better toxicity profiles. Trials of paclitaxel in combination with platinum drugs have demonstrated improvement in both response rates and survival [7]. While subsequent studies have provided contradictory results [8–10], there is little doubt that platinum-taxane combinations are regarded by most ovarian cancer specialists as the gold standard for chemotherapy of this disease [11].

Intraperitoneal Therapy

The attraction of intraperitoneal therapy for ovarian carcinoma stems from three facets of this approach in this disease:

i.   Disease Characteristics — this is an illness that remains intraperitoneal for the majority of its natural history and for which optimal primary surgical therapy has been shown to have an impact on survival. Even when complete remission is obtained, however, microscopic peritoneal residual disease frequently remains.

ii.   Drug Characteristics — locoregional therapy offers the opportunity for localised dose intensification with a reduction in systemic side-effects. The intraperitoneal (IP) route is an acceptable alternative for systemic administration of soluble drugs (cisplatin and carboplatin), while for larger, water-insoluble chemotherapy such as paclitaxel, the pharmacokinetic advantage extends to a depot effect.

iii. Peritoneal Characteristics — The peritoneum is an active part of the immune system, with enormous numbers of macrophages and up to 2 percent of cells being dendritic cells [12]. If there is a role for immunotherapy in the management of this disease, this is the logical site for the administration of such treatment.

Intraperitoneal radioisotopes have been explored as a treatment for this disease since the 1950s. The initial use of ^{198}Au was superseded by ^{32}P, a pure β-emitter and the isotope with which most experience has been gained. Comparisons with chemotherapy that would be deemed inadequate by today's standards have shown no survival differences although there is greater toxicity in those patients receiving radiocolloid [4,13] and as chemotherapy has developed the routine use of IP radioisotopes has followed the "demise" of external beam radiotherapy.

Intraperitoneal administration of chemotherapy has been explored in numerous phase I and II trials as salvage therapy [14–20]. These trials confirmed that IP chemotherapy is possible with a wide range of drugs and that there is a degree of anti-tumour activity for most agents. The single most important trial of IP chemotherapy is the randomised phase III study performed in America by the Gynaecologic Oncology Group [21]. Here, patients were randomised to intravenous or intraperitoneal cisplatin 100mg/m^2, both given in combination with intravenous cyclophosphamide. This study, which took 10 years to complete, showed clear advantages for the intraperitoneal regimen, including lower toxicity, a median survival of 49 months (compared with 41 months) and pathological complete remission in 40 percent compared with 31 percent respectively. The intervening years since the inception of this study have seen major changes in the agents used for conventional therapy of ovarian cancer, notably the substitution of carboplatin for cisplatin and the emergence of paclitaxel as first-line therapy. Both these drugs can be given intraperitoneally and future trials of these agents are awaited.

The Immune Environment of the Peritoneum

Studies on human peritoneal tissue invariably rely upon tissue collected from patients undergoing invasive abdominal procedures for other medical reasons. The findings from these studies may not, therefore, be directly applicable to the normal human peritoneum, nor to its response to the presence of malignant ovarian tissue. A combination of immunocytochemistry and fluorescent staining with flow cytometry has shown that approximately 45 percent of peritoneal cells are of monocyte/macrophage lineage, a similar proportion are T lymphocytes, with around 2 percent B lymphocytes and up to 8 percent natural killer (NK) cells [12].

Antigen Presenting Cells (APCs)

Dendritic cells are present in much smaller numbers than macrophages, comprising no more than 2 percent of all peritoneal cells. These cells are, however, the most potent of antigen presenting cells, (APCs) and this proportion represents a major reservoir of APCs. The macrophage population differs from that in peripheral blood, demonstrating a more mature phenotype that includes increased expression of MHC class II antigens and Fcγ Receptors types II and III [22]. The collaborative role of peritoneal macrophages and dendritic cells (at that time poorly characterised as "reticular cells") in antigen presentation, particularly of antigen-antibody complexes, was first identified in 1971 [23]. Radiolabelled immune complexes were found to be ingested by peritoneal macrophages which then moved into intimate contact with reticular cells, clustering and extending pseudopodia. Radioactivity thereafter appeared within the reticular cells. It has been postulated that this facility for antigen presentation may reflect frequent antigenic challenge brought about by the connection of the peritoneal cavity to the exterior via the Fallopian tubes, uterus and external female genitalia.

Lymphocytes

The majority T cell population has a CD4/CD8 ratio of 0.4, which is the inverse of what is seen in the peripheral blood [12,24]. The CD8+ population has some unusual characteristics, notably a high proportion also possess CDw60 which characterises T-helper function [24,25]. Analysis of the cytokine patterns produced by peritoneal T cell clones has shown a higher than expected frequency of a T helper type 2 pattern (producing IL-4, IL-5 and Interferon γ) amongst CD8+ lymphocytes. This, together with reduced cytolytic activity by these T cells, is indicative of their involvement in supporting humoral immune responses in the peritoneum.

The B cell population of the peritoneum is largely composed of the CD5+ subset, designated B-1 [26,27]. These B cells possess surface-bound low-affinity immunoglobulin and as such they are thought to have a key role in the primary immune response. They have also been shown to be able to respond to antigenic stimulation by affinity maturation and immunoglobulin class switching, changing from the blunt instrument of first-line response to a more refined, antigen-specific defence mechanism. The proliferation of B-1 cells is enhanced in the peritoneum not only by T helper 2 function but also by selective support provided by peritoneal stromal cells [27].

Intraperitoneal Immunization

Experimental animals are often immunized via the intraperitoneal route. This is not only a matter of convenience, but also of the strength of the immune response obtained. Antigen-antibody complexes have been shown to be more efficient immune stimulators than either alone [28]. Studies of the human immune response to intraperitoneal immunization are fewer, but there is convincing evidence that IP immunization leads to both a local and a systemic immune response [26]. The features of the local response include the generation of relatively large numbers of cells which produce surface and/or secretory IgG or IgA.

Immunotherapy of Ovarian Cancer

No immunotherapeutic manipulation has yet emerged as an accepted part of ovarian cancer management. Many trials have, however, been conducted, often with clearly documented tumour responses.

Non-specific Immune Stimulants

The immune stimulants most often used in cancer have been BCG (Bacillus Calmette-Guérin) and *Corynebacterium parvum (C. parvum)*. The use of BCG has produced disappointing results. Two large randomised trials failed to show any benefit from the addition of BCG to combination platinum-based chemotherapy [29,30].

The experience with C. *parvum* in ovarian cancer has been particularly extensive, both intraperitoneally and systemically; alone and in conjunction with cytotoxic chemotherapy. There is no doubt that ovarian cancer responds to C. *parvum* therapy. Bast et al. reported a surgically-confirmed response rate of 45 percent to intraperitoneal treatment, while Berek et al. [91] documented a more modest 31 percent response rate, but with 10 percent pathological complete remission. Initial studies of combination chemoimmunotherapy with intravenous C. *parvum* plus alkylating agents showed improved responses and survival for chemoimmu-notherapy [31]. Most of these trials were not randomised, however, and they date from the pre-cisplatin era. One study from that period which used a more aggressive chemotherapy regimen (cyclophosphamide plus high dose methotrexate) found no advantage to the addition of *C. parvum* [32] and extrapolating these results to the present-day use of less toxic, more efficacious platinum chemotherapy, it would seem that any benefit to the addition of *C. parvum* in advanced ovarian cancer is unlikely. The toxicity profile, particularly of intraperitoneal *C. parvum*, has also mitigated against its continued use [33] although there have been no trials studying it in combination with platinum-based chemotherapy.

Other non-specific immunotherapeutics have been used in ovarian cancer, although the literature is less extensive. These include the use of the streptococcal antigen OK-432 [34], sizofiran (a beta-1,3-glucan) and thymopentin (a pentapeptide derived from the thymopoetin amino acid sequence [35]. Sizofiran has generated the most clinically relevant results of these three, with improved survival for patients receiving platinum-based chemotherapy combined with sizofiran compared with those receiving chemotherapy alone [36]. The survival advantage may be due in some way to activation of peritoneal macrophages [37], a similar mechanism having been demonstrated for OK-432 [38]. The majority of the work on these immune stimulants emanates from the Japanese literature and these results have failed to be reproduced in the Western literature.

Cytokines

The many and varied actions of the cytokines has made them attractive agents either for combination with chemotherapy or for consolidation or salvage therapy where there is chemo-insensitive disease.

Interferon-α

Intraperitoneal IFN-α. has been shown to stimulate peritoneal NK activity [39] and its ability to induce complete remissions where there is residual disease is clear with overall response rates varying between 30 and 70 percent [40,41], with small volume disease (<0.5 cm) most likely to be eradicated [42]. Unfortunately no survival advantage has been demonstrated where intraperitoneal IFN-α has been used as consolidation therapy for patients in complete remission [43]. IFN-α has been combined with most of the active cyotoxics, principally carboplatin, both drugs being given intraperitoneally. Whilst there is no doubt that such regimens are active against residual peritoneal disease [44,45], a randomised trial has failed to show any benefit from the addition of IP IFN-α to IP carboplatin [46].

Interferon-β

IFN-β has a better side effect profile than IFN-α, but the only small study of intraperitoneal IFN-β in ovarian cancer failed to demonstrate worthwhile additional anti-tumour activity [47].

Interferon-γ

The key trial of intraperitoneal IFN-γ reported an overall response rate of 31 percent in 98 patients with residual peritoneal disease following platinum-based chemotherapy [48]. The pathological complete remission rate was an exceptional 23 percent although the results of follow-up trials are awaited.

A more recent trial compared chemotherapy (cisplatin plus cyclosphamide – a rather outdated regimen) with and without sub-cutaneous IFN-γ as first-line therapy for patients who had already undergone debulking surgery for stages Ic to IIIc [49]. Both response rate and progression-free survival were improved in the experimental arm, although any overall survival difference has yet to reach statistical significance.

Interleukin-2

IL-2 has been used both alone and in combination with tumour-infiltrating lymphocytes (TIL) or lymphokine-activated killer (LAK) cells [50–55]. It has been used both intraperitoneally, intravenously and sub-cutaneously. No consistent benefit has been shown in any of these small trials, although activation of an intraperitoneal cytokine cascade and associated cytotoxicity has been demonstrated [56]. The best clinical response rates remain only of the order of 20 percent and given the alternatives for salvage therapy, this level of activity does not warrant the associated toxicity.

Cellular Vaccines

The use of irradiated autologous or allogeneic tumour cells (with or without various adjuvants) as cancer vaccines has become well-established in melanoma therapy and even has a precedent in non-immunogenic tumours such as colon cancer. There are only two such trials in ovarian cancer. The earlier of the two trials used allogeneic tumour cells with BCG as an adjuvant [57]. Ten patients with either recurrent disease or "advanced" disease at presentation received monthly intradermal vaccination in addition to chemotherapy. No details about chemotherapy in this trial are provided. An apparent survival advantage was seen when patients were compared with historical controls who received chemotherapy alone. (The reader should note that this trial dates from 1976, prior to the introduction of platinum-based chemotherapy). The second trial used autologous tumour and C. parvum as adjuvant [58]. The vaccine was again combined with chemotherapy, eleven of 14 patients receiving a cisplatin-based regimen that would be considered acceptable today. This trial details very little about the efficacy of the addition of the vaccine, although it describes the use of autologous tumour skin testing as a useful marker of immunisation. These are small, non-randomised studies and therefore although the scientific information remains relevant, the clinical results should be viewed with caution. It is also difficult relating these trials to modern practice due to the changes that have taken place in all areas of ovarian cancer management.

The use of genetically-modified tumour cells as cancer vaccines illustrates the cross-over between cancer "vaccinology" and gene therapy. Manipulation of cells to express either co-stimulatory molecules or cytokines should result in tumour cells that are more immunogenic (vide infra).

Non-cellular Vaccines

Candidate antigens for cancer vaccination include the carbohydrate Thomsen-Freidenreich (TF) antigen, peptides derived from tumour associated antigens (eg,

MUC^{-1}) and cruder preparations of tumour antigens derived from lysed tumour cells. A phase I/II trial using intraperitoneally administered viral oncolysates of two ovarian cancer cell lines showed some evidence of clinical activity in patients with measurable disease [56]. Similarly, a small phase I trial of TF conjugated to Keyhole Limpet Haemocyanin (KLH) and administered with the adjuvant DETOX recorded two minor responses (i.e. less than a partial remission) out of 11 patients with bulky disease [59]. Although laboratory evidence of immune activation can be demonstrated [60], it is too soon to say whether this will result in a vaccine of clinical value.

Immune Gene Therapy

This term serves to distinguish gene therapy with immunotherapeutic intent from the host of other cancer gene therapy maneuvers. The subject of genetic immunopotentiation in cancer where there is T cell receptor dysregulation is discussed in Chapter 12. The purpose of such therapy here may be to render ovarian tumour cells more immunogenic by transfection with co-stimulatory molecules or cytokine genes, or to transfect genes encoding tumour-associated antigens into immunocompetent antigen presenting cells.

Theoretically either approach could lead to the host mounting an immune response against autologous cells incorporated into the vaccine. There are a number of reasons why this may fail in practice, including variable expression of tumour-associated antigens and down-regulation of MHC antigens by tumour cells in advanced cancer [61]. The postulated mechanisms of escape by solid epithelial malignancies from immune elimination are discussed in Chapter 9. There are as yet no published clinical studies applying these approaches in ovarian cancer.

Monoclonal Antibodies in Ovarian Cancer Therapy (Mab)

Three approaches to MAb therapy of ovarian cancer have been the subject of extended research. These include the use of Mab alone, re-targeting of effector cells (lymphocytes, monocytes or NK cells) using bi-specific antibodies and radioimmunotherapy. A single trial of intraperitoneal immunotoxin produced no clinical responses in 23 patients [62].

Unlabelled Monoclonal Antibody Therapy

A list of tumor-associated antigens (over)-expressed on the surface of ovarian cancer cells is shown in Table 16.1.

A perceived problem with early MAb therapy was the development of an immune response against the murine protein. It was assumed that Human Anti-Murine Antibodies (HAMA) would have a blocking effect on the therapeutic MAb or even produce immune complexes with harmful consequences, up to and including serum sickness directed against the murine Fc portion of immunoglobulin. Whilst both these worries proved to have some foundation [63], the production of certain types of HAMA has wider implications for the use of MAbs in different therapeutic strategies.

Jerne, in 1974, speculated on the regulatory mechanisms in the human immune system which limited the antibody response to an antigen [64]. His idiotypic

Table 16.1. Frequency of antigens expressed by ovarian carcinomas and the antibodies used to detect them.

Antigen	Frequency on malignant ovarian tissue	Available monoclonal antibodies
CA125	89%	OC125, B43.13, 145-9
MUC1	90%	HMFG1, HMFG2, SM3, NCRC48
TAG-72	100%	B72.3
PLAP	67%	H17E2, NDPG2, H317, H7
Folate Binding Protein (FBP)	98%	MOv18
OA3	100%	OV-TL3

network theory (elaborated by others [65] and simplified here) has already been discussed in Chapter 9. Briefly it states that where an antibody is produced by the immune system, a further level of antibodies is generated whose targets are epitopes within the antigen binding site of the first antibody. These are broadly referred to as "anti-idiotypic antibodies", and they in turn lead to the production of a further level of "anti-anti-idiotypic antibodies", whose targets are the antigen binding sites of the anti-idiotypic antibodies and (possibly) so on in a cascade of internally reacting antibodies. This theory has since been proven, not least in the HAMA response to MAb administration [66]. The anti-idiotypic (or Ab2) response to an administered Mab (Ab1) may include a species whose antigen binding site is the mirror image of that of the administered antibody, forming an "internal image" of the target antigen. The anti-anti-idiotypic antibodies (Ab3) may therefore contain species whose antigen binding site is similar to that of the administered MAb, targeting the same antigen, but of fully human phenotype. This has led to the use of MAbs specifically to generate idiotypic networks, effectively functioning as cancer vaccines. Typically small, non-tolerigenic doses (100μg to a few mg) are used and routes of administration have included intramuscular, sub-cutaneous and more logically, intradermal injection for dendritic APC activation.

Two German groups have published extensively on the use of unlabelled MAbs B43.13 directed against CA125 [67] and B72.3 directed against TAG-72 [92], both tumor-associated antigens expressed on ovarian carcinomas. Idiotypic networks have been generated by both antibodies [68,69] and following on from observations made when these MAbs were used for RIS, patients seem to have a better than expected prognosis [67,70]. A randomised phase II trial of B43.13 versus placebo was instituted in 1996 [71], but closed due to poor accrual. Trials of an anti-idiotypic antibody generated against B43.13 are currently underway [72]. The humanized anti-HER2 MAb Trastuzumab ("Herceptin") might be expected to have some activity in c-erbB2-expressing ovarian cancer, but no studies have been published at the time of writing.

Cellular Re-targeting Using Bi-specific Antibodies

Chemical or recombinant methods may be used to create hybrid MAb or F(ab)$_2$ composed of two Fab fragments each targeting different antigens. Bi-specific-antibodies (bsAb) have been used to attempt to redirect cytotoxic cells to tumour cells by combining an anti-tumour Fab with an antigen binding moiety directed against T-lymphocytes (usually CD3), the type 1 Fcγ-Receptor (CD64) which is found on macrophages and NK cells, or CD16 found on NK cells.

Canevari and colleagues have reported extensively on pre-clinical and clinical work re-targeting lymphocytes to ovarian cancer using intraperitoneal adminis-tration of both bi-specific antibodies and activated T-cells [73–75]. One phase II trial documented 4 complete remissions of peritoneal metastases in 27 patients with small volume disease. T-lymphocytes were activated ex vivo using IL-2 and 11 patients received intraperitoneal IL-2 as part of their regimen. The overall response rate was given as 27 percent, with partial remissions claimed in 3 patients, but objective laparoscopic measurement of partial remission is not strictly possible and a peritoneal complete response rate of 15 percent with this form of therapy is a more useful statistic. Pre-clinical models suggested improved efficacy with prior activation of autologous T-cells ex vivo followed by re-infusion of these T-cells after they have been pre-incubated with the bsAb. This group has now extended their work to activating T-cells using anti-CD28 co-stimulation [76]. Patients thus receive two bsAb, one which targets CD3 and the Folate Binding Protein (FBP) and the other targeting FBP and CD28. They are also focusing their efforts on treating patients in the adjuvant setting.

Intraperitoneal Radioimmunotherapy (RIT)

Ovarian carcinoma is intrinsically less radiosensitive than lymphoma (the para-digm for successful use of RIT). There is no doubt, however, that in the past some subsets of patients have benefited either from whole abdominal irradiation [5] or from intraperitoneal radiocolloids [13]. The rationale for intraperitoneal RIT of epithelial ovarian cancer is that targeting of radioactivity to tumour tissue will enable higher activities and/or dose rates to be delivered without concomitant damage to normal tissue. The established clinical algorithm for the management of ovarian cancer means that most patients will have undergone surgery followed by chemotherapy. Trial patients therefore fall into three categories; those with recurrent/persistent disease following chemotherapy; those with small volume peritoneal disease and those with microscopic or undetectable disease (the "minimal residual disease" or "adjuvant" setting).

Most investigators have used ^{131}I as the initial radioisotope, which combines β and γ emissions [77–79]. This allows direct labelling of the MAb (via tyrosine residues) and imaging of the progress of the MAb through the body due to the γ-emission. ^{131}Iodine-based RIT is complicated both by the unwanted irradiation of normal tissue (and attendant staff), by γ-radiation and by tissue dehalogenation (which produces free ^{131}I). This in turn requires prophylactic administration of unlabelled iodine to prevent selective uptake by and irradiation of the thyroid. RIT would be better accomplished using an isotope with only a β particle, and later studies have switched to such isotopes in the hope of refining the targeting process [77, 80–82]. The characteristics of the more popular β-emitters are shown in Table 16.2. Many of these isotopes cannot be conjugated directly to antibody

Table 16.2.   Characteristics of isotopes chosen for their beta-emissions

Isotope	β-energies (MeV)	Half-life (days)	γ-emission
[131]I	0.6063 0.3338 0.2479	8	Yes
[90]Y	2.2839	2.67	No
[177]Lu	0.149	6.7	Yes
[186]Re	1.076 0.939	3.78	Yes
[188]Re	2.118 1.962	0.7	No

but require a bifunctional chelator conjugated to the MAb first [83,84]. These chelating agents are based upon DTPA, usually having been engineered for greater stability of the chelation complex and some have associated side-effects. The MAbs used have targeted a wide range of tumour-associated antigens.

The use of intraperitoneal rather than intravenous administration adds a level of complexity to the procedure. A number of investigators have attempted to answer the question of whether the IP route is superior to IV administration for targeting of the peritoneum. The results are equivocal and deal mainly with patients who had tumour nodules. These results may not, therefore, be applicable to the setting that is considered to be the most appropriate use of RIT; namely as consolidation of complete remission after chemotherapy.

Several authors have reported resolution of malignant ascites following RIT and where objective assessment of response has been made, some macroscopic disease appears to regress following such treatment [79–81]. The question of true minimal residual disease (i.e. microscopic disease only in the peritoneum) has only been addressed in one trial — a phase I/II study of ^{90}Y-labelled HMFG1 [85]. A small group of patients in first complete remission was found to have a better than expected outcome after RIT when compared with historical controls. This has led to a randomised phase III trial for such patients, but preliminary evidence suggests that there is no survival advantage in this trial.

Controversies surround the mechanism of action of intraperitoneal RIT. Conventional dosimetry predicts that insufficient radioactivity can be delivered to the peritoneum, compared with external beam radiotherapy. There is no guarantee, however, that conventional dosimetry is applicable to this form of treatment [86], particularly where it is administered in the adjuvant setting. If radiation is truly targeted preferentially to microscopic deposits, the overall activity delivered to normal peritoneum may be reduced without loss of efficacy. Questions also arise from the immunological sequelae of RIT. The development of HAMA and anti-idiotypic antibodies following RIT is accompanied, (in the ^{90}Y-HMFG1 trial), by rashes, arthralgia, myalgia and in two cases, neuropathy [87]. These reactions were seen with much greater severity with a macrocyclic chelate "DOTA" than with the non-macrocyclic chelate "CITC", which was eventually chosen for the phase III trial. There is a suggestion that these large molecules may be functioning as haptens, particularly when stabilised by the addition of yttrium to the ring structure. If the delivered radiation cannot account for any response to treatment, the question arises whether responses are immunologically mediated and whether these therapies are truly functioning as idiotypic vaccines.

The Future

There are several new strategies on the horizon for the treatment of ovarian malignancy. Interest has recently been generated in the fusion of tumour cells and APCs, with responses seen in a recent clinical trial in renal cell cancer [86]. This is supported by recent evidence that patients with breast and ovarian cancer can be effectively vaccinated with autologous dendritic cells (DCs) pulsed with HER-2/neu or MUC-1-derived peptides, producing sustained peptide-specific cytotoxic lymphocytes (CTL's), although the immunodominant peptides involved are not yet known [89]. These effects have also recently been observed in patients with advanced ovarian cancer, where CD8+ lymphocytes were stimulated in vitro with autologous ovarian tumor lysate-pulsed DCs. This vaccination resulted in MHC-restricted CTL activity against short-term autologous ovarian carcinoma cell lines, with the T cells of patients exhibiting the Th1 cytokine bias necessary for cell kill [90]. These new therapies will contribute to the development of active and adoptive immunotherapy in patients with residual or resistant ovarian cancer following conventional cytoreductive surgery and chemotherapy.

References

1. Griffiths C. Surgical resection of tumour bulk in the primary treatment of ovarian carcinoma. NCI Monograph 1975;42:101.
2. Luesley D Lawton F Blackledge G Hilton, C Kelly, K Rollason, et al. Failure of second-look laparotomy to influence survival in epithelial ovarian cancer. Lancet 2 1988;(8611):599–603.
3. van der Burg M, van Lent M, Buyse M, et al. The effect of debulking surgery after induction chemotherapy on the prognosis in advanced epithelial ovarian cancer. N Engl J Med 1995;332:629–34.
4. Vergote I, Vergote-De Vos L, Abeler V, et al. Randomised trial comparing cisplatin with radioactive phosphorus or whole-abdomen irradiation as adjuvant treatment of ovarian cancer. Cancer 1992;69:741–5.
5. Dembo, AJ. Abdominopelvic radiotherapy in ovarian cancer. A 10-year experience. Cancer 1985;55 (9 Suppl):2285–90.
6. Lambert HE, Rustin GJ, Gregory WM, Nelstrop AE. A randomized trial comparing single-agent carboplatin with carboplatin followed by radiotherapy for advanced ovarian cancer: a North Thames Ovary Group study. J Clin Oncol 1993;11(3):440–8.
7. McGuire WP, Hoskins WJ, Brady MF, Kucera PR, Partridge EE Look, et al. Cyclophosphamide and cisplatin compared with paclitaxel and cisplatin in patients with stage III and stage IV ovarian cancer [see comments]. N Engl J Med 1996;334 (1):1–6.
8. Sandercock J, Parmar M, Torri V. First-line chemotherapy for advanced ovarian cancer: paclitaxel, cisplatin and the evidence. Br J Cancer 1998;78(11):1471–8.
9. Stuart G, Bertelsen K, Mangioni C, Trope C, James K, Cassidy J, et al. Updated analysis shows a highly significant improved overall survival (OS) for cisplatin-paclitaxel as first line treatment of advanced ovarian cancer: mature results of the EORTC-GCCG, NOCOVA, NCIC CTG and Scottish Intergroup trial. Los Angeles:American Society of Clinical Oncology, 1998.
10. Harper P. A Randomised Comparison of Paclitaxel (T) and Carboplatin (J) Versus a Control Arm of Single Agent Carboplatin (J) or CAP (cyclophosphamide, Doxorubicin and Cisplatin): 2075 Patients Randomised Into the 3rd International Collaborative Ovarian Neoplasm Study (ICON3). Atlanta, Georgeia: American Society of Clinical Oncology, 1999.

11. Adams M, Calvert A, Carmichael J, Clark P, Coleman R, Earl H, et al. Chemotherapy for ovarian cancer – a concensus statement on standard practice. Br J Cancer 1998;78(11):1404–6.
12. Kubicka U, Olszewski WL, Tarnowski W, Bielecki K, Ziolkowska A, Wierzbicki Z. Normal human immune peritoneal cells: subpopulations and functional characteristics. Scand J Immunol 1996;44(2):157–63.
13. Young RC, Walton LA, Ellenberg SS, Homesley HD, Wilbanks GD, Decker DG, et al. Adjuvant therapy in stage I and stage II epithelial ovarian cancer. Results of two prospective randomized trials. New Engl J Med 1990;322(15):1021–7.
14. Hacker NF, Berek JS, Pretorius RG, Zuckerman J, Eisenkop S, Lagasse LD. Intraperitoneal cis-platinum as salvage therapy for refractory epithelial ovarin cancer. Obstet Gynecol 1987;70(5):759–64.
15. Campora E, Bruzzone M, Chiara S, Alama A, Iskra L, Carnino F, et al. Intraperitoneal cytosine arabinoside administered in sequence with systemic cisplatin, doxorubicin, and cyclophosphamide in advanced ovarian cancer. Gynecol Oncol 1990;37(1):39–43.
16. Kirmani S, McVey L, Loo D, Howell SB. A phase I clinical trial of intraperitoneal thiotepa for refractory ovarian cancer. Gynecol Oncol 1990;36(3):331–4.
17. Pfeiffer P, Bennedbaek O, Bertelsen K. Intraperitoneal carboplatin in the treatment of minimal residual ovarian cancer. Gynecol Oncol 1990;36(3):306–11.
18. Dufour P, Bergerat JP, Barats JC, Giron C, Duclos B, Dellenbach P, et al. Intraperitoneal mitoxantrone as consolidation treatment for patients with ovarian carcinoma in pathologic complete remission. Cancer 1994;73(7):1865–9.
19. Markman M. Intraperitoneal paclitaxel in the management of ovarian cancer. Semin Oncol. Seminars in Oncology 1995;22(5):86–7.
20. Chambers SK, Chambers JT, Davis CA, Kohorn EI, Schwartz PE, Lorber MI, et al. Pharmacokinetic and phase I trial of intraperitoneal carboplatin and cyclosporine in refractory ovarian cancer patients. J Clin Oncol. Journal of Clinical Oncology 1997;15(5):1945–52.
21. Alberts DS, Liu PY, Hannigan EV, O'Toole R, Williams SD, Young JA, et al. Intraperitoneal cisplatin plus intravenous cyclophosphamide versus intravenous cisplatin plus intravenous cyclophosphamide for stage III ovarian cancer. New Engl J Med. New England Journal of Medicine 1996;335(26):1950–5.
22. Eischen A, Duclos B, Schmitt-Goguel M, Rouyer N, Bergerat JP, Hummel M, et al. Human resident peritoneal macrophages: phenotype and biology. Br J Haematol 1994;88(4):712–22.
23. Stuart AE, Davidson AE. The handling of antigen-antibody complexes and of antigen by human peritoneal cells in vitro. J Pathol 1971;104(1):37–43.
24. Hartman J, Maassen V, Rieber P, Fricke H. T lymphocytes from normal human peritoneum are phenotypically different from their counterparts in peripheral blood and CD3- lymphocyte subsets contain mRNA for the recombination activating gene RAG-1. Eur J Immunol 1995;25(9):2626–31.
25. Birkhofer A, Rehbock J, Fricke H. T lymphocytes from the normal human peritoneum contain high frequencies of Th2-type CD8+ T cells. Eur J Immunol 1996;26(4):957–60.
26. Lue C, van-den-Wall-Bake AW, Prince SJ, Julian BA, Tseng ML, Radl J, et al. Intraperitoneal immunization of human subjects with tetanus toxoid induces specific antibody-secreting cells in the peritoneal cavity and in the circulation, but fails to elicit a secretory IgA response. Clin Exp Immunol 1994;96(2):356–63.
27. Hardin JA, Yamaguchi K, Sherr DH. The role of peritoneal stromal cells in the survival of sIgM+ peritoneal B lymphocyte populations. Cell Immunol 1995;161(1):50–60.
28. Perkins KA, Chain BM. Presentation by peritoneal macrophages: modulation by antibody-antigen complexes. Immunology 1986;58(1):15–21.
29. Alberts D, Mason-Liddil N, O'Toole R, Abbott T, Kronmal R, Hilgers R, et al. Randomized phase III trial of chemoimmunotherapy in patients with previously untreated stages III and IV suboptimal disease ovarian cancer: a Southwest Oncology Group Study. Gynecol Oncol 1989;32(1):8–15.
30. Creasman W, Omura G, Brady M, Yordan E, DiSaia P, Beecham J. A randomized trial of cyclophosphamide, doxorubicin, and cisplatin with or without bacillus Calmette-Guerin in patients with suboptimal stage III and IV ovarian cancer: a Gynecologic Oncology Group study. Gynecol Oncol 1990;39(3):239–43.
31. Rao B, Wanebo H, Ochoa MJ, Lewis JJ, Oettgen H. Intravenous Corynebacterium parvum: an adjunct to chemotherapy for resistant advanced ovarian cancer. Cancer 1972;39 (2):514–26.
32. Barlow J, Piver M, Lele S. High-dose methotrexate with "RESCUE" plus cyclophosphamide as initial chemotherapy in ovarian adenocarcinoma. A randomized trial with observations on the influence of C parvum immunotherapy. Cancer 1980;46(6):1333–8.
33. Bast RJ, Berek J, Obrist R, Griffiths C, Berkowitz R, Hacker N, et al. Intraperitoneal immunotherapy of human ovarian carcinoma with Corynebacterium parvum. Cancer Res 193;43:1395–401.

34. Kawagoe K, Masuda H. Advanced ovarian cancer treated by intraperitoneal immunotherapy with OK-432. Jap J Clin Oncol 1986;16(2):137–42.
35. Mallmann P, Krebs D. Investigations on cell-mediated immunity in patients with breast and ovarian carcinomas receiving a combination of chemotherapy and immunotherapy with thymopentin. Methods & Findings Exp Clin Pharm 1990;12(5):333–40.
36. Inoue M, Tanaka Y, Sugita N, Yamasaki M, Yamanaka T, Minagawa J, et al. Improvement of long-term prognosis in patients with ovarian cancers by adjuvant sizofiran immunotherapy: a prospective randomized controlled study. Biotherapy 1993;6(1):13–8.
37. Chen J, Hasumi K. Activation of peritoneal macrophages in patients with gynecological malignancies by sizofiran and recombinant interferon-gamma. Biotherapy 1993;6(3):189–94.
38. Koelbl H, Micksche M, Gitsch G, Hanzal E, Nowotny C. Treatment with biologic response modifiers in patients with ovarian cancer. Eur J Obstet Gynecol Reprod Biol 1991;41(1):64–9.
39. Lichtenstein A, Spina C, Berek J, Jung T, J Z. Intraperitoneal administration of human recombinant interferon-alpha in patients with ovarian cancer: effects on lymphocyte phenotype and cytotoxicity. Cancer Res 1988;48(20):5853–9.
40. Nicoletta MO, Fiorentino MV, Vinante O, Prosperi A, Tredese F, Tumolo S, et al. Experience with intraperitoneal alpha-2a interferon. Oncology Switzerland 1992;49(6):467–73.
41. Berek J, Stonebraker B, Lentz S, Adelson M, DeGeest K, Moore D. Intraperitoneal alpha-interferon in residual ovarian carcinoma: a phase II gynecologic oncology group study. Am Soc Clin Oncol, Los Angeles, 1998.
42. Willemse P, de Vries E, Mulder N, Aalders J, Bouma J, Sleijfer D. Intraperitoneal human recombinant interferon alpha-2b in minimal residual ovarian cancer. Eur J Cancer 1990;26 (3):353–8.
43. Proietto A, Hacker NF. Intraperitoneal interferon-alpha-2b for patients with no macroscopic disease following second-look laparotomy. Int J Gynecol Cancer 1993;3(5):324–8.
44. Ferrari E, Maffeo DA, Graziano R, Gallo MS, Pignata S, De-Rosa L, et al. Intraperitoneal chemotherapy with carboplatin and recombinant interferon alpha in ovarian cancer. Eur J Gynaecol Oncol. European Journal of Gynaecological Oncology 1994;15(6):437–42.
45. Frasci G, Tortoriello A, Facchini G, Conforti S, Persico G, Mastrantonio P, et al. Carboplatin and alpha-2b interferon intraperitoneal combination as first-line treatment of minimal residual ovarian cancer. A pilot study. Eur J Cancer Part A Gen Top 1994;30(7):946–50.
46. Bruzzone M, Rubagotti A, Gadducci A, Catsafados E, Foglia G, Brunetti I, et al. Intraperitoneal carboplatin with or without interferon-alpha in advanced ovarian cancer patients with minimal residual disease at second look: a prospective randomized trial of 111 patients. G.O.N.O. Gruppo Oncologic Nord Ovest. Gynecol Oncol 1997;65(3):499–505.
47. Rambaldi A, Introna M, Colotta F, Landolfo S, Colombo N, Mangioni C, et al. Intraperitoneal administration of interferon beta in ovarian cancer patients. Cancer 1995;56 (2):294–301.
48. Pujade-Lauraine E, Guastalla JP, Colombo N, Devillier P, Francois E, Fumoleau P, et al. Intraperitoneal recombinant interferon gamma in ovarian cancer patients with residual disease at second-look laparotomy. J Clin Oncol 1996;14(2):343–50.
49. Windbichler G, Hausmaninger H, Stummvoll W, Graf A, Kainz C, Lahodny J, et al. Interferon-gamma in the first-line therapy of ovarian cancer: a randomized phase III trial. Br J Cancer 2000;82(6):1138–44.
50. Kamada M, Sakamoto Y, Furumoto H, Mori K, Daitoh T, Irahara M, et al. Treatment of malignant ascites with allogeneic and autologous lymphokine-activated killer cells. Gynecol Oncol 1989;34(1):34–7.
51. Steis RG, Urba WJ, VanderMolen LA, Bookman MA, Smith-JW II, et al. Intraperitoneal lymphokine-activated killer-cell and interleukin-2 therapy for malignancies limited to the peritoneal cavity. J Clin Oncol 1990;8(10):1618–29.
52. Stewart J, Hird V, Snook D, Dhokia B, Sivolapenko G, Hooker G, et al. Intraperitoneal yttrium-90-labeled monoclonal antibody in ovarian cancer. J Clin Oncol 1990;8(12):1941–50.
53. Freedman RS, Edwards CL, Kavanagh JJ, Kudelka AP, Katz RL, Carrasco CH, et al. Intraperitoneal adoptive immunotherapy of ovarian carcinoma with tumor- infiltrating lymphocytes and low-dose recombinant interleukin-2: A pilot trial. J Immunother 1994;16 (3):198–210.
54. Freedman RS, Gibbons JA, Giedlin M, Kudelka AP, Kavanagh JJ, Edwards CL, et al. Immunopharmacology and cytokine production of a low-dose schedule of intraperitoneally administered human recombinant interleukin-2 in patients with advanced epithelial ovarian carcinoma. J Immunother Emphasis Tumor Immunol 1996;19(6):443–51.
55. Edwards R, Lembersky B, Kunschner A. Intraperitoneal interleukin-2 (IL-2) produces durable responses for refractory ovarian cancer. Am Soc Clin Oncol 1995.
56. Freedman R, Edwards C, Bowen J, Lotzova E, Katz R, Lewis E, et al. Viral oncolysates in patients with advanced ovarian cancer. Gynecol Oncol 1988;29(3):337–47.

57. Hudson C, McHardy J, Curling O, English P, Levin L, Poulton T, et al. Active specific immunotherapy for ovarian cancer. Lancet 1976;ii:877–9.

58. Gusdon JJ, Homesley H, Jobson V, Muss H. Treatment of advanced ovarian malignancy with chemoimmunotherapy using autologous tumor and Corynebacterium parvum. Obstet Gynecol 1983;62(6):728–35.

59. Yacyshyn M, Poppema S, Berg A, MacLean G, Reddish M, Meikle A, et al. CD69+ and HLA-DR+ activation antigens on peripheral blood lymphocyte populations in metastatic breast and ovarian cancer patients: correlations with survival following active specific immunotherapy. Int J Cancer 1995;61(4):470–4.

60. Ioannides C, Platsoucas C, Freedman R. Immunological effects of tumor vaccines: II. T cell responses directed against cellular antigens in the viral oncolysates. In Vivo 1990;4(1): 17–24.

61. Bodmer WF, Browning MJ, Krausa P, Rowan A, Bicknell DC, Bodmer JG. Tumor escape from immune response by variation in HLA expression and other mechanisms. Ann N Y Acad Sci 1993;690:42–9.

62. Pai L, Bookman M, Ozols R, Young R, Smith Jd, Longo D, et al. Clinical evaluation of intraperitoneal Pseudomonas exotoxin immunoconjugate OVB3-PE in patients with ovarian cancer. J Clin Oncol 1991;9(12):2095–103.

63. Davies K, Hird V, Stewart S, Sivolapenko G, Jose P, Epenetos A, et al. A study of in vivo immune complex formation and clearance in man. J Immunol 1990;144:4613–20.

64. Jerne N. Towards a network theory of the immune system. Ann Immunol (Inst Pasteur) 1974;125C:373–89.

65. Bona C, Victor-Kobrin C, Manheimer A, Bellon B, Rubinstein L. Regulatory arms of the immune reponse. Immunol Rev 1984;79:25–44.

66. Courtenay-Luck NS, Epenetos AA, Sivolapenko GB, Larche M, Barkans JR, Ritter MA. Development of anti-idiotypic antibodies against tumour antigens and autoantigens in ovarian cancer patients treated intraperitoneally with mouse monoclonal antibodies. Lancet 1988;2(8616):894–7.

67. Baum R, Noujaim A, Nani A, Moebus V, Hertel A, Niesen A, et al. Clinical course of ovarian cancer patients under repeated stimulation of HAMA using MAb OC125 and B43.13. Hybridoma 1993;12(5):583–9.

68. Baum RP, Niesen A, Hertel A, Nancy A, Hess H, Donnerstag B, et al. Activating anti-idiotypic human anti-mouse antibodies for immunotherapy of ovarian carcinoma. Cancer 1994;73(3 Suppl):1121–5.

69. Madiyalakan R, Sykes T, Dharampaul S, Sykes C, Baum R, Hr G, et al. Anti-idiotype induction therapy: evidence for the induction of immune response through the idiotype network in patients with ovarian cancer after administration of anti-CA125 murine monoclonal antibody B43.13. Hybridoma 1995;14(2):199–203.

70. Wagner U. Antitumor antibodies for immunotherapy of ovarian carcinomas. Hybridoma 1993;12(5):521–8.

71. Medac. OVAREX (MAb-B43.13). A murine monoclonal antibody for the immunotherapy and immunoscintigraphy of epithelial ovarian tumours, medac Gesellschaft fur klinische 1996.

72. Reinartz S, Boerner H, Koehler S, Von Ruecker A, Schlebusch H, U W. Evaluation of immunological responses in patients with ovarian cancer treated with the anti-idiotype vaccine ACA125 by determination of intracellular cytokines–a preliminary report. Hybridoma 1999;18(1):41–5.

73. Bolhuis RL, Stoter G, Arienti F, Canevari S. Adoptive immunotherapy (Meeting abstract). Proc Annu Meet Am Assoc Cancer Res 1994.

74. Canevari S, Mezzanzanica D, Mazzoni A, Negri D, Ramakrishna V, Bolhuis R , et al. Bispecific antibody targeted T cell therapy of ovarian cancer: Clinical results and future directions. J Hematother 1995;4(5):423–7.

75. Canevari S, Stoter G, Arienti F, Bolis G, Colnaghi MI, Di RE, et al. Regression of advanced ovarian carcinoma by intraperitoneal treatment with autologous T lymphocytes retargeted by a bispecific monoclonal antibody. J Natl Cancer Inst 1995;87(19):1463–9.

76. Mazzoni A, Mezzanzanica D, Jung G, Wolf H, Colnaghi M, Canevari S. CD3-CD28 costimulation as a means to avoiding T cell preactivation in bispecific monoclonal antibody-based treatment of ovarian carcinoma. Cancer Res 1996;56(23):5443–9.

77. Stewart J, Hird V, Snook D, Sullivan M, Myers M, Epenetos A. Intraperitoneal 131I- and 90Y-labelled monoclonal antibodies for ovarian cancer: pharmacokinetics and normal tissue dosimetry. Int J Cancer Supp 1988;3:71–6.

78. Buraggi GL, Crippa F, Gasparini M, Seregni E, Gavoni N, Marini A. Radioimmunotherapy of ovarian cancer with 131I MOv18: preliminary results (Meeting abstract). Fourth Annual Symposium: Current Status and Future Directions of Immunoconjugates. Diagnostic and Therapeutic Applications in Benign and Malignant Disorders 1992.

79. Crippa F, Bolis G, Seregni E, Gavoni N, Scarfone G, Ferraris C, et al. Single-dose intraperitoneal radioimmunotherapy with the murine monoclonal-antibody i-131 mov18 - clinical-results in patients with minimal residual disease of ovarian-cancer. Eur J Cancer 1995;31A(5):686–90.
80. Stewart JA, Belinson JL, Moore AL, Dorighi JA, Grant BW, Haugh LD, et al. Phase I trial of intra-peritoneal recombinant interleukin-2/lymphokine-activated killer cells in patients with ovarian cancer. Cancer Res 1990;50(19):6302–10.
81. Jacobs AJ, Fer M, Su FM, Breitz H, Thompson J, Goodgold H, et al. A phase I trial of a rhenium 186-labeled monoclonal antibody administered intraperitoneally in ovarian carcinoma: Toxicity and clinical response. Obstet Gynecol 1993;82(4):586–93.
82. Alvarez R, Partridge E, Khazaeli M, Plott G, Austin M, Kilgore L, et al. Intraperitoneal radio-immunotherapy of ovarian cancer with 177Lu-CC49: a phase I/II study. Gynecol Oncol 1997;65:94–101.
83. Meares C, McCall M, Rearden D, Goodwin D, Diamanti C, McTigue M. Conjugation of antibodies with bifuncyional chelating agents:isothiocyanate and bromoacetamide reagents, methods of analy-sis and subsequent addition of metal ions. Anal Biochem 1984;142:68–78.
84. Meares C, Moi M, Diril H, Kukis D, McCall M, Deshpande S, et al. Macrocyclic chelates of radio-metals for diagnosis and therapy. Br J Cancer 1990;62(Suppl X):21–6.
85. Hird V, Maraveyas A, Snook D, Dhokia B, Soutter WP, Meares C, et al. Adjuvant therapy of ovarian cancer with radioactive monoclonal antibody. Br J Cancer 1993;68(2):403–6.
86. Myers M. Dosimetry for radiolabelled antibodies–macro or micro? Int J Cancer Suppl 1988;2:71–3.
87. Maraveyas A, Snook D, Hird V, Kosmas C, Meares CF, Lambert HE, et al. Pharmacokinetics and toxicity of an yttrium-90-CITC-DTPA-HMFG1 radioimmunoconjugate for intraperitoneal radio-immunotherapy of ovarian cancer. Cancer 1994;73(3 Suppl):1067–75.
88. Kugler A,Stuhler G, Walden P, Zoller G, Zobywalski A, Brossart P, et al. Regression of human metastatic renal cell carcinoma after vaccination with tumour cell-dendritic cell hybrids. Nature Med 2000;6(3):332–6.
89. Brossart P, Wirths S, Stuhler G, Reichardt VL, Kanz L, Brugger W. Induction of cytotoxic T-lym-phocyte responses in vivo after vaccinations with peptide-pulsed dendritic cells. Blood 2000;96:3102–8.
90. Santin AD, Hermonat PL, Ravaggi A, Bellone S, Pecorelli S, Cannon MJ, Parham GP. In vitro induction of tumor-specific human lymphocyte antigen class 1-restricted CD8 cytotoxic T lympho-cytes by ovarian tumor antigen-pulsed autologous dendritic cells from patients with advanced ovarian cancer. Am J Obstet Gynecol 2000;183:601–9.

17. The Immunology and Molecular Biology of Breast Cancer

Isha A. Mustafa and Kirby I. Bland

Introduction

Though often overlooked, the breast functions as part of the immune system. Normal breast tissue contains not only glandular epithelial cells, adipocytes and blood vessels, but also lymphocytes. There are cells of immune origin present within the breast at all times which continuously release IgA [1]. Additionally, immunoglobulin and possibly T-cell immunity is passed from mother to infant during the time of lactation [2].

It is widely known that breast parenchymal cells are affected by hormonal changes, including both proliferative and quiescent signals, however, it is less well appreciated that breast lymphocytes also react to hormonal stimulation and suppression. The immunologic and molecular biologic pathways which affect the inception and progression of breast cancer remain obscure despite decades of research. The processes of carcinogenesis and tumorigenesis are begun long before there is clinical evidence of disease. The degree of immune surveillance and molecular management during this period of clinical latency is not clear. Likewise, the immunologic changes which allow for tumor tolerance and progression are also ambiguous and most probably not constant throughout all stages of the disease.

It is far from certain what changes take place in the process from immune suppression to immune tolerance of tumors and their metastases. These issues are covered elsewhere in this book. Assuredly, there must be defined stages of immune response to and surveillance of breast cancer. It has been shown that the inflammatory response of patients to their own tumors declines as lesions progress from in situ, to invasive and finally to metastatic disease. Eighty two percent of patients with in situ disease show an immune response, compared with 47 percent and 20 percent in patients with invasive disease and those with nodal involvement, respectively [3].

Identification of specific genetic aberrations, as well as specified immunologic cell types and cytokine profiles associated with breast cancer have only begun to establish a foundation for an improved understanding of breast cancer immunology and molecular biology. It is in this context that the present and the future of breast cancer therapy are viewed.

Tumor Infiltrating Lymphocytes

Tumor infiltrating lymphocytes (TIL) from primary breast cancers have been compared with lymphocytes found in non-neoplastic sites with respect to function and type. Vose and Moore demonstrated that TIL from breast cancers were composed predominantly of T cells. Furthermore, they showed that breast cancer TIL were functionally inferior to other T cells. They also reported that these TIL could suppress the normal proliferative and cytotoxic abilities of peripheral lymphocytes [4].

Additional evidence of the depressed natural killer (NK) activity of TIL was provided by Eremin et al [5]. They were also able to demonstrate that, when added to peripheral lymphocytes, TIL significantly suppressed the NK activity of the peripheral cells. Taken together these findings are important because the presence of TIL has been thought to indicate a protective immune response and confer a more favorable prognosis. These data, however, would suggest that TIL may play a vital role in loss of immune surveillance and enhanced capability for tumor growth and metastases. Perhaps, depending on the stage of disease, TIL can be either beneficial or detrimental in their immune responsiveness to breast cancer.

When Whiteside and others analyzed TIL from breast cancer patients for cell type, CD8+ cells were more abundant than CD4+ cells [6]. Few of the cells expressed either receptors or antigens consistent with activation of these immune cells. Though response to stimulation was depressed, the investigators were able to isolate the clones which did respond. The majority were CD4+ cells with some cytolytic activity. This study showed that TIL in their native environment do not provide either adequate or effective immunity against breast cancer.

Recently, Wong and co-workers compared the functional ability of TIL in breast cancer patients with the functional ability of lymphocytes in axillary nodes (LNL) and peripheral blood (PBL) in the same patients [7]. The number of TIL was affected only by stage of disease and was not affected by size, grade or estrogen receptor (ER)/progesterone receptor (PR) status of the primary tumor. Synthesis of Th1 and Th2 cytokines by lymphocytes from each site was measured. In addition, the ability of the cells to mediate a cytotoxic response to breast cancer cell lines was assessed.

Lymphocytes from all sites demonstrated a predominantly Th1 response. TIL produced mainly INF-γ, compared with lymph node lymphocytes (LNL) and peripheral blood lymphocytes (PBL), which produced mainly IL-2. Stimulation with IL-2 resulted in much higher levels of tumoricidal activity in TIL from node-positive compared with node-negative patients and IL-2-stimulated tumoricidal activity was greatest by far in PBL, being approximately four times the activity stimulated in LNL and TIL. In all, the predominant immune response to breast cancer locally, regionally and systemically was effectively Type 1, however, immune cells appear to function differently in each of these different environments.

These data suggest that node-positive patients can be distinguished from node-negative patients by measurement of the level of IL-2-stimulated tumoricidal activity of local TIL. This information could therefore alter the need for surgical treatment of this disease. This type of analysis of the primary tumor may be used to determine which patients are node-positive vs. node-negative, thereby potentially eliminating the need for sentinel node biopsy and/or axillary node dissection, since therapy could be based on these characteristics of the primary tumor alone. Furthermore, if cytotoxic function in node-positive TIL is greater than that in node-negative TIL, then the suggestion is that the leukocytes in the tumors of these patients have been activated. This fact would have potential therapeutic implications when one considers the future role of immuno-modulatory therapy, including the use of various forms of tumor vaccines, in these patients.

Major Histocompatibility Antigens and Adhesion Molecules

Class I major histocompatability antigens must be expressed by tumors for immune cells to interact and for T-cell receptor stimulation. MHC class I and intercellular adhesion molecule (ICAM-1) expression must be present in order to have T-cell-mediated killing of breast cancer cells [8]. However, it may also be possible that the presence of these surface molecules results in immune-stimulated growth of the tumor.

One study from the Icelandic Cancer Society examined 59 breast carcinomas and found that 57.6 percent expressed MHC class I antigen, while 44.1 percent expressed ICAM-1. The growth-stimulatory response of these breast cancers to lymphocytes was significantly associated with the expression of MHC class I antigen [9]. Although there was a similar trend to the presence of ICAM-1, this did not reach statistical significance. These findings may be clinically relevant because according to the data in this study, those patients whose tumors heterogeneously express MHC class I antigen have a 71 percent incidence of nodal metastases and a 41 percent incidence of disease relapse. This compared with a 32 percent and 11 percent incidence of metastases and relapse respectively in patients whose tumors were negative for MHC class I antigen expression.

It has been hypothesized that MHC class I-positive cells may incite TIL to produce cytokines which in turn stimulate the growth of MHC class I-negative cells present within the same tumor. This would explain the apparent dichotomy in the role of the immune system in both the surveillance and stimulation of breast cancer. T-cell mediated killing of tumor cells would be possible in the "immunologically visible" MHC class I-positive cells, whilst cytokine and growth factor release from recruited immune cells would induce cell growth in the "immunologically invisible" MHC class I-negative cells.

MHC class I status in a single tumor surely has some influence on the immune response to that tumor, but does it affect the immune response to concurrent or subsequent tumors in the same tissue of origin? In a study from the Institute of Breast Diseases, New York Medical College, Black et al. analyzed survival among 129,394 patients with invasive breast cancer. Patients with no in situ disease were compared with patients who had in situ disease in addition to invasive disease. These authors found that survival was enhanced if patients had a prior simultaneous or subsequent in situ breast cancer [10]. It thus appears that better differentiated in situ breast cancers are able to express appropriate MHC and MHC-associated antigens, thus mounting a cell-mediated immunity against the tumor. These same surface antigens might be present on concurrent or subsequent invasive tumors making those tumors vulnerable to cell-mediated attack. These results must be viewed with caution, however, since the authors never demonstrated direct evidence of enhanced cell-mediated immunity, nor were other confounding variables (such as screening bias) eliminated.

The immune system also recognizes other cell surface markers and receptors in association with, or in addition to, the major histocompatibility antigens. CD44 is a cell surface receptor involved in adhesion of cells as well as between tumor cells and the extracellular matrix. Cancer cells often undergo changes in the expression or function of adhesion molecules. This may have profound effects on tumor cell differentiation, invasion, metastatic potential, apoptosis, wound healing and lymphocyte homing, depending on the specific isoform of the receptor constitutively expressed or down-regulated.

Early stages of breast cancer are associated with both qualitative and quantitative changes in CD44 expression. It is notable that normal breast duct and acinar epithelial cells completely lack CD44 expression. On the other hand, normal basal cells of the terminal duct lobular unit express almost all of the CD44 isoforms. In benign proliferative diseases of the breast, there is up-regulated expression of specific isoforms in luminal epithelium, suggesting that these isoforms participate in enabling the enhanced proliferative rates of breast cells. Neoplastic non-invasive lesions of the breast demonstrate a unique footprint of CD44 variants and isoforms compared with that seen in benign diseases. As well, the footprint changes as the grade of ductal carcinoma-in-situ (DCIS) increases and there are CD44 isoforms present in invasive breast cancer which are not present in non-invasive neoplasms of the breast [11].

Adhesion molecules may be useful as prognostic markers or therapeutic targets in women with breast cancer. There appears to be a correlation between the pattern of CD44 expression and other established prognostic markers such as tumor size, lymph node status and hormone receptor expression. Certain CD44 isoforms may serve as targets for antibody based breast cancer therapy. It seems that the CD44v3 and CD44v4 isoforms, which occur solely in neoplastic (both in situ and invasive) breast epithelial cells, would serve as the best markers and perhaps the most appropriate targets for proposed therapies.

Cytokines and Growth Factors

Lymphocytes and monocytes are the sources of many growth factor proteins and cytokines which function locally through both autocrine and paracrine mechanisms as well as systemically. Growth factors and cytokines can act as mitogens and they coordinate and stimulate cellular activity and proliferation. Steroid hormones, like estrogen and progesterone, influence normal breast cells and breast cancer cells through mechanisms intimately bound to these substances [12]. Selective estrogen receptor modulators like Tamoxifen have an additive inhibitory effect on the growth of breast tumors when given in conjunction with cytokines and certain growth factors [13].

The creation of a surgical wound puts into motion a series of wound healing cascades that include the recruitment of immune cells and the local release of both cytokines and growth factors from those cells. Matrix metalloproteinases are enzymes that degrade growth factors, cytokines and other wound-associated proteins. These enzymes help orchestrate the delicate dynamic profile of the healing wound. They are pivotal in remodeling the extracellular matrix, however, they also influence both normal mammary gland development and breast cancer formation [14]. Inhibitors of metalloproteinases have been used to halt cancer progression and may represent a viable future therapeutic option [15].

For many decades, surgeons have observed a high rate of cancer recurrence at surgical scar sites. The factors vital to normal wound healing, may act as stimulants to cancer cells [16]. Additionally, tumor cells shed into the circulation which might travel to distant sites or return to the surgical bed, may be stimulated to grow by cytokines and growth factors present both locally as well as in peripheral blood serum [17–19].

The impact of local environmental influences of the surgical wound bed is best demonstrated when one analyzes local cancer recurrence rates after breast-conservation therapy. In the National Surgical Adjuvant Breast and Bowel Project trial B-06 (NSABP-B06) there was a 40.9 percent in-breast failure rate at 10 years follow-up after treatment including only lumpectomy with negative margins [20,21]. This is compared to a rate of 12.4 percent after lumpectomy with adjuvant radiotherapy.

A study done by Holland et al. demonstrated that the probability of residual breast cancer decreases in proportion to increasing distance from the primary tumor [22]. The authors studied mastectomy specimens both microscopically and mammographically and found that removing 2 cm around the primary tumor left residual cancer in 42 percent of cases. When margins were increased to 4 cm, (the amount of tissue equivalent to a quadrantectomy), the incidence of residual tumor in the remaining breast dropped to 10 percent.

These two studies appear to corroborate each other with respect to residual cancer and the risk of in-breast recurrence. However, one must wonder why there was such a high rate of recurrence among patients with negative margins. More importantly, why did all the recurrences take place at the site of prior tumor extirpation and not elsewhere within the breast? Surgical site recurrence is common to both irradiated and non-irradiated patients, while recurrence in a different quadrant within the same breast is uncommon, at only 3-4 percent by 10 years [23–25].

Wound healing is dependent on neo-vascularization of the wound bed. In order for new vessel formation to begin, angiogenic factors must be released. In addition to stimulation by these growth factors in the wound, the primary tumor may also produce angiogenic factors like vascular endothelial growth factor (VEGF), transforming growth factor beta (TGF-β) and basic fibroblast growth factor (FGF). High levels of expression of tumor-derived angiogenic factors have been shown to correlate with a worse prognosis in breast cancer [26]. Any angiogenic factors present in the healing wound would thus theoretically enhance growth already stimulated by the release of the tumor's own angiogenic factors. Taken together, these studies suggest that the immunologic, cytokine and growth factor responses that occur in the normal process of wound healing are considerable factors impacting upon tumor recurrence rates [27].

Metastatic implantation and tumor cell growth is not a random phenomenon. Local cytokines and growth factors heavily influence the induction of metastatic deposits [28–30]. The establishment and growth of these tumor cells is encouraged by the presence of both the appropriate growth factors and the corresponding tumor-associated growth factor receptors. It is for this reason that organ-specific sites are preferred and the surgical wound is a common ground for tumor recurrence. The same chemo-attractants that recruit platelets, fibroblasts, endothelial cells and inflammatory cells into a wound and trigger those cells to proliferate and produce other growth factors and cytokines, also attract and stimulate cancer cells that contain similar receptors.

In a cytokine and growth factor-enhanced environment, fewer cells are needed to produce metastatic deposits. As well, non-implanted, free-floating cells rather than implanted cells not only survive, but are capable of forming a tumor nidus and propagating, given the correct cytokine/growth factor milieu. Tumor implantation has not been shown to occur in already healed wounds [31–32]. Thus, local wound recurrence of breast cancer is not likely due to a late phenomenon, but is most probably an event which takes place early during the post-operative wound-healing phase when residual cells, (or possibly cells which have returned to the wound via the circulation), are stimulated by the local environment [33–35].

In addition to the cytokines generated by the healing wound, there are particular cytokine profiles present at sites of malignant tumors that are distinct from the cytokine profiles present at the sites of benign growths. These cytokines are elaborated by cells in response to the tumor itself. Yamamura et al. have demonstrated a T_H1 type cytokine response to benign dermal tumors. This finding is in contrast to the T_H2 type response to malignant dermal tumors, where the cytokine milieu favors immunosuppression [36]. With respect to breast cancer in particular, both T_H1 and T_H2 cytokines have been demonstrated.

IL-10, (a T_H2-type cytokine), appears to be the most consistently observed of the cytokines in human breast tumors [37]. This is an important phenomenon because IL-10 may be associated with T-cell anergy [38,39]. This may explain the abundance of TIL within breast tumors, (especially early stage tumors), without any concomitant cell-mediated immune response to the tumor cells and is consistent with the work of Wong et al. (vide supra) where TIL produced mainly interferon gamma (INF-γ) and not IL-2, whilst LNL and PBL from the same patients produced mainly IL-2 and where the IL-2 producing lymphocytes generated the greatest tumoricidal activity.

The lack of IL-2 cytokine in human breast carcinoma notwithstanding, the presence of IL-2 mRNA in TIL of primary breast cancers is an intriguing phenomenon because, IL-2 is responsible for TIL activation and proliferation [40]. IL-10 may inhibit the production of IL-2, thereby creating a situation where there is a relative protection conferred on breast tumors by the intra-tumoral cytokine balance. The future of breast cancer therapy may focus on re-establishing the proper cytokine milieu, by definitive cytokine therapy in concert with conventional chemotherapy or hormonal therapy, or by adoptive immunotherapy, either of cytokine gene-modified lymphokine activated killer cells (LAK) or antigen (or peptide-primed) T-cell clones.

There is evidence to suggest that the T_H2 response may function to inhibit the growth or spread of cancerous cells in spite of its immunosuppressive effect. This cytokine profile may recruit antigen-presenting cells and enhance tumor antigen presentation to those cells [41]. Eventual growth and spread of malignant disease however, suggests that the tumor growth and metastatic control exerted by the T_H2 cytokine profile surrounding malignant tumors is not adequate. Antigen presenting cells may kill MHC class I positive tumor cells but stimulate MHC class I negative cells to grow. The time lag in selecting these MHC class I clones may explain the transition from tumor suppression to tumor growth enhancement. Treatment of malignant tumors with T_H1 cytokines like IL-2 and TNF-α, change cytokine profiles in favor of a cell-mediated immune-enhanced profile thereby tipping the balance back to one in which growth is arrested.

Another mechanism by which tumors manipulate the cytokine response of immune cells as well as the reaction of tumor cells to elaborated cytokines is by alteration of cell-associated cytokine receptors and receptor-associated molecules. IL-4 is a cytokine that has been demonstrated to be secreted by primary breast tumors and to be present in the peripheral blood of breast cancer patients [42]. This cytokine is normally released from activated NK cells and may be involved in the immune surveillance of breast cancer. Tumor cells may alter, down-regulate or lose molecules associated with IL-4 binding chains within IL-4 receptors to prevent this cytokine from exerting any effects. These types of changes appear to be independent of other prognostic indicators such as tumor stage, nodal status, ER status or grade.

Interleukin-4 receptor changes have been shown to correlate with differences in survival in breast cancer. One study by Kaklamanis et al. demonstrated a 92 percent survival in patients with unaltered IL-4 receptors compared with a 70 percent survival in patients with altered receptor-associated molecules, though this difference did not reach statistical significance [43]. These types of findings may have ramifications for systemic IL-4 therapy, including cytokine, vaccine and gene therapy for the treatment of breast cancer.

Breast Cancer Antigens

Certain antigens are associated with malignant breast tissue and may render a survival and/or proliferative advantage to breast tumors. These same antigens may also act as current or potential targets for breast cancer therapy. HER-2 protein also known as c-erbB-2 (human epidermal growth factor receptor-2) is a 185 kDa glycoprotein which has tyrosine kinase activity homologous to the epidermal growth factor receptor. This protein is over-expressed in 25–30% of breast cancers.

Epitopes of the HER-2 protein are recognized in association with MHC Class II HLA-DR4. This produces a T_H1 response to HER-2 receptors present on human breast tumors. Therefore, the presence of HER-2 breast cancer-associated antigen results in increased secretion of INF-γ and IL-4 cytokines which induce proliferation of peripheral blood monocytes [44]. These MHC Class II-restricted epitopes are targets for monoclonal antibody-binding to block the effects of the HER-2 protein. This T_H1 response to HER-2 antigen by cytotoxic lymphocytes (CTLs) suggests that CD4+ cells are involved in the immune reaction to breast cancer.

Humanized monoclonal antibody to an extracellular domain of HER-2 receptor has recently been used with success to treat women with tumors that over express c-erbB-2 protein [45–47]. Though growth of breast cancer cells may decrease when a single antibody is used alone, apoptosis may result when a combination of antibodies to distinct epitopes in separate domains which are independently functionally important are used [48,49]. The combination of monoclonal antibody therapy with conventional cytotoxic chemotherapy may also have an additive or synergistic tumor ablative effect.

References

1. Going JJ, Anderson TJ, Battersby S, MacIntyre CCA. Proliferative and secretory activity in human breast during natural and artificial menstrual cycles. Am J Pathol 1988;130:152–63.
2. Eglinton BA, Roberton DM, Cummings AG. Phenotype of T-cells, their soluble receptor levels, and cytokine profile of human breast milk. Immunol Cell Biol 1994;72:306–13.
3. Black MM, Leis HP. Cellular responses to autologous breast cancer tissue. Sequential observations. Cancer, 1973;32:384–9.
4. Vose BM, Moore M. Suppressor cell activity of lymphocytes infiltrating human lung and breast tumours. Int J Cancer 1979;24:579–85.
5. Eremin O, Coombs RRJ, Ashby. Lymphocytes infiltrating human breast cancers lack K-cell activity and show low levels of NK-cell activity. Br J Cancer 1981;44:166–76.
6. Whiteside TL, Miescher S, Hurlimann J, Moretta L, von Fliedner V. Clonal analysis and in situ characterization of lymphocytes infiltrating human breast carcinomas. Cancer Immunol Immunother 1986;23:169–78.
7. Wong PY, Staren ED, Tereshkova N, Braun DP. Functional analysis of tumor-infiltrating leukocytes in breast cancer patients. J Surg Res 1998;76:95–103.
8. Vanky F, Wang P, Patarroyo M, Klein E. Expression of the adhesion molecule ICAM-1 and major histocompatability complex class I antigens on human tumor cells is required for their interactions with autologous lymphocytes in vitro. Cancer Immunol Immunother 1990;31:19–27.
9. Ogmundsdottir HM, Petursdottir I and Gudmundsdottir I. Interactions between the immune system and breast cancer. Acta Oncologica 1995;34(5):647–50.
10. Black MM, Zachrau RE, Hankey BF, Feuer EJ. Prognostic significance of in situ carcinoma associated with invasive breast carcinoma. Cancer 1996;78:778–88.
11. Bankfalvi A, Terpe H-J, Breukelmann D, Bier B, Rempe D, Pschadka G, Krech R and Bocker W. Gains and Losses of CD44 expression during breast carcinogenesis. Histopathology 1998;33:107–16.
12. Lippman ME, Dickson RB. Mechanisms of growth control in normal and malignant breast epithelium. Recent Prog Horm Res 1989;45:383–440.
13. Toi M, Bicknell R, Harris AL. Inhibition of colon and breast carcinoma cell growth by IL-4. Cancer Res 1992;52:275–9.
14. Benaud C, Dickson RB, Thompson EW. Roles of the matrix metalloproteinases in mammary gland development and cancer. Breast Ca Res Treat 1998;50(2):97–116.
15. Wang M, Liu YE, Greene J, Sheng S, Fuchs A, Rosen EM, et al. Metalloproteinase inhibitors to treat cancer progresssion. Oncogene 1997;14(23):2767–74.
16. Sporn MB, Roberts AB. Peptide growth factors and inflammation, tissue repair and cancer. J Clin Invest 1986;78:329–32.
17. Brown DC, Purushotham AD, Birnie GD, George WD. Detection of intraoperative tumor cell dissemination in patients with breast cancer by use of reverse transcription and polymerase chain reaction. Surgery 1995;117:96–101.
18. Reid SE, Scanlon EF, Murthy MS. Do blood-borne cancer cells contribute to local recurrence? Clin Exp Metastasis 1994;12:91.
19. Mayhew E, Glaves D. Quantitation of tumorigenic disseminating and arrested cancer cells. Br J Cancer 1984;50:159–66.
20. Fisher B, Bauer M, Margolese R et al. Five-year results of a randomized clinical trial comparing total mastectomy and segmental mastectomy with or without radiation in the treatment of breast cancer. N Engl J Med 1985;312:665–73.
21. Fisher B, Redmond C, Poisson R, et al. Eight year results of a randomized clinical trial comparing total mastectomy and lumpectomy with or without irradiation in the treatment of breast cancer. N Engl J Med 1989;320:822–8.
22. Holland R, Veling SH, Mravunac M, Hendriks JHCL. Histologic multifocality of T_{is} and T_{1-2} breast carcinomas. Implications for clinial trials of breast-conserving surgery. Cancer 1985;56:979–90.
23. Clark RM, McCulloch PB, Levine MN, et al. Randomized clinical trial to assess the effectiveness of breast irradiation following lumpectomy and axillary dissection for node-negative breast cancer. J Natl Cancer Inst 1992;84:683–89.
24. Clarke DH, Martinez AA. Identification of patients who are at high risk for locoregional breast cancer recurrence after conservative surgery and radiotherapy: a review article for surgeons, pathologists, and radiation and medical oncologists. J Clin Oncol 1992;10:474–83.
25. Kurtz JM. Factors influencing the risk of local recurrence in the breast. Eur J Cancer 1992;28:660–6.
26. Relf M, LeJeune S, Scott PAE et al. Expression of the angiogenic factors vascular endothelial cell growth factor, acidic and basic fibroblast growth factor, tumor growth factor b-1, platelet-derived

endothelial cell growth factor, placenta growth factor, and pleiotrophin in human primary breast cancer and its relation to antiogenesis. Cancer Res 1997;57:963–9.

27. Reid SE, Scanlon EF, Kaufman MW, Murthy MS. Role of cytokines and growth factors in promoting the local recurrence of breast cancer. Br J Surgery 1996;83:313–20.

28. Radinsky R, Fidler IJ. Regulation of tumor cell growth at organ-specific metastases. In Vivo 1992;6:325–31.

29. Smith RR, Thomas LB, Hilberg AW. Cancer cell contamination of operative wounds. Cancer 1958;11:53–62.

30. Murphy P, Alexander P, Senior PV, Fleming J, Kirkham N, Taylor I. Mechanisms of organ selective tumour growth by bloodborne cancer cells. Br J Cancer 1988;57:19–31.

31. Davies DE, Farmer S, White J, Senior P, Warnes S, Alexander P. Contribution of host-derived growth factors to in vivo growth of a transplantable murine mammary carcinoma. Br J Cancer 1994;70:263–9.

32. Baker DG, Masterson TM, Pace R, Constable WC, Wanebo H. The influence of the surgical wound on local tumor recurrence. Surgery 1989;106:525–32.

33. Murthy MS, Goldschmidt RA, Rao LN, Ammirati M, Buchmann T, Scanlon EF. The influence of surgical trauma on experimental metastases. Cancer 1989;64:2035–44.

34. Simpson-Herren L, Sanford AH, Holmquist JP. Effects of surgery on the cell kinetics of residual tumor. Cancer Tret Rep 1976;60:1749–60.

35. Gunduz N, Fisher B, Saffer EA. Effect of surgical removal on the growth and kinetics of residual tumor. Cancer Res 1979;39:3861–5.

36. Yamamura M, Modlin RL, Ohmen JD, Moy RL. Local expression of antiinflammatory cytokines in cancer. J Clin Invest 1993;91:1005–10.

37. Venetsanakos E, Beckman I, Bradley J, Skinner JM. High incidence of interleukin 10mRNA but not interleukin 2 mRNA detected in human breast tumours. Br J Cancer 1997;75(12):1826–30.

38. Becker JC, Brabletz T, Czerny C, Termeer C, Brocker EB. Tumour escape mechanisms from immunosurveillance: induction of unresponsiveness in a specific MNC-restricted CD4+ human T cell clone by the autologous MHC class II+ melanoma. Int Immunol 1993;5:1501–8.

39. Becker JC, Czerny C, Brocker EB. Maintenance of clonal anergy by endogenously produced IL-10. Int Immunol, 1994:6:1605–12.

40. Coventry BJ, Weeks SC, Heckford SE, Sykes PJ Bradley J, Skinner JM. Lack of IL-2 Cytokine expression despite IL-2 messenger RNA transcription in tumor-infiltrating lymphocytes in primary human breast carcinoma. J Immun 1996;156:3486–92.

41. Golumbek, PT, Lazemby AJ, Levitsky HJ, Jaffee LM, Karusuyama H, Baker M, et al. Treatment of established renal cancer by tumor cells engineered to secrete interleukin-4. Science 1991;254:713–6.

42. Lorenzen J, Lewis CE, McCracken D, Horak E, Greenal M, McGee JOD. Human tumor-associated NK cells secrete increased amounts of interferon-gamma and interleukin-4. Br J Cancer 1991;64:457–62.

43. Kaklamanis L, Koukourakis MI, Leek R, Giatromanolaki A, Ritter M, Whitehouse R, et al. Loss of interleukin 4 receptor-associated molecule gp200-MR6 in human breast cancer: prognostic significance. Br J Cancer 1996;74:1627–31.

44. Tuttle TM, Anderson BW, Thompson WE, et al. Proliferative and cytokine responses to class II HER-2/neu-associated peptides in breast cancer patients. Clin Ca Res 1998;4:2015–24.

45. Cobleigh MA. Efficacy and safety of Herceptin (humanized anti-HER2 antibody) as a single agent in 222 women with HER2 overexpression who relapsed following chemotherapy for metastatic breast cancer. Proc Mer Soc Clin Oncol 1998;17:97a (abstract #376).

46. Slamon D. Addition of Herceptin (humanized anti-HER2 antibody) to first line chemotherapy for HER2 overexpressing metastatic breast cancer (HER2+/MBC) markedly increases anti-cancer activity: A randomized multinational controlled phase III trial. Proc Amer Soc Clin Oncol 1998;17:98a (abstract #377).

47. Pegram M, Hsu S, Lewis G, Pietras R, Beryt M, Sliwkowski M, et al. Inhibitory effects of combinations of HER-2/neu antibody and chemotherapeutic agents used for treatment of human breast cancers. Oncogene, 1999 Apr 1;18(13):2241–51.

48. Dougall WC, Greene MI. Biological studies and potential therapeutic applications of monoclonal antibodies and small molecules reactive with the neu/c-erbB-2 protein. Cell Biophys 1994;24-25:209–18.

49. Katsumata M, Okudaira T, Samanta A, Clark DP, Drebin JA, Jokicoeur P, et al. Prevention of breast tumour development in vivo by downregulation of the p185neu receptor. Nat Med 1995;1(7):644–8.

18. The Immunobiology of Malignant Melanoma

Daniel E. Speiser and Soldano Ferrone

Introduction

Human malignant melanoma is the most investigated of all solid malignancies by tumor immunologists. This somewhat surprising interest reflects, at least in part, the fact that several lines of evidence suggest that malignant melanoma can be considered as an "immunoresponsive tumor". During the past years, humoral and cellular anti-melanoma associated antigen (MAA) specific immune activity has been detected in patients with malignant melanoma [1,2]. Moreover, many studies have found associations between the level of expression of immunologically relevant molecules (such as HLA antigens and adhesion molecules) in primary lesions and their histopathological characteristics as well as with the clinical course of the disease [3,4], with further associations between primary lesion regression and lymphocyte infiltration or, in some cases, with an oligoclonal T cell-response [5–8].

The interest of the tumor immunologist in malignant melanoma together with the significant progress in immunological and recombinant DNA technology has accounted for the major progress in recent years in the identification and molecular characterization of human MAA [9–14]. The availability of these well-defined peptides and the lack of therapeutic efficacy of conventional chemotherapy and radiotherapy in metastatic melanoma, have spearheaded an increasing number of clinical trials designed to test new immunotherapeutic strategies in patients with malignant melanoma.

In this chapter, we describe the clinically relevant MAA identified in human melanoma cells and the strategies employed for their identification. This is followed by the clinical trials which have been or are currently being performed in patients with malignant melanoma and the methodology utilized to monitor the humoral and cellular immune responses in immunized patients along with potential future immunotherapeutic strategies.

Identification and Characterization of Human Melanoma Associated Antigens (MAA)

A major breakthrough in the identification of human MAA, as well as of other types of human tumor-associated antigens, has been the development of methodologies which do not require purified antigens to generate probes to detect the variable isoforms of MAA expressed by melanoma cells. With one exception, the probes, (whether they are the variable portion of an antibody or the variable portion of a T-cell receptor), are the product of a single cellular clone and therefore have a high discriminatory power.

Antibody-based Techniques To Identify Human MAA

Immunization of various animal species, (including non-human primates) and of patients with malignant melanoma, using human melanoma cells or antigen preparations at different stages of purification, was extensively utilized in the 1960s and early 1970s to develop antibodies to human MAA. These attempts were essentially unsuccessful because of the difficulties in identifying unknown MAA species with as yet uncharacterized antibodies and an inability to generate in a reproducible fashion antibody populations with well-defined specificity and with high association constants for MAA [1].

These limitations were largely overcome by the development of the hybridoma methodology to produce mouse monoclonal antibodies (mAb) [15] where mice are immunized with human melanoma cells or with MAA preparations. Individual antibody producing B cell clones are isolated from the spleen of immunized mice through hybridization with mouse myeloma cells (Figure 18.1), with the resulting hybridomas representing an unlimited source of individual antibody populations with defined and reproducible characteristics. These antibody populations can easily be screened with large panels of cell lines, normal tissues and benign or malignant lesions, to identify those which recognize MAA, i.e. antigens with selective expression by melanoma cells. Through the efforts of many investigators, this hybridoma technology has been successfully utilized to identify a number of MAA epitopes, which display a distinct molecular profile and tissue distribution [16]. The large majority of MAA are expressed on the cell surface, since mAb were screened in binding assays with viable cells.

Attempts have also been made to utilize human mAb in order to identify MAA [16]. These investigations have been prompted by the interest in identifying MAA recognized by the human immune system and in generating anti-MAA antibodies which would not generate an anti-mouse Ig response when injected into patients for diagnostic and/or therapeutic purposes. With a few exceptions [17–19], these approaches have failed mainly because of the difficulties in generating stable antibody-producing hybridomas. Furthermore, the practical difficulties in producing large amounts of high-affinity human anti-MAA mAb, (mainly as IgM), have imposed severe restrictions on the characterization of the corresponding MAA. Recently, two new approaches have been successful in identifying MAA recognized by human antibodies. One of these techniques is represented by the phage display antibody method, i.e. a collection of recombinant phage libraries, each displaying a different antigen-binding domain on its surface [20,21] (Figure 18.2). These libraries are constructed by fusing genes encoding the coat protein of a

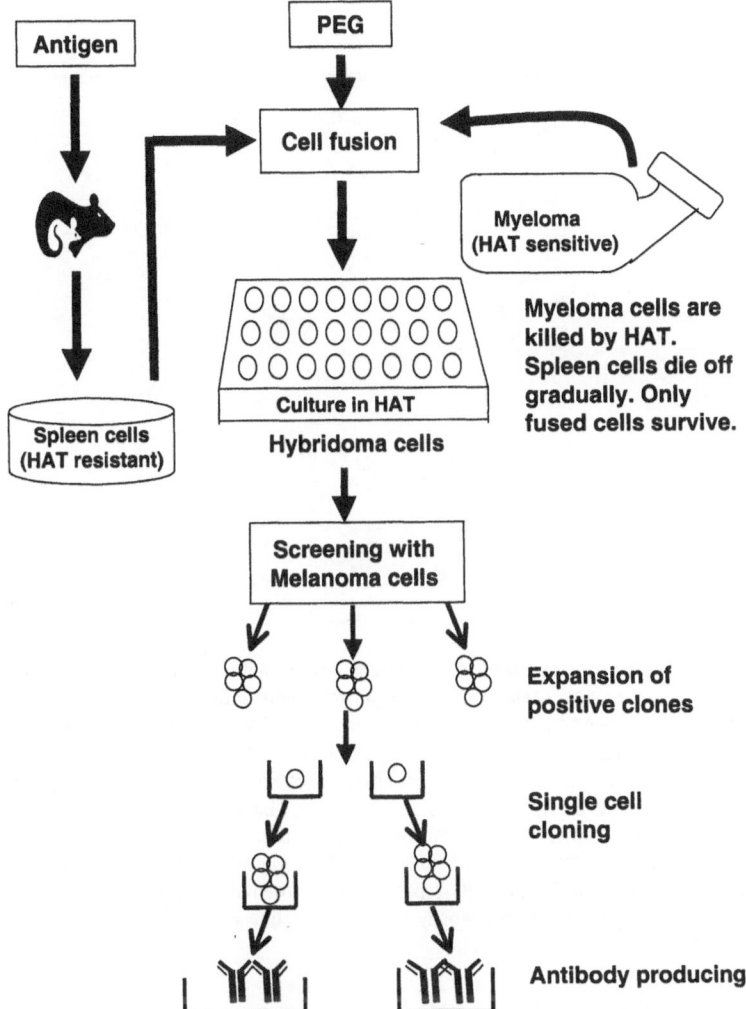

Figure 18.1. Schematic representation of the hybridoma methodology to identify human MAA. Mice are immunized with melanoma cells. Mice which produce high titer antibodies following immunizations with human melanoma cells or antigen preparation are sacrificed. Splenocytes and lymph node lymphocytes are isolated and fused in the presence of polyethylene glycol (PEG) with a myeloma cell line which lacks hypoxanthine-guanine phosphoribosyl transferase (HGPRTase). PEG promotes membrane fusion. Only a small proportion of the cells fuse successfully. Cells are cultured in medium supplemented with hypoxanthine, aminopterin and thymidine (HAT). Only fused cells survive in HAT medium since splenocytes die spontaneously following 1-2 weeks in culture and myeloma cells are killed by HAT. Hybridomas secreting antibodies reacting with melanoma cells are identified by testing spent medium with melanoma cells. Hybridomas secreting anti-MAA antibodies are subcloned. Antibody secreting clones are expanded and used as a source of antibodies.

phage to gene segments encoding antigen-binding domains of antibodies. The latter are cloned from B-lymphocytes of either naïve or immune hosts. Infection of bacteria with phage containing gene fusions, results in phage-expressing antigen-binding domains of antibody fragments on their outer surface so that antibodies recognizing MAA can be isolated by panning phage display antibody

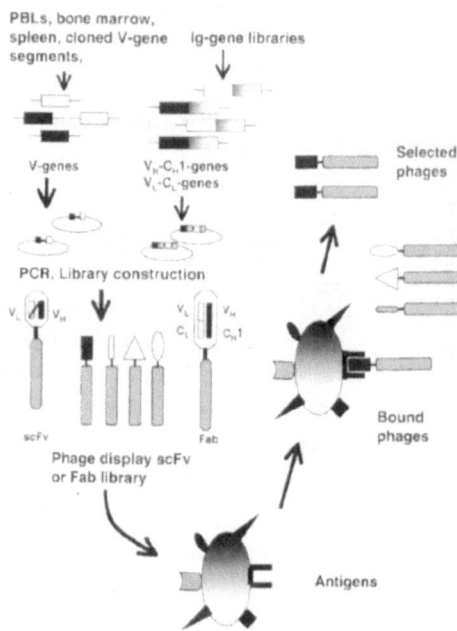

PBLs, bone marrow,
spleen, cloned V-gene   Ig-gene libraries
segments,

V-genes V_H-C_H1-genes
                 V_L-C_L-genes

PCR, Library construction

V_L V_H V_L V_H
                     C_L C_H1

scFv   Fab

Phage display scFv
or Fab library

Selected
phages

Bound
phages

Antigens

Figure 18.2. Schematic representation of the phage display antibody library methodology to identify human MAA. To produce single chain Fv (scFv) or Fab fragments antibodies, V_H and V_L genes or V_H–C_H1 and V_L-C_L genes are amplified by PCR from mRNA of peripheral blood lymphocytes, bone marrow cells or splenocytes or from cloned V-gene segments or Ig-gene libraries. The V_H–C_H1 and V_L-C_L genes or V_H and V_L genes which are joined together with a short linker sequence are inserted into phages. Phages replicate and express the scFv or Fab fragments on their tips. Phages displaying the antibody fragments which recognize antigens expressed on melanoma cells are isolated by incubating the phage antibody library with melanoma cells. Phages which bind specifically to melanoma cells are eluted and amplified by infecting an appropriate bacteria strain. By repeating this procedure, (which is referred to as panning), three or four times, phages expressing antibody fragments reacting with melanoma cells are isolated from the library.

libraries with melanoma cells. The possibility to utilize lymphocytes from naïve hosts as a source of antibodies eliminates the need to immunize patients and facilitates the identification of MAA which are not relatively immunogenic.

It was a general expectation that the diversity of MAA identified with this approach would be broader than that of those identified with the hybridoma methodology. Contrary to these expectations, the diversity of MAA identified with the phage antibody library has been relatively restricted and in most of the studies the antigen identified has been the high molecular weight MAA (HMW-MAA, [22,23] an antigen which is immunodominant in BALB/c mice. In the second approach, sera from patients with melanoma have been used as a source of antibodies for the serological analysis of recombinant cDNA expression libraries (SEREX) generated from melanoma cells [24]. This process is shown in Figure 18.3. Here, the library is cloned into phages which are secondarily transfected into Escherichia coli bacteria and recombinant proteins, (expressed during lytic infection of these bacteria), then transferred onto nitrocellulose membranes and tested for reactivity with patient serum. Positive clones are isolated and the nucleotide sequence of the inserted cDNA is determined.

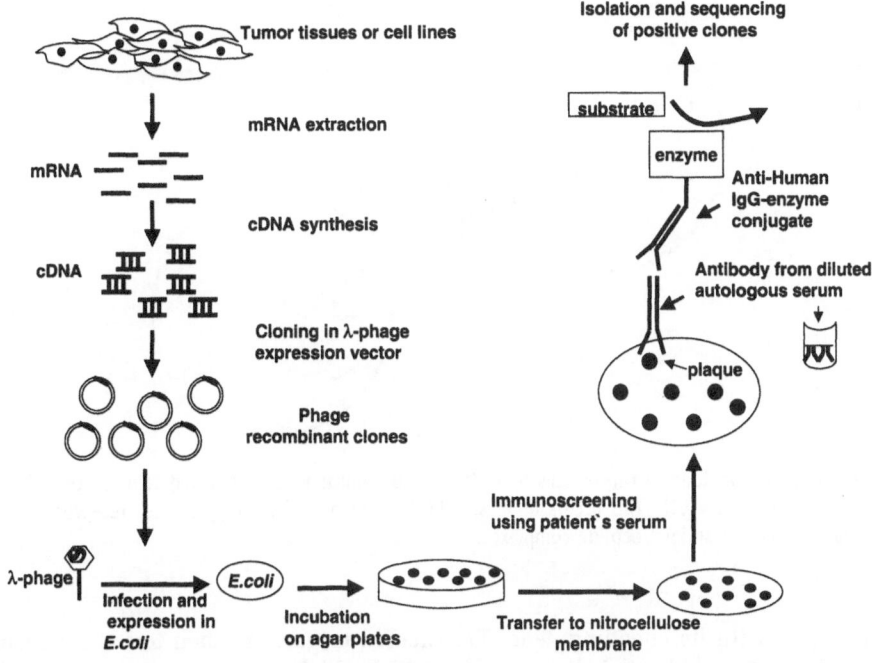

Figure 18.3. Schematic representation of the SEREX methodology to identify human MAA. mRNA is isolated from surgically-removed melanoma lesions or cultured melanoma cells and is converted to a double-stranded cDNA using the standard cDNA synthesis method. cDNA is cloned into λ-phage expression vector to construct a cDNA library. Phage recombinant clones are used to infect E. coli bacteria. Recombinant proteins expressed in E. coli are transferred to a nitrocellulose membrane. The membrane is sequentially incubated with serum from a patient with melanoma and with enzyme-conjugated anti-human Ig xeno-antibodies. Positive reactions are detected by the development of color following the addition of a substrate. Positive clones are isolated; the sequence of the inserted cDNA is determined and analyzed by DNA databank search. The distribution of the mRNA encoded by the identified clones in normal tissues and malignant lesions is analyzed by RT-PCR or Northern blot.

T Cell-based Techniques To Identify Human MAA

The development of T cell-based methodology to identify human MAA has greatly benefited from our understanding of the molecular basis of target cell recognition by T cells. At variance with antibodies, T cells recognize neither soluble antigens nor entire antigens. T cells recognize peptides which are derived from endogenous or exogenous proteins and are located in the groove of major histocompatibility complex (MHC) antigens on cell membranes [25,26]. As a result of this MHC restriction, peptides derived mostly from endogenously synthesized proteins are presented by MHC class I antigens to CD8+ T cells (Figure 18.4). On the other hand, peptides derived mostly from exogenous proteins are presented by MHC class II antigens to CD4+ T cells.

Several strategies have been applied to identify human MAA with T cells. In the one pioneered by Boon and his associates [9], cDNA libraries generated from melanoma cells are stably transfected into cells which do not express MAA, but which express the HLA class I restricting element either spontaneously or following

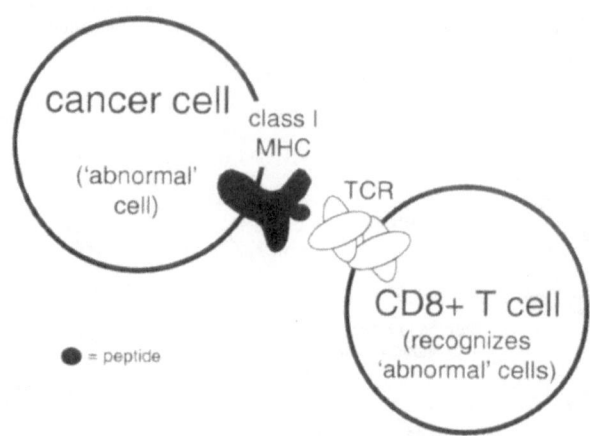

Figure 18.4. Recognition of cancer cells by CD8+ T cells. Similar to virus infected cells, cancer cells can be recognized by CD8+ CTL. This occurs upon specific binding of the clonotypic T cell receptor (TCR) to antigenic MHC class I antigen/peptide complexes.

transfection with its encoding gene. Transfected targets are then tested for recognition by tumor infiltrating lymphocytes (TIL) which are cytotoxic for the melanoma cells used to prepare the cDNA library. The cDNA clones that cause recognition of transfected cells are then isolated and sequenced for identification of the MAA and of the peptide presented by the HLA class I restricting element to cytotoxic T lymphocytes (CTL). In an alternative strategy pioneered by Hunt and his collaborators [10], peptides are eluted from MHC class I antigens expressed by melanoma cells and tested for recognition by CTL clones with specific reactivity against melanoma cells. The peptides recognized by CTL are sequenced utilizing mass spectrometry. A similar strategy has also been utilized to identify MAA recognized by CD4+ T cells [11].

Newer approaches have been developed by Rosenberg and colleagues [11,12], where a cDNA library generated from melanoma cells is fused to an Ii-leader sequence to facilitate proper loading to the HLA class II antigen compartment. The library is transfected to 293 bacteria engineered to express DMA, DMB, Ii and other components of the HLA class II antigen presentation and processing pathway. cDNA clones which stimulate proliferation of CD4+ T cells are isolated and sequenced.

Classification of Antibody and T Cell Defined MAA

Several types of MAA have been identified utilizing the strategies outlined in the previous section. Table 18.1 shows examples of MAAs classified into four major groups (for more complete reviews, see [13,14]. The first group includes cancer-testis antigens which are aberrantly expressed in tumor cells but are silent in normal cells, (with the exception of germ cells). Functionally, the peptides derived from these antigens, which are recognized by T cells, are tumor-specific. The germ cells which express these antigens do not express HLA class I antigens and therefore cannot present relevant immunogenic peptides to T cells.

The second group includes the tissue-specific antigens (so-called differentiation

Table 18.1. Melanoma associated antigens (MAA)

Group	Antigen	Peptide sequence	Presented by HLA-	Reference
1. CancerTestis(CT) Antigens [a]	MAGE-1	EADPTGHSY	A1, B35	Traversari C et al 1992 [28]
	NY-ESO-1	SLLMWITQC	A2.1	Jäger, E. et al 1998, [29]
	MAGE-10	GLYDGMEHL	A2.1	Huang, LQ et al 1999 [30]
2. Differentiation Antigens [b]	Melan-A/ Mart-1	(E)AAGIGILTV	A2.1	Kawakami Y et al 1994 [31]
	Tyrosinase	YMDGTMSQV	A2.1	Wölfel T et al 1994 [32]
	gp100	ITDQVPFSV	A2.1	Kawakami Y et al 1995 [33]
	TRP-1/gp75	MSLQRQFLR	A31	Wang R et al 1996 [34]
	HMW-MAA	——	——	
3. Overexpressed Antigens [c]	Gangliosides	——	——	
	PRAME	LYVDSLFFL	A24	Ikeda H et al 1997 [35]
4. Antigens encoded by mutated genes	CDK4	ACDPHSGHFV	A2.1	Wölfel T et al 1995 [36]
	β-Catenin	SYLDSGIHF	A24	Robbins P F et al 1996 [37]

Examples are given for each group of tumor-associated antigens. The peptides are presented by the indicated HLA class I molecules. This list is far from complete, because a large number of tumor-associated antigens have been identified, and more are likely to follow. a) Non-mutated self antigens with highly restricted tissue distribution (expressed by a significant proportion of tumors of different histological types but not expressed in most somatic tissue, usually with the exception of the testis and therefore called cancer testis (CT) antigens. b) Antigens specific for all the cells derived from the melanocyte lineage and therefore also expressed by normal melanocytes. c) Antigens expressed in normal cells, but expressed at much higher levels by melanoma cells. [For a complete listing of tumor antigens in malignant melanoma, consult http://www. cancerimmunity.org /peptidedatabase/Tcellepitopes.htm.]

antigens). The identification of these antigens has taken advantage of the ability of melanoma cells to activate CD8+ T cells. This property of melanoma cells has facilitated the search and identification of CD8+ T cell-defined, tumor-specific epitopes in melanoma cells. Several of the identified differentiation antigens have been characterized in detail with respect to antigenicity and binding capacity to HLA class I alleles and various T cell receptors.

The third group includes overexpressed antigens, i.e. moieties expressed at higher levels by tumor cells than by other types of cells. These antigens are derived from oncogenes, tumor suppressor genes, or various other non-mutated proteins.

Finally, the fourth group includes truly tumor-specific mutational antigens which result from specific mutations, abnormal transcription or aberrant translation. From a theoretical viewpoint, these antigens offer two advantages in the implementation of active specific immunotherapy. Firstly, it should be possible to elicit a robust immune response against these antigens, since they are foreign to the host whose immune system is unlikely to be tolerant. Secondly, the immune response elicited by mutated MAA is less likely to cause side-effects, since the target antigen is not expressed in normal tissues. On the other hand, from a practical standpoint there are at least two limitations in the use of mutated MAA as immunogens for the immunotherapy of melanoma. Here, the frequency of mutations which result in the generation of immunogenic epitopes is low in patients with melanoma and the mutations identified thus far in patients with melanoma are patient-specific. As a result, the immunotherapies ("vaccines") constructed with mutated MAA will also be patient-specific and are not applicable to the general population afflicted with melanoma.

Immunotherapy of Malignant Melanoma

The identification of markers expressed in a large number of melanoma lesions, but with restricted distribution in normal tissues has provided targets to implement the immunotherapy of melanoma. In the late 1970s and early 1980s, the development of anti-MAA monoclonal antibodies paved the way for trials of passive immunotherapy in patients with advanced disease [27]. More recently, passive immunotherapy has also been used for the adoptive transfer of activated lymphocytes [28]. The limited success of such passive immunotherapies in conjunction with the major progress in our understanding of the steps leading to an immune response and the development of adjuvants [40] and cytokines [41] has shifted the emphasis toward the development and application of active specific immunotherapy for the treatment of malignant melanoma.

The immunogens used in this approach range from whole melanoma cells to purified MAA. Clinical responses have been obtained in patients immunized with whole melanoma cells or with their fractions administered with or without immune stimulatory agents such as viruses, attenuated bacteria, bacterial extracts or cytokines [29]. Nevertheless, the results of these clinical trials which have been performed or are still being conducted utilizing cell lines or their fractions will not be reviewed in this chapter, since the multiplicity of the antigenic moieties administered to patients makes it difficult, if not impossible to identify the clinically relevant immune response(s) in immunized patients. Here we review the results of clinical trials performed with well-defined MAA, since the immune responses elicited by this strategy are better characterized and therefore, can be better analyzed in their clinical setting.

Immunotherapies Eliciting Humoral Anti-MAA Responses

Two types of immunogens have been utilized to implement antibody-based immunotherapy, notably ganglioside therapy and anti-idiotypic (anti-id) mAb which mimics MAA. The gangliosides used as immunogens include GM2 and GD3. The rationale underlying the use of GM2 ganglioside as an immunogen in trials of active specific immunotherapy is represented by the decreased risk of relapse in patients who were free of disease after complete surgical resection and who had natural anti-GM2 ganglioside antibodies [47]. The use of GD3 ganglioside as an immunogen in patients with melanoma [48] has been stimulated by the ability of murine anti-GD3 ganglioside mAb to inhibit the growth of melanoma cells and to mediate their complement-dependent lysis in vitro and to suppress the growth of human melanoma cells transplanted into nude mice [31]. GM2 ganglioside conjugated with keyhole limpet hemocyanin (KLH) and administered with the adjuvant QS21 has been found to induce anti-GM2 ganglioside antibodies in almost all the immunized patients [32]. In this clinical trial development of anti-GM2 ganglioside humoral immunity appeared to have a beneficial clinical effect since it was associated with survival prolongation. However, at an early time point in a phase III randomized multi-center trial, immunization with

GM2 ganglioside did not significantly improve the disease-free interval or patient survival [33]. Interestingly, sera derived from two of the immunized patients was also able to mediate complement-dependent lysis of melanoma cells in vitro. Whether this immunity has any effect on the clinical course of the disease remains to be determined.

Mouse anti-idiotyic (anti-id) mAb which mimics distinct determinants of HMW-MAA, GD2 ganglioside and GD3 ganglioside have been used to implement active specific immunotherapy in patients with melanoma [35]. The rationale underlying the use of anti-id mAb as immunogens is represented by the fact that they mimic MAA but are not identical to MAA which are for the most part self-antigens. Therefore anti-id mAb may be more effective than the original MAA in inducing an immune response to self-antigens, since they may stimulate B cell clones which have not been deleted during the establishment of self-identity. The in vitro and in vivo responses to anti-id mAbs have generally been enhanced by their administration with an adjuvant, without significant modification of their immunogenicity by conjugation with the carrier molecule. Despite this, the varying anti-id mAbs used have been found to differ markedly in their immuno-genicity, as measured by the percentage of the immunized patients who developed anti-MAA antibodies and by the level of these antibodies; with low titers developing in most of the immunized patients. This finding is likely to reflect the stimulation of B cell clones secreting antibodies with low reactivity to the MAA, directly resulting from differences between the epitopes recognized by anti-ids when compared with the primary MAA.

The humoral anti-MAA immunity elicited by anti-id mAb has been found to be associated with regression of metastases in a few patients and with survival prolongation in some clinical trials. Moreover, some patients had a favorable clinical course of the disease following immunotherapy with anti-id mAb in spite of the lack of a detectable immune response. This latter finding may reflect the development of an immune response below the sensitivity of the assays used. In contrast, other patients experienced disease progression whilst mounting significant detectable immune responses. Whether the latter finding reflects the lack of expression in the melanoma lesions of the MAA used as a target and/or other escape mechanisms remains to be determined.

Immunotherapies Eliciting MAA-specific CTL Responses

The molecular characterization of MAA identified with CTL [55] and the development of methodology to recognize peptides with HLA class I antigen-binding motifs [56] has provided well-defined moieties for the use of active specific immunotherapy of melanoma. Furthermore the significant progress in peptide biochemistry has greatly facilitated the preparation of clinically-graded peptides as pharmaceutical reagents for therapeutic use. As a result, during the last few years a number of clinical trials have been and are being performed at many institutions, using synthetic antigens (or DNA coding for them) as immunogens. The poor immunogenicity of peptides in conjunction with the "self nature" of the large majority of MAA have posed a major challenge to tumor immunologists [57]. The strategies utilized to overcome these difficulties have included the administration of peptides with adjuvants or cytokines, in vitro tumor cell lysate and peptide-stimulated dendritic cells for pulsed therapy [58,59], the utilization of T-helper epitopes, residue changes in the peptides to increase their affinity to

HLA class I antigens and the use of xenogeneic MAA with a high degree of human homology. The amount of peptide used is usually in the range of 50 µg/injection. Different immunization schedules have been utilized in many recent trials. It is generally agreed that immunizations have to be administered repetitively, since ongoing immune responses are usually not self-sustained.

The varying MAA used have differed markedly in their ability to induce MAA-specific CTL. For instance, the differentiation MAA, MART-1 and the cancer-testis antigen, NY-ES0-1 have been found to be more effective in eliciting MAA-specific CTL when compared with the cancer-testis antigens belonging to the MAGE family. These results are likely to reflect differences in the immunogenicity of the peptides used, although this has not been proven formally. We are not aware of any study which has compared different MAA-derived peptides in a controlled clinical setting. This phenomenon reflects in part the high cost of clinical trials and the practical difficulties in finding sufficient funds to support them and the result is that this constraint has generally restricted investigators to working with one or two peptides.

A beneficial effect of active specific immunotherapy on the clinical course of the disease has been observed in a variable percentage of the immunized patients, as measured by regression of metastatic lesions, stabilization of the disease and/or survival prolongation. It is noteworthy that there is not a close correlation between induction of MAA-specific CTL by active specific immunotherapy and clinical response [4]. Clinical evidence indicates that this finding reflects at least in part the mechanisms utilized by melanoma cells to escape from immune recognition and destruction [4]. These include structural and/or functional abnormalities in the antigen processing machinery and/or HLA class I antigens and/or in the MAA used as the target of immunotherapy. All these abnormalities cause the lack of presentation of MAA-derived peptides to CTL and as a result the lack of recognition of melanoma cells in vivo by CTL. However, escape mechanisms utilized by melanoma cells do not provide the complete explanation for the lack of clinical response and for the progression of the disease in spite of the induction and the persistence, respectively, of MAA-specific CTL. Ongoing trials of peptide-based immunotherapy in melanoma are shown in Table 18.2.

Before one can envisage phase III type studies in larger patient populations, these experimental immunotherapies need to be carefully evaluated in phase I and II clinical studies. Assessing the clinical outcome is not the major goal of such small scale studies. Rather, drug toxicity/safety, and therapy feasibility issues would be under investigation in such trials. These aims need to be coupled with a high level determination of biological immunoresponsiveness to specific agents or combinations. In immunotherapy, a major goal is to determine immune activation both quantitatively and qualitatively and this is done by laboratory immune monitoring during vaccination as described below.

Monitoring of MAA-specific Immune Responses in Patients Immunized with Active Specific Immunotherapy

A number of in vitro tests have been developed and applied to measure the humoral and cellular immune response elicited by active specific immunotherapy

Table 18.2.   Peptide-based immunotherapy trials in melanoma patients

Peptide(s)	HLA	Adjuvant	CTL	Tumor response	Reference
MAGE-3 $_{168-176}$	A1	None	Not detected	7/25 (28%)	Marchand, M. et al., 1998
Melan-A/Mart-1 $_{26-35}$					Jäger, E. et al., 1996
Tyrosinase $_{1-9}$		None	3/6		
Tyrosinase $_{368-376}$	A2	or	2/6		
gp100 $_{280-288}$		GM-CsF			
gp100 $_{457-466}$			0/6		
Influenza matrix $_{58-66}$			0/6	3/3	
Melan-A/Mart-1 $_{27-35}$	A2	IFA	12/18 15/18 by IFNγ release	0/23	Cormier, J. et al., 1997
gp100 $_{209-217}$		IFA	2/8	1/19	Rosenberg, S.A. et al., 1998
gp100 $_{209-217}$ (T210M)	A2	IFA	10/11	0/11	
gp100 $_{209-217}$ (T210M)		IL-2 + IFA	3/19	8/19 (42%) 5/12 (42%)	

The peptides were synthesized according to sequences representing melanoma-associated antigens (Table 18.1). One or multiple peptides were given either alone or together with immune adjuvant by intradermal, subcutaneous, or intramuscular injection. Clinical responses and detection of activated CTL varied from 0 to high percentages of response. Future immunotherapies include the use of new immunostimulatory drugs and/or antigen-stimulated dendritic cells (not shown).

in patients with melanoma. The assays which are most commonly used in clinical trials are discussed in the following sections [64].

Monitoring of Humoral Immune Responses

Monitoring of Anti-MAA Antibodies

The development or enhancement of anti-MAA antibodies in immunized patients is monitored by testing sera with melanoma cells and/or purified or recombinant MAA. The binding of antibodies to antigens may be detected in several ways; most notably by the development of colour in ELISA, the uptake of radioactivity in a binding assay with radio-labeled antibodies, the staining of targets in an immunofluorescence assay, the lysis of target cells in a complement- or cell-dependent cytotoxicity assay or by the rosetting of red blood cells with melanoma cells in an immune adherence assay [65–68]. The level of anti-MAA antibodies can be measured by titrating a patient's serum with the target antigen. When the target antigen is protein in nature, the specificity of a patient's antibodies can be confirmed by SDS-PAGE analysis of the antigens they immunoprecipitate from melanoma cells [68], or by Western blotting with a melanoma cell lysate [69]. When the target antigen is a ganglioside, the specificity of a patient's antibodies can be confirmed by immunostaining of gangliosides following separation of purified gangliosides or melanoma cell extracts by thin layer chromatography [48].

Monitoring of Anti-anti-Idiotypic Antibodies

When anti-id antibodies are used as immunogens, the development of anti-anti-id antibodies in immunized patients is monitored by testing sera with the immunizing anti-id antibodies (See Chapter 9). The binding of antibodies to the immunogen is detected by the development of colour in ELISA or the uptake of radioactivity in the binding assay with radio-labeled antibodies [70]. The specificity of anti-anti-id antibodies is assessed by testing a patient's sera with an isotype control. The level of anti-anti-id antibodies is measured by determining the ability of a patient's serum to inhibit the binding of the immunizing anti-id antibodies to the corresponding anti-MAA antibody. The specificity of the inhibition is tested utilizing an unrelated id-anti-id antibody complex.

Monitoring of Cellular Immune Responses

Monitoring of MAA Specific Cytotoxic CD8+ T Cell (CTL) Responses

The cytotoxicity assay measures the ability of a patient's CTL to lyse autologous melanoma cells or melanoma cells which express the restricting HLA class I element and the MAA used as a target. The extent of lysis is assessed by measuring the release of ^{51}Cr [71] or europium [72] following an in vitro incubation of ^{51}Cr- or europium-labeled melanoma cells with a patient's peripheral blood lymphocytes [67], purified T cells or CD8+ T cells. The specificity of the cytotoxicity is monitored utilizing target cells which do not express the relevant MAA and/or the restricting HLA class I molecule. The cytotoxicity assay has a low sensitivity and is only semi-quantitative, requiring functional competence, since the CTL must lyse the target cells in order to be detectable. A more quantitative assay is a variation of the cytotoxicity assay; the limiting dilution analysis (LDA) [73]. The latter assay which measures the extent of lysis of target cells by different numbers of CTL requires the CTL precursors to undergo a minimum of 10–11 cycles of replication over a one week period prior to being used as effectors in the cytotoxicity assay. Although LDA offers several advantages, its application to monitor a patient's cellular immune response is hampered by two limitations. Firstly, it requires a high cell viability and secondly, it does not detect activated CTLs (effector CTLs) during the peak of a CTL response, since effector cells may proliferate poorly in vitro and undergo apoptosis when stimulated in vitro, as may occur during the conduct of the LDA.

Monitoring of MAA-specific Cytokine-releasing Lymphocytes

This assay measures the number of a patient's T cells capable of producing cytokines following in vitro stimulation with the immunizing MAA. Although several cytokines have been assessed and detected, IFN-γ remains the most widely used. IFN-γ producing lymphocytes are enumerated by two techniques. In one, following in vitro stimulation for a few hours with the antigen, lymphocytes are fixed, permeabilized and stained intra-cellularly with fluorochrome-labeled anti-IFN-γ antibodies [74]. Cytokine-producing cells are then counted by flow cytometry. In the other technique, referred to as enzyme-linked immunospot (ELISPOT) assay [75], cell suspensions are cultured in microtiter plates on nitrocellulose filters (previously coated with anti-IFN-γ antibody) for 1–2 days in the presence of the

Inclusion criteria:
- Patient HLA-A2 positive
- Tumor Melan-A/Mart-1 positive

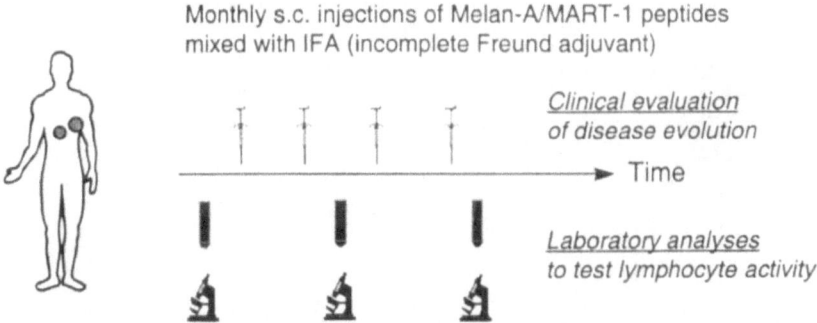

Monthly s.c. injections of Melan-A/MART-1 peptides
mixed with IFA (incomplete Freund adjuvant)

Clinical evaluation
of disease evolution

Time

Laboratory analyses
to test lymphocyte activity

Figure 18.5. Example of an immunotherapy trial with antigenic peptides. Melanoma patients may receive peptide-based immunotherapy, provided that they express the HLA class I molecule which can present the administered peptides to CD8+ T cells. For example, the Melan-A/Mart-1 peptide EAAGIGILTV is only appropriate for HLA-A2 patients. Furthermore, therapeutic benefit can only be expected when the patient's tumor cells express Melan-A/Mart-1. Patients who fulfill these inclusion criteria may receive monthly injections of Melan-A/Mart-1 peptides mixed with the immune adjuvant IFA. Tumor responses are assessed by clinical and radiological diagnostics. Immune responses are monitored by laboratory investigation of lymphocyte activation.

immunizing MAA. IFN–γ secreted in response to antigen stimulation is captured in the immediate surroundings of the activated cell. After the addition of an enzyme-conjugated anti-IFN–γ antibody and subsequent color development steps, discrete spots are generated, which can be quantitated microscopically, visually or electronically. Each spot represents one single cell secreting IFN–γ which is indicative of an antigen-specific T cell. Like cytotoxicity assays, ELISPOT possesses the advantage of detecting IFN–γ production at the single cell level. Therefore ELISPOT does not require expansion of antigen-specific T cells for their detection. An additional advantage of this method is the relatively short incubation time. An example of an immunotherapy trial with antigenic peptide therapy and immunologic monitoring is shown in Figure 18.5.

Monitoring of MAA-specific Lymphocytes with Soluble Fluorescent Multimeric MHC/ Peptide Complexes

To detect T cells recognizing the MAA of interest, attempts were made in the past to identify T-cell receptor (TCR) αβ gene segments encoding for the TCR with the antigen specificity under investigation, utilizing recombinant DNA methodology such as reverse transcription-polymerase chain reaction (RT-PCR). However, the results of these studies were disappointing as many CTL responses even against single antigen ligands were found to be highly diverse in terms of the repertoire of specific TCRs [76].

Attempts to label and visualize antigen-specific T cells have failed for many years, essentially because of the intrinsic low avidity of the clonotypic αβ TCR for the cognate MHC/peptide complex (the antigen ligand). The realization that multimers bind more stably and the production of soluble MHC class I and II/peptide

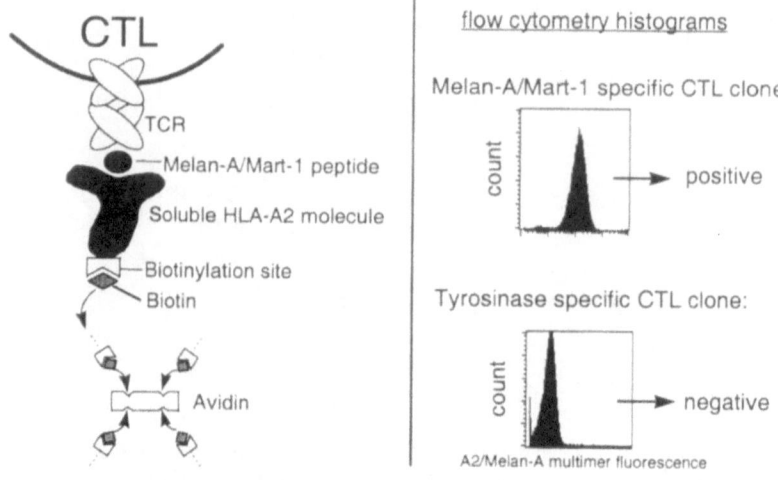

Figure 18.6. Direct visualization of specific CTL with fluorescent multimers. The left panel illustrates the components of a monomeric HLA-A2 antigen/peptide complex coupled to biotin. Due to the four biotin-binding sites of avidin, tetrameric (multimeric) complexes are formed, which are subsequently labeled with a fluorescent dye (not shown). The right panel shows histograms obtained by flow cytometry using the fluorescent multimers. To demonstrate specific binding, A2/Melan-A peptide multimers were used to stain an A2/Melan-A- (top right picture) and an A2/tyrosinase-specific T cell clone (bottom right picture) revealing positive staining by the former but not the latter.

multimeric complexes have constituted a technological breakthrough for the field of cell-mediated immunity. Indeed, by utilizing this new type of reagent a methodology has been developed to analyze antigen-specific T cell responses. T cells are stained with fluorescent conjugated multimers prepared with the restricting HLA class I molecule and with the antigen-derived peptide under investigation. The most widely used methodology takes advantage of the avidin molecule to generate multimeric (tetrameric) antigen ligand complexes (Figure 18.6) [77]. This technology has been previously discussed in the review commentary of Section 1 of this book as a method of determining CTL responsiveness during highly-active anti-retroviral therapy (HAART) in AIDS patients.

Alternatively, divalent MHC class I constructs have been generated using Ig as a scaffold [78]. The first study which utilized fluorescent multimers to quantitate antigen-specific T cells in tumor immunology focused on the analysis of Melan-A/MART-1- and tyrosinase-specific CD8+ T cells [2]. No tyrosinase-reactive T cells could be found in metastatic lymph nodes, but very high numbers of Melan-A/MART-1-reactive CD8+ T lymphocytes were present in all of a series of nine metastatic lymph nodes resected from six HLA-A2 melanoma patients. More recently, immunotherapy-induced T-cell responses were characterized by using fluorescent multimers to analyze lymphocytes ex vivo as shown in Figure 18.7 [79,80].

The assay to visualize antigen-specific T cells has several advantages. The major one is the possibility, for the first time in the 30 years since CTLs were first described, to enumerate these cells without the need to use complex indirect functional assays in vitro. In addition, this new technology enables rapid isolation and preparation of homogenous populations of antigen-specific T cells by cell

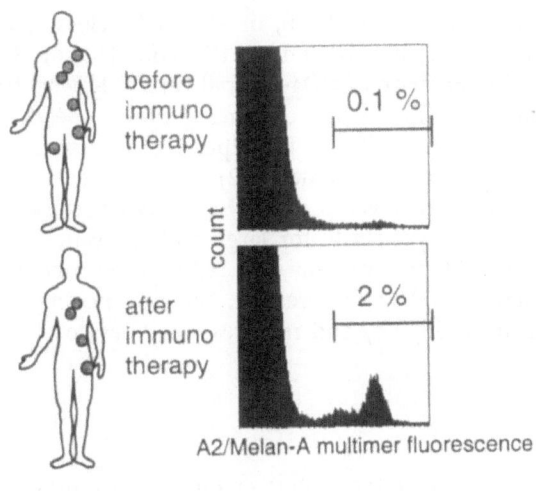

before immuno therapy

0.1 %

count

after immuno therapy

2 %

A2/Melan-A multimer fluorescence

● metastases

Figure 18.7. Peptide immunotherapy-induced regression of some metastases and expansion of Melan-A/Mart-1-specific CTL in a melanoma patient. The figure illustrates a melanoma patient with multiple skin and visceral metastases. In peripheral blood, Melan-A/Mart-1-specific T cells were few in number (0.1 percent of CD8+ cells), below the detection limit of 0.4 percent. After immunotherapy (that was scheduled as described in Figure 18.5), some metastases regressed and the number of Melan-A/Mart-1-specific CTL increased to about 2 percent. Such CTL were found to be activated and showed effector functions ex vivo, as well as being increased within melanoma metastases (not shown). For methods of CTL detection, see section Monitoring of MAA-specific lymphocytes with soluble fluorescent multimeric MHC/peptide complexes.

sorting. These populations are also a unique source of cells for TCR repertoire analysis and for antigen-targeted adoptive transfer therapy. Multimer staining also allows one to perform extensive phenotyping using the large panel of cell-surface markers available for human T cells including markers associated with cell activation status, homing, co-stimulatory receptors, killer activatory and inhibitory receptors, death receptors and integrins. In addition, intra-cellular proteins may also be analyzed by flow cytometry in conjunction with multimer staining. As a result, one can study the differentiation stage of antigen-specific T lymphocytes and obtain information about the extent to which T lymphocytes are activated and have responded to antigen challenge. Fluorescent multimers can also be utilized to detect and enumerate antigen-specific T cells in malignant lesions thus providing information about the interactions between CTL and malignant cells within a malignant deposit. The latter are likely to be the most informative site to characterize the interactions of tumor cells with the host's immune system and to provide much more accurate information concerning ongoing immune responses in patients than conventional in vitro cellular testing.

Monitoring of CD4+ Helper T-cell Responses

As CD8+ T cells are activated, CD4+ helper T cells are also stimulated to exert their effector functions upon engagement of the T cell receptor with MHC/peptide antigen complexes. As already discussed, while CD8+ T cells recognize antigenic peptides bound to HLA-A, -B, or -C (MHC class I) antigens, CD4+ T cells recognize antigenic peptides bound to HLA-DR, -DQ, or -DP (MHC class II) antigens. Although the majority of CD4+ T cells are only weakly (or non) cytolytic, they may provide immune "help" enhancing tumor-specific immune responses. For the monitoring of CD4+ T helper cells, assays that test cellular proliferation [81] or cytokine production [82] may be used. More recently, fluorescent multimers have been developed [83], although because of technical difficulties, this method is not yet ready for large scale investigation of CD4+ T cell responses. At any rate, at present only few MAA recognized by CD4+ helper T cells have been identified. For this reason, the monitoring of antigen-specific CD4+ T cells is still in its infancy and requires more development.

Conclusions

The information we have reviewed in this chapter clearly indicates that by taking advantage of the major progress made in immunology and recombinant DNA technology, a number of MAA with well-defined molecular characteristics have been identified. Most of them are shared by a large number of patients with melanoma. This characteristic in conjunction with their availability in a standardized and reproducible form has facilitated their use as immunogens to implement active specific immunotherapy in patients with melanoma and to monitor the immune response. Humoral and/or cellular anti-MAA immunity has been induced or enhanced in a variable percentage of immunized patients in a number of international clinical trials. In some patients the MAA-specific immune response is associated with regression of metastatic lesions, stabilization of the disease and/or survival prolongation.

Although there has been no report of complete recovery from the disease, these results indicate that the immune system has the potential to inhibit or at least to control tumor growth in patients with melanoma. Two results derived from the clinical trials performed thus far are noteworthy. In some patients, clinical responses have been documented following active specific immunotherapy although an MAA-specific immune response could not be detected. No mechanism(s) to explain this finding have been identified. In other patients a clinical response was not detected and disease progression was documented in spite of the development and persistence, respectively, of an MAA-specific immune response. These findings are likely to reflect at least in some patients, the multiple mechanisms utilized by malignant cells to escape from immune recognition and/or immune destruction. The latter observation suggests that multiple targets and multiple immunological effector mechanisms in combination with non-immunological modalities should be used to counteract the immune escape mechanisms utilized by malignant cells.

A number of immunization strategies have been utilized to implement active specific immunotherapy in patients with melanoma. The strategies differ in terms of the MAA used as an immunogen and of the conjugating adjuvant and/or cytokine and the immunization schedule. Therefore at present there is no objective information to assess which immunization strategy is more effective from a clinical standpoint. This represents one of the challenges which faces tumor immunologists and which requires a close collaboration between academic institutions and pharmaceutical companies given the high cost of clinical trials. The success of these investigations will very much depend on the identification of biological surrogate end points (as opposed to conventional classifications of clinical response), which can predict the clinical efficacy of any given immunization strategy.

Most, if not all of the clinical trials of active specific immunotherapy have been performed in patients with advanced disease. This is the least likely patient population to benefit from active specific immunotherapy, since these patients are likely to already have defects in their immune system. Furthermore an MAA-specific immune response is not likely to be able to control tumor growth in patients with a heavy tumor burden. Therefore future clinical trials should target patients with minimal residual disease or as a truly adjuvant strategy, especially since immunotherapy has not been found to be associated with troublesome side-effects in most of the patients immunized. To the best of our knowledge the various immunization strategies have not been compared in randomized double blind clinical trials.

References

1. Ferrone S, Pellegrino MA. Serological detection of human melanoma associated antigens. In: Herberman RB, McIntire R, editors. Cancer Immunodiagnosis, New York: MarcelDekker. 1979; 588–632.
2. Romero P, Dunbar PR, Valmori D, Pittet MJ, Ogg GS, Rimoldi D, et al. Ex vivo staining of metastatic lymph nodes by class I major histocompatibility complex tetramers reveals high numbers of antigen-experienced tumor-specific cytotoxic T lymphocytes. J Exp Med 1998;188:1641.
3. Natali P, Nicotra MR, Cavaliere R, Bigotti A, Romano G, Temponi M, et al. Differential expression of intercellular adhesion molecule 1 in primary and metastatic melanoma lesions. Cancer Res 1990; 50:1271.
4. Marincola FM, Jaffee EM, Hicklin DJ, Ferrone S. Escape of human solid tumors from T-cell recognition: molecular mechanisms and functional significance. Adv Immunol 2000;74:181.
5. Clark W H. Tumor progression and the nature of cancer. Br J Cancer 1991;64:631.
6. Mackensen A, Carcelain G, Viel S, Raynal MC, Michalaki H, Triebel F, et al. Direct evidence to support the immunosurveillance concept in a human regressive melanoma. J Clin Invest 199493:1397.
7. Shilyansky J, Nishimura MI, Yannelli JR, Kawakami Y, Jacknin LS, Charmley P, et al. T-cell receptor usage by melanoma-specific clonal and highly oligoclonal tumor-infiltrating lymphocyte lines. Proc Natl Acad Sci U S A 1994;91:2829.
8. thor Straten P, Becker JC, Seremet T, Brocker EB, Zeuthen J. Clonal T cell responses in tumor infiltrating lymphocytes from both regressive and progressive regions of primary human malignant melanoma. J Clin Invest 1996;98:279.
9. Hunt DF, Henderson RA, Shabanowitz J, Sakaguchi K, Michel H, Sevilir N, et al. Characterization of peptides bound to the class I MHC molecule HLA-A2.1 by mass spectrometry. Science 1992;255:1261.
10. Van Pel A, van der Bruggen P, Coulie PG, Brichard G, Lethé B, Van den Eynde B, et al. Genes coding for tumor antigens recognized by cytolytic T lymphocytes. Immunol Rev 1995;145:229.
11. Pieper R., Christian RE, Gonzales MI, Nishimura MI, Gupta G, Settlage RE, et al. Biochemical identification of a mutated human melanoma antigen recognized by CD4(+) T cells. J Exp Med 1999;189:757.
12. Wang RF, Wang X, Atwood AC, Topalian SL, Rosenberg SA. Cloning genes encoding MHC class II-restricted antigens: mutated CDC27 as a tumor antigen. Science 1999;284:1351.
13. Brinckerhoff LH, Thompson LW, Slingluff Jr CL. Melanoma vaccines. Curr Opin Oncol 2000;12:163.
14. Wang RF. The role of MHC class II-restricted tumor antigens and CD4+ T cells in antitumor immunity. Trends Immunol 2001;22:269.
15. Köhler G, Milstein C. Continuous cultures of fused cells secreting antibody of predefined specificity. Nature 1975;256:495.

16. Graf LH Jr, Ferrone S. Human melanoma-associated antigens. Human Immunogenetics. In: Litwin SD, editor. Basic Principles and Clinical Relevance. New York and Basel; Marcel Dekker, Inc., 1989; 643–79.

17. Irie RF, Sze LL, Saxton RE. Human antibody to OFA-I, a tumor antigen, produced in vitro by Epstein- Barr virus-transformed human B-lymphoid cell lines. Proc Natl Acad Sci USA 1982;79:5666.

18. Houghton AN, Brooks H, Cote RJ, Taormina MC, Oettgen HF, Old LJ.Detection of cell surface and intracellular antigens by human monoclonal antibodies. Hybrid cell lines derived from lymphocytes of patients with malignant melanoma. J Exp Med 1983;158:53.

19. Kan-Mitchell J, Imam A, Kempf RA, Taylor CR, Mitchell MS. Human monoclonal antibodies directed against melanoma tumor-associated antigens. Cancer Res 1986;46:2490.

20. Hoogenboom HR, Marks JD, Griffiths AD, Winter G. Building antibodies from their genes. Immunol Rev 1992;130:41.

21. Lerner RA, Kang AS, Bain JD, Burton DR, Barbas III CF. Antibodies without immunization. Science 1992;258:1313.

22. Noronha EJ, Wang X, Desai SA, Kageshita T, Ferrone S. Limited diversity of human scFv fragments isolated by panning a synthetic phage-display scFv library with cultured human melanoma cells. J Immunol 1998;161:2968.

23. Kupsch JM, Tidman NH, Kang NV, Truman H, Hamilton S, Patel N, et al. Isolation of human tumor-specific antibodies by selection of an antibody phage library on melanoma cells. Clin Cancer Res 1999;5:925.

24. Wang B, Chen YB, Ayalon O, Bender J, Garen A. Human single-chain Fv immunoconjugates targeted to a melanoma-associated chondroitin sulfate proteoglycan mediate specific lysis of human melanoma cells by natural killer cells and complement. Proc Natl Acad Sci USA 1999;96:1627.

25. Sahin U, Tureci O, Schmitt H, Cochlovius B, Johannes T, Schmits R, et al. Human neoplasms elicit multiple specific immune responses in the autologous host. Proc Natl Acad Sci USA 1995;92:11810.

26. Zinkernagel RM, Doherty PC. Restriction of in vitro T cell mediated cytotoxicity in lymphocytic choriomeningitis within a syngeneic or semiallogeneic system. Nature 1974;248:701.

27. Townsend ARM, Rothbard J, Gotch FM, Bahadur G, Wraith D, McMichael AJ. The epitopes of influenza nucleoprotein recognized by cytotoxic T lymphocytes can be defined with short synthetic peptides. Cell 1986;44::959.

28. Traversari C, van der Bruggen P, Luescher IF, Lurquin C, Chomez P, Van Pel A, et al. A nonapeptide encoded by human gene MAGE-1 is recognized on HLA-A1 by cytolytic T lymphocytes directed against tumor antigen MZ2-E. J Exp Med 1992;176:1453–7.

29. Jager E, Chen YT, Drijfhout JW, Karbach J, Ringhoffer M, Jager D, Arand M, Wada H, Noguchi Y, Stockert E, Old LJ, Knuth A. Simultaneous humoral and cellular immune response against cancer-testis antigen NY-ESO-1: definition of human histocompatibility leukocyte antigen (HLA)-A2-binding peptide epitopes. J Exp Med 1998;187:265–70.

30. Huang LQ, Brasseur F, Serrano A, De Plaen E, van der Bruggen P, Boon T, et al. Cytolytic T lymphocytes recognize an antigen encoded by MAGE-A10 on a human melanoma. J Immunol 1999;162:6849–54.

31. Kawakami Y, Eliyahu S, Sakaguchi K, Robbins PF, Rivoltini L, Yannelli JR, Appella E, Rosenberg SA. Identification of the immunodominant peptides of the MART-1 human melanoma antigen recognized by the majority of HLA-A2-restricted tumor infiltrating lymphocytes. J Exp Med 1994;180:347–52.

32. Wolfel T, Van Pel A, Brichard V, Schneider J, Seliger B, Meyer zum Buschenfelde KH, Boon T. Two tyrosinase nonapeptides recognized on HLA-A2 melanomas by autologous cytolytic T lymphocytes. Eur J Immunol 1994;24:759–64.

33. Kawakami Y, Eliyahu S, Jennings C, Sakaguchi K, Kang X, Southwood S, et al. Recognition of multiple epitopes in the human melanoma antigen gp100 by tumor-infiltrating T lymphocytes associated with in vivo tumor regression. J Immunol 1995;154:3961–8.

34. Wang RF, Parkhurst MR, Kawakami Y, Robbins PF, Rosenberg SA. Utilization of an alternative open reading frame of a normal gene in generating a novel human cancer antigen. J Exp Med 1996;183:1131–40.

35. Ikeda H, Lethe B, Lehmann F, van Baren N, Baurain JF, de Smet C, et al. Characaterization of an antigen that is recognized on a melanoma showing partial HLA loss by CTL expressing an NK inhibitory receptor. Immunity 1997;6:199–208.

36. Wolfel T, Hauer M, Schneider J, Serrano M, Wolfel C, Klehmann-Hieb E,et al. A p16INK4a-insensitive CDK4 mutant targeted by cytolytic T lymphocytes in a human melanoma. Science 1995;269(5228):1281–4.

37. Robbins PF, El-Gamil M, Li YF, Kawakami Y, Loftus D, Appella E, et al. A mutated beta-catenin gene encodes a melanoma-specific antigen recognized by tumor infiltrating lymphocytes. J Exp Med 1996;183:1185–92.
38. Natali PG, Fawwaz R, Ruiter DJ, Bigotti A, Kageshita T, Temponi M, et al. 1989. Immunodiagnostic and immunotherapeutic applications of anti human melanoma associated antigen monoclonal antibodies. In: Conti CJ, Slaga TJ, Klein-Szanto AJP, editors. Carcinogenesis — A comprehensive survey. Vol. 11 Skin Tumors: Experimental and Clinical Aspects. New York: Raven Press, Ltd., 1989; 133–64.
39. Yee C, Riddell SR, Greenberg PD. Prospects for adoptive T cell therapy. Curr Opin Immunol 1997;9:702.
40. Singh M, O'Hagan D. Advances in vaccine adjuvants. Nat Biotechnol 1999;17:1075
41. Villikka K, Pyrhonen S. Cytokine therapy of malignant melanoma. Ann Med 1996;28:227–33
42. Mitchell MS, Harel W, Groshen S. Association of HLA phenotype with response to active specific immunotherapy of melanoma. J Clin Oncol 1992;10:1158.
43. Hsueh EC, Gupta RK, Qi K, Morton DL. Correlation of specific immune responses with survival in melanoma patients with distant metastases receiving polyvalent melanoma cell vaccine. J Clin Oncol 1998;16:2913–20.
44. Bystryn J-C, Oratz R, Shapiro RL, Harris MN, Roses DF, Zeleniuch-Jacquotte A, et al. Double-blind, placebo-controlled, trial of a shed, polyvalent, melanoma vaccine in stage III melanoma. Proc Am Soc Clin Oncol 1999;18:434.
45. Hsueh EC, Nathanson L, Foshag LJ, Essner R, Nizze JA, Stern SL, et al. Active specific immunotherapy with polyvalent melanoma cell vaccine for patients with in-transit melanoma metastases. Cancer 1999;85:2160–2169.
46. Sosman JA, Unger JM, Liu P, Flaherty L, Kempf R, Thompson J, et al. Significant impact of HLA class I alleles on outcome in T3N0 melanoma patients treated with Melacine™ (MEL): an allogeneic melanoma cell lysate vaccine: Prospective Analysis of Southwest Oncology Group (SWOG)-9035. Proc Am Soc Clin Oncol 2001; 20, 351.
47. Livingston PO, Wong GY, Adluri S, Tao Y, Padavan M, Parente R, et al. Improved survival in stage III melanoma patients with GM2 antibodies: a randomized trial of adjuvant vaccination with GM2 ganglioside. J Clin Oncol 1994;12:1036.
48. Ragupathi G, Meyers M, Adluri S, Howard L, Musselli C, Livingston PO. Induction of antibodies against GD3 ganglioside in melanoma patients by vaccination with GD3-lactone-KLH conjugate plus immunological adjuvant QS-21. Int J Cancer 2000;85:659.
49. Cheresh DA, Honsik CJ, Staffileno LK, Jung G, Reisfeld RA. Disialoganglioside GD3 on human melanoma serves as a relevant target antigen for monoclonal antibody-mediated tumor cytolysis. Proc Natl Acad Sci U S A 198582:5155.
50. Hellstrom, I., Brankovan, V, Hellstrom, K.E. 1985. Strong antitumor activities of IgG3 antibodies to a human melanoma-associated ganglioside. Proc Natl Acad Sci USA 82:1499, 1985
51. Thurin J, Thurin M, Kimoto Y, Herlyn M, Lubeck MD, Elder DE, et al. Monoclonal antibody-defined correlations in melanoma between levels of GD2 and GD3 antigens and antibody-mediated cytotoxicityCancer Res 1987;47:1229.
52. Helling F, Zhang S, Shang A, Adluri S, Calves M, Koganty R, et al. G$_{M2}$-KLH conjugate vaccine: increased immunogenicity in melanoma patients after administration with immunological adjuvant QS-21. Cancer Res 1995;55:2783.
53. Kirkwood JM, Ibrahim JG, Sosman JA, Sondak VK, Agarwala SS, Ernstoff MS, et al. High-dose interferon alfa-2b significantly prolongs relapse-free and overall survival compared with the gm2-klh/qs-21 vaccine in patients with resected stage iib-iii melanoma: results of intergroup trial e1694/s9512/c509801. J Clin Oncol 2001;19:2370.
54. Wang X, Luo W, Foon KA, Ferrone S. Tumor associated antigen (TAA) mimicry and immunotherapy of malignant diseases. From anti-idiotypic antibodies to peptide mimics. Cancer Chemother. Biol. Resp. Modif. Annu. 2001;19 (in press).
55. Noronha EJ, Wang X, Ferrone S. Isolation of antibodies against tumor-associated cell surface antigens from a synthetic phage display scFv library. Methods Mol Biol 2001 (in press).
56. Melief CJM, Offringa R, Toes REM, Kast WM. Peptide-based cancer vaccines. Curr Opin Immunol 1996;8:651.
57. Speiser DE, Miranda R, Zakarian A, Bachmann MF, McKall-Faienza K, Odermatt B, et al. Self antigens expressed by solid tumors do not stimulate naive or activated T cells: implications for immunotherapy. J Exp Med 1997;186:645.
58. Thurner B, Haendle I, Roder C, Dieckmann D, Keikavoussi P, Jonuleit H, et al. Vaccination with mage-3A1 peptide-pulsed mature, monocyte-derived dendritic cells expands specific cytotoxic T cells and induces regression of some metastases in advanced stage IV melanoma. J Exp Med 1999;190:1669.

59. Nestle FO, Alijagic S, Gilliet M, Yuansheng S, Grabbe S, Dummer R, et al. Vaccination of melanoma patients with peptide- or tumor lysate-pulsed dendritic cells. Nat Med 1998;4:328.
60. Marchand M, Weynants P, Rankin E, Arienti F, Belli F, Parmiani G, et al. Tumor regression responsesin melanoma patients treated with a peptide encoded by gene MAGE-3. Int J Cancer 1995;63:883–5.
61. Jager E, Ringhoffer M, Arand M, Karbach J, Jager D, Ilsemann C, et al. Cytolytic T cell reactivity against melanoma-associated differentiation antigens in peripheral blood of melanoma patients and healthy individuals. Melanoma Res 1996;6:419–25.
62. Cormier JN, Salgaller ML, Prevette T, Barracchini KC, Rivoltini L, Restifo NP, et al. Enhancement of cellular immunity in melanoma patients immunized with a peptide from MART-1/MELAN A. Cancer J Sci Am 1997;3:37–44.
63. Rosenberg SA, Yang JC, Schwartzentruber DJ, Hwu P, Marincola FM, Topalian SL, et al. Immunologic and therapeutic evaluation of a synthetic peptide vaccine for the treatment of patients with metastatic melanoma. Nat Med 1998;4:321–7.
64. Speiser DE, Ohashi PS. Activation of cytotoxic T cells by solid tumors? Cell Mol Life Sci 1998;54:263.
65. Carey TE, Takahashi T, Resnick LA, Oettgen HF, Old LJ. Cell surface antigens of human malignant melanoma: mixed hemadsorption assays for humoral immunity to cultured autologous melanoma cells. Proc Natl Acad Sci U S A 1976;73:3278–3282.
66. McCabe RP, Quaranta V, Frugis L, Ferrone S, Reisfeld RA. A radioimmunometric antibody-binding assay for evaluation of xenoantisera to melanoma-associated antigens. J Natl Cancer Inst 1979; 62:455–463.
67. Imai K, Ferrone S. Indirect rosette microassay to characterize human melanoma associated antigens recognized by operationally specific xenoantisera. Cancer Res 1980; 40:2252–2256.
68. Matsui M, Temponi M, Ferrone S. Characterization of a monoclonal antibody-defined human melanoma-associated antigen susceptible to induction by immune interferon. J Immunol 1987; 139:2088–2095.
69. Desai SA, Wang X, Noronha EJ, et. al. Structural relatedness of distinct determinants recognized by mAb TP25.99 on β_2-μ associated and β_2-μ free HLA class I heavy chains. J Immunol 2000; 165:3275–3283.
70. Perosa F, Kageshita T, Ono R, Ferrone S. Serological methods to detect anti-idiotypic antibodies. Methods Enzymol 1989; 178:74–90.
71. Brunner KT, Mauel J, Cerottini JC, Chapuis B. Quantitative assay of the lytic action of immune lymphoid cells on 51-Cr-labelled allogeneic target cells in vitro; inhibition by isoantibody and by drugs. Immunology 1968; 14:181–196.
72. Blomberg K, Ulfstedt AC. Fluorescent europium chelates as target cell markers in the assessment of natural killer cell cytotoxicity. J Immunol Methods 1993; 160:27–34.
73. Sharrock CE, Kaminski E, Man S. Limiting dilution analysis of human T cells: a useful clinical tool. Immunol Today 1990; 11:281–286.
74. Maino VC, Picker LJ. Identification of functional subsets by flow cytometry: intracellular detection of cytokine expression. Cytometry 1998; 34:207–215.
75. Herr W, Schneider J, Lohse AW, Meyer zum Buschenfelde KH, Wolfel T. Detection and quantification of blood-derived CD8+ T lymphocytes secreting tumor necrosis factor alpha in response to HLA-A2.1-binding melanoma and viral peptide antigens. J Immunol Methods 1996; 191:131–142.
76. Casanova JL, Cerottini J-C, Matthes M, Necker A, Gournier H, Barra C, et al. H-2-restricted cytolytic T lymphocytes specific for HLA display T cell receptors of limited diversity. J Exp Med 1992;176:439.
77. Altman JD, Moss PAH, Goulder PJR, Barouch DH, McHeyzer-Williams MG, Bell JI, et al. Phenotypic analysis of antigen-specific T lymphocytes. Science 1996;274:94.
78. Greten TF, Slansky JE, KubotaR, Soldan SS, Jaffee EM, Leist TP, et al. Direct visualization of antigen-specific T cells: HTLV-1 Tax11-19-specific CD8(+) T cells are activated in peripheral blood and accumulate in cerebrospinal fluid from HAM/TSP patients. Proc Natl Acad Sci U S A 1998;95:7568.
79. Pittet MJ, Speiser DE, Liénard D, Valmori D, Guillaume P, Dutoit V, et al. Expansion and functional maturation of human tumor antigen-specific CD8+ T cells following vaccination with antigenic peptide. Clin Cancer Res 2001;7:796.
80. Speiser DE, Migliaccio M, Pittet MJ, Valmori D, Liénard D, Lejeune F, et al. Human CD8+ T cells expressing HLA-DR and CD28 show telomerase activity and are distinct from cytolytic effector T cells. Eur J Immunol 200131:459.
81. Clay TM, Hobeika AC, Mosca PJ, Lyerly HK, Morse MA. Assays for monitoring cellular immune responses to active immunotherapy of cancer. Clin Cancer Res 2001; 7:1127–1135.

82. Brosterhus H, Brings S, Leyendeckers H, et al. Enrichment and detection of live antigen-specific CD4(+) and CD8(+) T cells based on cytokine secretion. Eur J Immunol 1999; 29:4053–4059.

83. Novak EJ, Kiu AW, Nepom GT, Kwok WW. MHC class II tetramers identify peptide-specific human CD4(+) T cells proliferating in response to influenza A antigen. J Clin Invest 1999; 104:R63–R67.

Commentary on Section III

Andrew P. Zbar

The aim of this review section is to highlight important areas covered in the chapters concerning tumor immunology and to introduce potential future immunotherapeutic strategies in specific malignancies raised in these chapters.

In Chapter 10, Killion and Fidler discuss the immunobiology of the metastatic process and the nature of the host response in cancer dissemination. Recently, there has been great emphasis on the detection of low burden circulating and sequestered (mostly bone marrow) tumor cells in solid epithelial malignancies such as gastric, colonic, breast and lung carcinoma [1–3]. This finding will probably define the need for systemic therapy when conventional staging suggests that disease is localized and it may also act as a new surrogate end-point for the determination of adjuvant responses.

Although the specificity of this technique varies, its sensitivity is extremely high and it appears to be an independent prognostic variable in cancer-related outcome in these tumors. Despite the fact that the assay has not yet been standardized, both RT-PCR and immunomagnetic cell separation permit the detection of 1 tumor cell/10^7–10^8 mononuclear cells [4]. These new techniques will only be limited by illegitimate transcription of tumor-associated or epithelial-specific genes in haematopoetic cells or by the deficient (or heterogeneous) expression of the marker gene on the micrometastatic tumor cell [5]. How important the detection of these rogue cells is seems unclear at present, however, in theory, they can be characterized with respect to oncogene and tumor suppressor gene expression and the expression of angiogenic markers and growth receptors as well as act as ideal targets for immunotherapy [6].

As stated in this chapter, the prognosis of many tumors has been shown to correlate independently with the extent of tumor infiltrate [7], although it is the ability of these cells to be functional as cytotoxic lymphocytes (CTLs) capable of recognizing tumor-associated antigens or tumor-suppressive gene products, that is important [8]. In this context, paradoxically, immune interaction with specific tumor-related epitopes may allow selection of neoplastic phenotypic variants which could encourage the clonal development of a metastatic deposit following an incomplete immunological response [9].

The recent interest in tumor angiogenesis and angiogenesis inhibitors in clinical practice as well as the role of adhesion molecules, such as intercellular adhesion molecule-1(ICAM-1); vascular cell adhesion molecule-1 (VCAM-1) and the selectins, is part of an improved understanding of the metastatic process whereby tumor cells express specific endothelial adhesion receptors which link to endothelial ligands on the tumor neovasculature. Malignant cells detached from the primary tumor must penetrate into blood or lymph vessels, survive in the circulation, arrest in the capillary endothelium of distant organs and then extravasate and grow as secondary lesions. Therefore, adhesion interactions between endothelial and cancer cells appear to be crucial for the successful development of metastases. Selectins mediate the binding of leukocytes to the microvascular endothelium and experimental studies have suggested that the efficiency of the E-selectin-mediated binding of certain cancer cell lines to endothelial cells correlates with their metastatic potential. ICAM-1 is constitutively expressed by endothelial cells and by some leukocytes and serves as a ligand for the leucocyte $\beta 2$ integrin receptors LFA-1 and Mac-1. VCAM-1 is found mainly on activated endothelial cells and provides a ligand for the $\alpha 4\beta 1$ integrin receptor VLA-4. Both ICAM-1 and VCAM-1 are involved in firm leucocyte-endothelial adhesion, which facilitates leukocyte transmigration through the vascular wall. The expression of all three adhesion receptors has been demonstrated on the endothelial cells of small vessels at the invasive margin of many solid tumors, suggesting an important interaction between endothelial and tumor cells involved in metastatic spread.

Recently the soluble forms of these adhesion molecules have been recognized. They have been detected in the supernatants from cytokine-activated cultured endothelial cells and in the serum of healthy subjects where they have been shown to be elevated in patients with gastric, hepatobiliary, breast and colonic cancer and where high circulating levels have been associated with locally advanced and metastatic disease [10,11]. The association in gastrointestinal cancers between immunohistochemical adhesion molecule expression, tumor vascularity and leukocytic infiltration suggests an important role for these molecules in host immune response. Since leukocyte LFA-1 is also involved in the initial steps of adhesion of CTL's to target tumor cells, it is possible that ICAM-1 shedding from tumor cells could block the binding of CTL's to the cancer. Additional loss of adhesion molecules from activated endothelium could inhibit counterligands on the tumor cells themselves, preventing their adhesion to endothelial sites and thereby promoting metastasis [12,13]. ICAM-1 expression in the tumor microvasculature thus appears to have a dual effect, where it favours cytotoxic lymphocyte trafficking towards the cancer, enhancing tumor angiogenesis. Circulating ICAM-1 on the other hand, interferes with NK and LAK cell reactivity against tumor cells [14] and thus, the shedding of adhesion molecules by endothelial or tumor cells might block counterligands on immunocompetent recognition lymphocytes, promoting metastasis formation. An improved understanding of the mechanisms of membrane shedding of these adhesion mediators, their effect on the host immune response and the role of angiogenesis inhibitors on their expression is required to delineate their place in tumor progression and metastasis.

The demonstration by Folkman that solid tumor growth and metastasis is angiogenesis-dependent, [15] suggests a potential value of blood and tissue angiogenic markers as prognostic and survival determinants. Vascular endothelial growth factor (VEGF) is a dimeric heparin-binding glycoprotein which functions as a potent mitogen of vascular endothelial cells, providing an opportunity for their migration and organization for the neovascularization of micrometastases.

An important role for VEGF in tumor biology is suggested by its extensive immunohistochemical staining in different solid epithelial malignancies including stomach, lung, colon, breast, kidney, bladder and ovary. VEGF expression at both the mRNA and protein level, has been demonstrated in vivo in a variety of gastrointestinal tumors, with the intensity of its immunohistochemical expression reflecting intra-tumoral microvessel density, the presence of lymph node and hepatic metastases and cancer-specific survival [16] Recently, serum VEGF concentrations have been shown to be increased in a range of epithelial cancers, with the most elevated levels being found in disseminated cancer. Several groups have shown that pre-operative serum VEGF levels correlate with tumor stage and cancer-specific survival [17,18] as well as predict for the development of distant metastases.

The association of VEGF expression in gastrointesinal tumors with other important angiogenic markers such as platelet-derived endothelial growth factor suggests that such tumors may be prognostically divisible based upon their angiogenic profile, perhaps permitting their categorization in phase III trials with angiogenesis inhibitors. An improved understanding of circulating VEGF dynamics in solid cancer will assist in the development of new anti-angiogenesis therapies and perhaps best define those patients with potentially chemosensitive tumors. Such treatments could take the form of anti-sense gene delivery systems designed to inhibit transcription of pro-angiogenesis factors or strategies to disrupt vital receptor/ligand connections for these tumors where VEGF is almost exclusively expressed on the tumor microvasculature.Moreover, detectable VEGF binding capacity by both tumor-infiltrating lymphocytes and tumor-specific antigen-presenting dendritic cells is likely to influence treatments directed specifically at angiogenic proteins and their receptors.The inhibitory effect of local VEGF expression on the maturation of dendritic cells from their CD34+ precursors suggests an important role for VEGF in host immune response and a new strategy for VEGF-directed therapies [19]. In this sense VEGF expression (and detection) may reflect many neoplastic variables including tumor mass, angiogenesis index, dissemination capacity and specific anti-tumor immune dysfunction.

References

1. Cote RJ, Beattie EJ, Chaiwun B, Shi SR, Harvey J, Chen SC, et al. Detection of occult bone marrow micrometastases in patients with operable lung carcinoma. Ann Surg 1995;222:415–25.
2. Calaluce R, Miedema BW, Yesus YW. Micrometastases in colorectal carcinoma: a review. J Surg Oncol 1998;67:194–202.
3. Muller P, Schlimok G. Bone marrow " micrometastases" of epithelial tumors: detection and clinical relevance. J Cancer Res Clin Oncol 2000;126:607–18.
4. Zhong XY, Kaul S, Lin YS, Eichler A, Bastert G. Sensitive detection of micrometastases in bone marrow from patients with breast cancer using immunomagnetic isolation of tumor cells in combination with reverse transcriptase/polymerase chain reaction for cytokeratin-19. J Cancer Res Clin Oncol 2000;126:212–8.
5. Zippelius A, Kufer P, Honold G, Kollermann MW, Oberneder R, Schlimok G, et al. Limitations of reverse-transcriptase polymerase chain reaction analyses for detection of micrometastatic epithelial cancer cells in bone marrow. J Clin Oncol 1997;15:2701–8.
6. Fox SB, Leek RD, Bliss J, Mansi JL, Gusterson B, Gatter KC, et al. Association of tumor angiogenesis with bone marrow micrometastases in breast cancer patients. J Natl Cancer Inst 1997;89: 1044–9.

7. Murphy J, O'Sullivan GC, Lee G, Madden M, Shanahan F, Collins JK, et al. The inflammatory response within Dukes' B colorectal cancer: implications for progression of micrometastases and patient survival. Am J Gastroenterol 2000;95:3607–14.
8. Hilburger Ryan M, Abrams SI. Characterization of CD8+ cytotoxic lymphocyte/tumor cell interactions reflecting recognition of an endogenously expressed murine wild-type p53 determinant. Cancer Immunol Immunother 2001;49:603–12.
9. Seymour K, Pettit S, O'Flaherty E, Charnley RM, Kirby JA. Selection of metastatic tumor phenotypes by host immune systems. Lancet 1999;354(9194):1989–91.
10. Yoo NC, Chung HC, Chung HC, Park JO, Rha SY, Kim JH, et al. Synchronous elevation of soluble intercellular adhesion molecule-1 (ICAM-1) and vascular cell adhesion molecule-1 (VCAM-1) correlates with gastric cancer progression. Yonsei Med J 1998;39:27–36.
11. Velikova G, Banks RE, Gearing A, Hemingway I, Forbes MA, Preston SR, et al. Serum concentrations of soluble adhesion molecules in patients with colorectal cancer. Br J Cancer 1998;77:1857–63.
12. Sanchez-Rovira P, Jimenez E, Carracedo J, Barneto IC, Ramirez R, Aranda E. Serum levels of intercellular adhesion molecule 1 (ICAM-1) in patients with colorectal cancer: inhibitory effect on cytotoxicity. Eur J Cancer 1998;34:394–8.
13. Koyama S. Immunosuppressive effect of shedding ICAM-1 antigen on cell-mediated cytotoxicity against tumor cells. Jpn J Cancer Res 1994;85:131–4.
14. Becker JC, Termeer C, Schmidt RE, Bröcker E-B. Soluble intercellular adhesion molecule 1 inhibits MHC-restricted specific T cell/tumor interaction. J Immunol 1993;151: 7224–32.
15. Folkman J. What is the evidence that tumors are angiogenesis dependent? J Natl Cancer Inst., 1990;82:4–6.
16. Salven P, Mäenpää H, Orpana A, Alitalo K, Joensuu H. Serum vascular endothelial growth factor is often elevated in disseminated cancer. Clin Cancer Res 1997;3:647–51.
17. Kumar H, Heer K, Lee PWR, Duthie GS, MacDonald AW, Greenman J, et al. Preoperative serum vascular endothelial growth factor can predict stage in colorectal cancer. Clin Cancer Res 1998;4:1279–85.
18. Takeda A, Shimada H, Imaseki H, Okazumi S, Natsume T, Suzuki T, et al. Clinical significance of serum vascular endothelial growth factor in colorectal cancer patients: correlation with clinicopathological factors and tumor markers. Oncol Rep 2000;7:333–8.
19. Gabrilovich DI, Chen HL, Girgis KR, Cunningham HT, Meny GM, Nadaf S, et al. Production of vascular endothelial growth factor by human tumors inhibits the functional maturation of dendritic cells. Nat Med 1996;2:1096–103.

In Chapter 11, Professors Behr and Béhé discuss their latest results of radioimmunotherapy with novel anti-CEA antibody constructs as well as new work utilizing high linear energy transfer α-emitter therapy in nude mice bearing human colon cancer xenografts. The final part of the chapter describes peptide immunoscintigraphy in specialized neuroendocrine tumors and non-small cell carcinoma of the lung.

It appears that the role of radioimmunoscintigraphy particularly in the diagnosis of recurrent colorectal cancer following conventional external beam radiotherapy, (where traditional imaging with CT and MRI may be difficult to interpret), is diminishing. This is partly because of the sensitivity of newer modalities such as positron emission tomography in specialized centers. New antibodies such as Arcitumomab (developed by Immunomedics, Morris Plains, NJ) appear highly sensitive and specific for both colorectal and breast cancer and may permit the acquisition of information valuable in selecting cases for potentially curative second-look surgery, although randomized prospective trials using such imaging in discriminant function analysis are required [1,2]. These findings are correlated with enhanced uptake by this and other anti-CEA antibodies in CEA-transgenic mice bearing CEA-transfected syngeneic colorectal tumors [3] and have been translated to other tumors (most notably carcinoma of the ovary using murine monoclonal antibodies directed against the polymorphic epithelial mucin

MUC-1 or human antibodies against placental alkaline phosphatase). This has been enhanced further with radioimmunoscintigraphy using biotinylated monoclonal antibodies and avidin-streptavidin-biotin injection [4]. It would appear that FDG-PET SPECT imaging (and more recently, immuno-PET combining the specificity of monoclonal antibodies with the high sensitivity and resolution of PET scanning), is superior in the diagnosis of coincident distant metastases (liver, bone and lung) as well as in regional lymph node involvement when compared with CEA immunoscintigraphy in those patients with rising serum CEA levels [5].

This area has been significantly improved of late by the use of antibody phage display libraries which recognize tumor-specific epitopes. These antibody libraries are now derived from hybridoma cells, lymphocytes from immunized humans and mice and from fully human antibody repertoires which are produced in IgG-transgenic mice. Differential affinities can be pre-clinically tested using random or site-specific mutations of binding peptide domains from various scFv fragments. These may be covalently or non-covalently linked as dimers (so-called "diabodies") which show improved targeting and clearance properties as well as increased tumor avidity. Other mini-bodies (scFv-CH3 fusion proteins) have also been developed for this use.

In RIT, large single administration regimens using a short-range emitting radionuclide would be the most appropriate form of therapy for microscopic residual disease, provided that uptake of the radiopharmaceutical is relatively homogeneous. In order to improve the target/non-target uptake ratio, the therapeutic efficacy of RIT could be enhanced by the development of new targeting molecules (through genetically-engineered monoclonal antibodies, antibody fragments, single-chain antibodies, fusion toxins and peptides), improvements in radiolabeling chemistry, radionuclide fractionation for slowly growing macroscopic disease, locoregional RIT, pre-targeting and combination of RIT with biologic response modifiers or gene transfer techniques designed to increase target epitope and receptor expression [6].

The factors which inhibit radioimmunolocalization to some extent also affect the potency of radiopharmaceuticals used in therapy. Such radiolabeled antibodies emit continuous exponentially-decreasing low-dose radiation designed to induce local DNA strand breaks. The physical barriers to the effective delivery of RIT are the same as those of the attendant monoclonal antibody, including the heterogeneous tumor neovasculature, slow diffusion and convection rates towards the center of large tumor deposits which may be relatively poorly vascularized and high intra-tumoral pressures within the deposit which impede antibody influx into the neoplasm [7]. The main problems of such agents; namely the induction of host anti-Ig responses and the relatively slow plasma clearance of unbound antibody (leading particularly to bone marrow toxicity) has been recently partially solved by the use of a recombinant Ig with a CDR-grafted humanized antibody and a CH2 domain deletion. Such an antibody combines more rapid blood clearance (as compared with an intact humanized Ig), equivalent antigen-binding affinity and a reduced potential for eliciting HAMA responsiveness [8].

What is clear is that RIT in hematological malignancies has an established role using genetically-engineered chimeric and humanized antibodies against lymphoma and leukemia in both myeloablative and non-myeloablative regimens with minimal attendant radiation toxicity to normal tissues. Many new proteins are being developed to act as leukemia- and lymphoma-specific agents, inducing MHC-restricted T cell cytotoxicity; including idiotype-specific proteins, break point cluster region (bcr)-abl fusion oncoproteins, myeloid-specific differentiation antigens and antibodies directed against minor histocompatibility antigens over-expressed in myeloid malignancies [9].

As discussed in this chapter, RIT is a novel new method in the treatment of certain thyroid malignancies. Although thyroid cancer, in general, has a good prognosis, up to 30 percent of tumors can de-differentiate into relatively anaplastic variants. These tumors can lose their thyroid-specific functions rendering them effectively resistant to both radioiodide therapy and thyroxine mediated thyrotropin suppression [10]. Along with RIT, several other strategies have been employed recently in these de-differentiated tumors including, p53 gene reintroduction, suicide gene therapy using gancyclovir and HSV thymidine kinase transduction, gene therapy with an adenovirus-delivered IL-2 gene, DNA vaccination in MTC against the tumor marker calcitonin, *c-myc* blockade with anti-sense oligonucleotide therapy and transduction of the thyroid sodium/iodide transporter gene to re-render tumor tissue capable of accumulating iodide for re-introduction of radio-iodine therapy [11].

A further use for radiopharmaceuticals in surgical practice is in the area of radio-immunoguided surgery, colloquially referred to as RIGS. This has found particular value in both primary colorectal cancer and in CEA-driven second-look surgery and has also been reported in pancreatic, breast, ovarian, thyroid and prostate cancer. Radioactivity is detected intra-operatively with a gamma-detecting probe (Neo-probe 1000) with several studies suggesting that RIGS data may change the operative extent of resection in recurrent disease in up to one-third of cases [12-14]. Agents used include In- or Tc-labelled antibodies, antibody fragments and scFv's, biotinylated monoclonal antibody for pre-targeting and more recently, supplemented interferon administration designed to up-regulate tumor antigen expression by residual disease deposits. Additional RIGS-positive tissues may in some series be detected in up to 50 percent of patients, with RIGS-positive lymph node disease being microscopic in over two-thirds of nodes examined. In most such studies, patients who have RIGS-positive tissue remaining at the end of the procedure appear to have a worse cancer-specific outcome than those patients deemed to be RIGS-negative [15]. Moreover, the RIGS system may be used to define clinical target volume in specialized centers for intra-operative radiotherapy [16].

Similar approaches using such radiopharmaceuticals intra-operatively have been employed for sentinel node mapping in malignant melanoma, breast, vulvar and penile cancer as well as in the intra-operative detection of parathyroid adenomas and certain bone tumors such as osteoid osteomas [17]. The recent use of sentinel lymph node detection in colorectal cancer is designed to provide the pathologist with tissue samples which may be targeted for more comprehensive immuno-histological examination [18].

The authors discuss the advantages of equitoxic doses of Auger electron therapy over β-emitting radiometals in colon cancer in particular. The lower toxicity of the former new agents is probably a result of their short path length and relatively low energy, which necessitates that the antibody be internalized in order to reach the nuclear DNA. Such an effect is not detectable in the stem cells of red marrow, perhaps making this a safer form of radiopharmaceutical for therapeutic use [19].

References

1. Lechner P, Lind P, Goldberg DM. Can postoperative surveillance with serial CEA immunoscinti-graphy detect respectable cancer recurrence and potentially improve tumor-free survival? J Am Coll Surg 2000;191:511–8.
2. Lunniss PJ, Skinner S, Britton KE, Granowska M, Morris G, Northover JM. Effect of radioimmunoscintigraphy on the management of recurrent colorectal cancer. Br J Surg 1999;86:244–9.
3. Szalai G, Williams LE, Primus FJ. Tumor targeting with radiolabeled antibodies in a human carci-noembryonic antigen transgenic mouse model. Int J Cancer 2000;85:751–6.
4. Magnani P, Fazio F, Grana C, Songini C, Frigerio L, Pecorelli S, et al. Diagnosis of persistent ovarian carcinoma with three-step immunoscintigraphy. Br J Cancer 2000;82:616–20.
5. Wilkomm P, Bender H, Bangard M, Decker P, Grunwald F, Biersack HJ. FDG PET and immu-noscintigraphy with 99mTc-labeled antibody fragments for detection of the recurrence of color-ectal carcinoma. J Nucl Med 2000;41:1657–63.
6. Buchsbaum DJ. Experimental radioimmunotherapy. Semin Radiat Oncol 2000;10:156–67.
7. Jain RK. Vascular and interstitial barriers to delivery of therapeutic agents in tumors. Cancer Met Rev 1990;9:253–66.
8. Slavin-Chioriniu DC, Kashmiri SV, Lee HS, Milenic DE, Poole DJ, Bernon E, et al. A CDR-grafterd (humanized) domain-deleted antitumor antibody. Cancer Biother Radiopharm 1997;12:305–16.
9. Jurcic JG, Cathcart K, Pinilla-Ibarz J, Scheinberg DA. Advances in immunotherapy of hematologic malignancies:cellular and humoral approaches. Curr Opin Hematol 2000;7:247–54.
10. Zbar AP, O'Higgins NJ. The use and abuse of TSH suppression therapy for benign and malignant thyroid neoplasms. In Surgery of the Thyroid and Parathyroid. OH Clark, Q-Y Duh, A Siperstein eds. WB Saunders San Francisco 1997;54–68.
11. Schmutzler C, Koehrle J. Innovative strategies for the treatment of thyroid cancer. Eur J Endocri-nol 2000;143:15–24.
12. Roselli M, Buonomo O, Piazza A, Guadagni F, Vecchione A, Brunetti E, Cipriani C, Amadei G, Nieroda C, Greiner JW, Casciani CU. Novel clinical approaches in monoclonal antibody-based management in colorectal cancer patients: radioimmunoguided surgery and antigen augmentation. Semin Surg Oncol 1998;15:254–62.
13. Martinez DA, Barbera-Guillem E, LaValle GJ, Martin EW Jr. Radioimmunoguided surgery for gas-trointestinal malignancies: an analysis of 14 years of clinical experience. Cancer Control 1997;4:505–16.
14. Avital S, Haddad R, Troitsa A, Kashtan H, Brazovsky E, Gitstein G, et al. Radioimmunoguided surgery for recurrent colorectal cancer manifested by isolated CEA elevation. Cancer 2000;89:169–28.
15. Martin EW Jr, Thurston MO. Intraoperative radioimmunodetection. Semin Surg Oncol 1998;15:205–8.
16. Nag S, Martinez-Monge R, Nieroda C, Martin E Jr. Radioimmunoguided-intraoperative radiation therapy in colorectal carcinoma: a new technique to precisely define the clinical target volume. Int J Radiat Oncol Biol Phys 1999;44:133–7.
17. Schneebaum S, Even-Sapir E, Cohen M, Shacham-Lehrman H, Gat A, Brazovsky E, et al. Clinical applications of gamma-detection probes — radioguided surgery. Eur J Nucl Med 1999;26 (4 Suppl):S26–35.
18. Merrie AEH, van Rij AM, Phillips LV, Rossaak JI, Yun K, McCall JL. Diagnostic use of the sentinel node in colon cancer. Diseases Colon Rectum 2001;44:410–7.
19. Behr TM, Behe M, Lohr M, Sgouros G, Angerstein C, Wehrmann E, Nebendahl K, et al. Thera-peutic advantages of Auger electron- over beta-emitting radiometals or radioiodine when con-jugated to internalizing antibodies. Eur J Nucl Med 2000;27:753–65.

In Chapter 12, Whiteside explains in detail the subcellular mechanisms of impaired T cell receptor signaling which occur in many solid tumors and which appear to be stage related. There is substantial evidence supporting the view that patients with advanced solid malignancies have by diminished TcR-ζ chain and protein kinase expression which correlates with clinical course [1]. Recent research has centred more on tumor-infiltrating lymphocyte (TIL) function showing a general impairment of ex vivo lymphocyte stimulation in a range of solid cancers including colorectal cancer [2]. Moreover, although tumor-draining lymph node lymphocytes nearby progressively growing tumors are sensitized to tumor-associated antigens, they are incapable in most animal experiments of mediating tumor regression when adoptively transferred into secondary syngeneic tumor-bearing hosts.

A variety of signal transduction defects in the T cell receptor pathway have been described in TIL's with a reduction of ζ and ε chain and NF-κB expression; the latter functioning as a down-line nuclear transcription factor regulating a large number of genes involved in the immune response to foreign antigen. This cell-mediated impairment may be associated with the presence of tumor-directed apoptosis shown by the different T cell populations involved in tumor recognition, an effect which is in part mediated by the Fas/FasL apoptotic pathway. These mechanisms are normally involved in immunoelimination and T cell maturation [3].

Whiteside and others have written extensively about alterations in the expression and function of signal-transducing proteins in tumor-associated and draining lymph node T cells and NK cells in a range of tumors including ovarian cancer, head and neck tumors, melanoma, renal cell carcinoma and intracranial tumors. These effects are represented as variations in CD3-ε expression on T cells and FcγRIIIa expression on NK cells in both peripheral blood and tumor-associated lymphocytes, with defects in T cell receptor assembly as manifest by depressed tyrosine kinase p56 (lck) activity; both of which have been shown to correlate in some cases with impaired cancer-specific survival [4]. These changes are associated with excessive caspase-dependent apoptosis of T cells as shown by co-localization studies in in vivo apoptosis assays and by in vitro co-culture of T cells with tumor-specific cancer cell lines [5,6]. Preliminary evidence has shown that this mechanism may be supported by Fas ligand (FasL) expression by the tumor and that abnormal zeta-chain T cell receptor expression may be partially restored by ex vivo treatment with IL-2 [7–10]. This represents a further mechanism whereby tumors escape immunoelimination through the disabling of infiltrating lymphocytes expressing Fas. Here tumor cells have been shown in situ and in vitro (from cultured cell lines) to express FasL mRNA which induce apoptosis in Fas-sensitive Jurkat T cells and in mitogen-stimulated peripheral blood T cells undergoing activation-induced cell death [11]. A better delineation of these mechanisms will provide a molecular basis for new strategies which target caspase-independent pathways in apopotosis-resistant cancers [12].

Recently, chimeric immune receptors consisting of extracellular antigen-binding domains of individual tumor-associated antigens have been linked by retroviral transduction to the CD3-zeta signalling domains of the T cell receptor and these have been shown to bind to tumor antigens and to be specifically cytotoxic to tumor cell lines bearing the antigen. These receptors kill by Fas-mediated mechanisms and are protective in intra-peritoneal and subcutaneous tumor xenograft models [13]. Such a system will effectively bypass the normal mechanism of T cell receptor activation through MHC restriction [14]. Improved understanding of this important T cell dysregulation has paved the way for new Ig-TcR-based anti-tumor therapies in cancers where the primary tumor-associated antigen is weakly immunogenic.

References

1. Reichert TE, Rabinowich H, Johnson JT et al. Immune cells in the tumor microenvironment: mechanisms responsible for signaling and functional defects. J Immunother 1998,21:295-308.
2. Choi SH, Chung EJ, Whang DY et al. Alteration of signal-transducing molecules in tumor-infiltrating lymphocytes and peripheral blood T lymphocytes from human colorectal carcinoma patients. Cancer Immunol Immunopathol 1998,45:299-305.
3. Uzzo RG, Rayman P, Kolenko V et al. Mechanisms of apoptosis in T cells from patients with renal cell carcinoma. Clin Cancer Res 1999,5:1219-29.
4. Reichert TE, Day R, Wagner EM, Whiteside TL. Absent or low expression of the zeta chain in T cells at the tumor site correlates with poor survival in patients with oral carcinoma. Cancer Res 1998;58:5344-7.
5. Reichert TE, Rabinowich H, Johnson JT, Whiteside TL. Mechanisms responsible for signalling and functional defects. J Immunother 1998;21:295-306.
6. Menne C, Lauritsen JP, Dietrich J, Kastrup J, Wegener AK, Andersen PS, et al. T-cell receptor downregulation by ceramide-induced caspase activation and cleavage of the zeta chain. Scand J Immunol 2001;53:176-83.
7. Scaffidi C, Fulda S, Srinivasan A et al. Two CD95 (APO-1/Fas) signaling pathways. EMBO J 1998, 17:1675-87.
8. Whiteside TL. Immune cells in the tumor microenvironment. Mechanisms responsible for functional and signalling defects. Adv Exp Med Biol 1998;451:167-71.
9. Bukowski RM, Rayman P, Uzzo R, Bloom T, Sabdstrom K, Peereboom D, et al. Signal transduction abnormalities in T lymphocytes from patients with advanced renal carcinoma: clinical relevance and effects of cytokine therapy. Clin Cancer Res 1998;4:2337-47.
10. Gratama JW, Zea AH, Bolhuis RL, Ochoa AC. Restoration of expression of signal-transduction molecules in lymphocytes from patients with metastatic renal cell cancer after combination immunotherapy. Cancer Immunol Immunother 1999;48:263-9.
11. Uzzo RG, Rayman P, Kolenko V, Clark PE, Bloom T, Ward AM, et al. Mechanisms of apoptosis in T cells from patients with renal cell carcinoma. Clin Cancer Res 1999;5:1219-29.
12. Kolenko VM, Uzzo RG, Buzowski R, Finke JH. Caspase-dependent and — independent death pathways in cancer therapy. Apoptosis 2000;5:17-20.
13. McGuiness RP, Ge Y, Patel SD, Kashmiri SV, Lee HS, Hand PH, et al. Anti-tumor activity of human T cells expressing the CC49-zeta chimeric immune receptor. Hum Gene Ther 1999;20:165-73.
14. Abken H, Hombach A, Heuser C, Reinhold U. A novel strategy in the elimination of disseminated melanoma cells: chimeric receptors endow T cells with tumor specificity. Rec Results Cancer Res 2001;158:249-64.

Chapters 13 through 18 are devoted to the immunology and immunotherapy of some important solid tumors; including colorectal, renal cell, bladder, ovarian and breast cancer and malignant melanoma. These tumors were deliberately chosen for discussion as they are cancers with defined tumor-associated antigens against which specific immunotherapies have been designed and for which there is some preliminary clinical phase II and even phase III data available. I have highlighted the areas successively discussed in this section and mention novel immunotherapeutic approaches either currently in use or awaited in clinical practice.

In Chapter 13, Durrant and her colleagues outline new advances in the immunotherapy of colorectal cancer, both in advanced cases and as an adjuvant. Their interest has principally been in the area of monoclonal antibody immunotherapy using a human anti-idiotypic antibody 105AD7 derived from a hyperimmune subject who received radioimmunoscintigraphy [1]. Although a recent prospective Phase II trial using the antibody failed to show significant survival advantage in the adjuvant setting, they have characterized the antibody and shown that it alters cell-mediated immunocyte function affecting tumor infiltrates and CTL activity against autologous and allogeneic colorectal cancer cell lines. This work has been supplemented by that of Foon and his coworkers using a murine syngeneic anti-idiotypic antibody (3H1) which also produces a derived idiotypic network in patients with advanced colorectal cancer, despite the fact that there appears to be no effect on survival [2,3]. This latest data is commensurate with our recent work using a novel murine monoclonal (Ab1) antibody directed against the cell-based epitope of CEA, where survival was unaffected although anti-idiotypic activity was produced along with improvements in ex vivo peripheral T cell function. This was associated with a conversion of PBMC Th2 to Th1 cytokine profile during immunotherapy and the induction of IL-2 receptor expression by peripheral CD4+ lymphocytes when exposed in vitro to the immunizing antibody [4].

We must await the trials of newer active immunotherapeutic regimens using vaccination with native or cytokine gene-transduced tumor cells, tumor cell lysates, novel tumor-related peptides and carbohydrates and gene constructs encoding for these epitopes [5-7]. The ability to produce functional "auto-antibodies" to naturally occurring developmental antigens such as carcinoembryonic antigen and α-fetoprotein is still uncertain [8]. These have been recently demonstrated against recombinant-vaccinia-CEA and polynucleotide vaccine [9,10] although it is at present uncertain whether multiple-epitope vaccines are superior to genetically engineered recombinant single-epitope vaccines or human or xenogeneic antibodies directed against isolated epitopes of the tumor-associated antigen [11]. It is possible that the paratopes required for the induction of idiotypic networks, cellular immune responses and protective immunity against lethal tumor burden challenge are different.

Recently, new strategies have been aimed at colorectal cancer including active specific immunotherapy using irradiated autologous tumor cell-BCG combinations, where in an adjuvant setting, substantial risk reduction in the recurrence-free period in treated groups has been demonstrated [12,13]. Dendritic cells, (which are the most potent professional antigen presenting cells) would appear to be attractive vehicles to act as novel anti-cancer vaccines. The relative lack of efficient tumor antigen presentation on mature dendritic cells may be able to be bypassed by direct loading of these cells in vitro with oncoproteins. The use of dendritic cells harvested from cytokine-enriched peripheral blood mononuclear cells with ex vivo exposure to tumor antigens as pulsed therapy has been shown to be safe in Phase I/II trials of patients with advanced colorectal cancer, although the best type of dendritic cell, degree of maturity, choice of antigen, route and schedule of administration or the need for additional adjuvants or cytokines are not yet established [14]. The use of extracorporeal photopheresis where the transition of immature monocytes to dendritic cells by their cell surface CD molecule expression can be tracked, may provide a new means of developing loading for tumor cells without the complex need for ex vivo cytokine exposure, excessive cellular manipulation and purification [15,16]. Other types of dendritic cells may be able to be transfected with polynucleotides, tumor antigen DNA or RNA or with DNA encoding immunostimulatory cytokines or co-stimulatory molecules or by tumor cell-dendritic cell fusion [17]. The effects of these potential new therapies in colorectal cancer are awaited.

References

1. Durrant LG, Buckley TJD, Denton GWL, Hardcastle JD, Sewell HF, Robins RA. Enhanced cell-mediated tumor cell killing in patients immunized with human monoclonal anti-idiotypic antibody 105AD7. Cancer Res 1994;54:4837–80.
2. Foon KA, John WJ, Chakraborty M, Sherratt A, Garrison J, Flett M, et al. Clinical and immune responses in advanced colorectal cancer patients treated with anti-idiotype monoclonal antibody vaccine that mimics carcinoembryonic antigen. Clin Cancer Res 1998;3:1267–76.
3. Pervin S, Chakraborty M, Bhattacharya-Chatterjee M, Zeytin H, Foon KA, Chatterjee SK. Induction of anti-tumor immunity by an anti-idiotype antibody mimicking CEA. Am Assoc Cancer Res 1996;37:473–4(A # 3231).
4. Zbar AP, Snary D, Thomas H, Kmiot WA, Allen-Mersh TG. Immunoresponsiveness in metastatic colorectal cancer during anticarcinoembryonic antigen vaccination. Br J Surg 2000; 87:627(A).
5. Zbar AP, Lemoine NR, Wadhwa M, Thomas H, Snary D, Kmiot WA. Biological therapy: approaches in colorectal cancer. Strategies to enhance carcinoembryonic antigen (CEA) as an immunogenic target. Br J Cancer 1998;77:683–93.
6. Foon KA. Immunotherapy for colorectal cancer. Curr Oncol Rep 2001;3:116–26.
7. Syrigos KN, Karayiannakis AJ, Zbar A. Mucins as immunogenic targets in cancer. Anticancer Res 1999;19:5239–44.
8. Conry RM, Allen KO, Lee S, Moore SE, Shaw DR, LoBuglio AF. Human autoantibodies to carcinoembryonic antigen (CEA) induced by a vaccinia-CEA vaccine. Clin Cancer Res 2000;6:34–41.
9. Tsang KY, Zaremba S, Nieroda CA, Zhu MZ, Hamilton JM, Schlom J. Generation of human cytotoxic T cells specific for human carcinoembryonic antigen epitopes from patients immunized with recombinant vaccinia-CEA vaccine. J Natl Cancer Inst 1995;87:982–90.
10. Conry RM, Widera G, LoBuglio AF, Fuller JT, Moore SE, Barlow DL, et al. Selected strategies to augment polynucleotide vaccination. Gene Ther 1996;3:67–74.
11. Maruyama H, Zaloudik J, Li W, Sperlagh M, Koido T, Somasundaram R, et al. Cancer vaccines: single-epitope anti-idiotype vaccine versus multiple-epitope antigen vaccine. Cancer Immunol Immunother 2000;49:123–32.
12. Vermorken JB, Claessen AM, van Tinteren H, Gall HE, Ezinga R, Meijer S, et al. Active specific immunotherapy for stage II and stage III human colon cancer: a randomized trial. Lancet 1999;353(9150):345–50.
13. Hanna MG, Hoover HC, Vermorken JB, Harris JE, Pinedo HM. Adjuvant active specific immunotherapy of stage II and stage III colon cancer with autologous tumor cell vaccine: first randomized phase III trials show promise. Vaccine 2001;19(17-19):2576–82.
14. Chen W, Rains N, Young D, Stubbs RS. Dendritic cell-based cancer immunotherapy: potential for treatment of colorectal cancer? J Gastroenterol Hepatol 2000;15:698–705.
15. Berger CL, Xu AL, Hanlon D, Lee C, Schechner J, Glusac E, et al. Induction of human tumor-loaded dendritic cells. Int J Cancer 2001;91:438–47.
16. Song W, Tong Y, Carpenter H, Kong HL, Crystal RG. Persistent, antigen-specific, therapeutic anti-tumor immunity by dendritic cells genetically modified with an adenoviral vector to express a model tumor antigen. Gene Ther 2000;7:2080–6.
17. Bubenik J. Genetically engineered dendritic cell-based cancer vaccines-review. Int J Oncol 2001;18:475–8.

Nathan and Gore discuss the immunotherapeutic approach towards renal cell carcinoma in Chapter 14. Despite extensive reports with many different immunotherapeutic modalities, metastatic renal cancer appears to be highly resistant to systemic therapies, with only a few patients exhibiting complete responses to interferon or IL-2 therapy and with few long-term survivors [1]. Nevertheless, the recognition of immunological mediators involved in cases of spontaneous regression (even in the face of high tumor burdens) makes this cancer an attractive model for potential biotherapy. Moreover, the demonstration of infiltrating T cell dysregulation in this tumor (as outlined in Chapter 12) and an improved understanding of the molecular genetics of renal cell carcinoma, have suggested a role for such therapy. New cytokine approaches have utilized liposome-encapsulated depot formulations [2], GM-CSF therapy [3,4] and combined erythropoietin and IL-2 [5].

Active specific immunotherapy using irradiated autologous or allogeneic tumor cells combined with an adjuvant (such as Newcastle disease virus) has been unsuccessful at inducing tumor-specific humoral or cellular responses, although immunoactivity is directed against target cells transfected with the adjuvant protein [6].

More recently, antigen-pulsed dendritic cells have been employed using cell lysates from short-term autologous tumor cultures in the presence of keyhole limpet haemocyanin (KLH), with an improvement in in vitro responsiveness both to the adjuvant and to the tumor antigen [7]. This kind of approach needs to be tested, however, in the clinical setting of metastatic disease, since it appears that the adjuvant acts as a tracer molecule for the DC, determining the magnitude and dominance of the Th cytokine pattern of the response. This approach has been supplemented by transfection of isolated DCs with tumor mRNA, producing superior responses against autologous targets [8].

Recent improvements in renal cell cancer vaccines have been developed in animal models, transfecting tumor cells with cytokine genes such as IL-12 [9] or by creating hybrid cell vaccines where tumor cells are fused with class I and II matched or unmatched activated allogeneic lymphocytes [10]. Intra-tumoral therapy with IL-2 cDNA lipid complexes represents an attractive alternative which does not require the complex production of autologous or allogeneic vaccines and which does not have the attendant toxicity of systemic cytokine administration [11]. Further new forms of therapy include the use of non-myeloablative allogeneic peripheral blood stem-cell transplantation in order to induce graft-vs-tumor effects in patients with advanced renal cell carcinoma where there is already limited response to conventional immunotherapies [12]. Future aspects of such treatment will need to address low toxicity-conditioning regimens combined with specific tumor-associated antigen targeting where the degree of immunosuppression will vary with the closeness of transplant matching [13].

References

1. Coppin C, Porszolt F, Kumpf J, Coldman A, Wilt T. Immunotherapy for advanced renal cell cancer (Cochrane review). Cochrane Database Syst Rev 2000;3:CD001425.
2. Krup OC, Kroll I, Bose G, Falkenberg FW. Cytokine depot formulations as adjuvants for tumor vaccines. I. Liposome-encapsulated IL-2 as a depot formulation. J Immunother 1999;22:525–38.
3. Ryan CW, Vogelzang NJ, Dumas MC, Kuzel T, Stadler WM. Granulocyte-macrophage-colony stimulating factor in combnination immunotherapy for patients with metastatic renal cell carcinoma: results of two phase II clinical trials. Cancer 2000;88:1317–24.
4. Westermann J, Reich G, Kopp J, Haus U, Dorken B, Pezzutto A. Granulocyte/macrophage-colony-stimulating-factor plus interleukin-2 plus interferon alpha in the treatment of metastatic renal cell carcinoma: a pilot study. Cancer Immunol Immunother 2001;49:613–20.
5. Lissoni P, Rovelli F, Baiocco N, Tangini G, Fumagalli L. A phase II study of subcutaneous low-dose interleukin-2 plus erythropoietin in metastatic renal cell carcinoma progressing on interleukin-2 alone. Anticancer Res 2001;21(1B):777–9.
6. Zorn U, Duensing S, Langkopf F, Anastassiou G, Kirchner H, Hadam M, et al. Active specific immunotherapy of renal cell carcinoma: cellular and humoral immune responses. Cancer Biother Radiopharm 1997;12:157–65.
7. Holtl L, Reiser C, Papesh C, Ramoner R, Herold M, Klocker H, Radmayr C, Stenzl A, Bartsch G, Thurnher M. Cellular and humoral immune responses in patients with metastatic renal cell carcinoma after vaccination with antigen pulsed dendritic cells. J Urol 1999;161:777–82.

8. Heiser A, Maurice MA, Yancey DR, Coleman DM, Dahm P, Vieweg J. Human dendritic cells transfected with renal tumor RNA stimulate polyclonal T-cell responses against antigens expressed by primary and metastatic tumors. Cancer Res 2001;61:3388–93.

9. Hara I, Nagai H, Miyake H, Yamanaka K, Hara S, Micallef MJ, et al. Effectiveness of cancer vaccine therapy using cells transduced with the interleukin-12 gene combined with systemic interleukin-18 administration. Cancer Gene Ther 2000;7:83–90.

10. Kugler A, Seseke F, Thelen P, Kallerhoff M, Muller GA, Stuhler G, et al. Autologous and allogeneic hybrid cell vaccine in patients with metastatic renal cell carcinoma. Br J Urol 1998;82:487–93.

11. Daniels GA, Galanais E. Immunotherapy of renal cell carcinoma by intratumoral administration of an IL-2 cDNA/DMRIE/DOPE lipid complex. Curr Opin Mol Ther 2001;3:70–6.

12. Childs RW, Clave E, Tisdale J, Plante M, Hensel N, Barrett J. Successful treatment of metastatic renal cell carcinoma with a nonmyeloablative allogeneic peripheral-blood progenitor-cell transplant: evidence for a graft-versus-tumor effect. J Clin Oncol 1999;17:2044–9.

13. Barrett AJ. Conditioning regimens for allogeneic stem cell transplants. Curr Opin Hematol 2000;7:339–42.

In Chapter 15, Syrigos and Karayiannakis outline the use of intra-vesical therapies acting as non-specific immunostimulants, for particular use in superificial bladder cancer (Ta,T1 and some T2 disease), designed to reduce local recurrence or the new growth of papillary lesions. These lesions represent between 70–80% of all newly diagnosed bladder cancers and this tumor is discussed in a general surgical text because it appears to be the most responsive of solid tumors towards immunotherapy [1]. It would appear that these new therapies are affecting the overall prevalence of superificial bladder tumor recurrence, particularly where the initial presentation was with multiple intra-vesical tumors [2]. Direct comparisons between BCG immunotherapy and other intra-vesical chemotherapeutic agents such as thiotepa, doxorubicin and mitomycin C has shown superiority for BCG in cases at high risk for local recurrence [3]. Since bladder cancer is a multi-step process, it is a cancer potentially susceptible to chemoprevention with modest recent success with retinoid therapy, where the potent apoptosis-inducing retinoid fenretinide is currently undergoing phase III trials. [4,5] Despite the impact that BCG has on local tumor recurrence, there is, as yet, no demonstrated effect on tumor progression or cancer-specific survival.

The local and systemic immunological response towards intra-vesical BCG is contentious. Patients undergoing such therapy produce more urinary washout CD3+ and CD4+ cells with an increase in mucosal T cell expression of the γδ receptor and an increased peripheral cytotoxicity towards allogeneic bladder cancer cell lines which is somewhat dose-dependent [6]. In these patients there is evidence for MHC-restricted urothelial antigen expression as well as non-MHC-restricted cytotoxicity through NK and LAK cell activity, [7,8] with disease recurrence correlating with urinary cytokine (high IL-8 and low IL-18) measurement [9]. New perspectives in BCG therapy include the use of genetically-modified BCG strains which are capable of producing cytokines or the use of purified BCG sub-component therapy [10] such as BCG cell wall, plasma membrane, cytosolic, purified polysaccharides (glucan and arabinomannan), culture filtrate purified native proteins, recombinant 22kDa subfractions and the phosphate transporter proteins, PstS-2 and PstS-3. Moroever, there is recent evidence that polymorphism in the BCG host resistance gene (NRAMP1) can be identified, showing an inherent genetic variation in the response by macrophages to the intracellular growth of mycobacteria and perhaps creating an in vitro test for the likely responsiveness to BCG immunotherapy in patients with bladder cancer [11].

A range of other immunotherapeutic agents have successfully been reported, (as described in this chapter), including interferons, interleukin-2 and keyhole limpet haemocyanin (KLH). The optimal anti-tumor regimen, either of single instillated cytokines or chemoimmunotherapeutic combinations, with the least toxicity as well as the optimal method of assessment of response for specific tumor types is the challenge for the future. Clinical human trials of other agents administered intra-vesically such as levamisole, Rubratin (a *Nocardia rubra* cell wall skeleton protein), OK-432 (a streptococcal peptide) or *Lactobacillus casei* are awaited. The use of the orally active interferon inducer Bropirimine, (which is fully discussed in the chapter), is often reserved for patients with carcinoma-in-situ which has either failed BCG therapy or in those patients who are BCG-intolerant. Its primary role in BCG-naïve patients for in-situ disease has limited data at present [12].

References

1. Duque JL, Loughlin KR. An overview of the treatment of superficial bladder cancer. Intravesical chemotherapy. Urol Clin Nth Am 2000;27:125–35.
2. Kurth KH, Bouffioux C, Sylvester R, van der Meijden AP, Oosterlinck W, Brausi M. Treatment of superificial bladder tumors: achievements and needs. The EORTC Genitourinary Group. Eur Urol 2000;37 Suppl 3:1–9.
3. Malmstrom P. Improved patient outcomes with BCG immunotherapy vs. chemotherapy — Swedish and worldwide experience. Eur Urol 2000;37 Suppl 1:16–20.
4. Sabichi AL, Lerner SP, Grossman HB, Lippman SM. Retinoids in the chemoprevention of bladder cancer. Curr Opin Oncol 1998;10:479–84.
5. Clifford JL, Sabichi AL, Zou C, Yang X, Steele VE, Kelloff GJ, et al. Effects of novel phenylretina-mides on cell growth and apoptosis in bladder cancer. Cancer Epidemiol Biomarkers Prev 2001;10:391–5.
6. Gan YH, Mahendran R, James K, Lawrencia C, Esuvaranathan K. Evaluation of lymphocytic responses after treatment with Bacillus Calmette-Guerin and interferon-alpha 2b for superficial bladder cancer. Clin Immunol 1999;90:230–7.
7. Patard JJ, Saint F, Velotti F, Abbou CC, Chopin DK. Immune response following intravesical bacil-lus Calmette-Guerin instillations in superficial bladder cancer: a review. Urol Res 1998;26:155–9.
8. Brandau S, Riemensberger J, Jacobsen M, Kemp D, Zhao W, Zhao X, et al. NK cells are essential for effective BCG immunotherapy. Int J Cancer 2001;92(5):697–702.
9. Thalmann GN, Sermier A, Rentsch C, Mohrle K, Cecchini MG, Studer UE. Urinary Interleukin-8 and 18 predict the response of superficial bladder cancer to intravesical therapy with bacillus Calmette-Guerin. J Urol 2000;164:2129–33.
10. Zlotta AR, van Vooren JP, Denis O, Drowart A, Daffe M, Lefevre P, et al. What are the immunolo-gically active components of bacille Calmette-Guerin in therapy of superficial bladder cancer? Int J Cancer 2000;87:844–52.
11. Buu N, Sanchez F, Schurr E. The BCG host-resistance gene. Clin Infect Dis 2000;31 Suppl 3:S81–5.
12. Witjes WP, Konig M, Boeminghaus FP, Hall RR, Schulman CC, Zurlo M, et al. Results of a Eur-opean comparative randomized study comparing oral bropirimine versus intravesical BCG treat-ment in BCG-naïve patients with carcinoma in situ of the urinary bladder. European Bropirimine Study Group. Eur Urol 1999;36:576–81.

In Chapter 16 Nicolson examines the role of immunotherapy in ovarian cancer. This cancer is an ideal candidate for an immunotherapeutic approach, particu-larly with the use of intraperiotneal (IP) naked monoclonal antibodies directed against the well established tumor-associated antigens MUC-1, CA-125 and HER2/neu (cerb-B2) or with radiolabeled IP therapy [1]. These monoclonal antibodies (either alone or linked to toxins, biospheres or chemotherapeutic agents) frequently induce human anti-mouse antibodies (HAMA) which affect routine radioimmunometric assays of tumor markers such as CA-125, requiring specialist epitope analysis of serum for the follow-up of patients treated with murine products [2].Treatment relies on the natural history of recurrent or residual ovarian cancer which disseminates in the peritoneal cavity without visceral metastases and which may present to the general surgeon with small bowel obstruction or ascites of unknown origin. Here, locoregional delivery of therapeutic agents is desirable with less bone marrow toxicity and with laparosocopic assessment of recurrent disease being an essential adjunct to therapy. Newer IP agents have been utilized recently, including cisplatin, liposomal muramyltripeptide phosphatidylyethanolamine, recombinant cytokines (IL-2 and IFN-γ) and granulocyte-monocyte colony-stimulating factor; GM-CSF [3,4].

Latterly, pulsed adoptive dendritic cell (DC) or native tumor-infiltrating lymphocyte (TIL) immunotherapies have been used in collaboration with cytoreductive surgery in minimally residual disease (assessed laparoscopically) as well as in advanced cases. These strategies have employed autologous and allogeneic dendritic cells exposed in vitro to ovarian tumor antigens and lysates [5], resulting in the induction of MHC-restricted CTL activity directed against autologous ovarian cancers. These newer modalities may be supplemented by cell fusions between human ovarian carcinomas and DCs, producing heterokaryons which express the tumor-associated antigen CA-125 or by DC-derived co-stimulatory and adhesion molecule expression. These cells have been shown in recent animal models to lyse autologous ovarian tumor cells by an MHC class I-restricted mechanism [6]. The population expansion of autologous T lymphocytes which are genetically modified by transduction with chimeric antigen receptors derived from murine monoclonal antibodies directed against folate binding protein, (a protein overexpressed on ovarian cancers), is a new technique which is aimed at redirection of diverse non-specific T lymphocytes in peripheral blood to react specifically against ovarian cancer cells [7].

Although radioimmunotherapy has been shown in ovarian cancer to improve cancer-specific survival in patients treated with cytoreduction and platinum-based chemotherapy, there is a need for more controlled prospective randomized studies in subgroups of patients with minimal residual intraperitoneal disease (8,9).

References

1. Fleckenstein G, Osmers R, Puchta J. Monoclonal antibodies in solid tumors: approaches to therapy with emphasis on gynaecological cancer. Med Oncol 1998;15:212–21.
2. Baum RP, Niesen A, Hertel A, Nancy A, Hess H, Donnerstag B, et al. Activating anti-idiotypic human anti-mouse antibodies for immunotherapy of ovarian carcinoma. Cancer 1994;73(3 Suppl): 1121–5.
3. Klimp AH, DeVries EG, Scherphof GL, Daemen T. Chemo-immunotherapy of ovarian cancer in a murine tumor model. Anticancer Res 2000;20:2585–92.
4. Freedman RS, Kudelkla AP, Kavanagh JJ, Verschraegen C, Edwards CL, Nash M, et al Clinical and biological effects of intraperitoneal injections of recombinant interferon-gamma and recombinant interleukin 2 with or without tumor-infiltrating lymphocytes in patients with ovarian or peritoneal carcinoma. Clin Cancer Res 2000;6:2268–78.
5. Santin AD, Hermonat PL, Ravaggi A, Bellone S, Pecorelli S, Cannon MJ, et al. In vitro induction of tumor-specific human lymphocyte antigen class I-restricted CD8 aytotoxic lymphocytes by ovarian tumor antigen-pulsed autologous dendritic cells from patients with advanced ovarian cancer. Am J Obstet Gynecol 2000; 183:601–9.

6. Gong J, Nikrui N, Chen D, Koido S, Wu Z, Tanaka Y, et al. Fusions of human ovarian carcinoma cells with autologous or allogeneic dendritic cells induce antitumor immunity. J Immunol 2000;165:1705–11.
7. Parker LL, Do MT, Westwood JA, Wunderlich JR, Dudley ME, Rosenberg SA, et al. Expansion and characterization of T cells transduced with a chimeric receptor against ovarian cancer. Hum Gene Ther 2000;11:2377–8.
8. Epenetos AA, Hird V, Lambert H, Mason P, Coulter C. Long term survival of patients with advanced ovarian cancer treated with intraperitoneal radioimmunotherapy. Int J Gynecol Cancer 2000;10(S1):44–6.
9. Syrigos KN, Epenetos AA. Radioimmunotherapy of ovarian cancer. Hybridoma 1995;14:121–4.

In Chapter 17, Mustafa and Bland assess the immunological markers believed to be important in the assessment of patients with breast cancer. Although tumor-associated antigens, (most notably CEA, the polymorphic epithelial mucin MUC-1 and the growth factor receptors EGF-r and HER-2/neu), have been well characterized in breast carcinoma, prospective data of clinical trials using monoclonal murine and more recently, recombinant humanized antibodies directed against these antigens are still awaited. In some cases, these antibodies and their second generation products (such as the Fab' fragment Arcitumomab used in colorectal cancer detection) have been employed in the radioimmunoscintigraphic diagnosis of primary and recurrent breast cancer cases. These newer antibody fragments hold promise in the development of techniques such as immunoPET which could combine the specificity of immunoscinitgraphy with the sensitivity and resolution of PET scanning.

In 1998, Trastuzumab (Herceptin; Genetch, San Franscisco) became the second monoclonal antibody approved for the treatment of a malignant solid tumor. This antibody is a chimeric murine/human monoclonal which blocks the HER-2/neu receptor and which produces anti-idiotypic antibody networks in immunized patients [1]. The product of the HER-2/neu proto-oncogene, HER2, is a member of the human epidermal growth factor receptor family of tyrosine kinase receptors. Amplification of the HER2 gene and over-expression of the HER2 protein has been demonstrated in approximately 40 percent of breast carcinomas and appears to correlate with hormonal and chemo-responsiveness. Herceptin has been shown in early trials to prolong survival in metastatic breast cancer patients whose tumors overexpress the HER-2/neu protein, where when compared with patients receiving chemotherapy alone,there appears to be a longer time to progression and a longer response duration [2]. Recently, peptide-based vaccines based on the HER-2/neu protein have been shown to induce delayed-type hypersensitivity and peripheral T cell responses in immunized cases [3]. This work has been supplemented with new technology developing active and passive specific anti-HER-2/neu immunity using HER-2/neu transgenic (rNEU-TG) mice which develop spontaneous breast tumors after pregnancy [4]. These models have, however, shown that both a specific T-cell mediated and neu-specific IgG humoral response are required for the eradication of subcutaneous neu-expressing tumor explants and that limited responses by either arm of the immune response are insufficient for tumor elimination [5]. Recently, the humanized form of trastuzumab has been approved for clinical use in metastatic breast cancer [6].

MHC-restricted cytotoxic lymphocytes directed against MUC-1-expressing breast tumors has also been demonstrated when patients are immunized with whole murine or humanized anti-MUC-1 antibody (HMFG-1) combined with adjuvants such as mannan [7]. Polymorphic epithelial mucin (PEM), encoded by the MUC-1 gene is present at the apical surface of glandular breast epithelium and is over-expressed or aberrantly glycosylated in >90 percent of breast tumors, producing a novel immunotherapeutic target. This trans-membrane protein is released into the circulation as the cleaved marker of disease stage and progression, CA 15.3 frequently used in diagnosis and follow-up. This is of considerable importance, since the presence of pre-existing anti-MUC-1 IgG and IgM antibodies in early breast cancer prior to treatment, is associated with an improved cancer-specific survival [8]. Such an approach is being developed with antibody phage display libraries which provide unique single-chain Fv fragments directed against the MUC-1 mucin molecule (from hyperimmunized BALB/c mice), creating an antibody repertoire for single or multiple epitope recognition in future clinical use [9]. These antibody therapies are being developed in collaboration with new cytotoxic drugs, (such as the taxanes, vinorelbine, capecitabine, folate and topoisomerase-1 antagonists, multi-drug resistance inhibitors and liposomal anthracyclines) and molecular approaches which genetically inhibit intracellular signal transduction (tyrosine kinase inhibition therapy, heat-shock protein signal inhibition, dominant negative mutant inhibition of cerb-B2 and angiogenesis/telomerase inhibition).

The increasing trend towards high-dose chemotherapy with stem cell rescue in patients with locally advanced disease or high nodal burden, requires an understanding of the immunological reaction to breast cancer and the dynamics of immunocyte reconstitution, where there appears to be prolonged T cell dysfunction manifest as abnormal mitogenic T cell proliferation in vitro. This has important implications for the timing and type of immunotherapy when used in combination with high-dose chemotherapy, progenitor cell support or GM-CSF [10].

In the last few years, the concept of targeted resection of a limited set of axillary lymph nodes (so-called sentinel node biopsy) has been advanced over routine complete axillary dissection in selected cases, based on lymphoscintigraphic marking [11,12]. This approach appears to be at least 90 percent accurate in the identification and isolation of involved axillary nodes and may be assisted by immunolymphoscintigraphic marking [13], thus avoiding the morbidity associated with standardized axillary dissection [14].

References

1. Dillman RO. Perceptions of Herceptin: a monoclonal antibody for the treatment of breast cancer. Cancer Biother Radiopharm 1999;1:5–10.
2. Stebbing J, Copson E, O'Reilly S. Herceptin (tastuzamab) in advanced breast cancer. Cancer Treat Rev 2000;26:287–90.
3. Disi ML, Schiffman K, Gooley TA, McNeel DG, Rinn K, Knutson KL. Delayed-type hypersensitivity response is a predictor of peripheral blood T-cell immunity after HER-2/neu peptide immunization. Clin Cancer Res 2000;6:1347–50.
4. Cefai D, Morrison BW, Sckell A, Favre L, Balli M, Leunig M, Gimmi CD. Targeting HER-2/neu for active-specific immunotherapy in a mouse model of spontaneous breast cancer. Int J Cancer 1999;83:393–400.
5. Reilly RT, Machiels JP, Emens LA, Ercolini AM, Okoye FI, Lei RY, et al. The collaboration of both humoral and cellular HER-2/neu-targeted immune responses is required for the complete eradication of HER-2/neu-expressing tumors. Cancer Res 2001;61:880–3.
6. Kurebayashi JJ. Biological and clinical significance of her2 overexpression in breast cancer. Breast Cancer 2001;8:45–51.
7. Pietersz GA, Li W, Osinski C, Apostolopoulos V, McKenzie IF. Definition of MHC-restricted CTL

epitopes from non-variable number of tandem repeat sequence of MUC-1. Vaccine 2000;18:2059–71.

8. von Mensdorff-Pouilly S, Verstraeten AA, Kenemans P, Snijdewint FG, Kok A, Van Kamp GJ, et al. Survival in early breast cancer patients is favourably influenced by a natural humoral immune response tp polymorphic epithelial mucin. J Clin Oncol 2000;18:574–83.

9. Winthrop MD, DeNardo SJ, DeNardo GL. Development of a hyperimmune anti-MUC-1 single chain antibody fragments phage display library for targeting breast cancer. Clin Cancer Res 1999;5(10 Suppl):3088s–3094s.

10. Avigan D, Wu Z, Joyce R, Elias A, Richardson P, McDermott D, et al. Immune reconstitution following high-dose chemotherapy with stem cell rescue in patients with advanced breast cancer. Bone Marrow Transpl 2000;26:169–76.

11. Veronesi U, Galimberti V, Zurrida S, Pigatto F, Veronesi P, Robertson C, Paganelli G, Sciascia V, Viale G. Sentinel lymph node biopsy as an indicator for axillary dissection in early breast cancer. Eur J Cancer 2001;37:454–8.

12. Lucci A Jr, Kelemen PR, Miller C 3rd, Chardkoff L, Wilson L. National practice patterns of sentinel lymph node dissection for breast carcinoma. J Am Coll Surg 2001;192:453–8.

13. Britton KE, Jan H, al-Yasi AR, Biassoni L, Carroll MJ, Granowska M. Efficacy of immunoscintigraphy for detection of lymph node metastases. Recent Results Cancer Res 2000;157:3–11.

14. Kuehn T, Klauss W, Darsow M, Regele S, Flock F, Maiterth C, et al. Long-term morbidity following axillary dissection in breast cancer patients-clinical assessment, significance for life quality and the impact of demographic, oncologic and therapeutic factors. Breast Cancer Res Treat 2000;64:275–86.

In Chapter 18, Speiser and Ferrone discuss the identification and characterization of human melanoma-associated antigens (MAA's) and the immune monitoring of patients receiving ganglioside and anti-idiotypic monoclonal antibody therapy or "naturally occurring" peptide-based therapy.

In general, non-specific approaches using immune stimulants such as BCG and cytokines have met with very limited success as have the more specific regimens employing vaccines derived from tumor cells and their lysates. The longer term responsiveness to the approaches as outlined which impart either humoral or MHC-restricted cell-based responses may be impaired in emerging antigen-negative tumor variants [1].

The authors refer to new techniques such as SEREX, where spontaneous antibody responses develop to novel tumor-associated antigens. This has been designed to identify new CT type antigens such as NY-ESO-1 which are capable of inducing NY-ESO-1-specific spontaneous humoral and cellular immune responses in NY-ESO-1-expressing tumors [2]. These techniques may be supplemented by alteration of the immunogenicity of peptides by specific replacement of amino acids at primary anchor residues for peptide/MHC binding. Other techniques such as cDNA expression cloning with T cells, cDNA subtraction with representational differential analysis (RDA) and serial analysis of gene expression (SAGE) will be able to identify novel melanocytic lineage antigens which are capable of being recognized by immunocompetent T and B cells [3].

For strategies like immunotherapy, not anticipated to induce major tumor regression, surrogate T cell mediated markers of immune responsiveness are required. This field has undergone a recent explosion of activity particularly in the evaluation and monitoring of functional antigen-specific CTL (CD8+) responses, including in vitro functional measures, phenotypic assays and functional assays. A simple in vivo measure of activity is the delayed-type hypersensitivity (DTH) response. The problems encountered here include the antigen specificity of DTH analysis, whether the DTH is an "all-or-none" phenomenon or is capable of gradation and whether it is correlative in a discriminant analysis with other more quantitative in vitro functional T cell assays. Future aspects of the DTH response will be the ability to phenotypically isolate infiltrating T cells from DTH biopsies for functional assessment [4].

Semiquantitative in vitro phenotypic assays of antigen-specific cell-mediated immunity include flow cytometric TCR ($\alpha\beta$ subtype expression), peptide tetramer complex flow cytometry (see below) and PCR technology of T cells designed to detect restricted TCR repertoires through CDR3 sequencing. Functional in vitro measures of antigen-specific T cell reactivity have traditionally been performed using lymphoproliferation assays of purified T cell populations in the presence of purified or recombinant antigen and irradiated autologous or HLA-matched antigen-presenting cells. This may be influenced by non-specific immune stimulation and high proliferation may be produced by low levels of activated cells providing falsely high stimulation indices. This technique has been supplemented (as described in this chapter) with cytokine detection during lymphocyte activation either by ELISA or ELISPOT testing for individual cell assessment. The ELISPOT test provided now with computerized counting results in a relatively simple and accurate determination of activated lymphocytic response with the recent introduction of dual color methods to evaluate different cytokines simultaneously or with pre-loading of PBMC with poxvirus vectors which encode the antigen of interest as a stimulator [4]. Other functional in vitro assays include the detection of intra-cellular cytokines using multi-parameter flow cytometry, quantitative cytokine mRNA measurement using real-time PCR technology, direct cytotoxicity assays (with ^{51}Cr or Europium target cell lysis against purified tumor-associated antigen or where appropriate HLA-matched allogeneic tumor cell lines), flow cytometric CTL assays (using Propidium iodide for determination of cell viability) and limiting dilution assays for the detection of stimulated precursor cell frequency.The intra-cellular cytokine technique obviously assesses non-viable cells and this precludes the ability to clone them, although new techniques using magnetofluorescent liposomes conjugated to individual cytokine monoclonal antibodies, permits the detection of the surface expression of cytokines. This allows cells to remain viable since traditional permeabilization is not required [6]. All of these assay systems are difficult to perform, requiring specialized immunology laboratories, with poor inter-institutional standardization and an uncertain correlation between their detection and overall tumor-specific outcome [7].

The majority of recent work has been directed at inducing specific CTL production for peripheral blood monitoring during immunotherapy as assessed by tetramer-peptide flow cytometry. Although this intentional targeting of normal proteins is of speculative importance in human melanoma, it has resulted in inflammatory responses in tumors circumscribing pigmented areas of skin during peptide-specific CD8+ T cell clonal therapy which on tetrameric identification are identical to the cellular infusates [8]. Newer strategies against melanoma have included gene therapy using allogeneic melanoma cell vaccines which have been transfected with an IL-2 plasmid or autologous irradiated melanoma cells transfected with IL-6, IL-6 receptor, IL-7 or IL-12 [9-11]. These regimens have resulted in local regression and histological apoptosis of tumor cells in subcutaneous metastases. Other approaches have used adenoviral-encoded melanoma peptide therapy [12], grafting of T cells with a recombinant T-cell receptor [13] and peptide-generated dendritic cells [14,15]. The TCR grafting technique contains the antigen-binding domain as an extra-cellular single chain Fv fragment derived from a monoclonal antibody which is specific for HMW-MAA. The intra-cellular receptor moiety contains the cellular activation domain which consists of the gamma signaling chain of the Fc-ε receptor. This technique is designed to effectively bypass the presentation of MAA-associated peptides by MHC molecules to the TCR. The latter technique of dendritic cell therapy results in MHC-restricted peptide-specific CTL, although the dendritic cells may be pulsed with peptide, protein or tumor cell lysate or transfected with viral vectors or naked nucleic acid. Other techniques include the generation of tumor/dendritic cell hybridomas [16]. Such approaches have been shown variably to induce cross-priming of T cells against autologous tumors expressing the full gamut of MAA's. Such a capacity validates approaches where irradiated allogeneic tumor cells could be used in human studies to deliver tumor antigens to dendritic cells for less personalized vaccination protocols [17].

Improved characterization of tumor-specific peptides will permit the construction of peptide-HLA tetrameric complexes for user-friendly estimation of peripheral levels of antigen-specific CTL. These newer techniques as described, provide greater cell populations than limiting dilution analysis (LDA), which requires quite a high proliferative potential. Balanced against this, however, tetrameric technology reflects the relative promiscuity of peptide-MHC class I ligands, with a significant potential for cross-reactivity in the identification of antigen-specific CTLs. These tetramers will assist in the dissection of the reacting T cell population, assessing the TCR activation state, apoptosis susceptibility and expression of inhibitory receptors by T cells. The true functional status of these T cell subpopulations remains to be identified. Improved understanding of the existence and significance of hypofunctional populations of CD8+ cells and CD4+ helper cell function using MHC class II tetramers (as suggested in this chapter) during tumor-specific immunotherapy is, however, required [18].

Finally, in melanoma and other solid malignancies encountered by the general surgeon, improved understanding of apoptotic mechanisms amongst potentially immunocompetent infiltrating lymphocytes and delineation of new markers such as death receptors may have a great impact on therapy in the future. These two areas are inter-linked with the FasL expressed by many tumors being a member of the TNF receptor family incorporating death receptors [19]. The intra-cytoplasmic death domains of these receptors will then activate a series of cysteine proteases (the caspases) through specific adaptor molecules [20,21]. The expression and signaling of this family of trans-membrane proteins is highly regulated and divisible into separate entities. These include apoptosis triggers (such as Fas ligation or the TNF-related apoptosis-inducing ligand — TRAIL), apoptosis modulators (most notably members of the Bcl-2 family and Bcl-2 interacting proteins) and Fas/FasL modulators including FLICE, FADD (Fas-associated death domain-like IL-1 beta converting enzyme inhibitors) and FLICE-inhibitory (FLIP) proteins, each of which are potential targets for immune activation in many solid malignancies including melanoma [22,23].

References

1. Saida T. Recent advances in melanoma research. J Dermatol Sci 2001;26:1–13.
2. Jager D, Jager E, Knuth A. Vaccinatiuon for malignant melanoma: recent developments. Oncology 2001;60:1–7.
3. Kawakami Y, Suzuki Y, Shofuda T, Kiniwa Y, Inozume T, Dan K, et al. T cell immune responses against melanoma and melanocytes in cancer and autoimmunity. Pigment Cell Res 2000;13 Suppl 8:S163–9.

4. Waanders GA, Rimoldi D, Lienard D, Carrel S, Lejeune F, Dietrich PY, et al. Melanoma-reactive human cytotoxic T lymphocytes derived from skin biopsies of delayed-type hypersensitivity reactions induced by injection of an autologous melanoma cell line. Clin Cancer Res 1997;3:685–96.
5. Larsson M, Jin X, Ramratnam B, Ogg GS, Engelmayer J, Demoitie MA, et al. A recombinant vaccinia virus-based ELISPOT assay detects high frequencies of Pol-specific CD8 T cells in HIV-1-positive individuals. AIDS 1999;13:767–77.
6. Schefford A, Assenmacher M, Reiners-Schramm L, Lauster R, Radbruch A. High-sensitivity immunofluorescence for detection of the pro- and anti-inflammatory cytokines γ-interferon and interleukin-10 on the surface of cytokine-secreting cells. Nat Med 2000;6:107–110.
7. Clay TM, Hobeika AC, Mosca PJ, Lyerly HK, Morse MA. Assays for monitoring cellular immune responses to active immunotherapy of cancer. Clin Cancer Res 2001;7:1127–35.
8. Yee C, Thompson JA, Roche P, Byrd DR, Lee PP, Pipekorn M, et al. Melanocyte destruction after antigen-specific immunotherapy of melanoma: direct evidence of t cell-mediated vitiligo. J Exp Med 2000;192:1637–44.
9. Osanto S, Schiphorst PP, Weijl NI, Dijkstra N, Van Wees A, Brouwenstein N, et al. Vaccination of melanoma patients with an allogeneic, genetically-modified interleukin 2-producing melanoma cell line. Hum Gene Ther 2000;11:739–50.
10. Moller P, Moller H, Sun Y, Dorbic T, Henz BM, Wittig B, et al. Increased non-major histocompatibility complex-restricted activity in melanoma patients vaccinated with cytokine gene-transfected autologous tumor cells. Cancer Gene Ther 2000;7:976–84.
11. Nawrocki S, Murawa P, Malicki J, Kapcinska M, Gryska K, Izycki D, et al. Genetically modified tumor vaccines (GMTV) in melanoma clinical trials. Immunol Lett 2000;74:81–6.
12. Perricone MA, Claussen KA, Smith KA, Kaplan JM, Piraino S, Shankara S, et al. Immunogene therapy for murine melanoma using recombinant adenoviral vectors expressing melanoma-associated antigens. Mol Ther 2000;1:275–84.
13. Abken H, Hombach A, Heuser C, Reinhold U. A novel strategy in the elimination of disseminated melanoma cells: chimeric receptors endow T cells with tumor specificity. Rec Results Cancer Res 2001;158:249–64.
14. Ribas A, Butterfield LH, Hu B, Dissette VB, Chen AY, Koh A,et al. Generation of T-cell immunity to a murine melanoma using MART-1-engineered dendritic cells. J Immunother 2000;23:59–66.
15. Lau R, Wang F, Jeffery G, Marty V, Kuniyoshi J, Bade E, et al. Phase I trial of intravenous peptide-pulsed dendritic cells in patients with metastatic melanoma. J Immunother 2001;24:66–78.
16. Hadzantonis M, O'Neill H. Review: dendritic cell immunotherapy for melanoma. Cancer Biother Radiopharm 1999;1:11–22.
17. Berard F, Blanco P, Davoust J, Neidhart-Berard EM, Nouri-Shirazi M, Taquet N, et al. Cross-priming of naïve CD8 T cells against melanoma antigens using dendritic cells loaded with killed allogeneic melanoma cells. J Exp Med 2000;192:1535–44.
18. Waldrop SL, Davis KA, Maino VC, Picker LJ. Normal human CD4+ memory T cells display broad heterogeneity in their activation threshold for cytokine synthesis. J Immunol 1998;161:5284–95.
19. Rathmell JC, Thompson CB. The central effectors of cell death in the immune system. Annu Rev Immunol 1999;17:781–828.
20. Saikumar P, Dong Z, Mikhailov V, Denton M, Weinberg JM, Venkatachalam MA. Apoptosis: definition, mechanisms and relevance to disease. Am J Med 1999;107:489–506.
21. Utz PJ, Andeson P. Life and death decisions: regulation of apoptosis by proteolysis of signaling molecules. Cell Death Differ 2000;7:589–602.
22. Konopleva M, Zhao S, Xie Z, Segall H, Younes A, Claxton DF, et al. Apoptosis. Molecules and mechanisms. Adv Exp Med Biol 1999;457:217–36.
23. Nguyen T, Thomas W, Zhang XD, Gray C, Hersey P. Immunologically-mediated tumor cell apoptosis: the role of TRAIL in T cell and cytokine-mediated responses to melanoma. Forum (Genova) 2000;10:243–52.

SECTION IV

IMMUNOLOGY AND THE GASTROINTESTINAL TRACT

19. The Gastrointestinal Immune System — An Overview

Stefan Schreiber and Susanna Nikolaus

Epithelial Cells and Barrier Function of the Intestinal Mucosa

The intestinal barrier function is based on a complex interaction between the mechanical barrier imposed and the immune system of the gut. The mechanical barrier is formed by the mucous layer and the epithelial wall. A continuous, intact epithelial layer is pivotal for the integrity as well as the mechanical barrier function of the mucosa in order to prevent an uncontrolled invasion of bacterial, exogenous dietary or other luminal antigens.

The most important task of the mucosa-associated immune system of the gut (Gut Associated Lymphoid Tissue (GALT)) is the complete exclusion of intestinal toxic and infectious pathogens. This is shown in Figure 19.1. To fulfill its role, the GALT is considerably different in its functional and regulative characteristics from the normal peripheral blood immune system.

About 90 percent of the immune cells of the entire body are located in the mucosa-associated immune system and the intestine produces more than two thirds of the body's immunoglobulin, influencing and directing the intestinal immune system by specific presentation of antigens. Epithelial cells can express class-I histocompatibility antigens (HLA, MHC) and thus induce cytotoxic (CD8) T-suppressor-cells. During intestinal inflammation MHC class-II molecules are expressed on epithelial cells as well and appear to present antigens to CD4 T-helper cells. In vitro, epithelial cells secrete cytokines that stimulate or regulate inflammation (including IL-6, IL-8 and TGF-β), although the in vivo evidence for epithelial cell cytokine production seems less clear. Epithelial cells thus contribute to local intestinal immunoregulation to a considerable degree.

Tolerance against "normal" fecal flora is an important part of the barrier function. In the normal intestine, microbial stool flora appears to be only weak stimulators for the mucosa-associated immune system. There are valid indicators though, that this tolerance against endogenous flora is impaired in chronic inflammatory conditions like inflammatory bowel disease (IBD). This results in the loss of the normal inflammation-free immunoregulation in the intestinal lamina propria. An exaggerated immunologic reaction against physiologic stool

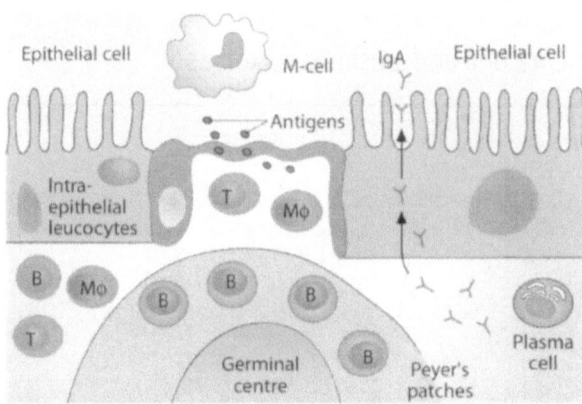

Figure 19.1. The mucosa-associated immune system of the gut (also called "Gut Associated Lymphoid Tissue" — GALT) is located in the intestinal lamina propria and within the Peyer's patches. An epithelial layer forms a mechanical barrier against the intestinal lumen. Within the epithelial layer a population of intra-epithelial lymphocytes (IEL) can be found. In the stroma of the lamina propria, mast cells, macrophages, B and T-lymphocytes are present to fulfill complex defence tasks. Predominantly, antibodies of isotype IgA are produced. Peyer's patches are structures similar to lymph follicles, which can be detected in only a few places. They have a germinal center that is surrounded by B cells. Above the Peyer's patches specialized epithelial cells with a flat cell surface without villi or microvilli can usually be found. They are called M-(microfold)-cells and select antigens of the intestinal lumen by glycoprotein receptors, which they forward to the lymphocytes of the Peyer's patches by transcytosis. The cytoplasm of the M-cells covers only a few nanometers in contrast to neighboring cells. The basal cell membrane on the apex of the M cell forms a domed cavity. Mononuclear phagocytes and T-lymphocytes very often can directly contact cell membranes of the M-cells by depositing themselves at the basal M-cell membrane. The M-cells constitute a selective filter for antigen exposure of the GALT, which allows controlled stimulation of immune cells in the Peyer's patches. Thus a controlled immune reaction can proceed, which guarantees the continuous exposure of the GALT to characteristic antigens of the intestinal lumen. (Originally published in Foelsch UR, Kochsiek K, Schmidt RF. Pathophysiologie, Chapter 19, pp. 284–293. Springer Verlag).

flora then could contribute to an intensified inflammation. Genetically-determined disturbance in immune tolerance thus comprises one attractive hypothesis for the etiopathogenesis of IBD where the inflammatory response might progress independently from antigenic exposure and characterized by a genetically dysregulation of local anti-microbial tolerance (See Chapter 20).

T- and B-lymphocytes in the Intestinal Lamina Propria

T- and B-lymphocytes are important elements of the specific immunologic response of the intestinal mucosa-associated immune system. Antigen specifity is determined by the T-cell antigen receptor and the specifity of the immunoglobulin molecules, respectively. Immune cells are mainly found in three anatomic regions of the intestinal wall: within the epithelium, in the lamina propria and submucosally in structures similar to lymph follicles, the Peyer's patches (Figure 19.1).

While T-cells constitute the main part of the immunocompetent cells of the lamina propria, other immunocytes comprise the infiltrating population, including approximately 10–15% macrophage/monocyte lineages, 20–30% B-cells and up to 30–50% T-cells. In comparison with the peripheral blood there is a significantly larger share of B-lymphocytes. The Peyer's patches are built similarly to lymph follicles in that they have a germinal center which mainly consists of activated T-cells and is surrounded by a dense rim of B-cells. This anatomic structure and the make-up of the immunocyte populations do not appear to alter during acute inflammatory attacks. M-cells which control the introduction of antigens into the intestinal lumen can often be detected in a close anatomical relationship to the Peyer's patches.

Antigens are presented to CD4$^+$ ("helper") or CD8$^+$ ("cytotoxic") T-cells by phagocytes on class-I or II MHC molecules involving further accessory molecules. In this process, only those T-cells are stimulated which are specific for the antigen presented. This T-cell specificity is determined by the T-cell antigen receptor where if the "right" antigen is contacted, an immunologic activation and clonal expansion of the specific stimulated T-lymphocyte will result. Apart from contact between MHC-bound antigen and antigen receptor, a variety of accessory molecules (including ICAM-1) as well as further soluble mediators, such as Interleukin 1-β (IL-1β) or Tumor Necrosis Factor alpha (TNF-α), are involved. The analysis of the clonal distribution of T-cell antigen receptors (by repertoire studies) in the expanded T-cell population frequently permits insights into the inherent nature of the stimulated antigens in particular disorders (e.g. autoimmune diseases).

Intestinal T-lymphocytes even show a limited repertoire of antigen receptors in the normal, non-inflamed intestinal mucosa, i.e. the number of antigens that may act as immunologic stimulators is clearly limited. The domino effect of T-cell-bound activation processes secondarily aids T cell/B cell cooperation and resultant activation leads to clonal expansion and expression of cell surface molecules, such as MHC class-II, CD23 (the Fc receptor for IgE) and the Interleukin-2 receptor. Influenced by T-cell cytokines such as transforming growth factor β (TGF-β) and Interleukin 4 and 5, B-cell maturation processes lead to plasma cells which locally produce immunoglobulin of the correct isotype for immuno-regulation.

A large number of investigations indicate a physiological state of increased immune activation in the normal intestinal immune system in comparison with the peripheral blood. Apart from the biological qualities of this cell population, the continuous stimulation of the intestinal mucosa by antigens may contribute to the "constant state" of activation of lymphocytes in a healthy intestinal lamina propria. However, this stimulation does not provoke an inflammatory process that would damage the integrity and the function of the intestinal mucosa. On the contrary, it appears to contribute to a spontaneous and steady secretion of immunoglobulins (mainly the A isotype) by intestinal B-lymphocytes and plasma cells.

In the healthy lamina propria, a spontaneous production of immunoglobulins can already be found in comparison with the peripheral blood as a product of a low level continuous immunologic activation. The immunoglobulin isotype A (IgA) represents up to 90 percent of the immunoglobulins produced in the intestinal lamina propria (Figures 19.2 and 19.3), whereby 61 percent of the IgA is secreted by the colonic mucosa as the IgA2 isoform. IgA2 is highly resistant to

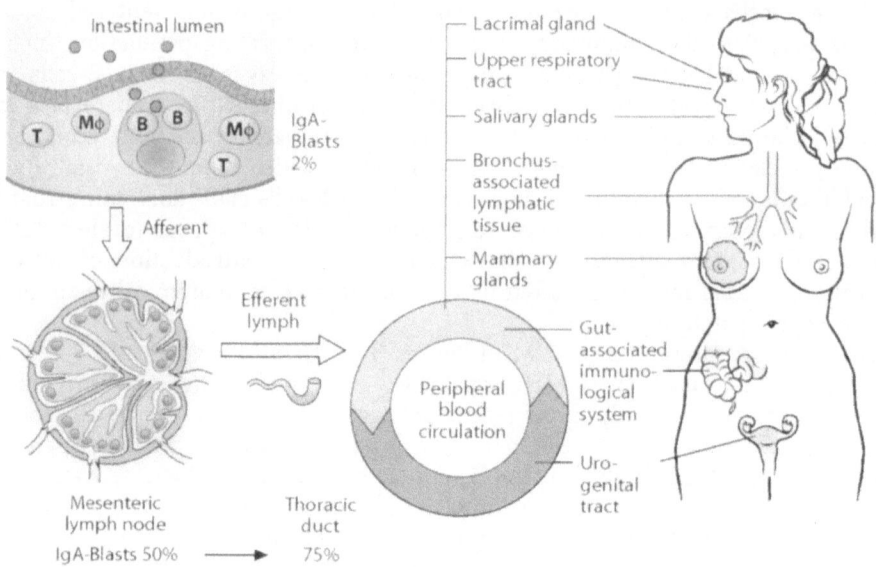

Figure 19.2. Homing of IgA-B-lymphocytes into the intestinal mucosal surfaces. After an initial antigen contact, IgD/IgM-positive B cells leave the Peyer's patches to mature into IgA producing B-lymphocytes in the periphery. This so-called maturational journey ends for the majority of the B cells after producing the IgA isotype and by re-entering the mucosal compartment. Homing receptors, which are expressed on high endothelial venules anatomically closely connected to the mucosal lamina propria, play an important role here. Accumulation of IgA-producing B cells can be seen in the mucosal tissue of the gut, in the bronchial apparatus, the urogenital tract, mammary, lacrimal and salivary glands, as well as in the oral mucosa. The IgA produced in the mucosa is important for safeguarding the integrity of the mucosal barrier. It should be noted that a genetically-determined IgA deficiency does not lead to severe clinical symptoms. (Originally published in Foelsch UR, Kochsiek K, Schmidt RF. Pathophysiologie, Chapter 19, pp. 284–293. © Springer Verlag).

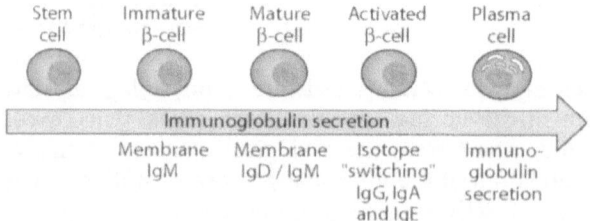

Figure 19.3. B cell differentiation and immunoglobulin secretion. While stem cells are maturing into B cells, membrane expression of IgM and IgD is seen. IgD/IgM positive B-lymphocytes leave the bone marrow. In this phase they already show their fully developed antigen specificity defined by light chains, whereas heavier chains define the immunoglobulin isotype. A complicated genetic rearrangement results in the change of isotype of D/M to IgA and further to IgE via various G-subclasses. The process known as isotype switching is irreversible (so-called "downstream switching") and accomplished by rearrangement of the coding genes for the heavier chains in 3'-5' direction. B-lymphocytes secrete only little immunoglobulin during this differentiating process finally maturing as plasma cells. During this process they lose the membrane expression of immunoglobulins in exchange for high secretion rates. (Originally published in Foelsch UR, Kochsiek K, Schmidt RF. Pathophysiologie, Chapter 19, pp. 284–293. © Springer Verlag).

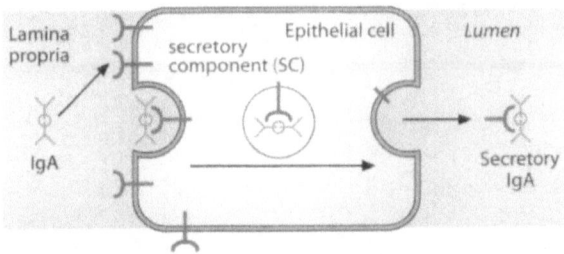

Figure 19.4. IgA secretion in the gastrointestinal tract. IgA forms polymeric complexes consisting of two or more molecules using a joining (J) chain. Although the exact mechanism of this molecular interaction has not been fully explained yet, it appears clear that binding to the J-chain is a necessary precondition for the subsequent secretion of IgA into the intestinal lumen. A glycoprotein (secretory component (SC)), is expressed on the surface of epithelial cells and the IgA-dimer bound to the SC is transported from the basal to the luminal surface of the epithelial cells by transcytosis. There, the transmembrane domain of the SC is cleaved and the IgA-dimer is released into the intestinal lumen as secretory IgA covalently bound to the remaining SC. (Originally published in Foelsch UR, Kochsiek K, Schmidt RF. Pathophysiologie, Chapter 19, pp. 284–293. © Springer Verlag).

the effects of bacterial enzymes of the intestinal lumen. IgA has unique characteristics when compared with IgG. IgA is largely unable to activate complement and cannot activate other immune cells because of its lack of Fc receptors, resulting in the elimination of antigens without attendant cell-dependent effector events or inflammatory responses normally linked to other Ig isotypes. On the luminal surface of the colonic epithelium, IgA is partly integrated into the mucus matrix (Figures 19.4). IgA is therefore an important component of the intestinal immune system and its barrier function to exclude pathogens without inducing inflammation which would have a deleterious effect on resorptive functions.

Endothelial Cells

The immigration of immune cells into the intestinal lamina propria is mediated by adhesion molecules that can be found on leucocytes as well as on endothelial cells (Figure 19.5). Adhesion molecules can be divided into three groups: the immunoglobulin super-family (e.g. Intercellular Adhesion Molecule (ICAM)-1 expressed on monocytes and endothelial cells, Vascular Cell Adhesion Molecule (VCAM) expressed on endothelial cells of smaller vessels), the integrins (e.g. the Very Late Antigen (VLA) on lymphocytes or the Lymphocyte Function-associated Antigen (LFA)-1 on leucocytes) and the selectins (e.g. the Endothelial Leucocyte Adhesion Molecule (ELAM)-1 expressed on endothelial cells).

Selectins control the primary contact between leucocytes and the endothelial surface. The group of E and P-selectins are expressed on cytokine-activated endothelial cells. In contrast to this, L-selectin is formed permanently on leucocytes during their circulation between the periphery and the GALT.

Adhesion molecules control the selection of immune cells that tend to migrate from blood vessels into the tissue compartments. This process has been well characterized (Figure 19.6). If the adhesive power of the non-covalent bond between selectins and their ligands on the one hand and the shearing powers of the bloodstream on the other hand are in equilibrium, leucocytes will slow down

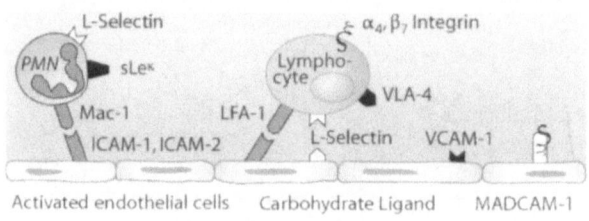

Figure 19.5. Adhesion molecules. The adhesion process is mediated by potential interaction of a variety of carbohydrate ligands. Binding to selectins induces signaling which leads to an increased expression of integrins (e.g. VLA-1 or VLA-4) on leucocytes. Subsequently, interaction with molecules of the immunoglobulin superfamily takes place. The intercellular adhesion molecules (ICAM) 1 and 2, which are expressed on activated endothelial cells, appear to be of particular importance during inflammatory processes to mediate immigration of leucocytes. The molecules MAC-1 and the lymphocyte function associated antigen-1 (LFA-1) are ligands for ICAM-1 on granulocytes and lymphocytes. Molecules similar to ICAM-1 such as the Mucosal Addressed Cell Adhesion Molecule-1 (MAdCAM-1) target other cell populations to the intestinal lamina propria, by binding T-cells via the ligands $\alpha4$, $\beta7$-integrin, which is expressed on activated lymphocytes). sLe^x = Sialyl Lewis x antigen. (Originally published in Foelsch UR, Kochsiek K, Schmidt RF. Pathophysiologie, Chapter 19, pp. 284–293. © Springer Verlag).

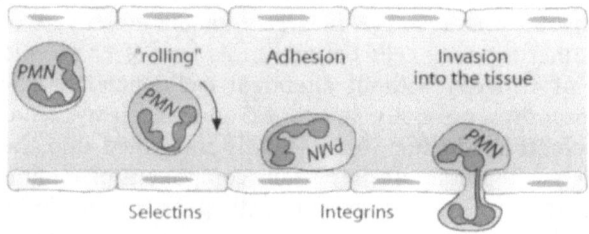

Figure 19.6. Leucocyte migration into inflamed tissue is mediated by adhesion molecules in various steps. The rolling motion of the cells alongside the vascular walls is dependent upon the equilibrium of adhesion powers of the non-covalent bond of selectins and their ligands on the one hand and the shearing powers of the bloodstream on the other. The much stronger bond of integrins to molecules of the immunoglobulin superfamily is known as secondary adhesion ("sticking") and induces the transmigration of adhering leucocytes through the endothelial cell layer into the tissue below. (Originally published in Foelsch UR, Kochsiek K, Schmidt RF. Pathophysiologie, Chapter 19, pp. 284–293. © Springer Verlag).

from the blood flow and will start moving in a "rolling" motion along the vascular walls. The selectin-mediated bond induces an increased expression of integrins on leucocytes, which consequently leads to interaction with ligands of the immunoglobulin superfamily (ICAM-1 binds the antigen LFA-1 and VCAM-1 binds the integrin VLA-4). This bond, which is also called secondary adhesion or "sticking", is much stronger than the initial selectin bonds, inducing the transmigration of adherent leucocytes through the endothelial cell layer into the underlying extra-cellular matrix.

During the process of immune cell maturation (which is an important part of the learning experience of the immune system where näive lymphocytes are anergized or apoptosed), B cells (and T cells) will be first exposed to antigens in the Peyer's patch. The selection of antigen exposure is controlled through the M cells as described above. After egress from the Peyer's Patch, the B cells mature though different stages by isotype switching through downstream rearrangements of the immunoglobulin genes (See Chapter 1). IgA or IgE-producing plasma cells result as late maturational B cell forms with their entry into the appropriate tissues such as the lamina propria being mediated by a combination of adhesion molecules constitutively expressed on small endothelial venules and lymphocytes, (most notably the alpha-4-beta-7 integrin and MAdCAM-1 up-regulated on lymphocytes).

Monocytes, Macrophages and Granulocytes

Macrophages and monocytes can be identified by their specific ultra-structural characteristics and by surface markers in the intestinal lamina propria. Those so-called mononuclear phagocytes play an important role in the phagocytosis of potential pathogens, as well as in antigen presentation and in the local synthesis of proteases, oxygen- free radicals, nitrous-oxide (NO), eicosanoids and cytokines (Figure 19.7). These cells are most likely involved in secondary immune defenses and in the continuation of inflammatory reactions. During acute inflammation, granulocytes are the prevailing cell populations within the lamina propria. They account for most of the local tissue destruction in infectious or immune conditions such as IBD by their release of acute-phase mediators and proteins. Together with the granulocytes, monocyte/macrophage lineages constitute the main

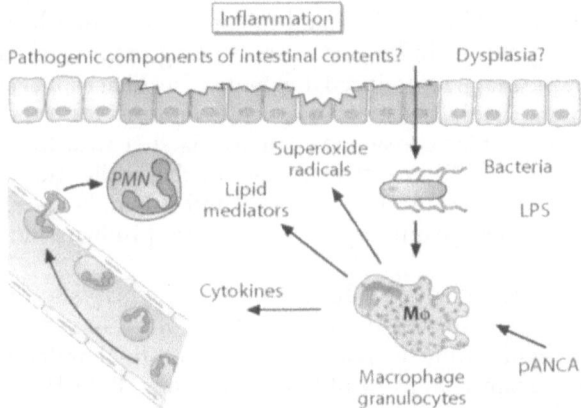

Figure 19.7. Phagocytes and inflammation mediators are the central elements of the pathophysiology of intestinal inflammation. It must be assumed, though, that the pathogenic components of the stool (bacterial LPS) add to the amplification of intestinal inflammation. Macrophages and granulocytes are then able to release a host of mediators. Superoxide radicals lead to toxic destruction of the tissue and potential pathogens in the immediate surroundings of the phagocytes. At the same time, lipid mediators (prostaglandins, leukotrienes, thromboxanes, platelet activating factors) are released in large quantities. Although lipid mediators have an amplifying effect on inflammation, they do not seem to play a key role in the control of inflammatory reaction. Cytokines released by granulocytes and macrophages have directly toxic effects and regulate the complex network of immunologic processes of the mucosa. In chronic intestinal inflammation the production of pro-inflammatory cytokines appears to be the overriding event, resulting in activation of the vascular endothelium and prompting a further influx of inflammatory cells. Mφ = macrophage/monocyte. (Originally published in Foelsch UR, Kochsiek K, Schmidt RF. Pathophysiologie, Chapter 19, pp. 284–293. © Springer Verlag).

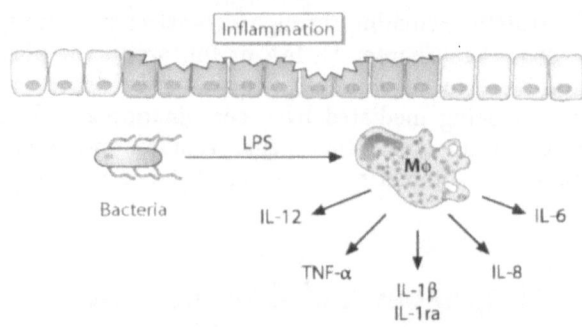

Figure 19.8. The immunologic activation of lymphocytes by monocytes and macrophages is controlled by the T-cell antigen receptor and accessory molecules activated through cell-to-cell contact and the accessory pro-inflammatory cytokines such as IL-1β and TNF-α. Macrophages and granulocytes secrete not only IL-1β and TNF-α, but also IL-8 and IL-6. It appears that IL-12 also plays a prominent role in the initiation of the inflammation process. Interleukin-1 receptor antagonist (IL-1ra) is the endogenous antagonist of IL-1β, competing for the IL-1 receptor and blocking stimulation. (Originally published in Foelsch UR, Kochsiek K, Schmidt RF. Pathophysiologie, Chapter 19, pp. 284–293. © Springer Verlag).

producers of pro-inflammatory cytokines in the inflamed intestinal lamina propria.

Pro-inflammatory cytokines are important mediators for initiation and perpetuation of acute inflammatory events. Tumor necrosis factor α (TNF-α), Interleukin 1β (IL-1β), Interleukin 8 (IL-8) and to some extent Interleukin 6 (IL-6) are key players in this group of inflammation-enhancing mediators. Tumor Necrosis Factor α (TNF-α) is mainly produced by monocytes/macrophages and by activated T-cells (Figure 19.8). It causes fever and induces the synthesis of acute-phase proteins (in particular C-reactive protein) together with IL-6 as a secondary mediator. Furthermore, TNF-α activates endothelial cells (to up-regulate the expression of adhesion molecules) as well as T and B-lymphocytes. During intestinal inflammation, large quantities of TNF-α are produced in the intestinal mucosa.

Interleukin 1β (IL-1β) displays effects which are synergistic or identical with those of TNF-α. The secretion of IL-1β as well as TNF-α in inflamed and healthy mucosal tissue is significantly increased during intestinal inflammation in contrast with the non-inflamed mucosa of healthy persons. Both IL-1β and TNF-α re generally produced by the same immune cell lineages.

Interleukin 2 (IL-2) is produced exclusively by T-cells and represents a powerful growth factor for T and B-cells as well as for natural killer (NK) cells. Increased levels of IL-2 and its soluble receptor (sIL-2R) can be found in the intestinal mucosa and in circulation during acute inflammatory conditions. Interleukin 6 (IL-6) also belongs in the group of pro-inflammatory cytokines, although its biological effects differ in some respects from those of TNF-α and IL-1β, at times being also involved in anti-inflammatory processes. Like IL-1β, IL-6 is generated by mononuclear cells of the lamina propria, with the secretion significantly increased during acute and chronic inflammatory processes and mirroring their state of activity.

Interleukin-8 plays an important role in the chemotaxis of neutrophils, lymphocytes and monocytes although its role in intestinal inflammation has not

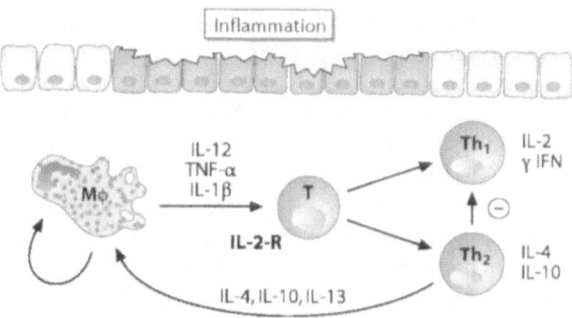

Figure 19.9. Pro-inflammatory cytokines and their antagonists. Pro-inflammatory cytokines (IL-1β, TNF-α, IL-8) and inflammation-augmenting T-cell cytokines (Interleukin 2; IL-2, Interferon-gamma, IFN-γ) are in equilibrium with anti-inflammatory cytokines (Interleukins 4, 10 and 13), which antagonistically counteract immunologic activation. These balances, which can be found on the monocyte/macrophage lineage as well as on the T-helper cells, (TH1 versus TH2), are crucial for maintenance of a normal, non-inflammatory state of the mucosa in the presence of many exogenous pathogens. (Originally published in Foelsch UR, Kochsiek K, Schmidt RF. Pathophysiologie, Chapter 19, pp. 284–293. © Springer Verlag).

yet been fully determined. IL-8 is especially elevated during acute mucosal inflammation where it functions as a potent chemo-attractor for acute-phase immunocytes. Interferon γ (IFN-γ) comprises an important cytokine which predominantly activates macrophages and where it up-regulates MHC class I and II expression for antigenic processing and T cell co-stimulation. Interleukin-12 (IL-12) constitutes a messenger substance that is produced mainly by type 1 T-helper lymphocytes. Apart from the central role IL-12 plays in initiating inflammatory actions, it primarily induces the production of IFN-γ. An increased production of IL-12 and its crucial impact on the regulation of intestinal inflammation has been shown in both Crohn's Disease and ulcerative colitis (See Chapter 20).

Anti-inflammatory cytokines and receptor antagonists are locally required in order to limit inflammatory reactions. These mediators are in equilibrium in a healthy immune system as they can counteract immunologic activation in many instances. Mononuclear phagocytes, epithelial cells, endothelial cells and fibroblasts can all produce anti-inflammatory factors, including Interleukin-1-receptor-antagonist (IL-1ra) and soluble Interleukin receptors. They are able to interact with pro-inflammatory mediators and to inhibit them either by blocking the respective soluble cytokines or by blocking the respective receptors.

In mice, T-helper cells can be divided into type 1 (TH1) and type 2 (TH2) cells by their cytokine patterns and characteristic surface markers. TH2 cells produce Il-4, IL-5, IL-10, IL-13 whereas TH1 cells produce the pro-inflammatory cytokines IL-2, IL-12 and IFNγ. In humans, T-helper cells cannot be divided so easily into these archetypal subpopulations. Characteristic surface markers are lacking and the functional differentiation by their cytokine patterns is not as clear. The production of Interleukin 4 can be traced back to a few particular subpopulations, but Interleukin 10 is mainly produced by activated monocytes and macrophages. TH1 cytokines (particularly IL-12) are involved in most inflammatory diseases as essential mediators, whereas TH2 cells are preferential mediators in allergic reactions.

Interleukin 4 (IL-4), Interleukin-13 (IL-13) and Interleukin-10 (IL-10) are the main important anti-inflammatory cytokines in the mucosa so far identified. In addition to their specific influence on B-cell differentiation and maturation, they have clearly defined anti-inflammatory qualities. The main producers of these cytokines are the type 2 T-helper cells and cells of the monocyte/macrophage lineage. Il-4, IL-13 and IL-10 have enormous anti-inflammatory potential, which is demonstrated by the in vitro inhibition of pro-inflammatory cytokine secretion by T-cells, monocytes, macrophages and neutrophils.

The anti-inflammatory effect of IL-10 was first investigated in animal models. Mice, in which the IL-10 gene has been functionally destroyed by mutation (so-called "IL-10-knock-out" mice), develop a colitis that is similar to chronic inflammatory diseases recognized in humans. In Il-10-knock-out mice and other animal experimental systems (e.g. mice with severe combined immunodeficiency, "SCID mice", in which colitis is caused by an adoptive transfer of syngeneic T-helper cell populations), IL-10, but not IL-4 has a clearly outlined anti-inflammatory effect. In these models as well as in recent preliminary human trials, both in vitro and in vivo release of IL-1β and TNF-α by monocytes/macrophages can be dose-dependently reduced in experimental colitis and IBD respectively by the administration of recombinant human IL-10. Taken together, these findings indicate that the delicate balance of pro and anti-inflammatory factors and their influence on each other plays a pivotal role in the pathogenesis of chronic intestinal inflammation. The equilibrium of pro- and anti-inflammatory factors merges in the regulation of the transcription of immune and inflammation-style genes in immune cells.

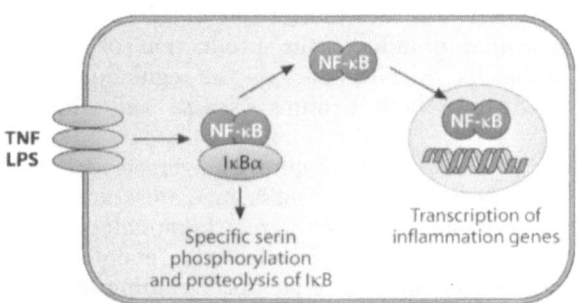

Figure 19.10. Nuclear factor kappa B (NFκB) comprises a molecule that is present in the cytoplasm of nearly all mammalian cells. In most cases it can be found as a dimer from a 50 kDa (p50) and a 65 kDa (p65) protein. It is either bound to a specific inhibitor (IκB) or a large NFκB precursory molecule (e.g. p105). Its expression is up-regulated by various stimulating factors (TNF-α and LPS), with a specific serine-phosphorylation of IκB occurring through the action of several kinases (IKK1 and IKK2 and well as NIK). IκB then is marked for degradation by the addition of ubiquitin and is degraded by the proteasome complex within minutes. Released NFκB presents a nuclear target sequence which, formerly covered by IκB., results in the rapid translocation of the molecule into the nucleus. There it can bind to defined DNA sequences in the promoter areas of inflammation genes. The transactivating factor NFκB can then initiate or amplify other transcription processes. NFκB regulation has been shown for a host of inflammation genes, including Interleukin-8, ICAM-1, TNF-α, Interleukin-1β and class-II MHC molecules as well as for viral pathogens such as the human immunodeficiency virus (HIV) and the cytomegalovirus (CMV). (Originally published in Foelsch UR, Kochsiek K, Schmidt RF. Pathophysiologie, Chapter 19, pp. 284–293. © Springer Verlag).

Nuclear factors, which control the transcription process by binding to DNA elements in gene promoter regions, may also be important in normal mucosal defense mechanisms. In particular, nuclear factor Kappa B (NFκB), which regulates the transcription of almost all pro-inflammatory cytokines, plays a significant role in the regulation of immune activation in granulocytes, monocytes/macrophages and T cells (Figure 19.10). In resting, unstimulated cells, molecules of the NFκB family are constitutively bound to inhibitors in the cytoplasm. These inhibitors include I kappa B alpha (IκBα) or large NFκB precursor molecules such as p105. A host of activating stimuli, (in particular lipopolysaccharids, LPS and TNF-α), act as principal initiators in the phosphorylation of IκBα resulting in rapid proteolytic dissociation of the NFκB-IκBα complex and leading to an activation of NFκB. Upon activation, NFκB transmigrates from the cytoplasm into the nucleus, where it binds to specific DNA sequences in the promoter area of inflammation genes including interferons, IL-1β, IL-8, HLA class II and ICAM-1, synergistically amplifying the transcription of almost all pro-inflammatory cytokines. It would appear then that both TNF-α and NFκB act as final common denominators in the mucosal inflammation/regulation cycle.

Many anti-inflammatory drugs appear to work via inhibition of nuclear factor kappa B activation. Anti-inflammatory molecules like Interleukin-10 or substances like glucocorticoids and to a smaller degree even 5-aminosalicylate, stabilize or induce constitutive inhibitors of NFκB activation (Figure 19.11). In addition to NFκB several different transcription factors are involved in the intra-cellular regulation of inflammation gene transcription. Important members include STAT proteins (signal transducers and transcription activators) which are dormant cytoplasmatic factors normally phosphorylated by Janus kinases (JAK) following the activation of cytokines and growth factors. These secondary proteins can then initiate the transcription of specific groups of cytokine-inducible genes.

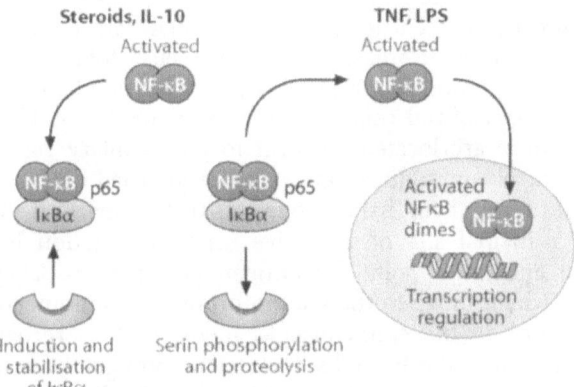

Figure 19.11. Inhibition of NFκB. Activation of transcription factors by cytokines is a hallmark of inflammation. Many drugs empirically characterized as immunosuppressive in nature, work by influencing pro-inflammatory cytokine transcription factors. Thus NFκB is inhibited in its activation through different mechanisms by glucocorticoids, Interleukin-10 (IL-10) and to a lesser degree by 5-aminosalicylic acid. (see text). (Originally published in Foelsch UR, Kochsiek K, Schmidt RF. Pathophysiologie, Chapter 19, pp. 284–293. Springer Verlag).

Commentary on Chapter 19

Andrew P. Zbar and Anastasios J. Karayiannakis

Mucosal immunology is still poorly understood. Within gut-associated lymphoid tissues the mucosal barrier balances appropriate responsiveness to cognate antigen with physiological tolerance directed towards innocuous haptens and foreign peptides. Immune activity is controlled by the local cytokine micro-environment and by the production of large quantities of surface IgA (sIgA) designed to exclude antigen in the mucus layer.

Both humoral and cell-mediated abnormalities have been demonstrated in active inflammatory bowel disease (IBD), however, the pattern of response is not distinctive for each disease type [1,2]. The ontogeny, location and function of these different lymphoid compartments is in part determined by their cellular surface expression of adhesion molecules and is locally regulated by the cytokine microenvironment which controls their site-directed migration [3]. Some of these cells are destined to function as memory cells, others as non-professional antigen-presenting cells and still others as effector cells.

Gut-Associated Lymphoid Tissues (GALT) and Peyer's Patches

The Peyer's patches (PP) are organized areas of lymphoid tissue overlaid by a specialized epithelium called follicle-associated epithelium (FAE). The FAE [4,5] contains the epithelial M (microfold) cell which controls macromolecular transport across intact epithelium, thereby limiting antigen exposure to näive and memory T cells located in the lamina propria [6,7]. The PP are devoid of crypts and villi and lie directly adjacent to lymphoid follicles with germinal centres containing centrocytes and centroblasts, dendritic cells, follicular dendritic cells (which retain antigen in immune complexes by Fc and complement receptors) and macrophages. These specialized cells of monocyte/macrophage lineage present in the dome of the follicle are located adjacent to postcapillary venules (PCV) permitting lymphovascular communication. They are guarded by specific endothelial addressin molecules recognizing lymphocyte cell-surface markers [8,9].

The PP is the principal site of inductive immune function in the intestine, acting as the first encounter point for antigen presentation. They serve as the storehouse of cells which move to the lamina propria as immunocompetent effectors and which return to the epithelium as memory IEL's recognizing cognate antigen. As inductive sites, the PP links professional antigen-presenting cells with näive T lymphocytes and stimulates the proliferation of cells committed to surface production of IgA [10]. The principal cell of the PP is the CD4+MHC class II+(T helper cell) capable of high affinity PCV binding, antigen processing and cytokine-induced assistance for B cell maturation. Evidence for these functions comes from the absence of competent effector cells in germ-free rodents and SCID mice [11,12]. It remains unknown whether the GALT-associated M cells are also capable of rudimentary antigen processing but it is unlikely in humans since they neither express MHC class II molecules on their surface (as opposed to the rodent M cell) [13] nor do they contain the lysosomal machinery necessary for antigenic degradation [14,15]. These cells have, however, been shown to selectively bind reovirus [16], *E.coli* [17], lectins and protozoa [18] and thus contribute towards the selective entry of macromolecular antigen.

Surface-IgA (sIgA) Production and Mucosal Defence

The main humoral end product of the mucosal immune system is sIgA. The system of surface delivery of this immunoglobulin is complex and requires globulin polymerization, surface receptor recognition of the polymer and attendant transporter molecules (a secretory component and a J peptide stabilizing chain). Uncommitted cells of the B and pre-B lineage which have the machinery to produce (or already express) surface IgM are converted by a process referred to as class switching towards committed IgA-producing plasma cells. This phenomenon occurs within the GALT after antigen exposure and is driven by regulatory T cells which selectively switch off IgG and IgM production by B-lymphocytes homing from the circulation back to GALT tissues. It is driven by the local cytokine microenvironment, (principally by IL-2, IL-5 and TGF-β produced by local CD4+ cells), which permit uncommitted B cells containing the cellular machinery for the V region of immunoglobulin gene expression and rearrangement to undergo antigen-specific clonal expansion [19–21].

Mucosal IgA is synthesized at a very high rate, (about 3 grams per day) and exists in two allotypic forms. The principal mucosal IgA is IgA_2 which differs from circulating IgA (IgA_1) in that it is activated by bacterial proteases and only produced by B cells which have returned to GALT tissues. The release of IgA first requires polymerization (pIgA) and complexing with a stabilizing connecting J glycoprotein which attaches to the penultimate cysteine residues of the two alpha heavy chains of the polymer. This complex is then recognized by a pIgA receptor located on the basolateral surface of the epithelial cell after preliminary attachment of a secretory component which is believed to stabilize the compound and to resist surface proteolysis. The secretory component is unique as a ligand in that its production is independent of that of pIgA and in that it can function as a separate membrane-based receptor molecule. It is not recycled and is referred to as a "sacrificial receptor".

Surface IgA itself will also secondarily control pIgA expression by gut epithelium as well as the population of T cells with Fc receptors for sIgA recognition [22]. The function of local sIgA at the gut mucosa is principally to inhibit microbial attachment in the mucus layer and this phenomenon, referred to as "immune exclusion" is well suited to an immunoglobulin isotype with poor effector Fc function where non-specific and relatively harmless antigens or those with epitope resemblance to self are prevented epithelial entry or inflammatory cell support.

Lamina Propria (LP) Lymphocytes

The cells which traffic to the lamina propria are heterogeneous but the main cell of the region is the CD4+ T cell designed for effector cross-talk following antigen exposure. Fifty percent of the lamina propria cells are CD4+ with less CD8+ cells and minimal antibody-dependent cellular cytotoxicity (ADCC) or lymphokine activated killer (LAK) cell function. Cell-mediated cytolytic activity is not a feature of the lamina propria lymphocyte and these cells display poor proliferative capacity in vitro on exposure to standard mitogens [23,24]. Natural killer (NK) cell function by these cells although demonstrable in vitro against specific targets (for example K562 cells of myelogenous leukaemia, Daudi Burkitt lymphoma cells and HT-29 colonic cancer cells) is generally fairly limited [25,26].

Within the lamina propria, the function of the CD4+ lymphocyte is that of immunoregulation and "immune assist". Cells in this immunological compartment are involved in antigen presentation, local cytokine production and site-specific migration dependent upon complex interactions between endothelial recognition addressins and cell-surface immunocyte adhesion molecules.

Intra-epithelial Lymphocytes [27]

These cells have been recognized as specialized lymphocytes for many years, although their ontogeny and rôle in mucosal defence still remains unclear. They are CD8+ MHC class II-negative differentiated T cells many of which contain the $\gamma\delta$T cell receptor isoform. (TCR) These cells are weakly functional as cytotoxic lymphocytes (CTL's) and poorly proliferative on exposure to mitogens in vitro. Most are basally located in the epithelium and will vary from 20 per 100 epithelial cells in the jejunum to as little as 5 per 100 epithelial cells in the colon.

There is much debate about their origin, since they are found in germ-free rodents, SCID mice and thymectomized radiation bone marrow chimaeras, all models which fail to express the $\alpha\beta$TCR isoform [28,29]. This would imply that these cells are primarily extrathymic in origin. It may well be that if IEL's are not presented with TCR ligands early in development, they either tolerize or die. It has been suggested that they are PP-derived, recognizing highly conserved antigen and are involved as front line memory cells which have a primary immunoregulatory role in mucosal tolerance. Although the mechanisms of mucosal tolerance are poorly understood, antigen presentation and processing by the gut is similar to other tissues elsewhere in the body in that it is MHC-restricted. Mucosal tolerance is believed to require the induction of a subset of T suppressor cells, the formation of antigen/antibody and possibly antigen-anti-idiotypic complexes and subset clonal anergy or deletion [30,31]. This phenomenon may also require the downregulation of circulating "contrasuppressor cells" which reverse T-regulated suppression by providing helper T cell support but which are devoid of conventional Th cell surface markers [32].

The 20 percent of IEL's which are $\alpha\beta$ TCR + are also CD45R0+, a surface marker for cells with prior antigen exposure, giving IEL's a role in immunological memory. The $\gamma\delta$TCR is capable of response to an atypical group of enterocyte antigens such as the enterocyte-expressed CD1d isoforms and non-classical MHC protein groups. The $\gamma\delta$ IEL is thus capable of recognition of partly processed viral and/or bacterial antigen in an MHC-unrestricted fashion. These cells are probably long-lived immunoregulators which equates well with the observation of selective increases in CD4+populations and relative reductions in CD8+ populations only in epithelia covering areas of active antigen absorption, such as the FAE.

It has been speculated that $\gamma\delta$ T cells also function in immune surveillance, maintaining mucosal integrity by eliminating epithelial cells which have become damaged through contact with surface bacteria and heat shock proteins [33]. IEL's also express the surface integrin αEβ7 which is a promoter of TCR activation and also a ligand of the epithelial restitution molecule E-Cadherin. It is possible that the presence of this unusual receptor is important for cells with surveillance capacity and is designed to limit surface inflammatory activity and migration, maintain epithelial continuity and control the selective colonization and stability of autochthonous microbial flora in different parts of the gut.

Lymphocyte Trafficking and Endothelial/Effector Interactions in the LP: the Role of Adhesion Molecules

The extent of migration of lymphocytes in different immune compartments of the gut differs, with lymphocyte movements being substantially greater near the PCV of GALT when compared with the remaining absorptive surface of the gut. The exchange in the system is high with an estimated 2×10^8 cells passing across the GALT daily [34].

The process requires availability of cell type in the circulation, delivery of antigen-specific cells to the intestinal vasculature, endothelial PCV attachment, transendothelial transit, stromal adhesion and release and translymphatic departure. Homing of lymphocytes will vary in accordance with their state of activation, cellular phenotype (CD4+ vs. CD8+) and stromal interactions. In the complicated cell/endothelial interactions which occur near the PCV, several major groups of molecular determinants have been implicated. These include lymphocyte-specific integrins, selectins and carbohydrate determinants and endothelial-specific adhesins, addressins and selectins. Integrins and immunoglobulin-like molecules are constitutively expressed on the lymphocyte surface and include very-late-activation antigens (VLA) whose ligands are VCAM-1 and fibronectin, LFA-1 (lymphocyte function-associated antigen) and CD11a/CD18 (ligands ICAM-1 and ICAM-2 respectively), L-Selectins (ligands mucosal endothelial cell antigens (MECA) determinants) and Sialyl-Lewis X antigens (ligands E (endothelial)-selectins).

Mucosal endothelial addressins include MadCAM-1 (which is also a major integrin ligand and which is strongly constitutively expressed on PP and lamina propria venules), ICAM-1, ICAM-2 and E-Selectin. The selectins are important ligand molecules in the adhesion of lymphocytes to the specialized high endothelial venules of the PP epithelium and mesenteric lymph nodes [35,36].

Cytokine Microenvironment in the LP

Local cytokine production within this lymphoid compartment will either trigger or suppress acute cellular responses, induce chemotaxis of the monocyte/macrophage lineage, stimulate effector mitogenesis, cell differentiation and epithelial restitution and (as already mentioned), control local sIgA production. The generated Th1 cell referred to above has been implicated in coeliac disease [37], cow's milk allergy syndrome [38], specialized food sensitivities [39] and graft vs. host disease (GVHD) following small bowel transplantation [40,41]. Although much is

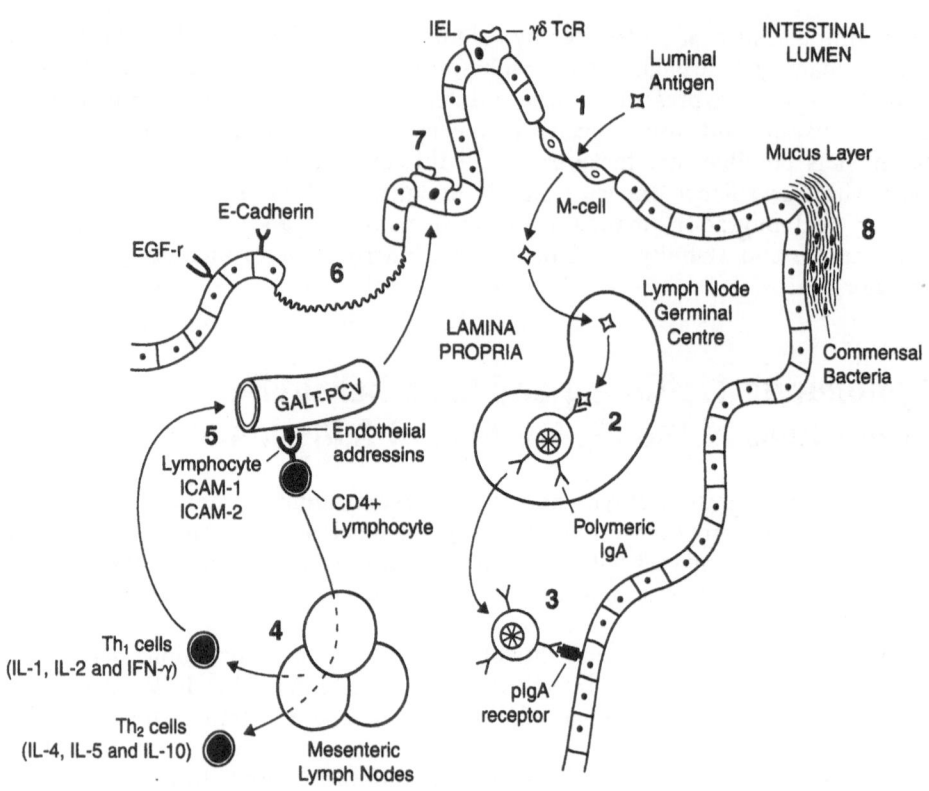

Figure 19c.1. An overview of mucosal immunology and defence in a Peyer's patch. Legend: EGF-r: Epidermal growth factor receptor; IEL: Intra-epithelial lymphocyte; $\gamma\delta$ TcR: $\gamma\delta$ T-cell receptor; M cell: M (microfold) cell; pIgA: Polymeric surface IgA; GALT: Gut-associated lymphoid tissue; PCV: Post-capillary venule. The mucosal barrier represents a balance between tolerance towards innocuous haptens and local defence directed against harmful antigen. A number of specific immunological activities are directed by the mucosal border: (1). Antigen presentation occurs at the specialized M (microfold) cell. (2). Antigen processing occurs in the germinal centres of lymphoid accumulations with B cell immunoglobulin switching towards surface IgA production. (3). Surface IgA adheres antigen to the luminal surface in polymeric form binding to specific polymeric IgA receptors located on the basal surface of epithelial cells. (4). Lymphocyte trafficking occurs from the GALT through mesenteric lymph nodes and via the systemic circulation. Lymphocytes in draining lymph nodes are divisible into Th1 cells producing IL-1, IL-2 and IFN-γ. These cells are responsible for cell-mediated immunity in the lamina propria. Th2 lymphocytes produce immunoregulatory IL-4,IL-5 and IL-10 and direct humoral responsiveness. (5). Homing of CD4+ (T helper) lymphocytes occurs in the GALT tissues directed by GALT-PCV expression of specific endothelial addressins. These are recognized by CD4+ lymphocytes in the lamina propria expressing ICAM-1, ICAM-2 and MadCAM receptors. (6). Initiation of epithelial restitution is under the partial direction of E-Cadherin and trefoil peptides. Restitution will limit the entry of potentially harmful antigens. (7). A small percentage of CD4+ lymphocytes migrate to the epithelial surface as intra-epithelial lymphocytes (IEL's). These express $\gamma\delta$ T-cell receptors and have limited proliferative capacity. They are believed to be involved in the generation of immunological memory and mucosal lymphoid downregulation (tolerance) towards innocuous haptens and peptides. (8). Non-immunological physical defence mechanisms against injury include the mucus barrier itself, intermittent peristalsis and the competitive effects of commensal bacteria trapped in the mucus layer.

known about cytokines and their complex reactions, there has been relatively little research on the importance for mucosal immunology of the cytokine receptors necessary for their function. They are divisible into the haematopoietic receptors, the interferon receptors and the TNF/Nerve growth factor receptors. These systems are related to apoptotic cell mechanisms operating by receptor/transducer molecule redundancies. The importance of both cytokine agonists and cytokine receptor antagonists such as IL-1 receptor antagonist (IL-1Ra) and humanized anti-TNF-α monoclonal antibodies are currently being investigated in experimental colitides [42,43].

Non-immune Mechanisms of Mucosal Defence

The induction by some antigens of anergy and other antigens of intense mucosal inflammation may in part also be a result of non-immune mechanisms. Physical barriers to antigen entry and processing include the mucus barrier itself, the presence of epithelial tight junctions and intermittent peristalsis. Chemical factors in the lumen may also modify antigen, altering epitopes presented to the lymphoid network. This "luminal processing" includes the action of salivary amylase and lysozyme, gastric acid and pepsin and intestinal/pancreatic proteases. Bacterial and viral commensal subpopulations will also alter the availability and possibly the conformation of harmful epitopes. Continuous epithelial renewal must be linked to the limitation of antigen presentation although it is unknown at present how luminal surveillance peptides and rapid response trefoils involved in epithelial restitution interrelate with mucosal immune defence [44].

A diagrammatic overview of the main mechanisms implicated in the mucosal immune network is shown in Figure 19c.1.

References

1. Toy LS, Mayer L. Basic and clinical overview of the mucosal immune system. Seminars in Gastrointestinal Disease 1996;7(1):2–11.
2. Elson CO, McCabe RP. The immunology of inflammatory bowel disease. In Shorter RG, edtiro. Inflammatory bowel disease 4th Ed. Baltimore: Williams & Wilkins, 1995; 203–52.
3. MacDonald TT, Spencer J. Lymphoid cells and tissues of the gastrointestinal tract. In Heaton RV, editor. Gastrointestinal and Hepatic Immunology. Cambridge Reviews in Clinical Immunology. Cambridge: Cambridge University Press, 1994; 1–23.
4. Brantzaeg P, Bjerke K. Immunomorphological characteristics of human Peyer's patches. Digestion 1990;46(Suppl 2):262–73.
5. Cornes JS. Number, size and distribution of Peyer's patches in the human small intestine. Part 1. The development of Peyer's patches. Gut 1965;6:230–3.
6. Trier S. Structure and function of intestinal M cells. Gastroenterology Clinics North America 1991;20(3):531–47.
7. Owen RL, Jones AL. Epithelial cell specialization within human Peyer's patches: an ultrastructural study of intestinal lymphoid follicles. Gastroenterology 1974;66:189–203.
8. Mayer L, So LP, Yio XY, Small G. Antigen trafficking in the intestine. Ann New York Academy Sciences 1996;778:28–35.
9. Ottaway CA. Lymphocyte migration to the gut mucosa. In Heaton RV, editor. Gastrointestinal and hepatic immunology cambridge reviews in clinical immunology. Cambridge: Cambridge University Press. 1994; 24–47.
10. Sanderson IR, Walker WA. Uptake and transport of macromolecules by the intestine:possible role in clinical disorders(an update).Gastroenterology 1993;104:622–39.

11. MacDonald TT, Spencer J. Cell-mediated immune injury in the intestine. Gastroenterology Clinics North America 1992;21(2):367-86.

12. Bandeira A, Mota-Santos T, Itohara S, Degermann S, Heusser C, Tonegawa S, et al. Localization of γ/δ T cells to the intestinal epithelium is independent of normal microbial colonization. J Exp Med 1990;172:239-44.

13. Allan CH, Mendrick DL, Trier JS. Rat intestinal M cells contain acidic endosomal-lysosomal compartments and express class II major histocompatibility determinants. Gastroenterology 1993;104:698-708.

14. Jarry A, Robaszkiewicz MN, Brousse N, Potet F. Immune cells associated with M cells in the follicle-associated epithelium of Peyer's patches in the rat: An electron and immunoelectron microscopic study. cell Tissue Research 1989;255:293-8.

15. Owen RL, Apple RT, Bhalla DK. Morphometric and cytochemical analysis of lysosomes in rat Peyer's patch follicle epithelium:their reduction involume fraction and acid phosphatase content in M cells compared to adjacent enterocytes. Anat Rec 1986;216:521-7.

16. Wolf JL, Rubin DH, Finberg R. Intestinal M cells: a pathway for entry of reovirus into the host. Science 1981;212:471-2.

17. Inman LR, Cantey JR. Specific adherence of escherichia coli (strain RDEC-1) to membranous (M) cells of the Peyer's patch in escherichia coli diarrhoea in the rabbit. J Clin Invest 1983;71: 1-8.

18. Marcial MA, Madara JL. Cryptosporidium:cellular localization,structural anlysis of absorptive cell-parasite membrane-membrane interactions in guinea pigs and suggestion of protozoan transport by M cells.Gastroenterology 1986;90:583-94.

19. Kawanishi H, Saltzman L, Strober W. Mechanisms regulating IgA class-specific immunoglobulin production in murine gut-associated lymphoid tissues.I. T cells derived from Peyer's patches that switch sIgM B cells to sIgA cells in vitro. J Exp Med 1983;157:433-50.

20. Lebman DA, Nomura DY, Coffman RL, Lee FD. Molecular characterization of germ line immunoglobulin A transcripts produced during transforming growth factor type β-induced isotype switching. Proc Natl Acad Sci USA 1990;87:3962-6.

21. Coffman RL, Seymour BWP, Lebman DA, Hiraki DD, Christiansen JA, Shrader B, et al. The role of helper T cell products in mouse B cell differentiation and isotype regulation. Immunol Rev 1988;102:5-28.

22. Mestecky J, McGhee JR. Immunoglobulin A (IgA) :molecular and cellular interactions involved in IgA biosynthesis and immune response. Adv Immunol 1987;40:153-245.

23. James SP, Graeff AS, Zeitz M. Predominance of helper-inducer T cells in mesenteric lymph nodes and intestinal lamina propria of normal non-human primates. Cell Immunol 1987;107:372-83.

24. MacDermott RP, Franklin GO, Jenkins KM, Kodner IJ, Nash GS, Weinrieb IJ. Human intestinal mononuclear cell.I.Investigation of antibody-dependent,lectin-induced and spontaneous cell-mediated cytotoxic capabilities. Gastroenterology 1980;78:47-56.

25. Targan S, Britvan L, Kendal R, Vimadalal S, Soll A. Isolation of spontaneous and interferon inducible natural killer-like cells from human colonic mucosa:lysis of lymphoid and autologous epithelial target cells. Clin Exp Immunol 1983;54:14-22.

26. Gibson PR, Jewell DP. The nature of the natural killer (NK) cell of human intestinal mucosa and mesenteric lymph node. Clin Exp Immunol 1985;61:160-8.

27. Barrett TA,Bluestone JA. Development of TCR γδ IELs. Seminars in Immunol 1995;7(5):299-305.

28. Cerf-Bensussan N, Guy-Grand D. Intestinal intraepithelial lymphocytes. In Mucosal Immunology: Basic Principles.Gastroenterol Clin Nth America 1991;20(3):549-76.

29. Guy-Grand D, Cerf-Bensussan N, Malissen B, Malassis-Seris M, Briottet C, Vassalli P. Two gut intraepithelial (CD8+) lymphocyte populations with different T cell receptors: a role for the gut epithelium in T cell differentiation. J Exp Med 1991;173:471-81.

30. Kruisbeek AM, Amsen D. Mechanisms underlying T-cell tolerance. Curr Opin in Immunol 1996;8:233-44.

31. Brandtzaeg P. History of oral tolerance and mucosal immunity. Ann NY Acad Sci 1996;778:1-27.

32. Kitamura K, Kiyono H, Fujihashi K, Eldridge JH, Beagley KW, McGhee JR. Isotype-specific immunoregulation. Systemic antigen induces splenic contrasuppressor cells which support IgM and IgG subclass but not IgA responses. J Immunol 1988;140:1385-92.

33. Musch MW, Chang EB. Heat shock proteins as physiological and clinically relevant mediators of intestinal epithelial protection. In: McLeod RS, Martin F, Sutherland LR, Wallace JL, Williams CN, editors. Trends in inflammatory bowel disease therapy. Dordrecht: Kluwer Academic Publishers, 1997; 3-7.

34. Ottaway CA. Lymphocyte migration to the gut mucosa. In: Heatley RV, editor. Gastrointestinal and

hepatic immunology. Cambridge Reviews in Clinical Immunology. Cambridge: Cambridge University Press, 1994; 24–47.

35. Haynes RO. Integrins: versatility, modulation and signalling in cell adhesion. Cell 1992;69:11–25.
36. Nakache M, Berg E, Streeter P, Butcher EC. The mucosal vascular adressin is a tissue-specific endothelial-cell adhesion molecule for circulating lymphocytes. Nature 1989;337:179–81.
37. Kontakou M, Przemioslo R, Sturgess R et al. Expression of TNF-γδIL-6 and IL-2 mRNA in the jejunum of patients with coeliac disease. Scand J Gastroenterol 1995;30:456–63.
38. Heyman M, Darmon N, Dupont C et al. Mononuclear cells from infants allergic to cow's milk secrete tumour necrosis factor-alpha altering intestinal function. Gastroenterology 1994;106:1514–23.
39. Walker-Smith J. Food sensitive enteropathies. Clin Gastroenterol 1986;15:55–69.
40. Holler E, Kolb HJ, Hintermeier-Knabe R, Mittermuller J, Thierfelder S, Kaul M, Wilmanns W. Role of tumour necrosis factor alpha in acute graft versus host disease and complications following allogeneic bone marrow transplantation. Transplantation Proceedings 1993;25:1234–6.
41. Dallman M, Larsen C, Morris C. Cytokine gene transcription in vascularized organ grafts:analysis using semi-quantitative polymerase chain reaction. J Exp Med 1991;174:493–6.
42. Barrett KE. Cytokines: sources,receptors and signallings. Bailliere's Clinical Gastroenterology 1996;10(1):1–15.
43. Przemioslo RT, Ciclitira PJ. Cytokines and gastrointestinal disease mechanisms. Bailliere's Clinical Gastroenterology 1996;10(1):17–32.
44. Poulsom R. Trefoil Peptides. Bailliere's Clinical Gastroentreology 1996;10(1):113–34.

20. The Immunology of Inflammatory Bowel Disease

N. Chadwick and D.P. Jewell

Introduction

Inflammatory bowel disease (IBD), encompassing Crohn's disease and ulcerative colitis, is an immune-mediated condition of unknown aetiology. It is possible that a single infectious agent is responsible for these diseases, however, it is generally believed that chronic intestinal inflammation results from an inability to down-regulate the host immune response against enteric bacteria following an initial breach of the intestinal mucosal barrier. It is likely that a range of environmental and genetic factors also result in this host immune dysfunction. Complex combinations of such factors may give rise to chronic intestinal inflammation, which is subsequently characterised clinically as Crohn's disease or ulcerative colitis (Figure 20.1). Therefore, characterising disease heterogeneity within IBD patients is important in our understanding of the aetiology and pathogenesis of this condition.

Evidence that IBD is the result of a systemic immune dysfunction comes from a number of sources, most notably the various animal models of colitis. In attempts to determine the function of various genes involved with the immune system, researchers have generated transgenic and knockout mice with the result that many have developed chronic intestinal inflammation. Other studies have shown that immunodeficient mice reconstituted with naïve T cells develop chronic colitis characterised by a T helper 1 (Th1) T cell pathology, suggesting that human IBD may result from an unchecked Th1 response. The importance of enteric bacteria in these rodent models is underlined by the finding that similar animals grown in a germ-free environment either fail to develop colitis or develop a milder form of the disease. These animal models of colitis show us that disruption of distinct genes involved with the immune system can lead to a phenotypically similar disease, but whether any of the genes involved with colitis in these rodent models are relevant to human IBD remains to be seen. In any case, these animal models allow us to understand the pathogenesis of chronic intestinal inflammation and provide a convenient system for testing potentially therapeutic drugs.

Evidence of a systemic immune dysfunction in human IBD has come from a report of patients with active CD given allogeneic marrow transplantation for

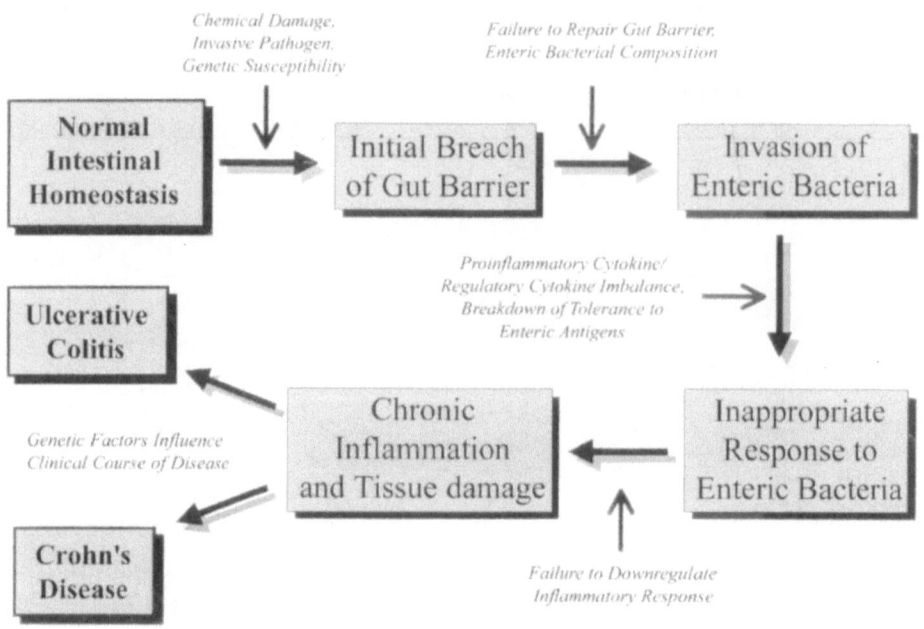

Figure 20.1. Influences involved with the development of IBD.

leukaemia [1]. The replacement of host immune cells with donor cells led to long-term remission in the majority of these patients, suggesting that the host immune system may have been responsible for the original disease. However, immunosuppressive therapies may also have contributed to the control of disease activity, somewhat confusing the overall picture of response.

Genetics of IBD

Recent studies on the familial nature of ulcerative colitis and Crohn's disease have shown that the familial incidence is between 12–18% and that first-degree relatives are the most commonly affected [2]. Furthermore, within a multiply-affected family, there is a high degree of concordance with respect to disease type (UC or CD) and to disease behaviour. This suggests a role for genetic susceptibility and is supported by the failure to find an increased incidence of inflammatory bowel disease in adopted children within an affected family or in the spouses of probands. However, the strongest epidemiological evidence for a genetic factor comes from twin studies. Studies in Sweden [3] and the UK [4] have shown that disease concordance is much higher for monozygotic twins than dizygotic twins. Since members of both types of twins shared similar environments during childhood, this difference in disease incidence is almost certainly genetic. Furthermore, for monozygotic twins, concordance rates are higher if one member of a pair has

Crohn's disease suggesting a higher genetic component for Crohn's disease than for ulcerative colitis. Even so, the concordance rate was still only 45 percent in Sweden and less in the UK, indicating a relatively minor role for susceptibility genes. The mode of inheritance is not clear and the difficulties are compounded by the fact that ulcerative colitis and Crohn's disease may not be distinct diseases; there may well be considerable disease heterogeneity.

Nevertheless, the use of microsatellite markers, which are distributed throughout the genome, has allowed genome-wide searches to be made to determine linkage between disease type and candidate loci on specific chromosomes. These linkage analyses have identified loci on chromosomes 1, 2, 3, 5, 6, 7, 12, 14 and 19 which appear to contain susceptibility genes. These regions of linkage are large and attempts are now being made to narrow them to less than 1 CM in order to attempt gene isolation. Even then, the genetic region may contain a hundred or more genes, many of which may not yet have been sequenced and characterised.

The most widely replicated linkage region has been a peri-centromeric locus on chromosome 16 which is specific for Crohn's disease and is not shared with ulcerative colitis. Recently, a gene has been identified (NOD2) in this region which is mutated in about 20 percent of Crohn's patients compared with only 2 percent of the normal population [5,6]. The gene encodes for a protein which acts as an intra-cellular receptor for bacterial lipopolysaccharide with the subsequent activation of NF-kB.

Within the other loci of linkage there are known genes, many of which may be relevant to a generalized chronic inflammatory response. These include genes for mucins (chromosome 7), chemokine receptors (chromosome 3), integrins (chromosome 12), growth factors (chromosome 12), interleukin (IL)-4 receptor (chromosome 16) and E-cadherins (chromosome 16). Many of these are polymorphic and studies are in progress to determine whether specific polymorphisms are associated with particular diseases.

So far, the candidate gene approach has been most productive in terms of HLA-Class I and II alleles. Studies from Japan [7] and Los Angeles [8] have suggested that HLA-DR2 is more frequently represented in ulcerative colitis patients although this has not been so for European populations. However, HLA genes may influence the clinical characteristics of the disease. Thus HLA-DRB1*0103 (a rare allele of DR1) is associated with severe disease and the frequent need for colectomy. Similarly, the HLA-DR3, DQ2 haplotype appears to be associated with extensive disease, especially in females and is also associated with primary sclerosing cholangitis. HLA alleles also seem to determine whether or not a patient with either ulcerative colitis or Crohn's disease will develop some of the other extra-intestinal manifestations. Thus, patients who have HLA-B27, -B35, and -DR103 are much more likely to develop an acute, reactive arthropathy in association with a relapse of their disease, whereas those who are HLA-B44 are more likely to develop a persistent small joint arthropathy. It is interesting that only about 60 percent of IBD patients who develop ankylosing spondylitis are positive for HLA-B27 compared with more than 90 percent of sporadic ankylosing spondylitis. Thus, both Crohn's disease and ulcerative colitis are polygenic disorders that share some genes which appear to confer an overall susceptibility to developing a chronic inflammatory disease of the intestine in response to a variety of environmental factors. The precise disease that develops appears to be influenced by "disease-specific" genes and yet other genes may control the course and behaviour of the disease.

Animal Models of Colitis

In recent years, many models of colitis have been reported, some bearing closer resemblance to human IBD than others. Four types of animal models exist: i) spontaneous models, ii) chemically-induced models, ii) knockout and transgenic models, and iv) reconstituted models. These are summarised in Table 20.1.

Spontaneous Models

A well-studied spontaneous model is the cotton-top tamarin model, which bears a close resemblance to ulcerative colitis in humans, resulting in the formation of crypt abscesses, neutrophil infiltration and mucin depletion [9]. Interestingly, the

Table 20.1. Some important experimental models of IBD

Rodent Model	Pathology	Possible Mechanisms	Bacterial Influence
IL-2 KO	Acute and chronic colitis	Inhibition of development of regulatory T cells Inhibition of epithelial restitution	Yes
IL-2R KO	Colitis	Inhibition of development of regulatory T cells Inhibition of epithelial restitution	?
IL-10 KO	Enterocolitis	Lack of important regulatory cytokine → Th1 response	Yes
TGF-β1 KO	Multi-organ inflammation, ileitis and colitis	Lack of important regulatory cytokine → Th1 response	?
HLA-B27 Tg	Gastritis and enterocolitis	Mechanism of presentation of luminal antigens → immunopathogenic response	Yes – Bacteriodes vulgatus
β2-microglobulin Tg	Gastritis and enterocolitis	Defective antigen processing and presentation	Yes
TCRα / TCRβ KO	Colitis	Inhibition of development of regulatory T cells	?
MHC class II KO	Acute colitis	Inhibition of development of regulatory T cells Lack of tolerance-inducing antigen presentation mechanisms	?
CD45 RB[hi] reconstituted SCID	Chronic colitis	Unregulated Th1 response to enteric bacteria	Yes – Helicbacter hepaticus
N-cadherin dominant-negative KO	Focal enteritis	Defective gut barrier function → repeated bacterial invasion	?
TNBS-induced colitis	Colitis	Haptenisation of host antigens → immunopathogenic response	Yes

monkeys only appear to develop disease in captivity and not in the wild. As in human disease, the types of colitis are phenotypically diverse and inheritance of disease is not Mendelian. Increased faecal tumour necrosis factor (TNF)-α levels have been reported, similar to human IBD and the inflammation is responsive to current therapies for human IBD, such as prednisolone.

Chemically-induced Models

Many chemically-induced models of colitis are characterised by a self-limiting acute disease from which the animals recover and are therefore not strictly models of *chronic* human IBD. These models include the acetic acid-induced model, the dextran sodium sulphate model and the trinitrobenzene sulphonic acid (TNBS) model. Of these, the TNBS model has been used to study the phenomenon of oral tolerance.

The normal gut encounters a vast array of foreign antigens (from food and enteric bacteria) and yet remains in a state of low level inflammation without developing a chronic inflammatory response. The term "oral tolerance" has been used to describe this phenomenon although the mechanisms behind this tolerance to frequently encountered non-pathogenic foreign antigens are not well understood (See Chapter 19).

Rats given an intra-rectal instillation of TNBS develop an acute colitis (characterised by a massive neutrophil infiltrate and crypt abscesses) resulting from the host immune response against self antigens haptenised by TNBS. However, rats fed these potentially immunogenic proteins prior to TNBS injection do not develop colitis [10].

Further rodent studies have shown that large and small doses of orally administered antigens induce tolerance through different mechanisms. It is thought that large doses of soluble antigen lead to "clonal anergy" whereby antigen-specific T cells become unable to proliferate in response to subsequent exposure to the same antigen. Alternatively, apoptosis (programmed cell death) of antigen-specific T cells may occur, preventing responses to further antigen challenge. Tolerance to low doses of antigen is thought to be mediated by specific cytokines such as, IL-10, transforming growth factor (TGF)-β and monocyte chemotactic protein (MCP)-1. These cytokines are released by antigen-specific T cells within the Peyer's patches and lamina propria and prevent the development of an immunopathogenic response driven by Th1 CD4+T cells specific for the same antigen [11]. This is shown diagrammatically in Figure 20.2. As well as preventing activation of antigen-specific T cells, this secretion of tolerance-inducing T cells may have a "bystander effect," whereby several different T cell clones are affected, inducing tolerance to a wider range of antigens. This is particularly important in the gut mucosa where a vast array of bacterial antigens are encountered in close proximity.

Knockout and Transgenic Models

In contrast to acute models of colitis, models involving manipulation of an animal's immune system often results in a chronic wasting disease, bearing a closer resemblance to human IBD and are therefore of more use in terms of dissecting the immunopathogenic mechanisms involved with chronic colitis [12]. Knockout (KO) mice have provided some intriguing insights into mechanisms involved with

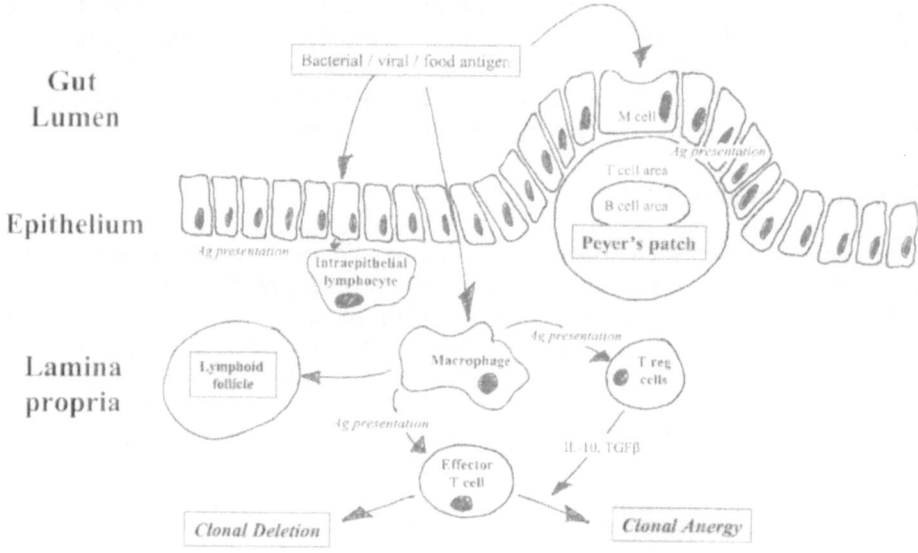

Figure 20.2. Antigen presentation and oral tolerance within the small intestinal mucosa.

the development of chronic colitis. These mice contain a particular genetic deletion leading to the absence of the respective gene product. The IL-10 and TGF-β knockout mice develop colitis that can be explained by the absence of these immunoregulatory cytokines leading to an uncontrolled immunopathogenic response. The colitis that develops in IL-2 and IL-2R knockout mice is more difficult to explain given that IL-2 is involved with T cell activation. However, T cell activation via the IL-2R has been shown to be necessary for proliferation of a T cell subset involved with regulating the immune response (regulatory T cells). In addition, IL-2 is also involved with epithelial cell proliferation and so an IL-2 or IL-2R deficiency may prevent restitution of the epithelium following an initial breach, leading to repeated bacterial invasion and chronic inflammation.

The importance of gut barrier function is highlighted in the case of the N-cadherin transgenic mouse, which has been manipulated to develop patches of intestinal mucosa lacking this cell adhesion molecule [13]. Inflammation develops in these regions of deficient gut barrier function presumably due to the repeated invasion of luminal bacteria and poor epithelial restitution.

T cell receptor (TCR) α or β chain knockout mice have also been shown to develop colitis as do MHC class II knockout mice. These deletions are thought to lead to abnormalities in T cell development resulting in a failure to delete auto-antigen-reactive effector T cells populations or a failure to expand regulatory T cell populations. Alternatively, MHC class II knockout mice may fail to present antigen in a tolerance-inducing manner to mucosal T cells, eliciting an immune response to luminal antigens and subsequent inflammation.

Rats transgenic for human HLA-B27 have also been shown to develop colitis. HLA-B27 has been shown to be a risk factor for a number of human diseases, such as ankylosing spondylitis. Presumably, the manner in which antigen is presented via HLA-B27 on antigen presenting cells elicits a pro-inflammatory response. In addition, rats transgenic for β2-microglobulin also develop colitis, probably due to defective antigen processing and presentation mechanisms leading to inappropriate immune responses.

Reconstituted Model

A reconstituted mouse model of colitis has provided valuable insights into which cell types are responsible for the development of intestinal inflammation. This model involves the isolation of T cell subsets from the spleen of normal mice that are then reconstituted into severe combined immunodeficient (SCID) mice [14]. Reconstitution of SCID mice with CD45RB^{hi} CD4+ T cells (naïve T cells) results in the development of chronic wasting colitis characterised by mononuclear cell infiltration, epithelial hyperplasia and goblet cell depletion. Experiments have shown that these naïve T cells differentiate into Th1 CD4+ T cells following reconstitution and are responsible for the development of colitis. This disease can be prevented by the concurrent addition of the CD45RB^{low} subset of CD4+ T cells (memory T cells) which contain the CD4+ regulatory T cell population (characterised by expression of the IL-2 receptor, CD25).

Th1 cells mediate disease via the production of pro-inflammatory cytokines such as TNFα and IFNγ, leading to a cell-mediated response, while cytokines such as IL-10 and TGFβ produced by regulatory T cells within the CD45RB^{low} T cell population inhibit this cell-mediated response

Role of Bacteria

In all of these animal models, it has been shown that growth in germ-free conditions prevents or attenuates the development of colitis. In some models, the specific bacterial pathogen responsible for the development of intestinal inflammation has been sought. For instance, *Bacteriodes vulgatus* has been shown to be important in the development of colitis in the HLAB27 transgenic rat, while *Helicobacter hepaticus* has been shown to be important in the CD45RB^{hi} reconstituted model. The emerging picture from these various models of colitis is that different types of intestinal inflammation are mediated by different bacterial pathogens. Moreover, the genetic background of the animal may also influence which bacterial species modulate disease activity. The complexity of the relationship between the enteric flora and the development and progression of colitis in these models may have important implications in the treatment of human disease.

These experimental models of colitis improve our understanding of normal gut immunology and provide insights into which molecules and which cell subsets may be responsible for the development of human disease. In particular, models show that distinct defects in T cell regulation, activation and development as well as antigen presentation, can lead to the development of phenotypically similar chronic intestinal inflammation.

Cytokine Profiles in Human IBD

Is the development of human IBD mediated by Th1 or Th2-type inflammation, or a combination of both? Much research has focused on the type of ongoing T cell response in human IBD by analysing material for Th1 and Th2 cytokines. However, many studies have used end-stage diseased intestinal tissue for cytokine analysis (because of the problems associated with obtaining early-stage IBD tissue), revealing high levels of most cytokines (both pro-inflammatory and regulatory). These cytokine profiles of end-stage disease probably result from secondary inflammatory events and may have little bearing on the type of immune response involved in the initial development of IBD. Nonetheless, there are several studies analysing cytokine production in IBD tissue which provide insights into the disease immunopathogenesis.

There are several lines of evidence suggesting that Crohn's disease is driven by an unregulated immunopathogenic Th1 response to luminal bacterial antigens [15]. Similarly, ulcerative colitis may result from an unregulated Th2 response, although there is little evidence for this at present other than an a murine model of colitis which is mediated by IL-4 [16]. Several studies have attempted to overcome the problems with using end-stage disease tissue by using biopsies from ulcerative colitis from patients who have undergone colectomy and ileo-anal pouch formation. A small proportion (about 20%) of these patients develop inflammation of the newly formed pouch which resembles the original colitis. Therefore follow-up biopsies of ulcerative colitis patients after ileo-anal anastomosis (IAA) generates a tissue bank containing (in some cases) early-stage disease tissue. This tissue can be used to analyse the early immunological events associated with the development of chronic intestinal colitis. A summary of cytokine levels in human IBD is shown in Table 20.2.

Recently, markers of T cell subsets have been identified (such as certain chemokine receptors) which may permit the identification of immune response types in IBD. These markers have been used to indicate the presence of Th1 CD4+ T cells in the inflammatory lesions of patients with rheumatoid arthritis and ulcerative colitis [17]. Perhaps more importantly, the IL-12R β2 chain has been identified as a key Th1 T cell marker and is involved with Th1 cell development via IL-12 released from antigen-presenting cells such as macrophage and dendritic cells.

Th1 and Th2 Cell Development

The fate of T cell development (following antigen presentation) appears to be dependent upon the type of antigen presenting cell. Recent work has shown that at least 2 functionally distinct dendritic cell subsets are present (termed DC1 and DC2 cells) which can mediate T cell development towards the Th1 and Th2 phenotype, respectively [18.19].

In humans, the DC1 cells are derived from the myeloid lineage and express CD11c whereas DC2 cells are thought to be lymphoid-derived and express CD123 (the IL-3 receptor). DC1 and DC2 cells are capable in vitro of presenting antigen to T cells and inducing the development of Th1 and Th2 cells, respectively. Expression of particular cytokines and costimulatory molecules by dendritic cells determines the fate of T cell development.

Pro-inflammatory Cytokines

Many studies have sought to determine the relative expression of various pro-inflammatory cytokines in human IBD. Not surprisingly, most pro-inflammatory cytokines have been shown to be upregulated in active disease compared with

Table 20.2: Selected cytokine profiles in human IBD

Cytokine	Predominant cell types	Function	Status in IBD
Proinflammatory			
IFNγ	NK cells, Th1 CD4+ T cells, CD8+ T cells	Induces HLA class II expression on epithelial cells, promotes leukocyte infiltration. Decreases IL-10 production	↑ in IBD
TNFα	Monocytes, Th1 T cells macrophages,	Activation of endothelium. Induction of proinflammatory cytokines	↑ in Crohn's
IL-1	Macrophages	Induction of IL-6 and IL-8 synthesis	↑ in IBD
IL-2	T cells	T cell proliferation	↑ in IBD
IL-5	Th2 T cells	Eosinophil activation. IgA synthesis	↑ in UC ↓ in Crohn's
IL-6	Monocytes	B cell differentiation. Induction of acute phase proteins	↑ in IBD
IL-12	Dendritic cells, macrophages	Th1 T cell differentiation	↑ in Crohn's ? in UC
IL-15	Epithelial cells, macrophages	Early T cell activation and poliferation	↑ in IBD ↑ in inactive UC
IL-18	Dendritic cells	Th1 T cell differentiation	↑ in Crohn's
Regulatory			
IL-4	TCRγδ T cells, regulatory T cells	Inhibition of Th1 cell function and differentiation	↓ in Crohn's
IL-10	Th2 T cells, regulatory T cells	Inhibits IL-12 production and Th1 T cell differentiation. Inhibition of proinflammatory cytokine expression	↑ in IBD
TGFβ	Regulatory T cells, epithelial cells	Inhibition of Th1 cell function and differentiation. Epithelium restitution. Mediates fibrosis. Decrease IgG and IgM secretion	↑ in IBD

inactive disease and normal control tissue. These include interferon (IFN)-γ, TNF-α and interleukins 1, 2, 4, 6, 12, 13, 15 and 18.

IL-12 is an important Th1 cytokine, expressed by activated macrophages and dendritic cells inducing naïve T cell differentiation towards the Th1 phenotype. Mechanistically, IL-12 and IL-18 synergise to induce IFNγ expression by naïve T cells which leads to their differentiation into Th1 cells [20]. In addition, IL-12 also inhibits Th2-cell polarisation, further promoting a cell-mediated immune response. High levels of IL-12 and IL-18 have been demonstrated in Crohn's disease tissues [15,21] although the expression levels in ulcerative colitis patients have not been well characterised at this time.

IFNγ is produced by natural killer (NK) cells, Th1 CD4+ T cells and CD8+ T cells in response to IL-12 and IL-18 stimulation and high expression has been demonstrated in Crohn's disease tissue [22]. IFN-γ induces HLA class II expression on epithelial cells (and other cell types), and adhesion molecule expression on circulating leukocytes, leading to increased leukocyte infiltration into inflammatory lesions.

Increased TNF-α levels have been observed in inflamed IBD tissue (particularly in Crohn's disease tissue) compared with inactive and control tissue [23]. TNF-α in produced by activated monocytes, macrophages and Th1 CD4+ T cells and induces various pro-inflammatory events such as cytokine and chemokine release from epithelial cells and endothelial cells, resulting in increased leukocyte trafficking and activation. As well as inducing typical cell-mediated Th1 responses, TNF-α also induces Th2 responses such as histamine release by mast cells and basophils. Since TNF-α is able to non-specifically induce pro-inflammatory events, it represents an important target and a final common pathway for immunotherapeutic strategies.

IL-2 and IL-15 share several pro-inflammatory effects since they share a common receptor subunit. IL-15 is believed to be produced at the early stages of inflammation by epithelial cells and macrophages, inducing IL-2 expression by T cells and inhibiting T cell apoptosis. IL-2 expression induces T cell activation and proliferation in an autocrine fashion and also downregulates IL-15 expression. Several studies have shown increased IL-15 production in active IBD and more interestingly, in inactive ulcerative colitis when compared with normal control tissue [24]. Therefore it may be the case that an unregulated overproduction of IL-15 in ulcerative colitis may induce abnormal T cell activation, leading to chronic inflammation.

IL-1 expression has also been shown to be altered in IBD with increased circulating and tissue levels in active disease. IL-1 is produced by activated macrophages whereas its natural inhibitor, IL-1 receptor antagonist (IL-1ra) is produced by monocytes, macrophages and neutrophils. An imbalance between IL-1 and IL-1ra expression levels has been reported in IBD [25], although this phenomenon may well be a result of the ongoing chronic inflammatory processes.

Increased IL-6 expression by activated monocytes has been demonstrated in IBD patients when compared with control patients [26]. IL-6 is a multi-potent cytokine which mediates the differentiation of B cells into mature immunoglobulin-secreting cells. The expression of IL-5, (a typically Th2 cytokine involved in eosinophil activation), has been shown to be up-regulated in ulcerative colitis tissue but not in Crohn's disease tissue [22], supporting the hypothesis that ulcerative colitis may be mediated by a Th2-dominant response.

Two recent papers have shown that mutations in the NOD2 gene may play an important role in the development of Crohn's disease [5,6]. NOD2 is thought to regulate the activity of the transcription factor Nuclear Factor-κB (NF-κB) in response to lipopolysaccharide, a component of the bacterial cell wall. NF-κB is important in inflammation as it transcribes several pro-inflammatory cytokines and therefore mutations in NOD2 may prevent the normal regulation of NF-κB, leading to an inappropriate inflammatory response against normal enteric bacteria.

In summary, the levels of most pro-inflammatory cytokines are increased during active disease, probably as a result of positive feedback mechanisms within the mucosal immune system, given the redundancy of the cytokine network. Of special interest are cytokines which are differentially expressed in Crohn's disease and ulcerative colitis tissue; most notably, IL-5, IL-12 and IL-15, as these findings may represent different and relatively disease-specific underlying immunopathogenic mechanisms.

Regulatory Cytokines

The expression of regulatory cytokines in IBD has also been the subject of intense interest. Many of these cytokines play a role in the development of Th2-type inflammation but they also downregulate cell-mediated responses and are considered regulatory. For instance, IL-4, IL-10 and IL-13 are produced by Th2 CD4+ T cells and are involved with their development, as well as inhibiting Th1 CD4+ cell development and activation. Indeed, a low level of IL-4 expression by resident intestinal T cells of the TCRγδ phenotype may be essential in preventing Th1 responses and maintaining homeostasis within the intestinal mucosa. Decreased IL-4 expression has been shown within the lamina propria of Crohn's disease tissue [15] (compared with control tissue) although this may be a consequence of the different cell types present within the inflamed mucosa when compared with normal tissue.

IL-10 is produced both by Th2 and regulatory CD4+ T cells as well as epithelial cells and is a potent inhibitor of Th1-type immune responses, inhibiting IL-12 production by dendritic cells and macrophages. No striking differences have been found, however, between IBD and control tissue in terms of IL-10 expression, possibly reflecting a failure of the host immune system to down-regulate an inflammatory response once established.

TGF-β is a key regulatory cytokine produced by a range of cell types including epithelial cells and regulatory CD4+ T cells. In the CD45RB^{hi}-reconstituted murine model colitis, treatment with anti-TGF-β antibodies abolished the protection of colitis by the CD45RB^{low} subset of CD4+ T cells, indicating that TGF-β production by the regulatory population of CD4+ T cells is essential in down-regulating Th1 cell responses. TGF-β inhibits pro-inflammatory cytokine production and it has been postulated that a reciprocal relationship between IFN-γ and TGF-β responses regulates the occurrence and activity of mucosal inflammation. In this regard, TGF-β expression has been shown to be increased in active IBD, suggesting a regulatory response to established disease [27]. This cytokine has also been shown to play a role in epithelial restitution following injury, therefore high TGF-β levels may represent an attempt to repair damaged epithelium. Interestingly, TGF-β induces fibrin and collagen deposition by fibroblasts and so the production of TGF-β as an attempt to switch off a Th1 response may give rise to fibrosis of surrounding tissue leading an important secondary complication which is the *sine qua non* of Crohn's disease.

Chemokines

Several studies have sought to determine the role of various chemokines in IBD. Chemokines are a rapidly expanding group of chemotactic cytokines which co-ordinate leukocyte trafficking. Several pro-inflammatory cytokines, such as IL-1 and TNF-α induce chemokine expression by a range of cell types, including epithelial and endothelial cells. Different chemokines have chemo-attractant effects on different cell types depending on their chemokine receptor expression.

IL-8 (originally described as a cytokine) predominantly attracts neutrophils via its receptor CXCR1 and has been shown to be up-regulated in IBD tissue [28]. Also, epithelial neutrophil-activating peptide 78 (ENA-78) has been shown to be up-regulated on the epithelium in active and inactive IBD tissue compared with control tissue [29]. Therefore, IL-8 and ENA-78 may play an important role in neutrophil infiltration in IBD. RANTES (Regulated upon Activation, Normal T-Expressed and Secreted) has been shown to be up-regulated in IBD tissue, inducing T cell infiltration via its receptors CCR3, CCR4 and CCR5. Similarly, increased expression of monocyte chemotactic protein-1 (MCP-1) has been demonstrated in active IBD tissue, accounting for monocyte infiltration via its receptor CCR2 [30].

Infiltration of different T cell subsets may be determined by chemokine expression within inflammatory lesions. For instance, secondary lymphoid tissue chemokine (SLC) may predominantly attract Th1 CD4+ T cells via the CXCR3 and CCR7 receptors, while thymus and activation-regulated chemokine (TARC) may predominantly attract Th2 CD4+ T cells via the CCR4 and CCR8 receptors. Interestingly, SLC activates $\alpha 4\beta 7$ integrin (the ligand for the intestinal mucosa-specific receptor mucosal addressin adhesion molecule (MAdCAM)-1) on circulating leukocytes, emphasising the potential importance of this chemokine in intestinal inflammation. (See Chapter 19) Chemokines are also able to co-ordinate the infiltration of different cell types within an inflammatory lesion and may play a role in the development of Th1 and Th2 responses, but much remains to be discovered about their role in IBD.

Humoral Responses in IBD

Immunoglobulin Production

Secretory IgA (sIgA) is produced by a subset of B cells within the intestinal lamina propria and binds to antigen within the gut lumen, providing a first line of defence by preventing invasion of microbes. In addition, these sIgA/antigen complexes may be taken up by Peyer's Patches within the small bowel as a mechanism of sampling antigen within the gut lumen.

Decreased sIgA production has been shown in IBD patients [31] although this may be due to a displacement of resident sIgA-producing B cells by activated IgG-producing plasma cells during chronic inflammation. An increase in IgG_1 and IgG_2-producing plasma cells has been observed in ulcerative colitis and Crohn's disease, respectively [32]. IgG_2 is a less effective complement-fixing immunoglobulin than IgG_1 and the production of this subtype in Crohn's disease may lead to defective antigen clearance and a persistence of immunopathogenic antigens.

Auto-antibodies

Antibodies against host antigens have been widely described in IBD patients. Antibodies against colonic epithelial cell antigens have been described [33] and may result from cross-reactivity with enteric bacterial antigens. Such antibodies could lead to immune-mediated damage to the gut barrier and the development of chronic inflammation. However, the evidence for such a mechanism remains controversial and the presence of such antibodies may be a secondary phenomenon resulting from exposure of epithelial antigens not usually encountered by the host immune system following damage to the epithelium.

The same explanation could be used for the presence of antibodies against the 40kD antigen described by Das and colleagues, and anti-neutrophil cytoplasmic antibodies (ANCA) in IBD patients. The 40kD antigen is expressed in several tissues including the intestinal epithelium where it has been shown to be reactive with IgG and complement in patients with ulcerative colitis and antibodies to this antigen have been detected in the sera of ulcerative colitis patients [34]. It is possible that an autoimmune reaction against this antigen may precipitate a breakdown in gut barrier function, although the evidence for this remains controversial. The exact nature of the antigen is also uncertain and its identification as an isoform of tropomyosin has yet to be confirmed.

A perinuclear distribution of ANCA termed pANCA has been described in the sera of patients with ulcerative colitis, colonic Crohn's disease, sclerosing cholangitis and autoimmune hepatitis [35]. At least one target antigen of pANCA is a nuclear histone protein but the role of these antibodies in chronic inflammation is still unclear, although it is possible that they play a role in the resolution of inflammation by inducing neutrophil apoptosis.

The presence of pANCA has been used in combination with other criteria as a diagnostic test for ulcerative colitis. Similarly, the presence of anti-*Saccharomyces cerevisiae* antibodies (ASCA) can be used to improve the diagnostic accuracy of Crohn's disease and the ratio of ANCA to ASCA has recently been used as a diagnostic tool to help differentiate ulcerative colitis from Crohn's disease [36].

Complement

Complement activation is an integral part of the humoral immune system, however, inappropriate activation may lead to tissue damage and chronic inflammation. Antibody-antigen interactions induce complement activation, leading to the opsonisation of invading microbes (See Chapter 1). In addition, components of the complement pathway also activate cells of the innate immune system (eg. basophils, neutrophils and mast cells) as well as non-immune cells, (most notably, smooth muscle cells and endothelial cells).

Increased levels of complement components have been described in IBD. Serum levels of the C3 product C3c, have been shown to be significantly higher in Crohn's disease than in ulcerative colitis [37] and activated C3b products have been detected on the inflamed surface epithelium in ulcerative colitis tissue [38]. Deposits of complement components have also been shown on the endothelium in IBD tissue, possibly involved with the secondary vasculitis believed to perpetuate some of the inflammatory events. It is likely that abnormal complement activation results from on-going chronic inflammatory events and a generalised increase in immunoglobulin production.

Apoptosis and IBD

The importance of apoptosis in intestinal inflammation has only recently been revealed. The intriguing differences between ulcerative colitis and Crohn's disease, in terms of the cell types and their frequency undergoing apoptosis, suggest that this phenomenon plays an important role in IBD.

Apoptosis occurs in normal gut tissue as part of the general turnover of cells. Here, epithelial cells constantly migrate from the crypts to the surface epithelium where they undergo apoptosis and are phagocytosed by macrophages or shed into the lumen. During immune responses, T cells undergo apoptosis when activated unless they receive a specific set of molecular signals preventing the triggering of apoptosis. Apoptosis of activated T cells is thought to play a major role in the resolution of inflammation in the gut, preventing the development of chronic intestinal inflammation. Also, apoptosis of effector T cells within the lamina propria may be a mechanism involved with the generation of oral tolerance.

Although apoptosis is mediated by a complex combination of molecules, two molecules in particular, Fas and Fas ligand (FasL), play a major role. The intestinal epithelium constitutively expresses Fas and when FasL is also present, epithelial cells undergo apoptosis. In ulcerative colitis, high levels of FasL have reproducibly been shown to be expressed by T cells within the lamina propria, inducing a high frequency of epithelial cell apoptosis [39].

This high frequency of epithelial cell apoptosis may disrupt mucosal barrier function leading to a chronic inflammatory response to invading luminal bacteria. Additionally, lamina propria phagocytes may be unable to deal with this high level of apoptosis resulting in the uncontrolled release of intracellular molecules which can invoke a particular inflammatory response.

It is possible that peripheral blood T lymphocytes produce more FasL than resident lamina propria lymphocytes and increased levels of FasL production in inflamed gut may be explained by the infiltration of peripheral T cells. This would indicate that epithelial cell apoptosis in ulcerative colitis is a secondary phenomenon important in the perpetuation of chronic inflammation. However, increased levels of apoptosis have been demonstrated in uninvolved colonic tissue from ulcerative colitis patients, suggesting that epithelial cell apoptosis is an early event in the development of chronic intestinal inflammation [40].

In contrast, no increase in lamina propria lymphocyte apoptosis or FasL expression is observed in Crohn's disease tissue when compared with normal tissue [39]. This may reflect a decreased susceptibility of infiltrating T cells to undergo apoptosis following activation, leading to a prolonged and self-perpetuating inflammatory response. In addition, this may represent a breakdown in tolerance to luminal antigens, such that reactive T cells continue to proliferate and secrete cytokines rather than undergo clonal deletion.

From this evidence, it appears that apoptosis plays a major role in the perpetuation of chronic intestinal inflammation. The clear differences between ulcerative colitis and Crohn's disease in terms of apoptosis may indicate different underlying immunopathogenic mechanisms. However, evidence against a primary role for apoptosis in the development of IBD comes from the observation that Fas or FasL-deficient mice do not develop chronic colitis. Whether or not apoptosis is important in the actual early development of IBD is uncertain, although the molecular pathways involved with apoptosis may represent novel targets for immunotherapeutic strategies.

Gut Barrier Function

The intestinal epithelium is a key component of the gut barrier. As well as physically preventing the influx of bacteria, goblet cells of the epithelium secrete mucin which provides a first line of defence against invasive bacteria. Mucin is a complex glycoprotein and its composition and expression has been the focus of much interest in terms of ulcerative colitis. Nicotine has been shown to induce colonic mucin synthesis [41], an interesting finding given that smoking confers protection against ulcerative colitis (but not Crohn's disease).

Intestinal epithelial cells express adhesion molecules such as E-cadherin which plays a key role in gut barrier function by providing tight junctions between epithelial cells. In addition, E-cadherin forms junctions between epithelial cells and CD8+ intraepithelial lymphocytes via αEβ7 integrin. In an elegant series of experiments, a dominant negative E-cadherin transgenic mouse was produced which develops focal chronic inflammation in areas where expression of the E-cadherin gene has been switched off [14]. This underlines the importance of an intact epithelial barrier in maintaining the homeostasis of the underlying mucosa.

The epithelium of the small intestine is also composed of "M cells" which overlay lymphoid follicles forming Peyer's Patches and play a specialised role in the uptake and presentation of particulate antigen (such as bacterial antigens) to underlying lymphocytes. Epithelial cells are also capable of antigen uptake and presentation via MHC class II molecules. Class II expression is up-regulated by pro-inflammatory cytokines, suggesting that in inflamed tissue, class II expression by epithelial cells may partially direct an inflammatory response.

Epithelial cells are also capable of presenting antigen to intra-epithelial cells (IELs) in non-classical pathways via the cell surface molecule, CD1d. IFNγ upregulates CD1d expression on the intestinal epithelium and increases antigen presentation to lamina propria lymphocytes. However, the particular groups of antigens presented by these pathways remains to be determined in IBD.

Intestinal epithelial cells have been shown to express a ligand for CD8+ IELs termed gp180. IELs activated by gp180 have been shown to have a regulatory function and levels of gp180 expression in active and inactive IBD tissue have been shown to be lower than in normal tissue [42]. These data are supported by results showing that intestinal epithelial cells from IBD patients preferentially activate CD4+ T cells, whereas cells isolated from normal patients activate suppresser CD8+ T cells [43]. This has led to the hypothesis that a reduced gp180 expression pattern in the epithelium of IBD tissue may prevent regulatory CD8+ lymphocytes from suppressing immunopathogenic responses within the intestinal mucosa, leading to the development of chronic inflammation.

It has been shown that intestinal epithelial cells can produce a wide range of cytokines upon bacterial invasion and also upon exposure to pro-inflammatory cytokines [44]. Among the most widely studied of these are IL8 and MCP-1, which induce neutrophil and monocyte chemotaxis, respectively. Of interest, it has been shown that invasion of epithelial cells with different bacterial species induces different patterns of chemokine and cytokine expression, underlining the complex relationship between enteric bacteria and the intestinal epithelium.

TGF-β, epidermal growth factor (EGF) and hepatocyte growth factor (HGF) can mediate epithelial cell restitution following epithelial injury and it is possible that an abnormal expression of these molecules may prevent healing following injury, leading to repeated bacterial invasion and the development of chronic inflammation [45]. In support of this, it has been shown that treatment of rats with EGF protects against TNBS-induced colitis. Trefoil peptides are also important in epithelial cell differentiation and proliferation and increased expression has been shown in areas of ulceration within Crohn's disease tissue [46]. Mice lacking intestinal trefoil factor suffer from extensive colitis when given a chemical assault such as dextran sodium sulphate [47] suggesting an importance for these peptides in human IBD.

Short chain fatty acids (SCFAs) play an important role in the function of the intestinal epithelium. SCFAs are produced by luminal bacteria and are thought to provide an energy source for colonic epithelial cells where a metabolic defect in SCFA oxidation may be involved with the development of ulcerative colitis. The most widely studied SCFA is butyrate which has been shown to influence the biology of the colonic epithelium by modulating the expression of Bax, (a molecule which induces Fas-mediated apoptosis). It has been shown that butyrate prevents the expression of Bax, protecting the colonic epithelium against excessive Fas-mediated apoptosis [48]. Butyrate also modulates chemokine and cytokine production by physically interacting with epithelial cell DNA, inducing the expression of IL-8 while suppressing the expression of MCP-1 [49]. Therefore, abnormal butyrate levels in the colon may induce an inappropriate immune response to invading bacteria. Sulphate-reducing bacteria within the intestinal lumen metabolise butyrate and may be involved with altered butyrate levels possibly leading to the development of colitis. Dietary changes which increase the levels of enteric sulphate-reducing bacteria may therefore influence disease susceptibility. So far, attempts to treat ulcerative colitis patients with SCFAs have, however, proved largely unsuccessful.

Oligoclonal T Cell Responses

As discussed earlier, it has been shown that lamina propria T cells have a limited T-cell receptor (TCR) repertoire when compared with peripheral T cells. This ability to recognise only a limited number of foreign antigens may be due to the restricted presentation of these antigens by the intestinal epithelium. In attempts to define the lamina propria TCR repertoire in IBD, researchers have used a PCR-based methodology. PCR amplification of the gene sequence encoding the variable region of the TCR (the Vβ chain) leads to products of different sizes, reflecting the different T cell specificities in a given sample of cells. Therefore, if many T cell clones were expanded, PCR products of many sizes would be produced, whereas if only a few T cell clones were expanded, a smaller number of PCR product sizes would be produced. The latter case would presumably reflect a T-cell response to a single antigen or a group of similar antigens. This has been shown to be the case in ulcerative colitis and Crohn's disease with a restricted number of PCR product sizes when compared with normal controls [50].

Sequencing of the PCR products enables the amino acid sequence of the T-cell receptor to be determined. Comparison of these sequences between expanded T-cell clones within the same individual has revealed close similarities. More importantly, sequences from different individuals have also showed similarities, suggesting that in IBD there may be a limited T-cell repertoire response against a single antigen, or group of closely related (possibly bacterial) antigens. It may be possible in the future to use these TCRs to elucidate the antigen or antigens driving the T cell response in patients with IBD.

Current Therapeutic Strategies

Steroids

Corticosteroids have been used successfully to treat IBD for many years although the mechanisms of steroid action have only recently been elucidated. Steroids bind to steroid receptors on the cell surface and this steroid/receptor complex is internalised and migrates to the cell nucleus where it can modulate gene expression directly via steroid-responsive elements. These elements are associated with many genes with immunological functions and activation of these elements prevents the expression of many pro-inflammatory cytokines.

Steroid/receptor complexes may also interact with transcription factors in the cell cytoplasm. NF-kB is a transcription factor which induces the transcription of several pro-inflammatory cytokines and is usually bound to its inhibitor, ikB, in the cell cytoplasm. In response to certain pro-inflammatory stimuli, NF-kB dissociates from ikB and migrates to the nucleus. There is evidence to suggest that steroids stabilise ikB and prevent its degradation, thus preventing the migration of NF-kB to the nucleus and the transcription of pro-inflammatory cytokines. There is also evidence to suggest that steroids may induce apoptosis of leukocytes, (although the mechanisms remain obscure) and that they may regulate the synthesis of colonic mucin [41].

The serious side effects of long-term steroid usage limit the efficacy of this treatment. To overcome this problem, a modified steroid, budesonide, has been produced which has a 90 percent first-pass metabolism, limiting the systemic effects of steroid treatment. Additionally, steroids are often administered in enema form to treat colonic disease and reduce the systemic dosage. In some cases of chronic inflammation, the disease becomes resistant to steroid treatment. This steroid-refractory disease may arise due to a down-regulation of steroid receptors on the cell surface or may be due to inflammatory mechanisms which are independent of steroid modulation.

Other Therapies

Other commonly used treatments for IBD include the immunomodulatory drugs cyclosporin, 6-mercaptopurine, azathioprine, and methotrexate [51]. Cyclosporin is a selective, reversible immunosuppressor of T lymphocytes via its action on the transcription factor, nuclear factor of activated T cells (NFAT: See Chapter 6). 6-Mercaptopurine and azathioprine are steroid-sparing agents, both causing immunosuppression by interfering with nucleic acid metabolism in the immunological sequence which follows antigenic stimulation. The mechanisms of action of methotrexate involve the inhibition of thymidylate, purine and methionine synthesis with the accumulation of adenosine; a potent anti-inflammatory mediator. These actions inhibit cellular proliferation, decrease the formation of antibodies and inhibit the production of specialized mediators of inflammation such as the interleukins and eicosanoids.

Monoclonal antibodies to TNF have been recently developed for clinical use in steroid-resistant Crohn's disease and a chimeric IgG1 antibody (Infliximab: Centocor, Malvern Pa) is now licensed for the treatment of chonic active Crohn's disease unresponsive to steroids and immunosuppressives and for the management of fistulae [52,53]. About two-thirds of patients treated for either indication appear to respond to this new therapy. However, the duration respite is usually fairly limited and relapses are frequently seen over the subsequent few months. One trial has recently shown that infusions of antibody every 3 months are beneficial over the course of one year but at the end of that period there was little difference compared with the placebo-treated group. Side-effects have, however, been minimal. Acute hypersensitivity reactions can occur, especially in patients having repeat infusions when the time between infusions has exceeded one year and the reactions are associated with the development of high circulating titres of anti-chimeric antibodies. There is some concern about the 10-15% of patients who develop antibodies to dsDNA but the titres are low and they are transient. Of greater concern is the possibility of lymphoma, which seems exceptionally rare, as well as the potential for activation of tuberculosis. Patients who might have had TB in the past must therefore be screened before receiving antibody.

Future Therapeutic Strategies

Several new immunotherapeutic strategies are currently undergoing trials for the treatment of IBD. These include treatment with anti-α4β7 antibodies, new anti-TNF-α antibodies and agents, (such as Thalidomide), recombinant IL-10 and anti-sense therapy against intercellular adhesion molecule (ICAM)-1. Monoclonal antibodies specific for β7 integrin and mucosal addressin cell adhesion molecule-1 (MAdCAM-1) appear to reduce inflammation in the colon of the CD45RB^{hi} model of colitis [54]. Subsequently, it has been demonstrated that antibodies against the α4β7 integrin attenuate disease in the cotton top tamarin model of colitis [55]. In these studies, the short and long-term effects of single doses of antibody indicates that this antibody may somehow down-regulate immune responses within the mucosa as well as inhibit lymphocyte trafficking to the intestinal mucosa. Human trials with monoclonal antibodies directed against the α4β7 integrin are currently underway.

Anti-sense therapy is also undergoing trials for the treatment of IBD. This therapy involves the administration of short sequences of DNA (oligonucleotides) which have been chemically modified to increase their half-life. Such sequences are specific for target messenger RNA (mRNA) sequences and form hybrid oligonucleotide-RNA molecules within cells. This hybrid formation prevents translation of the mRNA into protein and also induces degradation of the target mRNA by host enzymes. In this manner, anti-sense therapy prevents the expression of specific proteins. Anti-sense therapy against ICAM-1 has been shown to be effective in preventing rejection of transplanted tissue in human trials and and promising results have been obtained using this approach to treat patients with steroid-refractory Crohn's disease [56].

Treatment with recombinant IL-10 (rIL-10) may also have therapeutic value in the management of IBD. In the TNBS model of colitis, treatment with rIL-10 attenuates disease severity and human trials are currently underway. Chemokines and their receptors represent good targets for future immunotherapeutic strategies. The relatively small size of chemokine molecules enables the ready design of pharmacological inhibitors and antagonists. The design of such molecules will permit the blocking of specific leukocyte infiltration pathways. Several molecules have already been synthesised to treat HIV-infected patients since the human immunodeficiency virus uses chemokine receptors such as CXCR4 and CCR5 as co-receptors for viral entry. Recently, modified RANTES molecules have been designed to bind to CCR5, but not to lead to uncontrolled intra-cellular signalling events. Since CCR5 is predominantly expressed on monocytes and Th1 CD4+ T cells, such antagonists may prove effective in blocking T cell and monocyte infiltration in IBD. Moreover, the rapidly expanding group of chemokines and their receptors represents a growing number of targets for this type of therapeutic strategy.

The recent findings showing a link between NOD2 and Crohn's disease [5,6] indicate that NF-κB is a key component of the inflammatory pathway in this disease. The importance of NF-κB is further underlined by the fact that several effective current therapeutic agents (including steroids) inhibit NF-κB, albeit non-specifically. Future treatments for Crohn's disease (at least for patients carrying NOD2 mutations) may involve the specific inhibition of NF-κB activity or alternatively, restoring the normal function of NOD2.

Conclusions

It is clear that the host immune system plays a central role in the progression of IBD. However, it remains unclear as to the overall importance of the immunological contribution to the aetiology of IBD. Genetically-manipulated murine models of colitis provide strong evidence that an underlying immunological dysfunction may play a major role in the development of chronic intestinal inflammation. However, the evidence for such a dysfunction in human IBD patients is so far uncertain. Data from genetic studies would suggest that combinations of susceptibility genes may give rise to phenotypically similar disease states. In this manner, the inheritance of specific genetic polymorphisms on their own may be insufficient to generate chronic inflammation. However, the inheritance of several of these polymorphisms may be sufficient to confer a significant degree of disease susceptibility. Work on NOD2 has shown how powerful genetic studies can point the finger of blame at particular components of inflammatory pathways. Similar complex immunogenetic studies will reveal other components of the inflammatory cascade that behave aberrantly in IBD and such knowledge will be essential for the design of future immunotherapeutic strategies directed against an increasing range of relatively disease-specific targets.

References

1. Lopez-Cubero SO, Sullivan KM, McDonald GB. Course of Crohn's disease after allogeneic marrow transplantation. Gastroenterology 1998; 114(3): 433–40.
2. Satsangi J, Jewell DP, Bell JI. The genetics of inflammatory bowel disease. Gut 1997; 40(5): 572–4.
3. Tysk C, Lindberg E, Jarnerot G, Floderus-Myrhed B. Ulcerative colitis and Crohn's disease in an unselected population of monozygotic and dizygotic twins. A study of heritability and the influence of smoking. Gut.1988; 29(7): 990–6.
4. Thompson NP, Driscoll R, Pounder RE, Wakefield AJ. Genetics versus environment in inflammatory bowel disease: results of a British twin study. BMJ 1996; 312(7023): 95–6.
5. Ahmad T, Satsangi J, McGovern D, Bunce M, Jewell DP. Review article: the genetics of inflammatory bowel disease. Aliment Pharmacol Ther 2001;15:731–748.
6. Ogura Y, Bonen DK, Inohara N, Nicolae DL, Chen FF, et al. A frameshift mutation in NOD2 associated with susceptibility to Crohn's disease. Nature. 2001; 411(6837): 603–6.
7. Hugot JP, Chamaillard M, Zouali H, Lesage S, Cezard JP, Belaiche J, et al. Association of NOD2 leucine-rich repeat variants with susceptibility to Crohn's disease. Nature 2001; 411(6837): 599–603.
8. Hugot JP, Laurent-Puig P, Gower-Rousseau C, Olson JM, Lee JC, Beaugerie L, et al. Mapping of a susceptibility locus for Crohn's disease on chromosome 16. Nature 1996; 379(6568): 821–23.
9. Asakura H, Tsuchiya M, Aiso S, Watanabe M, Kobayashi K, Hibi T, et al. Association of the

human lymphocyte-DR2 antigen with Japanese ulcerative colitis. Gastroenterology 1982; 82(3): 413-8.

10. Warren BF. Cytokines in the cotton top tamarin model of human ulcerative colitis. Aliment. Pharmacol. Ther.1996; 10 Suppl 2: 45-7.

11. Elson CO, Beagley KW, Sharmanov AT, Fujihashi K, Kiyono H, et al. Hapten-induced model of murine inflammatory bowel disease: mucosa immune responses and protection by tolerance. J Immunology 1996; 157(5): 2174-85.

12. Weiner HL. Oral tolerance: immune mechanisms and treatment of autoimmune diseases. Immunology Today 1997; 18(7): 335-43.

13. Powrie F, Leach MW. Genetic and spontaneous models of inflammatory bowel disease in rodents: evidence for abnormalities in mucosal immune regulation. Ther Immunol 1995;2(2):115-23.

14. Hermiston ML, Gordon JI. Inflammatory bowel disease and adenomas in mice expressing a dominant negative N-cadherin. Science 1995; 270(5239): 1203-7.

15. Leach MW, Bean AG, Mauze S, Coffman RL, Powrie F. Inflammatory bowel disease in C.B-17 scid mice reconstituted with the CD45RBhigh subset of CD4+ T cells. Am. J. Pathology 1996;148(5):1503-15.

16. Parronchi P, Romagnani P, Annunziato F, Sampognaro S, Becchio A, Giannarini L, et al. Type 1 T-helper cell predominance and interleukin-12 expression in the gut of patients with Crohn's disease. Am J Pathology 1997;150(3):823-32.

17. Boirivant M, Fuss IJ, Chu A, Strober W. Oxazolone colitis: A murine model of T helper cell type 2 colitis treatable with antibodies to interleukin 4. J Exp Med 1998;188(10):1929-39.

18. Qin S, Rottman JB, Myers P, Kassam N, Weinblatt M, Loetscher M, et al. The chemokine receptors CXCR3 and CCR5 mark subsets of T cells associated with certain inflammatory reactions. J Clin Invest 1998;101(4):746-54.

19. Moser M, Murphy KM. Dendritic cell regulation of TH1-TH2 development. Nat. Immunol 2000;1(3):199-205.

20. Reid SD, Penna G, Adorini L. The control of T cell responses by dendritic cell subsets. Curr Opin Immunol 2000;12(1):114-21.

21. Tominaga K, Yoshimoto T, Torigoe K, Kurimoto M, Matsui K, Hada T, et al. IL-12 synergizes with IL-18 or IL-1beta for IFN-gamma production from human T cells. Int Immunol 2000;12(2):151-60.

22. Pizarro TT, Michie MH, Bentz M, Woraratanadharm J, Smith MF Jr, Foley E, et al. IL-18, a novel immunoregulatory cytokine, is up-regulated in Crohn's disease: expression and localization in intestinal mucosal cells. J.Immunol 1999; 162(11):6829-35.

23. Fuss IJ, Neurath M, Boirivant M, Klein JS, de la Motte C, Strong SA, et al. Disparate CD4+ lamina propria (LP) lymphokine secretion profiles in inflammatory bowel disease. Crohn's disease LP cells manifest increased secretion of IFN-gamma, whereas ulcerative colitis LP cells manifest increased secretion of IL-5. J Immunology 1996;157(3):1261-70.

24. Breese EJ, Michie CA, Nicholls SW, Murch SH, Williams CB, Domizio P, et al. Tumor necrosis factor alpha-producing cells in the intestinal mucosa of children with inflammatory bowel disease. Gastroenterology.1994; 106(6):1455-66.

25. Sakai T, Kusugami K, Nishimura H, Ando T, Yamaguchi T, Ohsuga M, et al. Interleukin 15 activity in the rectal mucosa of inflammatory bowel disease. Gastroenterology 1998;114(6):1237-43.

26. Casini-Raggi V, Kam L, Chong YJ, Fiocchi C, Pizarro TT, Cominelli F. Mucosal imbalance of IL-1 and IL-1 receptor antagonist in inflammatory bowel disease. A novel mechanism of chronic intestinal inflammation. J Immunology 1995;154(5):2434-40.

27. Reinecker HC, Steffen M, Witthoeft T, Pflueger I, Schreiber S, MacDermott RP, et al. Enhanced secretion of tumour necrosis factor-alpha, IL-6, and IL-1 beta by isolated lamina propria mononuclear cells from patients with ulcerative colitis and Crohn's disease. Clin Exp Immunology 1993;94(1):174-81.

28. Babyatsky MW, Rossiter G, Podolsky DK. Expression of transforming growth factors alpha and beta in colonic mucosa in inflammatory bowel disease. Gastroenterology 1996;110(4):975-84.

29. Mazzucchelli L, Hauser C, Zgraggen K, Wagner H, Hess M, Laissue JA, et al. Expression of interleukin-8 gene in inflammatory bowel disease is related to the histological grade of active inflammation. Am J Pathology 1994;144(5):997-1007.

30. Z'Graggen K, Walz A, Mazzucchelli L, Strieter RM, Mueller C. The C-X-C chemokine ENA-78 is preferentially expressed in intestinal epithelium in inflammatory bowel disease. Gastroenterology 1997;113(3):808-16.

31. Mazzucchelli L, Hauser C, Zgraggen K, Wagner HE, Hess MW, Laissue JA, et al. Differential in situ expression of the genes encoding the chemokines MCP-1 and RANTES in human inflammatory bowel disease. J Pathology 1996;178(2):201-6.

32. MacDermott RP, Nash GS, Nahm MH. Antibody secretion by human intestinal mononuclear cells from normal controls and inflammatory bowel disease patients. Immunol Invest 1989; 8(1-4):449–57.

33. Kett K, Rognum TO, Brandtzaeg P. Mucosal subclass distribution of immunoglobulin G-producing cells is different in ulcerative colitis and Crohn's disease of the colon. Gastroenterology 1987;93(5):919–24.

34. Fiocchi C, Roche JK, Michener WM. High prevalence of antibodies to intestinal epithelial antigens in patients with inflammatory bowel disease and their relatives. Ann Intern Med 1989;110(10):786–94.

35. Biancone L, Mandal A, Yang H, Dasgupta T, Paoluzi AO, Marcheggiano A, et al. Production of immunoglobulin G and G1 antibodies to cytoskeletal protein by lamina propria cells in ulcerative colitis. Gastroenterology 1995;109(1):3–12.

36. Kallenberg CG, Mulder AH, Tervaert JW. Antineutrophil cytoplasmic antibodies: a still-growing class of autoantibodies in inflammatory disorders. Am J Med 1992;93(6):675–82.

37. Ruemmele FM, Targan SR, Levy G, Dubinsky M, Braun J, Seidman EG. Diagnostic accuracy of serological assays in pediatric inflammatory bowel disease. Gastroenterology 1998;115(4):822–9.

38. Elmgreen J, Both H, Binder V. Familial occurrence of complement dysfunction in Crohn's disease: correlation with intestinal symptoms and hypercatabolism of complement. Gut 1985;26(2):151–7.

39. Halstensen TS, Mollnes TE, Garred P, Fausa O, Brandtzaeg P. Surface epithelium related activation of complement differs in Crohn's disease and ulcerative colitis. Gut 1992;33(7):902–8.

40. Ueyama H, Kiyohara T, Sawada N, Isozaki K, Kitamura S, Kondo S, et al. High Fas ligand expression on lymphocytes in lesions of ulcerative colitis. Gut 1998;43(1):48–55.

41. Iwamoto M, Koji T, Makiyama K, Kobayashi N, Nakane PK. Apoptosis of crypt epithelial cells in ulcerative colitis. J Pathology 1996;180(2):152–9.

42. Finnie IA, Campbell BJ, Taylor BA, Milton JD, Sadek SK, Yu LG, et al. Stimulation of colonic mucin synthesis by corticosteroids and nicotine. Clin Sci Colch 1996;91(3):359–64.

43. Toy LS, Yio XY, Lin A, Honig S, Mayer L. Defective expression of gp180, a novel CD8 ligand on intestinal epithelial cells, in inflammatory bowel disease. J Clin Invest 1997;100(8):2062–71.

44. Mayer L, Eisenhardt D. Lack of induction of suppressor T cells by intestinal epithelial cells from patients with inflammatory bowel disease. J Clin Invest 1990;86(4):1255–60.

45. Jung HC, Eckmann L, Yang SK, Panja A, Fierer J, Morzycka-Wroblewska E, et al. A distinct array of proinflammatory cytokines is expressed in human colon epithelial cells in response to bacterial invasion. J Clin Invest 1995;95(1):55–65.

46. Podolsky DK. Healing the epithelium: solving the problem from two sides. J. Gastroenterology 1997;32(1):122–6.

47. Wright NA, Poulsom R, Stamp G, Van Norden S, Sarraf C, Elia G, et al. Trefoil peptide gene expression in gastrointestinal epithelial cells in inflammatory bowel disease. Scand J Gastroenterology Suppl 1992;193:76–82.

48. Mashimo H, Wu DC, Podolsky DK, Fishman MC. Impaired defense of intestinal mucosa in mice lacking intestinal trefoil factor. Science 1996;274(5285):262–5.

49. Hass R, Busche R, Luciano L, Reale E, Engelhardt WV. Lack of butyrate is associated with induction of Bax and subsequent apoptosis in the proximal colon of guinea pig. Gastroenterology 1997; 12(3):875–81.

50. Fusunyan RD, Quinn JJ, Ohno Y, MacDermott RP, Sanderson IR. Butyrate enhances interleukin (IL)-8 secretion by intestinal epithelial cells in response to IL-1beta and lipopolysaccharide. Pediatr Res 1998;43(1):84–90.

51. Probert CS, Chott A, Turner JR, Saubermann LJ, Stevens AC, Bodinaku K, et al. Persistent clonal expansions of peripheral blood CD4+ lymphocytes in chronic inflammatory bowel disease. J Immunology 1996;157(7):3183–91.

52. Targan SR, Hanauer SB, van Deventer SJ, Mayer L, Present DH, Braakman T, et al. A short-term study of chimeric monoclonal antibody cA2 to tumor necrosis factor alpha for Crohn's disease. Crohn's Disease cA2 Study Group. N Engl J Med 1997;337(15):1029–35.

53. Present DH, Rutgeerts P, Targan S, Hanauer SB, Mayer L, van Hogezand RA, et al. Infliximab for the treatment of fistulas in patients with Crohn's disease. N Engl J Med 1999;340(18):1398–405

54. Choi PM, Targan SR. Immunomodulator therapy in inflammatory bowel disease. Dig. Dis. Sci. 1994; 39(9): 1885–92.

55. Picarella D, Hurlbut P, Rottman J, Shi X, Butcher E, Ringler DJ. Monoclonal antibodies specific for beta 7 integrin and mucosal addressin cell adhesion molecule-1 (MAdCAM-1) reduce inflammation in the colon of scid mice reconstituted with CD45RBhigh CD4+ T cells. J Immunology 1997;158(5):2099–106.

56. Hesterberg PE, Winsor-Hines D, Briskin MJ, Soler-Ferran D, Merrill C, Mackay CR, et al. Rapid resolution of chronic colitis in the cotton-top tamarin with an antibody to a gut-homing integrin alpha 4 beta 7. Gastroenterology 1996;111(5):1373–80.
57. van Dullemen HM, van Deventer SJ, Hommes DW, Bijl HA, Jansen J, Tytgat GN, et al. Treatment of Crohn's disease with anti-tumor necrosis factor chimeric monoclonal antibody (cA2). Gastro-enterology 1995;109(1):129–35.
58. Yacyshyn BR, Bowen-Yacyshyn MB, Jewell L, Tami JA, Bennett CF, Kisner DL, et al. A placebo-controlled trial of ICAM-1 antisense oligonucleotide in the treatment of Crohn's disease. Gastro-enterology 1998;114(6):1133–42.

21. Lymphoproliferative Diseases of the Gastrointestinal Tract

Dorothy Pan, Carol S. Portlock and Martin S. Karpeh

Lymphoproliferative disorders of the gastrointestinal tract represent a diverse group of diseases, including many types of non-Hodgkin's lymphomas. The recognition of specific gastrointestinal lymphoproliferative disorders as discrete entities in newer non-Hodgkin's lymphoma classification schemes has improved diagnostic accuracy and has led to advances in therapy. The surgeon still has a role to play in the staging and diagnosis of lymphoma and in the management of acute complications related to gastrointestinal lymphoma in particular. The latter conditions are frequently secondary to chronic immunosuppression in high-risk patients.

In previous classifications of lymphoid neoplasms, as in the International Working Formulation [1] and Kiel classifications [2], histologic subtypes of non-Hodgkin's lymphomas were grouped according to clinical behavior and assigned specific grades [i.e. low-, intermediate-, or high-grade]. More recently, the Revised European-American Lymphoid [R.E.A.L.] classification [3] as described by the International Lymphoma Study Group and the World Health Organization [WHO] classification of Lymphoid Neoplasms [4,5] have supplanted these schemes. The R.E.A.L. classification stratifies lymphoid neoplasms according to lineage, cellular differentiation and clinical presentation. Through the use of morphologic, immunophenotypic, genetic and clinical features, the R.E.A.L. classification defines distinct entities that now collectively comprise the non-Hodgkin's lymphomas. Table 21.1 shows the WHO classification of non-Hodgkin's lymphomas.

Specific histologies of non-Hodgkin's lymphomas are associated with gastrointestinal tract involvement. The majority of these entities are of B-cell phenotype with T-cell lymphomas accounting for a minority of cases [6]. The more common entities involving the gastrointestinal tract include extranodal marginal zone lymphoma of MALT type, mantle cell lymphoma, diffuse large B-cell lymphoma, Burkitt's lymphoma and intestinal T-cell lymphoma. In the R.E.A.L. classification, two newly defined histologic entities with specific gastrointestinal tract involvement are the extranodal marginal zone lymphoma of MALT-type and the intestinal T-cell lymphoma [3]. Other histologies that involve the gastrointestinal tract less frequently include follicular lymphoma and very rarely Hodgkin's disease [7].

Table 21.1. WHO Classification of Non-Hodgkin's Lymphomas

1. B-cell neoplasms
    Precursor B-cell lymphoblastic leukemia/lymphoma
    Mature B-cell neoplasms
        B-cell chronic lymphocytic leukemia/small lymphocytic lymphoma
        B-cell prolymphocytic leukemia
        Lymphoplasmacytic lymphoma
        Mantle cell lymphoma
        Follicular lymphoma
        Marginal Zone B-cell lymphoma of mucosa-associated lymphoid tissues [MALT] type
        Nodal marginal zone lymphoma +/- monocytoid B cells
        Splenic marginal zone B-cell lymphoma
        Hairy cell leukemia
        Diffuse large B-cell lymphoma
        Burkitt's lymphoma
        Plasmacytoma
        Plasma cell myeloma
2. T-cell neoplasms
    Precursor T-cell lymphoblastic leukemia/Lymphoma
    Mature T-cell and NK-cell neoplasms
        T-cell prolymphocytic leukemia
        T-cell large granular lymphocytic leukemia
        NK-cell leukemia
        Extranodal NK/T-cell lymphoma, nasal type
        Mycosis fungoides
        Sezary Syndrome
        Angioimmunoblastic T-cell lymphoma [unspecified]
        Peripheral T-cell lymphoma [unspecified]
        Adult T-cell leukemia/lymphoma [HTLV-1]
        Systemic anaplastic large cell Lymphoma [T- and null-cell types]
        Primary cutaneous anplastic lage cell Lymphoma
        Subcutaneous panniculitis-like T-cell lymphoma
        Enteropathy-type intestinal T-cell lymphoma
        Hepatosplenic gamma/delta T-cell lymphoma

Harris NL et al. Blood 1994; 84:1361–92 [Reference 3]

The risk factors for non-Hodgkin's lymphoma involving the gastrointestinal tract include environmental causes, viral infections and chronic inflammatory states. Specific etiologies are correlated with subtypes of non-Hodgkin's lymphomas. i.e., Helicobacter pylori-associated chronic gastritis with extranodal marginal zone lymphoma of MALT type, chronic immunosuppression with viral etiologies and celiac disease with intestinal T-cell lymphoma. The mechanisms of pathogenesis will be considered below separately.

Diagnosis and Staging

While the diagnosis of non-Hodgkin's lymphoma is best made on evaluation of lymph node specimens, the use of new molecular tools has aided in the histopathologic evaluation of extranodal tissue specimens. As part of the initial diagnostic evaluation in suspected gastrointestinal tract lymphoma, a complete gastrointestinal evaluation is performed. This includes an upper gastrointestinal endoscopy, colonoscopy and small bowel series. Biopsy specimens should be taken of abnormal mucosa as well as random biopsies of macroscopically non-involved sites [8]. Endoscopic ultrasound of the upper gastrointestinal tract is often used to assess the depth of mucosal involvement [9].

Standard radiographic staging studies include CT scans of the chest, abdomen and pelvis. While CT scans often show little evidence of gastrointestinal abnormalities such as minimal gastric wall thickening in indolent non-Hodgkin's lymphomas, more pronounced findings such as bowel wall thickening, masses and adenopathy are frequently observed in aggressive lymphomas [10]. In the evaluation of aggressive non-Hodgkin's lymphomas, dynamic nuclear imaging tools such as PET scans (where available) [11,12] or gallium scans are also performed, although the PET scan has not been found to be a useful imaging tool for MALT lymphomas thus far [13]. A bone marrow biopsy is also performed as part of routine staging. Table 21.2 shows a recommended diagnostic evaluation protocol for non-Hogkin's lymphoma involving the gastrointestinal tract.

Non-Hodgkin's lymphomas are staged using the Ann Arbor classification for Hodgkin's disease [14] with modifications for non-Hodgkin's lymphomas [15] (Table 21.3). The staging systems frequently used for non-Hodgkin's lymphomas with gastrointestinal tract involvement are modifications of the Ann Arbor classification. The Musshoff staging system [16], the Blackledge staging system [17] and the TNM classification include sub-stages of limited stage disease that define more specifically regional extent of involvement. In the Musshoff staging system (Table 21.4), Stage IIE_1 disease is separated into two distinct subgroups. Stage IIE_1 identifies involvement of the gastric and regional perigastric nodes. Stage IIE_2 refers to gastric involvement with distant abdominal node involvement, such as nodes in the celiac axis. Stage IIE_1 appears to have a similar behavior as Stage IE, while Stage IIE_2 reflects more advanced stage disease with behavior similar to Stage IV [18].

Table 21.2. Diagnostic and staging evaluation of non-Hodgkin's lymphomas involving the gastrointestinal tract

1. Physical Examination: examine peripheral lymph nodes, Waldeyer's ring, spleen and liver
2. Blood work: complete blood count and differential, review of peripheral blood smear, LDH, renal function and liver function
3. Evaluation of the gastrointestinal tract
   a. Esophagogastroscopy; with multiple biopsies
   b. Colonoscopy
   c. Small bowel series
4. Radiographic Imaging
   a. CT scans of the chest/abdomen/pelvis
   b. Gallium scan for aggressive lymphomas
   c. PET scan if needed
5. Pathology review
   a. Histologic review, with classification according to the REAL or WHO classification
   b. Immunophenotyping
   c. Bone marrow biopsy

Table 21.3. Ann Arbor Staging Classification

Stage I	Involvement of a single lymph node region [I] or a single extranodal site [IE]
Stage II	Involvement of two or more lymph node regions on the same side of the diaphragm [II] or localized involvement of an extranodal site and of node or more lymph node regions on the same side of the diaphragm [IIE]
Stage III	Involvement of lymph node regions on both sides of the diaphragm [III], which may also be accompanied by involvement of the spleen or of an extranodal site [IIIE]
Stage IV	Diffuse or disseminated involvement of one or more extranodal organs or tissues, with or without associated lymph node involvement
Substage E	Localized, extranodal disease
Symptoms	"A" to designate absence of constitutional symptoms; "B" to designate presence of constitutional symptoms such as fevers, chills, night sweats, fatigue or weight loss

Table 21.4. Ann Arbor Classification modified by Musshoff

Stage I	Tumor confined to the GI tract without signs of dissemination
Stage II$_1$	Tumor confined to the GI tract with involvement limited to confluent locoregional lymph nodes [gastric or mesenteric]
Stage II$_2$	Tumor within the GI tract with involvement of distant subdiaphragmatic lymph nodes
Stage IV	Distant disease

Musshoff K: Strahlentherapie 1997; 153:218–21 [Reference 16]

MALT Lymphoma [Extranodal Marginal Zone Lymphomas of MALT Type]

Accounting for as much as 40% of lymphomas observed in the gastrointestinal tract [19], MALT lymphomas are classified as extranodal marginal zone lymphomas of MALT type in the R.E.A.L. classification [3]. These lymphomas were previously categorized as low grade small lymphocytic lymphomas in the International Working Formulation [1], but were not defined as a distinct clinicopathologic entity. MALT lymphomas behave as other indolent non-Hodgkin's lymphomas with prolonged survival if disease is confined to the gastrointestinal tract [20]. Compared to the nodal form of marginal zone lymphoma, MALT lymphomas of the gastrointestinal tract generally have longer overall survivals [21]. MALT lymphomas most frequently involve the stomach in areas devoid of endogenous mucosa-associated lymphoid tissue [i.e. "acquired" MALT]. Further discussion in this section will focus on gastric MALT lymphoma.

The development of MALT lymphoma has now been determined to be a multi-step process that first begins with chronic antigenic stimulation by Helicobacter pylori progressing to chronic gastritis. Helicobacter pylori stimulate both T- and B-lymphocytes to proliferate, leading to the development of an abnormal clone of B-lymphocytes. While clonal B-lymphocytes initially depend on T-lymphocytes to proliferate, the neoplastic B-cell population becomes independent of antigen stimulation with accumulation of sequential chromosomal aberrations [22].

Several lines of evidence support the role of Helicobacter pylori infection in the pathogenesis of MALT lymphomas. In clinical studies, Helicobacter pylori have been demonstrated in the gastric mucosa in 70–90% of patients with gastric MALT lymphoma. Further epidemiologic evidence from a large case control study by Parsonnet et al. identified 33 patients with low grade gastric MALT lymphoma and determined that these patients were more likely to have a history of Helicobacter pylori infection when compared with matched controls [23]. Regional studies demonstrate an increased incidence of MALT lymphomas in northeastern Italy and correlation of these lymphomas with an increased prevalence of Helicobacter pylori-associated gastritis [observed in 87 percent of biopsy specimens] [24].

In vitro studies have demonstrated that low grade MALT lymphomas proliferate in the presence of strain-specific Helicobacter pylori-derived T lymphocytes, but not in the presence of Helicobacter pylori alone [25]. Hussell et al. have subsequently demonstrated that tumor-infiltrating T-cells that are Helicobacter pylori-specific allow the growth of a malignant B cell clone that is responsible for MALT lymphoma [26]. More recently, patient-specific polymerase chain reaction [PCR] has been utilized to demonstrate that clonal B-cell populations exist prior to the development of MALT lymphoma. Using allele-specific PCR, histologically confirmed Helicobacter pylori gastritis specimens were shown to harbor clonal B-cell populations prior to the development of MALT lymphoma [27].

Multiple molecular events have been uncovered in MALT lymphomagenesis. (Table 21.5) The t(11;18)(q21;q21) reciprocal chromosomal translocation is observed in approximately 50% of MALT lymphomas and appears to be specific for extranodal marginal zone lymphoma, as it has not been identified in nodal or splenic marginal zone lymphomas or in other subtypes of non-Hodgkin's lymphomas. The t(11;18)(q21;q21) translocation represents the fusion of the apoptosis inhibitor gene, API2, on chromosome 11q21 with the novel MLT/MALT1 gene on chromosome 18q21. The function of MLT/MALT1 gene has not been elucidated, but the structure of the protein it encodes is known to contain several immunoglobulin–like C2-type domains. It is postulated that the MLT/MALT1 gene may play a role in normal hematopoiesis [28,29,30].

Late transforming events include the t(1;14)(p22;q32) translocation which results in dysregulation of the BCL-10 oncogene. The BCL-10 oncogene plays an

Table 21.5. Cytogenetic aberrations associated with histologic subtypes of non-Hodgkin's lymphomas

Extranodal marginal zone lymphoma	t[11;18][q21;q21]	MLT/MALT1
	t[1;14]	BCL-10
Mantle cell lymphoma	t[11;14]	PRAD1
Burkitt's lymphoma	t[8;14]	c-myc
	t[2;8] or t[8;22]	

important role in anti-apoptotic and proliferative signaling pathways [31,32,33] and it is postulated that BCL-10 induces autonomous growth of the neoplastic clone. Other molecular events include trisomy 3, p53 and *c-myc* mutations and genetic instability, as in the replication error repair [RER] phenotype. Inactivating mutations of the Fas gene have also been detected in relatively high numbers of extranodal marginal zone lymphomas.

The most common presenting symptoms of low grade gastric MALT lymphomas are dyspepsia and epigastric pain. Systemic symptoms are rarely associated with a primary MALT lymphoma. Endoscopy typically reveals non-specific gastritis or possibly an ulcerated lesion. Mass lesions within the stomach are uncommon in MALT lymphoma and portend a more aggressive histology. There is a continuous spectrum of lesions that are seen in the transition of Helicobacter pylori-associated gastritis to MALT lymphoma. The histologic features of lymphoid infiltrates in "acquired" MALT correlate with the histopathology of Peyer's Patches. Lymphoepithelial lesions are present, which represent lymphoid infiltrates invading gastric glands [34].

The typical phenotype of extranodal marginal zone lymphoma is characterized by expression of mature B-cell markers such as the CD19 and CD20 antigens and the absence of CD5, CD10 and CD23 antigen expression. Specific adhesion molecules have been identified that are implicated in the homing of these cells to mucosal tissue, including alpha-4 beta-7 integrin, which has been identified as a mucosal homing receptor [35] (See Chapter 20).

Recent studies have demonstrated that MALT lymphoma may be eradicated with antibiotic therapy [36]. Eradication of H. pylori infection with antibiotic therapy frequently results in regression of MALT lymphoma in patients who are H. pylori positive [37,38,39]. MALT lymphomas are often successfully treated with the combination of antibiotics and proton pump inhibitors, but it remains unclear whether this therapy alone will permit long-term regression of gastric MALT lymphoma. Isaacson has suggested that antibiotic therapy may sometimes suppress rather than eradicate the neoplastic clone responsible for MALT lymphoma [22].

When antibiotic therapy is inadequate in the treatment of MALT lymphoma, definitive therapy should be considered. The optimal treatment for primary gastric lymphomas has not been completely defined, but gastrointestinal-sparing [i.e. stomach-conserving] strategies are now routinely employed. In the past, MALT lymphomas localized to the gastrointestinal tract (as in the stomach) were treated surgically, but prospective series have demonstrated no difference in survival in patients undergoing gastrectomy when compared with those who were conservatively managed [40].

Because MALT lymphoma typically presents as a localized process often involving only the stomach, long-term remission can be achieved with local therapy. The use of low dose involved field radiation was evaluated in a prospective series of patients with low grade MALT lymphoma of the stomach. All 17 patients in this series achieved a biopsy-proven complete response after undergoing involved field radiotherapy with a cumulative dose of 3000 cGy [41]. Involved field radiotherapy is generally well-tolerated with no significant morbidity. Single-agent chemotherapy such as chlorambucil or oral cyclophosphamide also have demonstrated efficacy, although to date, there has been no prospective study demonstrating an improvement in survival with the use of chemotherapy in localized MALT lymphoma.

Diffuse Large B-cell Lymphoma

Diffuse large B-cell lymphomas are the most common form of non-Hodgkin's lymphomas accounting for 30 percent of NHL. Diffuse large B-cell lymphoma with gastrointestinal tract involvement most commonly involves the stomach, often presenting as either ulcerated or hemorrhagic lesions. Intestinal involvement is also fairly common. Disease often presents as limited stage with regional node involvement.

While most aggressive B-cell lymphomas were previously believed to arise from extranodal marginal zone lymphomas of MALT type or other indolent non-Hodgkin's lymphomas [42], recent evidence suggests that diffuse large B-cell lymphomas also arise de novo in the gastrointestinal tract. It is useful to consider aggressive large B-cell lymphomas with gastrointestinal tract involvement as usually arising de novo and more rarely as arising from a low grade MALT lymphoma.

In comparison to MALT lymphomagenesis, less cytogenetic data is known to characterize the molecular events in aggressive large B-cell lymphomas. Additional cytogenetic aberrations may induce the transformation of an indolent non-Hodgkin's lymphoma to a more aggressive histology. The transformation to an aggressive non-Hodgkin's lymphoma involves additional genetic mutations such as p53 deletions, p16 deletions and novel chromosomal translocations like t[8;14]. These p53 deletions have previously been described in aggressive lymphomas of primary gastrointestinal tract origin [43]. Partial gains of chromosome 11q and chromosome 12 have also been identified in many cases of primary gastrointestinal large cell lymphoma in a recent study [44].

Aggressive diffuse large B-cell lymphomas are highly treatable with curative outcomes observed in approximately half of the patients after first-line therapy. The standard first-line treatment is systemic chemotherapy with CHOP [cyclophosphamide, doxorubicin, vincristine and prednisone]. Several second-generation combination chemotherapy regimens have been compared to CHOP in prospective series, with no regimen proving to be superior to CHOP therapy [45].

In patients with regional disease such as primarily gastrointestinal tract involvement, combination chemotherapy may be administered followed by limited field radiotherapy. A randomized Phase II study comparing CHOP vs CHOP followed by involved field radiotherapy for early stage disease, demonstrated improved survival with the use of combined modality therapy [46]. Hence, short-course chemotherapy followed by involved field radiotherapy to the gastrointestinal tract for regional disease is often employed with good clinical outcomes and tolerance [47]. While surgery was employed as a therapeutic modality in the past [48], surgical resection is now reserved for acute presentations, such as bowel perforation or intractable gastrointestinal bleeding.

Mantle Cell Lymphoma

Mantle cell lymphoma is a separately recognized histologic entity incorporated into the R.E.A.L. and WHO classifications, previously termed diffuse small-cleaved cell lymphomas in the International Working Formulation. Because mantle cell lymphoma was not recognized as a distinct clinical entity prior to the R.E.A.L. classification, the disease and its therapy was not evaluated separately in reports of indolent and aggressive non-Hodgkin's lymphomas.

Mantle cell lymphomas typically present in advanced stage with generalized adenopathy, bone marrow involvement, peripheral blood and splenic involvement. Extranodal sites of disease, such as the gastrointestinal tract, are also frequently involved. Common symptoms at the time of presentation include weight loss, weakness, diarrhea, abdominal pain, rectal bleeding and anemia. However, a significant number of patients do not present with gastrointestinal symptoms, but will still have gastrointestinal tract involvement on biopsy [49].

Histologically, this entity is characterized by the diffuse presence of small-cleaved lymphocytes of intermediate differentiation. The characteristic immuno-phenotypic profile reflects the presence of B-lineage markers such as CD5, CD19, CD20, FMC7 in the absence of CD23 expression. The typical cytogenetic aberration involved in mantle cell lymphomas is a reciprocal t(11;14)(q13;q32) chromosomal translocation that results in the juxtaposition of the immunoglobulin heavy chain joining region on chromosome 14 with the BCL-1 region on chromosome 11 [50,51]. This reciprocal translocation causes dysregulation of the BCL-1 onco-gene and overexpression of cyclin D1. Cyclin D1 protein complexes with CD4 protein to move cells from the G1 phase into the S phase (Table 21.5).

A common presentation of mantle cell lymphoma involving the gastrointestinal tract is diffuse involvement, termed multiple lymphomatous polyposis. The term multiple lymphomatous polyposis [MLP] was originally coined by Cornes in 1961 to describe numerous polypoid lesions scattered throughout the gastrointestinal tract, while it was later determined that MLP was primarily a manifestation of mantle cell lymphoma. Whilst virtually all cases of multiple lymphomatous polyposis were previously ascribed to mantle cell lymphoma, recent reports show that indolent non-Hodgkin's lymphomas such as MALT lymphoma and follicular lymphoma may also present as multiple lymphomatous polyposis, albeit infrequently [52,53,54].

The Groupe D'Etude Lymphomes Digestifs reported the largest series of patients with multiple lymphomatous polyposis. In their cohort of 31 patients, clinical features included male preponderance, older age (>60 years) and evidence of a dominant tumor mass, typically in the ileocecal region. Disease often involved the jejunum and terminal ileum, but lesions were also seen to involve other sites such as the stomach and rectum. Patients treated with an anthracycline-based regimen in this series had better overall survival than patients treated without anthracyclines [55].

Mantle cell lymphomas behave in a pattern similar to other aggressive non-Hodgkin's lymphomas. The routine treatment of mantle cell lymphomas with gastrointestinal tract involvement is with combination chemotherapy. High dose therapy and autologous transplantation is being evaluated. Tumor lysis precautions and precautionary measures for gastrointestinal bleeding or perforation should be instituted.

Immunoproliferative Small Intestinal Disease [IPSID]

Immunoproliferative small intestinal disease [IPSID] is an indolent non-Hodg-kin's lymphoma that is characterized by the production of alpha heavy chain protein. IPSID is considered a form of MALT lymphoma, arising from native mucosa-associated lymphoid tissue [i.e. Peyer's Patches] within the small intestines. Originally described as "Mediterranean lymphoma", the term IPSID has now supplanted both alpha heavy chain disease representing the earlier stages of disease and "Mediterranean lymphoma" reserved for the later stages of disease.

IPSID is prevalent in the Mediterranean basin and Middle Eastern region. Additional sporadic cases of IPSID have been described in other parts of Europe, South America and in the United States. Common demographic features include lower socioeconomic status and poor sanitary conditions, poor personal hygiene with a peak incidence in the first through the third decades of life. Patients generally present with progressive malabsorption in the second and third decades. The clinical manifestations of disease include diarrhea, abdominal pain, malabsorption, weight loss, growth retardation and digital clubbing. IPSID remains localized to the small intestines for prolonged periods and patients who die usually do so as a consequence of severe malabsorption. The pattern of involvement may extend to mesenteric and retroperitoneal lymph nodes, however, extension to other intra-abdominal sites such as the liver and spleen is uncommon, occurring only late in the course of the disease [56,57,58].

IPSID has been described in stages of lymphoproliferative evolution. In the earlier stages of disease, a benign plasmacytic or lymphoplasmacytic infiltrate is found in the lamina propria causing broadening of the villi and separation of crypts. Gene rearrangements and light chain restrictions have been found in these earlier lesions, suggesting that neoplastic changes occur early in the course of disease despite the benign appearance of the mucosa. As the disease progresses to intermediate and later stages, there is villous atrophy and lymphomatous proliferation invading the depth of the intestinal wall.

While it is theorized that antigenic stimulation by intestinal bacteria or parasites is a causative factor, no specific organism has been identified. It is postulated that chronic stimulation of intestinal mucosa-associated lymphoid tissue by infection leads to proliferation of B-lymphocytes, which produce alpha heavy chain protein [a-CP]. The histologic findings of IPSID share similar features with MALT lymphoma with a pronounced plasma cell component within both the intestine and mesenteric lymph nodes, synthesizing large amounts of alpha heavy chains. It has been theorized that chronic antigenic stimulation of the intestinal IgA secretory immune system by intestinal microorganisms leads to hyperplasia of immunocytes with expansion of plasma cell clones. Mutations within neoplastic clones subsequently lead to deletions in the alpha-heavy chain and inability to synthesize light chains leading to the secretion of a-CP rather than intact IgA [56].

The treatment strategies for IPSID in earlier stages includes the use of broad spectrum antibiotics; notably tetracyclines or metronidazole to eradicate the purported antigen stimulus from the intestinal lumen. Supportive care measures are also instituted, as chronic diarrhea may require intravenous fluid and electrolyte repletion. The addition of corticosteroids to antibiotic therapy has also been reported to result in temporary remissions. For patients with later stages of IPSID or for patients with disease refractory to antibiotic therapy, combination chemotherapy with an anthracycline-based regimen is often employed. Total abdominal irradiation has previously been evaluated although this is now infrequently used.

Enteropathy-associated T-Cell Lymphoma [EATL]

Intestinal T-cell lymphomas are uncommon and may occur either with or without enteropathy. The most well-established entity is described as enteropathy-associated

T-cell lymphoma [EATL]. Originally, this was described as "malignant histiocytosis of the intestine". This entity was not separately defined in the International Working Formulation, Kiel, Rappaport or Luke-Collins classification schemes. However, in the present R.E.A.L. and WHO classifications, EATL is a separate entity now called Intestinal T-cell lymphoma.

EATL often appears as a rare, late complication of celiac disease. In different series, adult-onset celiac disease precedes the onset of EATL variably by an average of 2 to 10 years. It has been suggested that EATL results from a disordered response to gluten. Uncontrolled celiac sprue, in addition to advanced age, poor hygiene and male gender, are other risk factors for this disease, although in patients with celiac sprue, a gluten-free diet reduces the risk for development of non-Hodgkin's lymphoma [59].

The clinical features of EATL include male preponderance and typical symptoms of abdominal pain, weight loss and diarrhea. A substantial proportion of patients will present with clinical signs and symptoms of bowel obstruction or intestinal perforation. In a series of EATL patients described in England [59], surgery was performed emergently on nearly one-third of patients due to abdominal pain, bowel obstruction or evidence of peritonitis.

The characteristic lesions of EATL appear as circumferential ulcerated plaques. The jejunum is the most common site of involvement, with the colon and the rectum less frequently involved. The neoplastic cells of EATL have the immunophenotype of intraepithelial cytotoxic T cells and may exhibit epitheliotropism. The typical immunophenotype reveals expression of T-cell lineage markers such as CD3, CD45RO and cytotoxic T-cell markers. In addition, clonal rearrangements of the T-cell receptor $\alpha\beta$ gene are also identified. Specific HLA phenotypes such as DQA1*0501, DQB1*0201 and DR/DQ alleles associated with celiac disease predispose to the development of EATL.

The overall prognosis of Intestinal T-cell lymphomas is poor. The actuarial overall survival in one series was 20 percent. Combination chemotherapy typically used for aggressive non-Hodgkin's lymphomas was given to patients in one particular study, but treatment was often complicated by poor nutritional status requiring parenteral or enteral feedings and precluding completion of therapy. The complications of therapy included gastrointestinal bleeding, small bowel perforation and the development of enterocolic fistulae. Most patients succumb to illness with progressive disease caused by gastrointestinal complications such as bowel perforation [60,61].

Burkitt's Lymphoma

Burkitt's lymphoma has frequently been referred to as a high-grade lymphoma most often affecting children or young adults and to a lesser extent adults with immunodeficiency. In the R.E.A.L. classification, Burkitt's lymphoma is categorized as a peripheral B-cell lymphoma. The WHO classification includes both classic and variant [i.e. "Burkitt's-like"] forms of Burkitt's lymphoma in this category [5]. Three subcategories of Burkitt's lymphoma have been defined in the WHO classification: endemic, sporadic and immunodeficiency-associated. Both the endemic and sporadic forms of Burkitt's lymphoma present with extranodal sites of involvement, but it is the sporadic form that more often presents with gastrointestinal tract involvement particularly of the distal ileum and the cecum.

[The discussion of Burkitt's lymphoma in the setting of immunodeficiency is found in the following section.]

The typical chromosomal aberration in Burkitt's lymphomas is a reciprocal translocation of the immunoglobulin heavy chain promoter on chromosome 14 with the *c-myc* oncogene on chromosome 8, resulting in a balanced t[8;14][q24;q32] translocation (Table 21.5). This reciprocal translocation causes dysregulation of the *c-myc* oncogene, which encodes a basic Helix-Loop-Helix transcription factor involved in cell cycle progression and programmed cell death. Less frequent chromosomal translocations involve either the immunoglobulin light chain promoter on chromosomes 2 or 22 with the *c-myc* oncogene on chromosome 8, resulting in balanced t[2;8] or t[8;22] translocations [62].

Burkitt's lymphoma cells appear as monomorphic small lymphocytes with round nuclei and prominent nucleoli on morphologic review. The characteristic microscopic appearance of Burkitt's lymphoma is a diffuse "starry sky" pattern, often observed in the presence of numerous mitotic figures. The "starry sky" appearance is caused by benign macrophages, which have taken up apoptotic cell fragments. The typical immunophenotype of Burkitt's lymphoma exhibits expression of mature B-lineage markers such as CD10 and CD20 antigen. In addition, expression of Ki-67 antigen is detected, reflecting the high proliferative index of this tumor.

The differentiation of Burkitt's lymphoma from other types of aggressive non-Hodgkin's lymphomas is critical, as chemotherapeutic strategies for Burkitt's lymphoma differ. Burkitt's lymphomas have been effectively treated with intensive combination chemotherapy regimens given with intrathecal therapy [63,64].

Lymphoproliferative Disorders Associated with Immunodeficiency States

In the Setting of Human Immunodeficiency Virus (HIV) Infection

An increased incidence of lymphoproliferative disorders of the gastrointestinal tract are detected in the setting of an immunodeficiency state. With Human Immunodeficiency virus [HIV] infection, the typical non-Hodgkin's lymphomas encountered are aggressive histologies such as diffuse large B-cell lymphoma [immunoblastic subtype] or Burkitt's lymphoma. More than two-thirds of HIV-associated non-Hodgkin's lymphomas present with extranodal disease, however, the gastrointestinal tract is involved in 10–25% of cases [65]. In contrast to other forms of Burkitt's lymphoma, the usual sites of gastrointestinal tract involvement are in more unusual locations. The most common site in one series was the distal colon [66]. In addition to unusual sites of GI tract involvement, aggressive non-Hodgkin's lymphomas of the gastrointestinal tract in association with HIV infection tend to be disseminated with frequent bone marrow involvement [67]. The treatment involves the use of combination chemotherapy in conjunction with highly active anti-retroviral therapy [HAART] and the use of intrathecal therapy as indicated. (See Chapter 4)

In the Setting of Bone Marrow or Solid Organ Transplantation

Solid organ or allogeneic bone marrow transplantation-associated non-Hodgkin's lymphomas occur 50–100 times more frequently than in the general population. These post-transplant lymphoproliferative diseases [PTLD] are generally observed in association with Epstein-Barr virus infection. These lymphomas tend to be aggressive and frequently involve extranodal sites of disease including the gastrointestinal tract. Risk factors for the development of PTLD include the degree and length of immunosuppression, the type of immunosuppressive therapy, (in particular the use of cyclosporine), HLA compatibility and the presence of T-cell depletion (see Chapter 6).

The general approach to treating PTLD initially is to reduce the intensity of immunosuppression. Other approaches include immunotherapeutic agents such as alpha-interferon monoclonal antibodies, or cytotoxic chemotherapy if the previous measures fail. Recent evidence confirms the efficacy of Rituximab, (a monoclonal antibody targeting the CD20 antigen on B-lymphocytes), in treating post-transplantation lymphoproliferative disorders. Donor Leukocyte Infusion [DLI] may also be used, but it is often associated with significant toxicity and the development of graft versus host disease. (GVHD) In a subset of patients with localized PTLD, surgical resection or radiotherapy may control the disease effectively.

In the Setting of Immunosuppressive Therapy to Treat Other Diseases

Case reports of Hodgkin's lymphoma arising in the setting of chronic immunosuppressive therapy for the treatment of Crohn's disease and myaesthenia gravis have been reported. These patients had multifocal bowel involvement with classic Hodgkin's lymphoma. Hodgkin's lymphoma arising in this setting appears to be associated with Epstein-Barr virus lymphoproliferation [68].

Conclusions

The advent of new molecular diagnostic tools coupled with the re-classification of non-Hodgkin's lymphomas has led to advances in the pathogenesis and treatment of gastrointestinal tract lymphomas. Continuing efforts to elucidate the underlying clinico-pathologic features of gastrointestinal tract lymphomas will lead to identification of novel treatment approaches and may potentially change the management paradigms of these interesting diseases. The surgeon's role in these conditions appears to be ever-diminishing, with limited involvement in staging and diagnosis and an occasional place in the acute complications that accompany either specialized disease or definitive therapy.

References

1. National Cancer Institute. Summary and description of a working formulation for clinical usage. The non-Hodgkin's lymphoma pathologic classification project. Cancer 1982;49:2112–35.
2. Lennert K. The Kiel Classification, in Histopathology of Non-Hodgkin's Lymphomas [based on the updated Kiel Classification], edited by K Lennert, AC Feller: Springer, New York, 1992.
3. Harris NL, Jaffe ES, Stern H, et al. A Revised European-American Classification of Lymphoid Neoplasms: A Proposal from the International Lymphoma Study Group. Blood. 1994;84:1361–92.
4. Jaffe ES, Harris NL, Diebold J, et al. World Health Organization Classification of Neoplastic Dis-

eases of the Hematopoietic and Lymphoid Tissues: Report of the Clinical Advisory Committee Meeting — Airlie House, Virginia, November 1997. J Clin Oncol 1999;17:3835–49.

5. Harris NL, Jaffe ES, Diebold J, et al. Lymphoma Classification — from Controversy to Consensus: the R.E.A.L. and WHO Classification of Lymphoid Neoplasms. Ann Oncol 2000;11 Suppl 1: S3–S10.

6. AF List, Greer JP, Cousar JC, et al. non-Hodgkin's lymphoma of the gastrointestinal tract: an analysis of clinical and pathologic features affecting outcome. J Clin Oncol 6:1125–33.

7. Devaney K, Jaffe ES. The surgical pathology of gastrointestinal Hodgkin's disease. Am J Clin Pathol 1991;95:794–801.

8. de Jong D, Aleman BM, Taal BG, Boot H. Controversies and consensus in the diagnosis, work-up and treatment of gastric lymphoma: an international survey. Ann Oncol 1999;10:275–80.

9. Pavlick AC, Gerdes H, Portlock, CS. Endoscopic ultrasound in the Evaluation of Gastric Small Lymphocytic Mucosa Associated Lymphoid Tumors. J Clin Oncol 1997;15:1761–6.

10. Kessar P, Norton A, Rohatiner AZ et al. CT appearances of mucosa-associated lymphoid tissues [MALT] lymphoma. Eur Radiol 1999;9:693–6.

11. Zinzani PL, Magagnoli, M, Chierichetti F, et al. The Role of Positron Emission Tomography [PET] in the Management of Lymphoma Patients. Ann Oncol 1999;10:1181–4.

12. Jerusalem G, Beguin Y, Fassotte MF, et al. Whole-Body Positron Emission Tomography using 18F-Fluorodeoxyglucose for Post-treatment Evaluation of Hodgkin's Disease and Non-Hodgkin's Lymphoma has Higher Diagnostic and Prognostic Value than Classical Computed Tomography Scan Imaging. Blood 1999;94:429–33.

13. Hoffman M, Kletter K, Diemling M, et al. Positron emission tomography with fluorine-18-2-fluoro-2-deoxy-D-glucose [F18-FDG] does not visualize extranodal B-cell lymphoma of the mucosa-associated lymphoid tissue [MALT]-type. Ann Oncol 1999;10:1185–9.

14. Smithers DW. Summary of papers delivered at the Conference on Staging in Hodgkin's disease. Cancer Res 1971;31:1869–70.

15. Rosenberg SA. Validity of the Ann Arbor Staging Classification for the non-Hodgkin's lymphomas. Cancer Treat Rep 1977;61:1023–7.

16. Musshoff K. Clinical Staging Classification of non-Hodgkin's lymphomas. Strahlentherapie 1977;153:218–21.

17. Rohatiner A, D'Amore F, Coiffier B, et al. Report on a workshop convened to discuss the pathological and staging classifications of gastrointestinal tract lymphoma. Ann Oncol 1994;5:397–400.

18. d'Amore F, Brincker H, Gronbaek K, et al. Non-Hodgkin's lymphoma of the gastrointestinal tract: a Population-based analysis of incidence, geographic distribution, clinicopathologic presentation features, and prognosis. Danish lymphoma Study Group. J Clin Oncol 1994;12:1673–84.

19. Zucca E, Bertoni F, Roggero E et al. The Gastric Marginal Zone B-cell Lymphoma of MALT Type. Blood 2000;96:410–19.

20. Thieblemont C, Bastion Y, Berger F, et al. Mucosa-associated lymphoid tissue gastrointestinal and non-gastrointestinal lymphoma behavior: analysis of 108 patients. J Clin Oncol 1997;15:1624–30.

21. Nathwani BN, Anderson JR, Armitage JO, et al. Marginal Zone B-Cell Lymphoma: A Clinical Comparison of Nodal and Mucosa-Associated Lymphoid Tissue Types. Non-Hodgkin's Lymphoma Classification Project. J Clin Oncol 1999;17: 2486–92.

22. Isaacson PG. Gastric MALT lymphoma: From concept to cure. Ann Oncol 1999;10:37–645

23. Parsonnet J, Hansen S, Rodriguez L, et al. Helicobacter pylori infection and gastric lymphomas. N Engl J Med 1994;330:1267–71.

24. Doglioni C, Wotherspoon AC, Moschini A, et al. High incidence of primary gastric lymphoma in northeastern Italy. Lancet 1992;339:834–5.

25. Hussell T, Isaacson PG, Crabtree JE, et al. The response of cells from low-grade B-cell gastric lymphomas if mucosa-associated lymphoid tissue to Helicobacter pylori. Lancet 1993;342:571–4.

26. Hussell T, Isaacson PG, Crabtree JE, Spencer J. Helicobacter pylori-specific tumor-infiltrating T cells provide contact dependent help for the growth for malignant B cells in low-grade gastric lymphoma of mucosa-associated lymphoid tissue. J Pathol 1996;178:122–7.

27. Zucca E, Bertoni F, Roggero E, et al. Molecular analysis of the progression from Helicobacter pylori-associated chronic gastritis to mucosa-associated lymphoid tissue lymphoma of the stomach. New Engl J Med 1998;338:804–10.

28. Dierlamm J, Baens M, Wlodarska I, et al. The apoptosis inhibitor gene API2 and a novel 18q gene, MLT, are recurrently rearranged in the t[11;18][q21;q21] associated with mucosa-associated lymphoid tissue lymphomas. Blood 1999;93:3601–9.

29. Akagi T, Motegi M, Tamura A, et al. A novel gene, MALT1 at 18q21, is involved in t[11;18][q21;q21] found in low grade B-cell lymphoma of mucosa-associated lymphoid tissue. Oncogene 1999;18:5785–94.

30. Morgan JA, Yin Y, Borowsky AS, et al. Breakpoints of the t[11;18][q21;q21] in mucosa-associated

lymphoid tissue [MALT] lymphoma lie within or near the previously undescribed gene MALT1 in chromosome 18. Cancer Res. 1999;59:6205–6213.

31. Willis TG, Jayadel DM, Du MQ, et al. Bcl10 is involved in t[1;14][p22;q32] of MALT B cell lymphoma and mutated in multiple tumor types. Cell 1999;96:35–45.

32. Du MQ, Peng H, Liu H, et al. BCL10 gene mutation in lymphoma. Blood 2000;95:3885–90.

33. Zhang Q, Siebert R, Yan M, et al. Inactivating mutations and overexpression of BCL10, a caspase recruitment domain-containing gene, in MALT lymphomas with t[1;14][p22;q32]. Nat Genet 1999; 22:63–8.

34. Isaacson PG. Gastrointestinal Lymphomas of T- and B-cell Types. Mod Path 1999;12:151–8.

35. Drillenberg P, van der Voort R, Koopman G, et al. Preferential expression of the mucosal homing receptor integrin alpha-4 beta-7 in gastrointestinal non-Hodgkin's lymphomas. Am J Pathol 1997;150:919–27.

36. Wotherspoon AC, Doglioni C, Diss TC, et al. Regression of primary low-grade B-cell gastric lymphoma of mucosa-associated lymphoid tissue after eradication of helicobacter pylori. Lancet 1993;342:575–7.

37. Steinbach G, Ford R, Glober G, et al. Antibiotic treatment of gastric lymphoma of mucosa-associated lymphoid tissue: An Uncontrolled Trial. Ann Intern Med 1999;131:88–95.

38. Roggero E, Zucca E, Pinotti G, et al. Eradication of helicobacter pylori in primary low grade gastric lymphoma of mucosa associated lymphoid tissue. Ann Intern Med 1995;122:767–9.

39. Bayerdorffer E, Neubauer A, Rudolph B, et al. Regression of primary gastric lymphoma of mucosa-associated lymphoid tissue type after eradication of Helicobacter pylori. Malt Lymphoma Study Group. Lancet 1995;345:1591–4.

40. Koch P, Grothaus-Pinke B, Hiddemann W, et al. Primary lymphoma of the stomach: Three-year results of a prospective multicenter study. Ann Oncol 1997;8:S85–8.

41. Schechter NR, Portlock CS, and Yahalom J. Treatment of mucosa-associated lymphoid tissue lymphoma of the stomach with radiation alone. J Clin Oncol 1998;16:1916–21.

42. Chan JK, Ng CS, Isaacson PG. Relationship between high-grade lymphoma and low-grade B-cell mucosa-associated lymphoid tissue lymphoma. Am J Pathol 1990;136:1153–64.

43. Du M, Peng H, Singh N, et al. The accumulation of p53 abnormalities is associated with progression of mucosa-associated lymphoid tissue lymphoma. Blood 1995;86:4587.

44. Barth TFE, Dohner H, Werner CA, et al. Characteristic Pattern of Chromosomal Gains and Losses in Primary large B-cell Lymphomas of the Gastrointestinal Tract. Blood 1998;91:4321–30.

45. Fisher RI, Gaynor E, Dahlberg S, et al. Comparison of a Standard Regimen CHOP with three intensive chemotherapy regimens for advanced non-Hodgkin's lymphoma. New Engl J Med 1993;328:1002–6.

46. Yahalom J, Varsos G, Fuks Z, et al. Adjuvant cyclophosphamide, doxorubicin, vincristine, and prednisone chemotherapy after radiation in stage I low-grade and intermediate-grade non-Hodgkin's lymphoma. Cancer 1992;71:2342–50.

47. Miller TP, Dahlberg S, Cassady JR, et al. Chemotherapy alone compared with chemotherapy plus radiotherapy for localized intermediate- and high-grade non-Hodgkin's lymphoma. N Engl J Med 1998;339:21–6.

48. Shepard FA, Evans WK, Kutas G, et al. Chemotherapy following surgery for Stages IE and IIE Non-Hodgkin's lymphoma of the Gastrointestinal Tract. J Clin Oncol 1988;6:253–60.

49. Romaguera J, Dang N, Hagemeister FB et al. Evidence for need of upper and lower endoscopies with biopsy in staging of asymptomatic patients with aggressive mantle cell lymphoma. Proc Am Soc Hemat 2000: Abst #1440.

50. Tsujimoto Y, Yunis J, Onorato-Showe L, et al. Molecular cloning of the chromosomal breakpoint of B-cell lymphomas and leukemias with the t(11;14) chromosome translocation. Science 1984;224:1403.

51. Tsujimoto Y, Jaffe E, Cossman J, et al. Clustering of breakpoints on chromosome 11 in human B-cell neoplasms with the t(11;14) chromosome translocation. Nature 1985;315:340.

52. Kadayifci A, Benekli M, Savas MC, et al. Multiple Lymphomatous Polyposis. J Surg Oncol 1997;64:336–40.

53. Breslin NP, Urbanski SJ, Shaffer EA. Mucosa-Associated lymphoid Tissue [MALT] Lymphoma manifesting as Multiple Lymphomatous polyposis of the Gastrointestinal Tract. Am J Gastr 1999;94:2540–5.

54. Triozzi PL, Borowitz MJ, Gockerman JP. Gastrointestinal involvement and multiple lymphomatous polyposis in mantle-zone lymphoma J Clin Oncol 1986;4:866–73.

55. Ruskone-Fourmestraux A, Delmer A, Lavergne A, et al. Multiple Lymphomatous polyposis of the Gastrointestinal Tract: Prospective Clinicopathologic Study of 31 Cases. Gastroenterology 1997;112:7–16.

56. Fine KD and Stone MJ. Alpha-heavy chain disease, Mediterranean lymphoma, and immunoproliferative small intestinal disease: A Review of Clinicopathological Features, Pathogenesis, and Differential Diagnosis. Am J Gastroenterol 1999;94:1139–52.
57. Demirer T, Celebi H, Akcaglayan E, et al. Primary Low-Grade Lymphomas of the Intestine. J Clin Oncol 1999;17:3682–4.
58. Akbulut J, Soykan I, Yakaryilmaz F, et al. Five year results of the treatment of 23 patients with immunoproliferative small intestinal disease: a Turkish experience. Cancer 1997;80:8–14.
59. Gale J, Simmonds PD, Mead GM, et al. Enteropathy-type intestinal T-cell lymphoma; clinical features and treatment of 31 patients in a single center. J Clin Oncol 2000;18:795–803.
60. Wright DH. Enteropathy associated T cell lymphoma. Cancer Surv 1997;30:249–61.
61. Cellier C, Delabesse E, Helmer C, et al. Refractory sprue, coeliac disease, and enteropathy-associated T-cell lymphoma. French Coeliac Disease Study Group. Lancet 2000;356:203–8.
62. Hecht JL and Aster JC . Molecular biology of Burkitt's lymphoma. J Clin Oncol 2000;18:3707.
63. McMaster ML, Greer JP, Greco FA, et al. Effective treatment of small-cleaved cell lymphoma with high intensity brief-duration chemotherapy. J Clin Oncol 1991;9:941–6.
64. Magrath I, Adde M, Shad A, et al. Adults and children with small non-cleaved cell lymphoma have a similar excellent outcome when treated with the same chemotherapy regimen. J Clin Oncol 1996;14:925–36.
65. Heise W, Arasteh K, Mosterz P, et al. Malignant gastrointestinal lymphomas in patients with AIDs. Digestion 1997;58:218–24.
66. Beck PL, Gill MJ, Sutherland LR. HIV-associated non-Hodgkin's lymphoma of the gastrointestinal tract. Am J Gastroenterol 1996;91:2377–81.
67. Hernandez JA, Navarro JT, Ribera JM, et al. Primary gastrointestinal lymphoma in patients infected with HIV: Study of 15 cases in a series of 76 patients with non-Hodgkin's lymphoma and HIV infection. 1999 Med Clin [Barc] 1999;112:222–4.
68. Kumar S, Fend F, Quintanilla-Martinez L, et al. Epstein-Barr virus-positive primary gastrointestinal Hodgkin's disease: association with inflammatory bowel disease and immunosuppression. Am J Surg Path 2000;24:66–73.

COMMENTARY ON SECTION IV

Konstantinos N. Syrigos

In Chapter 19, Schreiber and Nikolaus discuss the immunology of the intestinal mucosal defence system. This is embellished by Zbar and Karayiannakis in their overview of the gut immune compartments, demonstrating the complex but ordered arrangement of adhesion molecules expressed by circulating effector cells and reciprocal addressins located on specialized post-capillary venules. It has been demonstrated both in pre-clinical models and in certain clinical conditions that gut stimulation may modulate the stress response, affecting both permeability and the mucosa-associated immune system. This intestinal barrier function is pivotal in order to prevent an uncontrolled invasion by foreign proteins and haptens, including microbial and dietary antigens. This barrier is based on the integrity of the epithelial layer and the effective exclusion of intestinal toxic and infectious pathogens by the mucosa-associated immune system of the gut known as the Gut Associated Lymphoid Tissue or GALT as described in this chapter.

The integrity and function of the GALT are regulated by the route and type of nutrition, in part through neuropeptides secreted by either the enteric nervous system or other neuropeptide-containing cells within the mucosa. It has been demonstrated that lack of enteral feeding (providing caloric intake via the intravenous route) results in a significant reduction in the GALT cell mass (mainly within the Peyer's patches, lamina propria and intraepithelial spaces) and consequent reduction of intestinal and respiratory IgA levels as well as in local CD4/CD8 ratios [1,2]. There is now a cumulative amount of data indicating that prolonged parenteral nutrition results in mucosal atrophy, reduced IgA production, increased bacterial overgrowth and loss of mucosal defenses against bacterial invasion, while extraintestinal sites (such as the peritoneal cavity and respiratory tract) are also adversely affected. The above observation becomes clinically relevant in critically ill intensive care unit patients, where the specifics of the enteral diet, (namely the supplementation with dietary arginine, trace elements and omega-3 fatty acids), preserves peripheral lymphocyte and monocyte function when compared with unsupplemented enteral feeding [3]. This pre-clinical effect has also translated into a reduced incidence of observed septic complications and nosocomial infections when both enteral and supplemented enteral feeds are used in the critically ill ICU patient [4-6]. Although these effects are also associated with improvements in subclinical lymphocyte parameters such as HLA-DR expression, this has not always correlated with reduced hospital stay or mortality in critically ill cases [7–9]. This effect of an enriched enteral formula has been shown in the clinic to improve the normal post-operative depression of lympho-cyte function (as measured by phagocytic indices and respiratory burst activity) as well as to preserve gut mucosal function, microperfusion and mucosal oxygen metabolism in patients undergoing major cancer surgery [10]. This has also been associated with a reduced hospital stay and infective complications in elective colonic, gastric and pancreatic cancer patients undergoing major resectional surgery who receive an immune-enhanced enteral diet [11]. These subtle effects on monocte function may act, however, as a two-edged sword, since over exuber-ant macrophage function may be central in the pathogenesis of adult respiratory distress syndrome (ARDS) and systemic inflammatory response syndrome (SIRS), with arginine-enhanced diets possibly priming otherwise down-regulated macro-phages. In these analyses, the timing of administration, the exact make-up of immune-enhanced enrichment diets, dosing and the clinical circumstances where these diets are most likely to be beneficial, require further study.

References

1. Li J, Kudsk KA, Gocinski B, Dent D, Glezer J, Langkamp-Henken B. Effects of parenteral and enteral nutrition on gut-associated lymphoid tissue. J Trauma 1995;39:44–51.
2. Heel KA, Kong SE, McCauley RD, Erber WN, Hall JC. The effect of minimum luminal nutrition on mucosal cellularity and immunity of the gut.J Gastroenterol Hepatol 1998;13:1015–10.
3. Mendez C, Jurkovich GJ, Wener MH, Garcia I, Mays M, Maier RV. Effects of supplemental dietary arginine, canola oil and trace elements on cellular immune function in critically injured patients. Shock 1996;6:7–12.
4. Engel JM, Menges T, Neuhauser C, Schaefer B, Hempelmann G. Effects of various feeding regimens in multiple trauma patients on septic complications and immune parameters. Anasthesiol Intensi-vemed Notfallmed Schmerzther 1997;32:234–9.
5. Stechmiller JK, Treloar D, Allen N. Gut dysfunction in critically ill patients: a review of the litera-ture. Am J Crit Care 1997;6:204–9.
6. Weimann A, Bastian L, Bischoff WE, Grotz M, Hansel M, Lotz J, et al. Influence of arginine, omega-3 fatty acids and nucleotide-supplemented enteral support on systemic inflammatory response syndrome and multiple organ failure in patients after severe trauma. Nutrition 1998;14:165–72.
7. Heyland DK, Cook DJ, Guyatt GH. Does the formulation of enteral feeding products influence infectious morbidity and mortality rates in the critically ill patient? A critical review of the evi-dence. Crit Care Med 1994;22:192–1202.
8. Braga M, Gianotti L, Radaeilli G, Vignali A, Mari G, Gentilini O, DiCarlo V. Perioperative immu-nonutrition in patients undergoing cancer surgery: results of a randomized double-blind phase 3 trial. Arch Surg 1999;134:428–33.
9. Galban C, Montejo JC, Mesejo A, Marco P, Celaya S, Sanchez-Segura JM, Farre M, Bryg DJ. An immune-enhancing enteral diet reduces mortality rate and episodes of bacteremia in septic inten-sive care unit patients. Crit Care Med 2000;28:643–8.
10. Braga M, Gianotti L, Cestari A, Vignali A, Pellegatta F, Dolci A, DiCarlo V. Gut function and immune and inflammatory responses in patients preoperatively fed with supplemented enteral for-mulas. Arch Surg 1996;131:1257–64.
11. McCarter MD, Gentilini OD, Gomez ME, Daly JM. Preoperative oral supplement with immunonu-trients in cancer patients. JPEN J Parenter Enteral Nutr 1998;22:206–11.

In Chapter 20, Chadwick and Jewell outline the cascade of inflammatory events presumably initiated by antigen in diverse animal models as an explanation of the aetiopathogenesis of inflammatory bowel disease (IBD). These processes effec-tively induce inflammation of both non-specific and specific types across the mucosa by the release of cytokines, chemokines and other pro-inflammatory markers as well as by activation of secondary antigen-presenting cells [1]. Although there is a relative polarization of Th1 and Th2 responses in animal models, the situation in humans is less distinct. In Crohn's disease there is a predominance of Th1 responsiveness, but although humoral immunity is more dominant in ulcerative colitis, there is less evidence for a Th2 pattern and it is also unclear whether cytokine profile at disease initiation differs from that in well-established disease as a primary or secondary phenomenon [2].

In IBD in general, a variety of autoantibodies have been differentially associated with the diagnoses of both Crohn's disease and ulcerative colitis, but although non-specific, they are more commonly encounterd in IBD than in other inflammatory diseases of the GI tract to suggest that they are entirely secondary. These agents include anti-*Saccharomyces cervisiae* antibody (ASCA) particularly noted in Crohn's disease which has familial aggregation and perinuclear anti-neutrophil cytoplasmic antibody (pANCA) which is detected in ulcerative colitis. Other colitis-associated antibodies include anti-endothelial cell antibody (AECA), antiepithelial autoantibody (the Das antibody) and anti-p40. Those detected in Crohn's disease include pancreatic autoantibody (PAB) and anti-erythrocyte autoantibody, AEA-15 [3]. It appears that combinations of antibodies are more specific for diagnoses particularly in difficult cases of isolated Crohn's colitis with atypical features in order to distinguish this from other colitides. Unfortunately the ASCA levels in many such cases are quite low with poor test sensitivity and it is unclear at present whether these tests are as useful in the early (as opposed to the established) stages of disease [4].

TNF appears to be a final common pathway mediator in Crohn's disease as discussed in this chapter, resulting in the activation of macrophages (which produce IL-12 and IL-18 necessary for Th1 cell differentiation), the provision of a co-stimulatory signal augmenting T cell responses, the induction of adhesion molecule expression and invoking pro-coagulant effects by the release of nitric oxide, platelet-activating factor and prostacyclin. It may also participate in metalloproteinase expression enhancing mucosal breakdown. Improved understanding of these pathogenic mechanisms has opened up new avenues for therapy and immune modulation in IBD. Recently healing of Crohn's-related fistulae has emerged as a particular goal of therapy worthy of separate consideration. In their chapter Chadwick and Jewell discuss the immune effects of conventional therapies. The use of metronidazole and the quinolones have significant immunomodulatory effects on peripheral lymphocyte cytokine production and corticosteroids equally diminish host production of the pro-inflammatory cytokines and chemokines as well as NF-κB, interfering with a variety of leukocyte functions; most notably adherence, chemotaxis and phagocytosis.

The thioguanine derivatives 6-Mercaptopurine (6-MP) and Azathioprine (AZA) have been discussed in Chapter 6 but these have specific effects on the proliferative activity of mitotically active lymphocyte populations as well as directly inhibiting cytotoxic T cell and NK cell function. In particular, the metabolism of the final active agent 6-thioguanine (6TG) is through thiopurine methyltransferase (TPMT) where heterozygous and recessive TPMT genetic variation results in a dose-dependent leukopenia despite high rates of remission [5]. In addition to pharmacogenomic testing of this type to determine drug sensitivity, it may be that TNF-resistant patients are predictable by the expression of TNF-α microsatellite haplotypes due to TNF promoter region polymorphism [6]. Methotrexate, which is occasionally used in steroid-resistant Crohn's disease as well as impairing DNA synthesis through inhibition of dihydrofolate reductase, also decreases the generation of IL-1 and induces T cell apoptosis [7]. The chemistry of Cyclosporine is well discussed in section 2, however, in IBD rapid response to this drug may act as a bridge to longer term immunomodulation with conventional agents such as 6-MP and AZA [8].

Recently a series of biological response modifiers have been approved for use particularly in complicated and steroid-resistant Crohn's disease. Given the fast-track approval of some of these agents, there is at present a surprising paucity of data concerning their safety and long-term effects as well as a clear guide to their clinical indications and use. These include Infliximab (Remicade), a chimeric IgG1 monoclonal anti-TNF antibody which has shown considerable recent success in fistulating Crohn's disease [9]. Its secondary effects may also be through complement fixation and inhibition of antibody-dependent cellular cytotoxicity (ADCC). Delayed-type hypersensitivity reactions experienced by some patients appears to correlate with circulating human anti-chimeric antibody levels, but somewhat worrisome is the reporting in a very small number of patients receiving Infliximab in clinical trials for both Crohn's disease and severe rheumatoid arthritis of a supervening lymphoproliferative disorder [10].

Because of the immunogeneicity of monoclonal antibody therapy, other anti-TNF strategies have therefore been employed. CDP571 is a humanized IgG4 anti-TNF-α antibody which has recently been studied in Crohn's disease. Its theoretical advantage is its humanized nature, however, its potential disadvantage is the fact that as an IgG4 isotype immunoglobulin it should not affect complement function or ADCC, which will possibly affect the durability of CDP571 therapy [11]. The recent success of anti-TNF strategies in Crohn's disease has led to an interest in Thalidomide, a drug infamous for its teratogenic potential. There have been two small studies of its use in Crohn's disease suggesting benefit, with its other immunomodulatory effects acting through inhibition of neutrophil function and the attenuation of angiogenesis [12-15]. Derivatives of Thalidomide (such as CC-3052) have recently been created with fewer adverse side-effects for selective anti-TNF efficacy [16]. Other methods of specific and non-specific TNF inhibition include the use of metalloproteinase inhibitors, antagonists of TNF convertase enzyme and etanercept, a genetically-engineered fusion protein combining the p75 TNF receptor isoform with an IgG1-Fc receptor [17]. Other antibody approaches include the use of humanized anti-α4-integrin antibody which is designed to disrupt the binding of α4β1 found on most monocytes and lymphocytes to VCAM-1 expressed on GALT endothelium. This has recently begun clinical trialling [18].

Cytokines have also been employed in clinical IBD practice with disappointing results using recombinant human IL-10, designed to suppress Th1 cytokine generation and differentiation of Th1 cells [19]. Recombinant human IL-11 has also shown benefit in patients with active Crohn's disease not receiving steroids. This cytokine is a member of the IL-6 family which promotes mucosal integrity in animal radiation and chemotherapy colitis models as well as in other traditional models of colitis [20,21]. Replication-deficient viral vectors which express immunoregulatory cytokines such as IL-4 and IL-10 as well as genetically-engineered molecules (IκB) which inhibit pro-inflammatory cytokine transcription are at present being developed [22].

There has been a recent explosion of new therapeutic approaches in IBD which

have included the use of conventional immunosuppressants in active inflammatory bowel disease; notably tacrolimus (FK506) and mycophenolate mofetil
[23,24] as well as anti-sense oligonucleotide therapy (such as ISIS-2302) directed
against the translation of ICAM-1 [24] and anti-sense anti-NF-κB therapies
[25,26]. Resistance to T cell apoptosis, (which has been demonstrated in active
Crohn's lesions), has been attributed to IL-6 signalling (either via its IL-6 receptor
or through trans-signaling without receptor recognition). Targeted anti-IL-6
receptor therapy and fusion proteins of the β-subunit (gp 130) of the IL-6 receptor with the Fc portion of human IgG1 appears to inhibit natural IL-6 signaling
via its receptor, stimulating local T cell apoptosis and potentially reducing the
chronicity of Crohn's lesions [27,28]. Current studies are assessing the rôle of
other specific immunomodulators such as growth hormone (GH) which promotes
healing of experimental colitis in GH-transgenic mice, G-CSF which is efficacious
in Crohn's perianal fistulae, proliferator-activated receptor (PPAR)-γ ligands
(which inhibit pro-inflammatory transcription factors and NF-κB) and matrix
metalloproteinase inhibitors designed to restrict T cell cytokine release [29].

The changing ecology of the human GI tract through the greater exposure to
antibiotics, improved hygiene and vaccination strategies may have relevance in
the progressive increase in immune-mediated gastrointestinal diseases in Western
society, including IBD. Probiotic therapy amounts to the administration of
healthy normal gut microflora to promote gut barrier function, provide maturational signals to the GALT and to balance pro-inflammatory and regulatory cytokine production at the mucosal level. This approach using *Lactobacillus* and
Bifidobacter strains has been successful in attenuating experimentally-induced IL-
10 knockout colitis [30], where it results in decreased intestinal myeloperoxidase
production and endotoxemia. Recent trials have suggested a role in human colitis
resistant to 5-ASA compounds and in post ileo-anal pouchitis [31,32]. It would
appear to be too simplistic to expect single probiotic therapy to be universally
successful in IBD, with a likelihood that its administration may need to be
changed in individual patients during the course of their disease. There are many
unresolved issues in their use; namely strain selection, dosage, frequency of
administration, optimal delivery and the most desirable delivery vehicle for use.
More recently, the scope of probiotic therapy has been advanced by the delivery
of genetically-modified bacteria in particular engineered to secrete IL-10, however,
the safety of such therapy and its ability to cross-infect the normal population,
needs careful study [33].

References

1. Mayer L, Eisenhardt D, Salomon P, Bauer W, Plous R, Piccinini L. Expression of class II molecules
   on intestinal epithelial cells in humans. Differences between normal and inflammatory bowel
   disease. Gastroenterology 1991;100:3–12.
2. Sartor RB. Review article: how relevant to human inflammatory bowel disease are current models
   of intestinal inflammation? Aliment Pharmacol Ther 1997;11:89–96.
3. Shanahan F. Antibody 'markers' in Crohn's disease: opportunity or overstatement? Gut
   1997;40:557–8.
4. Ruemmele FM, Targan SR, Levy G, Dubinsky M, Braun J, Seidman EG. Diagnostic accuracy of serological assays in pediatric inflammatory bowel disease. Gastroenterology 1998;115:822–9.
5. Dubinsky MC, Lamothe S, Yang HY, Targan S, Sinnett D, Theoret Y, et al. Optimizing and indivi-
   dualizing 6-MP therapy in IBD:the role of 6-MP metabolite levels and TPMT genotyping. Gastroenterology 1999;116:A702.

6. Plevy SE, Taylor K, DeWoody KL, Schaible TF, Shealy D, Targan SR. Tumor necrosis factor (TNF) microsatellite haplotypes and perinuclear anti-neutrophil cytoplasmic antibody (pANCA) identify Crohn's disease (CD) patients with poor clinical responses to anti-TNF monoclonal antibody (cA2). Gastroenterology 1997;112:A1062.

7. Seitz M. Molecular and cellular effects of methotrexate. Curr Opin Rheumatol 1999;11:226–32.

8. Fernandez-Banares F, Bertran X, Esteve-Comas M, Cabre E, Menacho M, Humbert P, Planas R, Gassull MA. Azathioprine is useful in maintaining long-term remission induced by intravenous cyclosporine in steroid-refractory severe ulcerative colitis. Am J Gastroenterol 1996;91:2498–9.

9. Present DH, Rutgeerts PJ, Targan S, Hanauer SB, Mayer L, van Hogezand RA, et al. Infliximab for the treatment of fistulas in patients with Crohns disease. N Engl J Med 1999;340:1398–405.

10. Bickston SJ, Lichtenstein GR, Arseneau KO, Cohen RB, Cominelli F. The relationship between infliximab treatment and lymphoma in Crohn's disease. Gastroenterology 1999;117:1433–7.

11. Stack WA, Mann SD, Roy AJ, Heath P, Sopwith M, Freeman J, Holmes G, Long R, Forbes A, Kamm MA. Randomised controlled trial of CDP571 antibody to tumour necrosis factor-alpha in Crohn's disease. Lancet 1997;349:521–4.

12. Barnhill RL, Doll NJ, Millikan LE, Hastings RC. Studies on the anti-inflammatory properties of thalidomide: effects on polymorphonuclear leukocytes and monocytes. J Am Acad Dermatol 1984;11:814–9.

13. Ehrenpreis ED, Kane SV, Cohen LB, Hanauer SB, Cohen RD. Thalidomide therapy for patients with refractory Crohn's disease: an open-label trial. Gastroenterology 1999;117:1271–7.

14. Vasiliauskas EA, Kam LY, Abreu-Martin MT, Hassard PV, Papadakis KA, Yang H, et al. An open-label pilot study of low-dose thalidomide in chronically active, steroid-dependent Crohn's disease. Gastroenterology 1999;117:1278–87.

15. Bauer KS, Dixon SC, Figg WD. Inhibition of angiogenesis by thalidomide requires metabolic activation, which is species-dependent. Biochem Pharmacol 1998;55:1827–34.

16. Marriott JB, Westby M, Cookson S, Guckian M, Goodbourn S, Muller G,et al. CC-3052: a water soluble analog of thalidomide and potent inhibitor of activation-induced TNF-alpha production. J Immunol 1988;161:4236–43.

17. Sandborn WJ, Hanauer SB. Antitumor necrosis factor therapy for inflammatory bowel disease: a review of agents, pharmacology, clinical results and safety. Inflamm Bowel Dis1999;5:119–33.

18. Gordon FH, Lai CWY, Hamilton MI, Allison MC, Fouweather M, Donoghue S, et al. Randomised double-blind placebo-controlled trial of recombinant humanized antibody to a4 integrin (antegren) in active Crohn's disease. Gastroenterology 1999;116:A726.

19. Schreiber S, Fedorak EN, Nielsen OH, Wild G, Williams NC, Jacyna M, et al. A safety and efficacy study of recombinant human interleukin-10 (rHuIL-10) treatment in 329 patients with chronic active Crohn's disease (CAD) Gastroenterology 1998;114:A1080.

20. Qiu BS, Pfeiffer CJ, Keith JC Jr. Protection by recombinant human interleukin-11 against experimental TNB-induced colitis in rats. Dig Dis Sci 1996;41:1625–30.

21. Sands BE, Bank S, Sninsky CA, Robinson M, Katz S, Singleton JW, et al. Prelminiary evaluation of safety and activity of recombinant human interleukin 11 in patients with active Crohn's disease. Gastroenterology 1999;117:58–64.

22. Jobin C, Panja A, Hellerbrand C, Limuro Y, Didonato J, Brenner DA, et al. Inhibition of proinflammatory molecule production by adenovirus-mediated expression of a nuclear factor κB superrepressor in human intestinal epithelial cells. J Immunol 1998;160:410–8.

23. Sandborn WJ. Preliminary report on the use of oral tacrolimus (FK506) in the treatment of complicated proximal small bowel and fistulizing Crohn's disease. Am J Gastroenterol 1997;92:876–9.

24. Neurath MF, Wanitschke R, Peters M, Krummenauer F, Meyer zum Buschenfelde KH, Schlaak JF. Randomised trial of mycophenolate mofetil versus azathioprinbe for treatment of chronic active Crohn's disease. Gut 1999;44:625–8.

25. Yacyshyn VR, Bowen-Yacyshyn MB, Jewell L, Taml JA, Bennett CF, Kisner DL, et al. A placebo-controlled trial of ICAM-1 antisense oligonucleotide in the treatment of Crohn's disease. Gastroenterology 1998;114:1133–42.

26. Neurath MF, Pettersson S, Meyer zum Buschenfelde KH, Strober W. Local administration of antisense phosphothioate oligonucleotides to the p65 subunit of NF-kappa B abrogates established experimental colitis in mice. Nat Med 1996;2:998–1004.

27. Sands BE. Therapy of inflammatory bowel disease. Gastroenterology 2000;118:S68–S82.

28. Atreya R, Mudter J, Finotto S, Müllberg J, Jostock T, Witz S, et al. Blockade of interleukin 6 *trans* signaling suppresses T-cell resistance against apoptosis in chronic intestinal inflammation, evidence in Crohn's disease and experimental colitis *in vivo*. Nature Med 2000;6:583–8.

29. Pender SL, Tickle SP, Docherty AJ, Howie D, Wathen NC, McDonald TT. A major role of matrix metalloproteinases in T cell injury in the gut. J Immunol 1997;158:1582–90.

30. Madsen KL, Doyle JS, Jewell LD, Tavernini M, Fedorak RN. *Lactobacillus* species prevents colitis in IL-10 gene-deficient mice. Gastroenterology 1999;116:1107–14.
31. Rembacken BJ, Snelling AM, Hawkey PM, Chalmers DM, Axon ATR. Non-pathogenic *Escherichia coli* versus mesalazine for the treatment of ulcerative colitis: a randomised trial. Lancet 1999;354:635–9.
32. Gionchietti P, Rizzello F, Venturi A, Brigidi P, Matteuzzi D, Bazzocchi G, et al. Oral bacteriotherapy as maintenance treatment in patients with chronic pouchitis: a double blind, placebo controlled trial. Gastroenterology 2000;119:305–9.
33. Steidler L, Hans W, Schotte L, Nelyrick S, Obermeier F, Falk W, Fiers W. Remaut E. Treatment of murine colitis by Lactococcus lactis secreting interleukin-10.Science 2000;289:1352–5.

In Chapter 21, Drs Pan, Portlock and Karpeh discuss the new classification systems of GI lymphoproliferative disorders and their presentation to the general surgeon particularly in the context of clinical immunosuppression. The classification of these tumors has been improved by standardization of a panel of monoclonal antibodies characterizing leukocyte antigens which are closely linked to cytologically distinct B cell phenotypes including the mantle zone, the extra-follicular compartment, the follicle center and plasma cell compartments [1]. Many studies have reported few cases of retrospective non-randomized patients and have lacked uniformity in histologic classification, clinicopathological variables or types of treatment. Equally they have been set in an era before the recognition of MALT as the origin of most GI lymphomas and the utilization of the Isaacson classification system following the general principles set up by the Kiel group [2,3]. The effectiveness of combination chemotherapy in advanced disease has forced a reconsideration and re-evaluation of the surgeon's role in early cases, perhaps affording a salvage in patients where complete remission is not achieved by initial chemotherapy and H. pylori eradication [4].

Non-Hodgkin's lymphoma (NHL) of the GI tract accounts for between 4–20% of all NHL and is the commonest site of extra-nodal presentation. As the stomach is the most frequently involved organ in the GI tract, the general surgeon will encounter this tumor particularly in complex patients with risk factors for GI lymphoma development, most notably immunosuppression after solid organ transplantation and HIV disease, as well as in patients with long-standing celiac and Crohn's disease. A significant proportion of these tumors are of relatively low grade histology arising from mucosa-associated lymphoid tissue and associated with H. pylori infection. In many cases, complete regression is possible following simple H.pylori eradication [5]. Distinct clinical entities encountered in the small bowel include primary intestinal T-cell lymphoma, immunoproliferative small intestinal disease and multiple lymphomatous polyposis which are described in this chapter. The latter in particular is a distinct clinical entity with a specific B cell phenotype (pan-B+,CD5+,CD10-) and genotype (Bcl-1 rearrangement) which is the intestinal counterpart of mantle cell lymphoma and which when recognized has an improved prognosis with aggressive therapy incorporating anthracycline-containing multi-drug regimens, high-dose radio-chemotherapy and stem cell autotransplantation [6].

High-grade B-cell NHL is the second commonest tumor affecting the HIV+ population and the incidence of the tumor is not declining despite the introduction of highly active anti-retroviral therapy (HAART). This has been accompanied, however, by a generally lower peripheral CD4 cell count at diagnosis, an increase in the diffuse large-cell variant and in primary CNS NHL in patients with clinical AIDS [7–9]. These tumors are almost always EBV-associated where in vivo infection of B lymphocytes with the EBV results in a broad expression of immunodominant viral latency genes as a viral reservoir in resting B cells. This opens up the prospect of EBV-directed T cell therapies in such patients as well as in post-transplant lymphomas particularly following bone marrow transplantation [10].

Post-transplant lymphoproliferative disorder (PTLD) as discussed in this chapter, is substantially increased in adults and children following a range of solid organ transplant types (kidney, heart, heart-lung and liver) and although many forms are non-EBV-associated, monitoring of EBV-infected lymphocytes (EBV DNA load) may identify some patients at risk for the development of PTLD [11–14]. The incidence of PTLD is not clearly associated with particular immuno-suppression régimes and many of these patients, despite monitoring, present with advanced disease and have a generally poor outcome. The optimal approach to therapy including immunosuppression reduction, anti-viral therapy (where appropriate), anti-CD20 monoclonal antibody administration and conventional chemotherapy is somewhat unclear. General surgeons have a diminished role today in the staging and management of NHL, but they are seeing more complicated presentations of lymphoma in severely immunocompromised patients who have undergone complex forms of chemoimmunotherapy.

References

1. Mielke B, Moller P. Histomorphologic and immunophenotypic spectrum of primary gastro-intestinal B-cell lymphomas. Int J Cancer 1991;47:334–43.
2. Rohatiner A, d'Amore F, Coiffier B, Crowther D, Gospodarowicz M, Isaacson P, et al. Report on a workshop convened to discuss the pathological and staging classifications of gastrointestinal tract lymphoma. Ann Oncol 1994;5:397–400.
3. Zucca E, Cavalli F. Gut lymphomas. Baillieres Clin Haematol 1996;9:727–41.
4. deJong D, Aleman BM, Taal BG, Boot H. Controversies and consensus in the diagnosis, work-up and treatment of gastric lymphoma: an international survery. Ann Oncol 1999;10:275–80.
5. Schmitt-Graff A. Immunological and molecular classification of mucosa-associated lymphoid tissue lymphoma. Recent Res Cancer Res 1996;142:121–36.
6. Ruskone-Fourmestraux A, Delmer A, Lavergne A, Molina T, Brousse N, Audouin J, et al. Multiple lymphomatous polyposis of the gastrointestinal tract: prospective clinicopathologic study of 31 cases. Group D'etude des lymphomas digestifs. Gastroenterology 1997;112:7–16.
7. Levine AM, Seneviratne L, Espina BM, Wohl AR, Tulpule A, Nathwani BN, et al. Evolving characteristics of AIDS-related lymphoma. Blood 2000;96:4084–90.
8. Hooper WC, Holman RC, Clarke MJ, Chorba TL. Trends in non-Hodskin lymphoma (NHL) and HIV-associated NHL deaths in the United States. Am J Hematol 2001;66:159–66.
9. Straus DJ. HIV-associated lymphomas. Curr Oncol Rep 2001;3:260–5.
10. Ambinder RF. Epstein-Barr virus associated lymphoproliferations in the AIDS setting. Eur J Cancer 2000;37:1209–16.
11. Swerdlow AJ, Higgins CD, Hunt BJ, Thomas JA, Burke MM, Crawford DH, Yacoub MH. Risk of lymphoid neoplasia after cardiothoracic transplantation, a cohort study of the relation to Epstein-Barr virus. Transplantation 2000;69:897–904.
12. Stevens SJ, Verschuuren EA, Pronk I, van der Bij W, Harmsen MC, The TH, et al. Frequent monitoring of Epstein-Barr virus DNA in unfractionated whole blood is essential for early detection of posttransplant lymphoproliferative disease in high-risk patients. Blood 2001;97:1165–71.
13. Tsai DE, Hardy CL, Tomaszewski JE, Kotloff RM, Oltoff KM, Somer BG, et al. Reduction in immunosuppression as initial therapy for posttransplant lymphoproliferative disorder: analysis of prognostic variables and long-term follow-up of 42 adults. Transplantation 2001;71:1076–88.
14. Dharnidharka VR, Sullivan EK, Stablein DM, Tejani AH, Harmon WE. North American Pediatric Renal Transplant Cooperative Study (NAPRTCS). Risk factors for posttransplant lymphoproliferative disorder (PTLD) in pediatric kidney transplantation: a report of the North American Pediatric Renal Transplant Cooperative Study (NAPRTCS). Transplantation 2001;71:1065–8.

Index